MALINS'
CLINICAL
DIABETES

D1631682

JOIN US ON THE INTERNET VIA WWW, GOPHER, FTP OR EMAIL:

WWW: http://www.thomson.com
GOPHER: gopher.thomson.com
FTP: ftp.thomson.com
EMAIL: findit@kiosk.thomson.com

A service of $\mathbf{I(T)P}$®

MALINS' CLINICAL DIABETES

Second edition

Malcolm Nattrass

Consultant Physician, Diabetes Resource Centre, Selly Oak Hospital, Birmingham

CHAPMAN & HALL MEDICAL

London · Weinheim · New York · Tokyo · Melbourne · Madras

Published by
Chapman & Hall, 2–6 Boundary Row, London SE1 8HN, UK

Chapman & Hall, 2–6 Boundary Row, London SE1 8HN, UK

Chapman & Hall GmbH, Pappelallee 3, 69469 Weinheim, Germany

Chapman & Hall USA, 115 Fifth Avenue, New York, NY 10003, USA

Chapman & Hall Japan, ITP-Japan, Kyowa Building, 3F,
2-2-1 Hirakawacho, Chiyoda-ku, Tokyo 102, Japan

Chapman & Hall Australia, 102 Dodds Street, South Melbourne,
Victoria 3205, Australia

Chapman & Hall India, R. Seshadri, 32 Second Main Road, CIT East,
Madras 600 035, India

First edition 1968
Second edition 1996

© 1996 Malcolm Nattrass

Typeset in 10/12pt Palatino by Photoprint, Torquay, Devon
Printed in Great Britain by Cambridge University Press, Cambridge

ISBN 0 412 30860 6

A catalogue record for this book is available from the British Library

Library of Congress Catalog Card Number: 96–85255

∞ Printed on permanent acid-free text paper, manufactured in
accordance with ANSI/NISO Z39.48–1992 and ANSI/NISO Z39.48–1984
(Permanence of Paper).

CONTENTS

PREFACE TO THE FIRST EDITION

This is a book about *clinical* diabetes and is intended primarily for those who encounter diabetic patients. It presents a picture of the disease derived from concentrated work in one of the largest clinics in Britain for a period of 24 years during which I have examined more than 12 000 newly diagnosed cases. A large experience is the justification for an attempt to set down a plain physician's view of diabetes. Having no qualification as a biochemist I have omitted a detailed discussion of much experimental and laboratory work which is already admirably summarized in a number of current texts and reports of symposia.

The more diabetic patients one sees the more difficult it becomes to present the simple picture that so many readers like. Diabetes is a disorder of such infinite variety that it becomes impossible to say that this always occurs or that never happens. We do see thin children with mild diabetes which can be controlled by dieting and fat women who develop severe ketosis.

At the present time clinicians are especially interested in the discovery of unsuspected cases of diabetes and the identification of those who have a high risk of developing the disease. Detection drives and attempts at preventive treatment may be undertaken with more enthusiasm than discretion and it is more than ever necessary that diabetic or 'prediabetic' patients should be under the care of physicians or general practitioners who will put their interests first and make balanced assessments of their needs.

Today a diabetic clinic provides the widest clinical range of any specialty in medicine with metabolic, vascular, neurological and psychiatric problems outstanding. In addition there is a chance to enjoy some of the pleasures of general practice which arise from long acquaintance with many of the patients. The chance, all too frequent, to ease the last years of those whose health is slowly failing calls for all the resources of the general physician.

The literature to which I have made reference is predominantly that of the scientifically English-speaking world. The reason for this provincialism is my inadequate knowledge of other languages. In compensation I conclude with a quotation from one of the greatest of all non-English sources, Don Quixote, *'No hay libro tan malo que no tenga algo bueno'* – there is no book so bad but there is something good in it.

1967 J.M.

PREFACE TO THE SECOND EDITION

When I was appointed as replacement for John Malins in 1979 he planted the seed in my mind that one day I should attempt a revision of his book *Clinical Diabetes Mellitus* which he had published in 1968. Each time we met thereafter he would enquire as to progress towards what he amusedly referred to as his immortality. I suspect that he was setting some sort of test in that he knew of the amount of work involved because he himself had done it. To the young, enthusiastic writer this was not known, but soon became apparent.

I had thought at the outset that taking the framework of Malins's textbook would make writing easier, if not quite make it a simple task. But like all, presumably, who have attempted to write a book I began with a profound and devastating underestimate of the amount of work to be done. While I envisaged a revision it soon became apparent that many areas would require completely rewriting. This was necessitated by developments and progress in the field. For example, with few exceptions diabetes mellitus was a single disease in Malins's 1968 book but in the interval to the rewriting this had become two different aetiological and pathogenic diseases with a similar manifestation.

One major area that did not change, of course, is the clinical description of the signs and symptoms of diabetes and its complications. These were a major attribute of the first edition and where appropriate they have been transcribed from the original for this volume. The preface to the first edition is also produced *verbatim* since much of what Malins wrote in 1968 remains true today – the diabetic clinic still provides the widest range of any specialty in medicine; diabetes remains a disorder of such infinite variety; and there is still the opportunity to enjoy some of the pleasures akin to general practice which arise from long acquaintance with many of the patients.

In this the second edition of Malins's textbook I have sought to maintain the original aim to produce a book primarily for those who encounter diabetic patients. Much of the experience quoted herein remains that of John Malins but the additions are my responsibility. The style of the original volume was uniquely that of Malins himself and while I have not aped this I hope that the volume retains an essentially readable quality and that not too many of the joins of past and present are visible.

M. N
Birmingham, January 1996

JOHN MELVILLE MALINS, 1915–1992

John Malins was educated at Shrewsbury and Birmingham University, qualifying in 1939. He was appointed Assistant Physician to the General Hospital, Birmingham in 1946 and from 1955 until his retirement in 1979 he was Consultant Physician and also Physician to Kidderminster Hospital. He was awarded a personal chair in Medicine by the University of Birmingham in 1971. When he was first appointed the specialist care of the diabetic patient was in its infancy and he set about developing the specialty with great energy and vigour. At his retirement in 1979 the Diabetic Clinic at the General Hospital was one of the largest in the UK and the fact that he achieved so much was due in no small part to his enthusiastic approach. To sit with him in the clinic was an education not only in the finer points of fact in diabetes but one was likely to be taken on an educational trip through the English Midlands as he talked with patients of the history and geography of their town or district. To the junior his feats of memory seemed prodigious as he enquired about patients' relatives whom he recalled had diabetes, or other aspects of family life; even the dog's name would not escape him. He could be infuriating as the junior hastened to finish the clinic only to be interrupted repeatedly as he recalled some detail of the patient's history or career that should be shared. Undoubtedly that was his secret; he found not only the disease an endless fascination but each and every patient was of interest to him both in their personalities and how this interacted with the disease.

In the development of the Diabetic Clinic at the General Hospital he was supported by a succession of talented senior registrars, notably Dr Michael FitzGerald, who went on to be Malins's colleague at Consultant level in the Clinic for more than 20 years, and a long line of clinical assistants, included among whom was his first wife Joanna. He was active in many areas of clinical research and in his textbook, *Clinical Diabetes Mellitus* (1968), was able to quote extensively from work done by him or under his supervision. This volume was the last substantive single-author textbook of diabetes.

Malins was not only a talented physician; he excelled in most things he turned his hand to. He played hockey for his county and the Midlands and his sporting career left him the legacy of a knee injury which affected a rather lop-sided walk. This walk was apparently unusually contagious, in that most of his Senior Registrars seemed to end up walking in a similar manner. He was also an amazing gardener, yet this is to understate his talent as he was as much a botanist as a plantsman, with a great love of trees. His knowledge is nowhere better displayed than in the second 'textbook' which he wrote in his retirement, *The Essential Pruning Companion* (1992), when, with his second wife, the gardening expert Penelope Hobhouse, he had custodianship of the National Trust property at Tintinhull House in Somerset.

Anyone who met Malins will have their own memories of him, whether they be his knowledge and wisdom or his mischievous smile or asides. All who knew or worked with him had their lives enriched by the experience.

ACKNOWLEDGEMENTS

While I am accountable for the content of this volume a number of people share the responsibility for my interest in diabetes and shaping my approach and views on the subject. I have been fortunate in working with, and therefore being in a position to learn from, a number of the most interesting and talented people in medicine. Professor Vincent Marks and Professor George Alberti shaped my career before my appointment as Consultant Physician in Birmingham and my colleagues in Birmingham, Dr Michael FitzGerald and Dr Alex Wright, continued my education. It is impossible to quantify my debt to Michael FitzGerald, who took me on as a registrar and later as a consultant colleague. Much of what is contained in this volume reflects his approach to the practice of diabetes, which he passed on to me.

I am grateful to Mrs Ruth Darling who typed numerous early editions of the manuscript with great patience. I am also grateful to Dr Peter Altman of the publishers Chapman & Hall, who has tolerated deadlines long past with encouragement rather than condemnation.

Finally, I am thankful that throughout the writing my wife has tolerated my retreats into the study, providing an endless source of sustenance and support.

Ancient views of the causation of diabetes were hardly formulated to the extent which would allow them to be called theories. Galen (AD 131–201) thought that diabetes was the result of a weakness of the kidneys, which attracted fluid and could not hold it back. His unquestioned authority perpetuated this idea for at least 1500 years in Western medicine. Avicenna (980–1037) may have suggested that a disturbance of liver function was the primary fault but Arab medicine in general followed and passed on the teachings of Galen. Later medieval writers named grief, diet, alcohol and venery as causes while Willis (1621–1675) blamed acid salts in the blood such as might result from immoderate drinking of cider, beer, or sharp wine but also from worry, sadness, grief and nervous ailments. Richard Mead (1673–1754) was the first in modern times to consider diabetes a disease of the liver. John Rollo (died 1809) made interesting observations but did not think deeply about the cause of diabetes and held that it was a disease of the stomach affecting digestion and assimilation in which the saccharine material was formed, chiefly from vegetable matter.

From this point the advances in science, and particularly those of the German chemists, in the first half of the 19th century lifted speculation to a higher plane and the new era culminated in the career of Claude Bernard (1813–1878), who made many fundamental observations. He observed that the kidney did not produce sugar but excreted the excess into the urine. More importantly, through careful experimental work, he observed that the liver normally stored starch and produced sugar which it secreted into the circulation. His idea of overproduction of sugar by the liver has persisted to the present day. Another discovery made by Claude Bernard, that puncture of the floor of the fourth ventricle caused glycosuria, was less constructive in its influence since it led to a widely held belief that diabetes was the result of disease of the nervous system. Naunyn (1839–1925) believed that disease of the nervous system and of the pancreas could produce diabetes but in most instances the diabetic constitution, or *Anlage*, was inherited. His views were vigorously endorsed for many years by Joslin (1869–1962).

The steps which led from the observations of Langerhans (1847–1888) to the discovery of insulin by Banting and Best are described elsewhere (Chapter 9). With the discovery of insulin the central position of the pancreas in the pathogenesis of diabetes seemed to be established. Yet it was soon apparent that changes in the islets of the diabetic were not striking; indeed the B-cells often appeared normal.

Meanwhile a distraction appeared in the form of the observations that hypophysectomy greatly ameliorated the diabetes produced in animals by pancreatectomy. This turned attention to the antagonism between the anterior pituitary and insulin, which culminated in the demonstration that crude extracts of the pituitary were diabetogenic in suitable animals and that this effect was due to pituitary growth hormone.

Another diabetogenic substance was reported in the 1940s which produced necrosis of the beta-cells of the islets. This compound was alloxan and its relationship to other simple compounds such as urea suggested the possibility that a chemical effect on the islets might initiate some cases of diabetes.

GENERAL POINTS OF AETIOLOGY

In searching for the aetiology of any human disease the starting point is the relative contributions of heredity and environment. Examples abound of diseases that are due entirely to one or other of these factors although, more commonly, each probably needs the other for full expression of the disease. It is appropriate to consider the aetiology of diabetes from these starting points but the history of the elucidation is instructive.

HEREDITY

The belief that diabetes is inherited is almost universal. The *Cikitsa Sthuana* of the Hindu Charaka (probably first century BC) mentions that the disease *madhumeha* (honey urine) could be transmitted from father to son. Richard Morton (died 1698) was the first European writer to refer to the inheritance of diabetes, but in more recent time its importance has been strenuously advocated by the two most influential experts of their time Naunyn (1839–1925) and Joslin (1869–1962). Perhaps because of their influence over many years the assumption was generally made that diabetes was inherited and that the only problem remaining was to elucidate the mode of inheritance. Recent trends in genetics go against an attempt to produce a simple and clear-cut pattern of inheritance.

IDENTICAL TWIN STUDIES

Studies in identical twins have a long tradition in diabetes and in other diseases where heredity is thought to be important in causation. They have been criticised in the past because of the tendency by some workers to over-extrapolate the findings, a human failing not restricted to twin studies.

There is a temptation to assume that high similarity rates between monozygous twin pairs are a consequence of their shared inheritance while conveniently forgetting that twins usually share the same environment for many years. Paradoxically, it is the differences between twin pairs that are more interesting and important. In studies of identical twins similarities can be due either to their identical genetic material or to their shared early environment but differences must be of environmental origin. In addition, if concordance rates are greater between identical twin pairs versus non-identical twin pairs in well matched groups, then assumptions can be made on the contribution of the genetic material.

Then-Berg (1938) reported 46 pairs of monozygous twins, 17 of whom were concordant with clinical diabetes and a further 13 concordant by a glucose tolerance test carried out on the second member of the pair. Of 87 pairs of non-identical twins nine were concordant and a further nine concordant by a glucose tolerance test. This finding, of greater concordance rates in identical versus non-identical twins, indicated the importance of heredity. Perhaps more importantly, Then-Berg reported that all identical twin pairs over the age of 43 years were concordant for diabetes. The work, which has been much quoted, should be read in the original before the significance of the results is assessed.

Other studies were in broad agreement with these findings. From Germany it was reported that 15 pairs were concordant out of 19 identical twin pairs and furthermore it was suggested that the severity of the diabetes was roughly the same in each pair. The results from the Joslin clinic were similar. In at least 16 out of 33 pairs of identical twins both had diabetes, whereas in only two out of 63 non-identical pairs was this the case, but not all twins thought to be non-diabetic were subjected to a glucose tolerance test. In Denmark, where there existed a twin registry, high concordance rates in monozygous pairs were

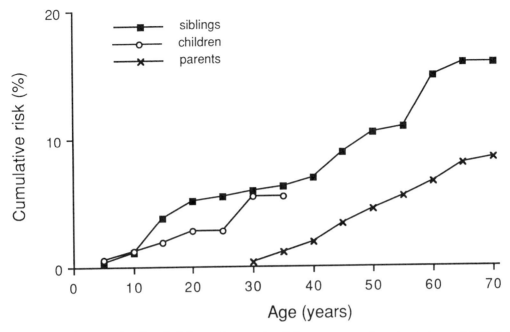

Fig. 1.1 Cumulative risk (%) of diabetes by age in different categories of relatives of 187 diabetic patients who were diagnosed before the age of 20 years. (Source: adapted from Degnbol and Green, 1978.)

noted which were more marked than in dizygous twins. Perhaps because the twin population which was studied was predominantly of older diabetics it was concluded that all identical twin pairs would eventually become concordant.

FAMILY STUDIES

Studies at the beginning of this century reported a family history of diabetes in 17–25% of patients. With increasing awareness of the disease, the figure has risen to 30–35%. Cammidge (1934) compared 1000 diabetics, of whom 39.6% gave a family history of diabetes, with 500 non-diabetic controls, with a family history of 3.4%. In our clinic 23% of patients gave a history of diabetes in the family at the time of diagnosis and this figure rose to 38% when the enquiry was repeated 15 years later. Virtually all of these studies have been performed in white populations

and many later studies have lacked adequate control data.

Harris (1950) noted that the siblings of diabetics with an onset of the disease in early life were much more likely to develop the disease themselves in early life than the siblings of those whose diabetes began in later life, an effect he thought was genetic rather than environmental.

These data were reanalysed by Degnbol and Green (1978) to compare them with their own data from the Steno Memorial Hospital. They calculated the cumulative risk of diabetes at specific ages of relatives of diabetics diagnosed aged 20 or less. Their results (Figure 1.1) were similar to those obtained by Harris (1950) in his early-onset diabetics. They drew attention to the cumulative risk for relatives of late-onset diabetes studied by Harris (1950), comparing these figures with those obtained in a study of the general population (FitzGerald *et al.*, 1961). There did not appear to be an

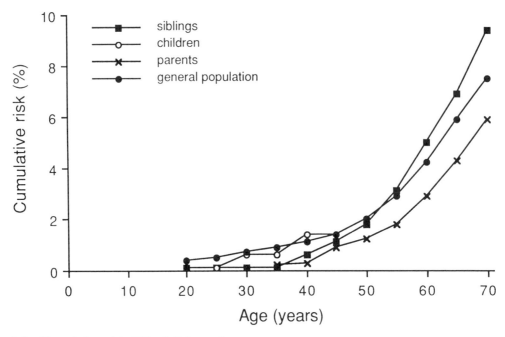

Fig. 1.2 Cumulative risk (%) of diabetes by age in different categories of relatives of 417 diabetic patients who were diagnosed before the age of 45 years. (Source: adapted from Harris, 1950. The cumulative risk for the general population is taken from FitzGerald *et al.*, 1961.)

increase in risk for parents, children or siblings of late-onset diabetics (Figure 1.2). From this difference between early- and late-onset diabetics they were led to the conclusion that 'early- and late-onset diabetes cannot have an identical genetic background', while generously acknowledging that Harris (1950) had been the first to show this.

Other evidence which was used to demonstrate the importance of heredity in diabetes was that derived from conjugal diabetes. Repeated attempts were made to demonstrate a simple mendelian inheritance of the disorder without any great success.

There were certain obvious difficulties in working out the possible genetic basis of diabetes from these early studies. Firstly, there was a tendency to regard diabetes as a single disease and this view persisted for many years despite the findings of Harris (1950). Although it was acknowledged that cases of pancreatic disease or haemochromatosis might

be different in character from those that arise for no apparent reason, the concept that diabetes might be a syndrome rather than a single disease is a relatively recent introduction. Secondly, the distinction between the normal and the slightly diabetic depends on tests of glucose tolerance which are interpreted in an arbitrary manner so that it may be difficult in population studies to segregate a diabetic and a non-diabetic population with absolute confidence. Thirdly, the age of onset of diabetes varies greatly and it presents most often in later life, with the result that many subjects who are normal today will be diabetic before they die or would become diabetic if they lived long enough.

In retrospect it is clear that interpretation of family history and identical twin studies was bound to fail so long as diabetes was considered one disorder. The concept of insulin-dependent diabetes as severe insulin deficiency while non-insulin-dependent diabetes was a milder degree of insulin deficiency, with the two conditions having a common aetiology, was a severe handicap to the emergence of a clear explanation of the genetics of diabetes.

CLASSIFICATION OF DIABETES

Substantial advances in recent years have clarified the aetiology of diabetes although the precise mechanism by which predisposing factors lead to manifest disease awaits elucidation. In part these developments have prompted a reclassification of diabetes, with the realization that a single aetiology could not explain the many forms of the disorder. Thus in aetiological terms, in addition to the well recognized clinical separation, diabetes mellitus cannot be considered a homogeneous disorder. Two major types exist, with numerous less well-defined syndromes. The classification of the World Health Organization (WHO, 1980, 1985) is widely accepted and is reproduced in Table 1.1. It is a simplified version of a classification from the Diabetes Data Group of the National Institutes of Health (National Diabetes Data Group, 1979). It is often forgotten or ignored that it was presented as an 'interim' classification and is therefore not fixed in tablets of stone. Indeed, even the apparently simpler aspects of the classification – the division into insulin-dependent and non-insulin-dependent, with subgroups of the latter based on the presence or absence of obesity – present problems. Is each of the two major groups homogeneous? and is a division of the second group based on obesity justified? Such questions will take time to resolve but as an interim classification upon which to base a consideration of aetiology the WHO classification will suffice.

AETIOLOGICAL CLASSIFICATION

The use of the terms 'type 1' and 'type 2' diabetes to describe the major forms of diabetes is based on aetiology. Many similarities exist between type 1 and insulin-dependent diabetes

Table 1.1 Classification of diabetes mellitus and other categories of glucose intolerance (WHO, 1985)

A. Clinical classes
  Diabetes mellitus
    Insulin-dependent – Type 1
    Non-insulin-dependent – Type 2
      (a) Non-obese
      (b) Obese
    Malnutrition-related
    Diabetes mellitus associated with certain
      conditions and syndromes
      (1) Pancreatic disease
      (2) Hormonal disease
      (3) Drug- or chemical-induced
      (4) Insulin or insulin receptor
          abnormalities
      (5) Genetic syndromes
      (6) Miscellaneous
    Impaired glucose tolerance
      (a) Non-obese
      (b) Obese
      (c) Associated with certain conditions or
          syndromes
    Gestational diabetes
B. Statistical risk classes (normal glucose tolerance
   with substantially increased risk of developing
   diabetes)
      Previous abnormality of glucose tolerance
      Potential abnormality of glucose tolerance

and type 2 and non-insulin-dependent diabetes but 'insulin-dependent' and 'non-insulin-dependent' are clinical terms. To use the terms of the aetiological and clinical classifications interchangeably or synonymously is a mildly dishonest approach since few insulin-dependent patients in the clinic, or even in important research studies, will have had the intensive investigation necessary to show that a patient who is clinically insulin-dependent is in fact aetiologically type 1.

AETIOLOGY OF TYPE 1 DIABETES

At the beginning of any aetiological investigation an attempt to identify a homogeneous group of patients can only be based on the clinical features of the disease. In clinical practice the features of insulin-dependent diabetes are abrupt onset, marked hyperglycaemia with a ready appearance of ketonuria or ketoacidosis, and insulin deficiency. The prevalence worldwide is presumed to be of the order of 0.1–0.5% although this cannot be ascertained with certainty and there exist populations in Africa and Asia where it is rare. Recent studies of distinct racial or specific geographical areas have shown marked differences in incidence. Figures range from the 0.8 per 100 000 of the population of Japan to 35 per 100 000 in Finland (Tuomilehto *et al.*, 1992) and approaching 30 per 100 000 in Sardinia (Green, Gale and Patterson, 1992). In the USA the incidence is of the order of 14 per 100 000 of the population (Diabetes Epidemiology Research International Group, 1988) and in the UK it is a similar figure (Karvonen *et al.*, 1993).

Although the clinical onset is usually sudden there is evidence of a long pre-diabetic, subclinical period in some individuals (Gorsuch *et al.*, 1981). A genetic tendency has been established although environmental precipitating factors, while acknowledged, have proved more difficult to ascertain with certainty.

GENETIC FACTORS

Population studies

Data on genetic factors implicated in the aetiology of type 1 diabetes are derived from studies of the human leucocyte antigens (HLA) of the major histocompatibility system (Singal and Blajchman, 1973). The genes that encode the antigens present on all nucleated cell surfaces (*HLA-A, HLA-B, HLA-C*) or some cells only (*HLA-D, HLA-DR*) are located on the short arm of chromosome 6. Near this location are genes that influence the immunological response, including antibody production and the cell-mediated immune response.

The HLA system is highly polymorphic, with each locus encoding a different cell surface antigen. But between the Class I,

HLA-A, HLA-B, HLA-C, and the Class II, HLA-D or HLA-DR, there is marked linkage disequilibrium. That is, certain of the antigens occur together more commonly than expected from their individual frequencies in the population. Early studies lacked this awareness, which has become clearer with developments in technique.

Current evidence points to a significant increase in relative risk of developing type 1 diabetes when possessing certain of the HLA antigens. The strongest associations in a caucasoid population are between the disease and HLA-DR$_3$ and -DR$_4$ while there is a negative association with HLA-DR$_2$ (Platz *et al.*, 1981). In early studies the association with HLA-A$_1$, HLA-A$_2$, HLA-B$_8$, HLA-B$_{15}$ and HLA-B$_{18}$ was noted but this now appears to be due to linkage disequilibrium of these antigens: A$_1$, B$_8$ and B$_{18}$ with DR$_3$ and A$_2$; B$_{15}$ with DR$_4$. Similarly the apparent decrease in association with B$_7$ is through linkage disequilibrium with DR$_2$.

There is evidence for heterogeneity within type 1 diabetes since DR$_3$ and DR$_4$ confer additive risk such that the heterozygote genotype *HLA-DR$_3$/HLA-DR$_4$* shows an increased relative risk even over the homozygotes. It should be stressed that the majority of studies have concentrated upon predominantly caucasoid populations. In other populations the frequency of a specific antigen in the normal population may differ markedly from Western populations. It is unclear therefore to what extent findings can be extrapolated from one population to another.

Further, if indirect, evidence of heterogeneity is apparent in the caucasoid populations. Patients with -DR$_3$ tend to have persistence of islet cell antibodies and occurrence of other clinical or subclinical organ-specific autoimmune disease while they also form low titres of insulin antibodies in response to treatment. Patients with -DR$_4$, however, have increased antibody production to viruses and heterologous insulin without other tendency to autoimmunity.

Table 1.2 HLA-DR frequencies (%) in controls and insulin-dependent diabetic patients from a caucasoid population (from Svejgaard *et al.*, 1986)

DR	Controls		Insulin-dependent diabetic patients	Relative risk
2	28.0		2.5	0.07
3	24.7		50.5	3.1
3/X		14.9	11.0	
3/3		4.8	9.5	
3/4		5.0	30.0	
4	34.2		71.9	4.9
4/X		21.2	20.0	
4/4		7.9	21.8	
9	1.4		4.6	1.3

Table 1.3 HLA-DR frequencies (%) in controls and insulin-dependent diabetic patients from a Japanese population (from Bertrams and Baur, 1986)

DR	Controls	Insulin-dependent diabetic patients	Relative risk
4/X	7.2	9.2	1.28
4/4	27.7	28.7	1.02
4/9	4.6	18.4	4.54
9/X	18.2	29.9	1.86
9/9	1.5	5.7	3.2

Most studies have demonstrated that more than 90% of caucasoid patients with insulin-dependent diabetes are positive for DR_3 or DR_4 (Bertrams and Baur, 1984). Typical of results is the study from Denmark (Svejgaard *et al.*, 1986) listed in Table 1.2. HLA-DR_2 is found only in very low frequencies in caucasian insulin-dependent patients. The relative risk is less than *HLA-DR* x/x, which has raised the suggestion that *HLA-DR$_2$* or a gene in linkage disequilibrium with *HLA-DR$_2$* may have a protective effect.

There are marked racial differences in the frequency of HLA antigens within populations. In Japan HLA-DR_3 is uncommon and is not associated with insulin-dependent diabetes (Bertrams and Baur, 1984). Here the antigen DR_9 shows a strong positive association, in contrast to the caucasoid population where it has a relative risk close to unity (Table 1.3). The positive association of DR_4 and negative association of DR_2 is maintained in this population.

In North Indians resident in England DR_3 and DR_4 are increased in frequency in insulin-dependent diabetic patients although the frequency of DR_4 is markedly lower in the control population than in a similar caucasoid population (Odugbesan *et al.*, 1987). In addition to a negative association with DR_2 a

further negative association was found with DR_7.

In a study of few patients the associations of DR_3 and DR_2 in caucasoid diabetics were repeated in black Nigerian diabetic patients but no association with DR_4 was found.

In contrast, the antigen associations in American black diabetics are similar to those of a caucasoid population which, it has been suggested, may reflect caucasoid pollution of the genetic pool. This suggestion finds support in studies of the black immigrant population of the UK, who show differences from the caucasoid population. This population is held to have less genetic admixture than the black American population. In insulin-dependent diabetic patients DR_4 is increased, with DR_2 and DR_5 decreased compared with black non-diabetic controls.

Despite the combined frequency, in the insulin-dependent diabetic patients of caucasoid origin, of DR_3 and DR_4 approaching 100%, their usefulness as genetic or predictive markers is extremely limited by the frequency of the antigens in the non-diabetic population (about 50%). In the search for more specific genetic markers the dominant approach has been by means of restriction fragment length polymorphism studies. HLA-DR antigens are made up of two alpha-chains and two beta-chains and are referred to as Class II antigens. Distinct from the DR antigen yet a Class II antigen is the DQ antigen, which is in strong linkage disequilibrium with DR, and a third Class II antigen, DP. The DQ region is composed of two alpha genes, DQ_{A1} and DQ_{A2} and two beta genes, DQ_{B1} and DQ_{B2}. Recent studies have identified certain amino acid sequences in DQ regions with links to type 1 diabetes.

Of critical importance would appear to be the identity of the amino acid at position 57 of the DQ_{B1} chain. Thus the DQ_{B1} aspartate 57 sequence in the DQ_{B1} gene appears to confer resistance to type 1 diabetes while DQ_{A1} arginine 52 in the DQ_{A1} gene results in susceptibility (Todd, Bell and McDevitt, 1987). To put this another way, people who express one Asp 57 positive allele have a risk of type 1 diabetes which is greater than those expressing two alleles. In the latter group there is almost complete resistance to the development of diabetes. People who do not express Asp 57 are at greatest risk of diabetes.

Somewhat against the importance of this finding is that a number of people express haplotypes that do not have Asp 57, for example DR_7, but they do not appear to be susceptible to diabetes. Conversely, 49% of Japanese type 1 diabetic patients are homozygous for Asp 57 and 49% are heterozygous.

Cloning and sequencing of the DQ and DR haplotypes linked with insulin-dependent diabetes have led to a hypothesis linking the individual features of the aetiology. The DQ molecule has a groove which has a beta-pleated sheet as the base of the groove with alpha helices forming the walls. One of these helices is coded for by the DQ_{A1} gene and the other by the DQ_{B1} gene. The absence of aspartate from position 57 of the DQ_{B1} gene and the presence of arginine at position 52 of the DQ_{A1} gene alter antigen presentation in a critical manner which confers susceptibility for insulin-dependent diabetes.

There is a potential pitfall in some of these studies. Clearly, to establish aetiological factors in this type of diabetes it was necessary to investigate a population in whom there could be no doubt of the type of clinical diabetes. Thus studies were conducted predominantly in children and young adults. With increas-

ing age insulin dependence is considerably more difficult to predict. Where this has been attempted it lends support to the heterogeneous nature of type 1 diabetes. Thus DR_3/DR_4 heterozygotes are increased in patients with onset below the age of 20 compared with older patients (Svejgaard *et al.*, 1986) and in our own study of patients aged 65 years and over and deemed to be insulin-dependent we found a preponderance of DR_3 but not of DR_4 (Kilvert *et al.*, 1986).

It should be stressed that the possession of DR_3, DR_4 or any other of the 'susceptibility' gene or genes does not, of course, imply certainty of the development of type 1 diabetes. Many normal people carry these antigens yet fail to develop diabetes. Nor does it currently point to the underlying defect, whether it is a direct effect of the antigen, a modification of the response to an environmental factor or a more distant effect. Similarly, the lower incidence of DR_2 does not have to point to a protective effect but may simply reflect that when there is a relative increase in DR_3 or DR_4 there must be a proportional decrease in the frequency of some antigen or antigens. The latter, a rather traditional view of the role of DR_2, may yet be shown to be erroneous and perhaps screening for protection will eventually be as important as, or more important than, screening for risk.

Twin studies

The work of Pyke and his colleagues from King's College Hospital in London lifted studies of identical twins to an altogether higher plane than previous twin studies. Careful studies of pairs of monozygous twins with either insulin-dependent or non-insulin-dependent diabetes have been performed by a succession of research registrars with results which have contributed significantly to our understanding of the inheritance and other aspects of aetiology and pathogenesis.

Their results show that when age of onset

is less than 45 years there is a concordance for diabetes of only 36% (Olmos *et al.*, 1988). HLA studies have shown an increase in the concordant pairs of HLA-B_8 although HLA-B_{15} was increased in both concordant and discordant pairs. Later studies found an increased prevalence of DR_3 and DR_4, with reduced prevalence of DR_5, DR_7 and DR_2, in both concordant and discordant pairs, but the heterozygote DR_3/DR_4 was most prevalent in concordant pairs (Johnston *et al.*, 1983).

Family studies

It would be tempting to conclude from population studies that there exists a particular diabetogenic gene which either is DR_3/DR_4 or is closely linked with the HLA type. Family studies, and particularly those including identical twins, are more useful in identifying this tendency. About 6–10% of type 1 diabetic patients have an affected first-degree relative and indeed when two siblings have the disorder an identical haplotype is found in 60% of cases. Rarely do diabetic siblings have completely different haplotypes.

Several large-scale family studies are under way in both the UK and the USA. The major handicap to useful data emerging appears to be the slow development of a second relative with insulin-dependent diabetes in the families. Currently a second case of diabetes would occur in a first-degree relative of an insulin-dependent diabetic at a rate of around 0.6–2.0 per 1000 families per year (Bingley and Gale, 1991).

Overlooked in the general enthusiasm for HLA-linked insulin-dependent diabetes is a difference in penetrance between familial and non-familial cases. The absolute risk of insulin-dependent diabetes for DR_3/DR_4 heterozygotes is 3% but for HLA identical siblings of an insulin-dependent diabetic it is 12%. This difference may be explained by additional genetic factors, environmental similarities or dilution of a specific subregion of HLA in non-familial cases.

Polymorphism of the insulin gene

The insulin gene lies on the short arm of chromosome 11. Closely linked to the insulin gene are the genes for tyrosine hydroxylase and insulin-like growth factor 2. These loci span 45 kb. The role of polymorphism of the 5′ flanking region of the human insulin gene has aroused considerable interest.

Genetic polymorphism can be detected by DNA digestion using restriction enzymes which cleave DNA at specific nucleotide sequences. Different-sized fragments indicate polymorphism and the use of probes with specific gene sequences allows identification of an individual's genotype. Polymorphism of the 5′ region of the insulin gene is due to a region of variable number of tandem repeats (VNTR). The three alleles identified are simply classed as 1, 2 or 3 and of these the class 2 allele is exceedingly rare. The class 1 allele with 50 repeats predisposes to insulin-dependent diabetes while the class 3 allele with 150–200 repeats protects. The susceptibility at the insulin gene region is localized to within the VNTR (Bennett *et al.*, 1995).

Direct evidence of alterations in function due to differences in the 5′ region is lacking yet it is clearly possible that a particular allele could alter insulin gene expression.

Other susceptibility genes

The degree of familial clustering of a disease is calculated from the ratio of the risk for siblings of patients to the population prevalence. For type 1 diabetes this is about 15 and it is clear that the genetic component cannot be accounted for in its entirety by a contribution from HLA antigens and the insulin gene. Davies *et al.* (1994) have calculated that the contribution from the HLA system is 42% and from the insulin gene 10% and in an effort to identify other susceptibility genes they have searched the human genome. Two further linkages were identified on chromosome 11q and 6q, with 16 other chromosome regions showing positive evidence of linkage to type 1 diabetes. None of these linkages has the power of even the insulin gene and it is likely that the remaining contribution to susceptibility is composed of a number of loci each contributing less than 6% – confirmation if it was needed of the polygenic nature of insulin-dependent diabetes mellitus.

ENVIRONMENTAL FACTORS

What emerges clearly from population studies is that a certain HLA haplotype may be associated with an increased relative risk of diabetes. Essential differences between members of families, particularly identical twins, and the widespread occurrence of the same haplotype in the normal population (when there is no justification for concluding that they are pre-diabetic) point with confidence to the important role of environmental factors in precipitating overt disease. Identifying specific environmental agents that precipitate type 1 diabetes has proved difficult and a critical approach to claims is desirable. The main factors identified as having potential for precipitating insulin-dependent diabetes are viruses, chemical toxins and stress.

Viruses

The role of viruses has received most attention. Viruses have been implicated on the basis of circumstantial evidence from population studies, more direct evidence from animal experiments, and some limited human information (Table 1.4). Gundersen (1927) drew attention to the possible relationship between mumps infection and insulin-dependent diabetes following an outbreak of mumps in Scandinavia which was followed by an upsurge in insulin-dependent diabetes. Gamble (1980) confirmed an association using data from the British Diabetic Association Childhood Diabetes Register. He reported a significant increase in consultations for mumps in the 6 months before the onset of diabetes.

Table 1.4   Evidence supporting a role for viruses in precipitating insulin-dependent diabetes

1. Population studies of incidence
2. Reports of antecedent viral infection and onset of diabetes (e.g. rubella, mumps)
3. Serological studies of antecedent viral illness
4. Animal models of virus-induced diabetes
5. Pancreatic insulitis and B-cell destruction following viral infection
6. Isolation of viruses from patients with acute onset diabetes and induction of diabetes in animals by these isolates
7. Development of islet-cell antibodies following viral infection

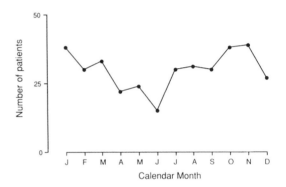

Fig. 1.3   Seasonal incidence of insulin-dependent diabetes diagnosed before 40 years of age in 357 patients. (Source: adapted from Gamble and Taylor, 1968.)

This register has provided other useful and interesting information on incidence of diabetes. It is clear from the data that there is a seasonal incidence of diabetes (Figure 1.3) as well as peaks of incidence of specific ages (Figure 1.4). In the UK the seasonal variation shows a broad peak from November to April and a narrower autumn peak from July to October. The age incidence shows a main peak at 12 years and a minor peak at 4–5 years. Both the seasonal and age incidence have been interpreted as indicating a role for viruses, usually explained through ages at which new schools are attended or times of

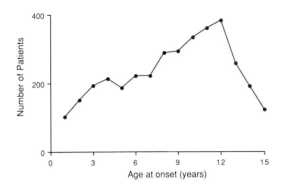

Fig. 1.4 Age incidence of insulin-dependent diabetes. (Source: adapted from Gamble, 1977.)

year of return to school with consequent exposure to a new or amended pool of viruses. These conclusions have depended upon the abrupt onset of type 1 diabetes, and the relationship to a longer prodromal period, now acknowledged in some patients (Gorsuch *et al.*, 1981), has not been considered in the explanation. Indeed, with regard to the seasonal variation it seems less likely that a child would report some symptoms when there is the prospect of a long summer holiday than when faced with the prospect of school.

In many of the children reported to the BDA register blood was obtained at diagnosis. Compared with non-diabetic controls a higher incidence of antibodies to Coxsackie B4 was observed (Gamble *et al.*, 1969). In contrast to this finding is a study from Sweden of children with newly diagnosed insulin-dependent diabetes where the prevalence of Coxsackie B virus IgM antibodies was similar in the diabetic children and their non-diabetic siblings (Frisk *et al.*, 1992).

In animals, a diabetic-like disease can be induced in mice by the M variant of the encephalomyocarditis virus (EMC) while in other rodents reovirus, Group B Coxsackie viruses and Venezualan equine encephalitis virus all produce diabetes. Not all strains of animals are susceptible to diabetes after viral infection, stressing the importance of genetic factors. To read the article by Notkins (1979)

is most instructive for although it cannot be doubted that viruses will produce diabetes it becomes apparent that considerable laboratory manipulation is necessary to produce the disease, often involving several passes of the virus through an animal strain. The histology of the lesion is more convincing. Macrophage and lymphocyte infiltration of the islet of Langerhans and even viral particles may be found in the B cells. The insulitis is similar to the findings in autopsy specimens from type 1 diabetic patients (Gepts and le Compte, 1981). After the observation of diabetes in children with congenital rubella Menser, Forrest and Bransby (1978) found similar changes in islet histology in experimental congenital rubella infection in rabbits.

Confirmation in the human islet has been more difficult to achieve since (hopefully) little autopsy material is available at diagnosis of type 1 diabetes. Insulitis is well-demonstrated but whether it represents recent infection or an immunological destruction is uncertain. Virus infection of the pancreas in humans has proved more elusive to demonstrate. The exception to this is the oft-quoted patient reported by Yoon *et al.* (1979). In a patient dying from a viraemia which precipitated acute diabetes mellitus, homogenates of pancreas added to mouse, monkey or human cell culture allowed recovery of the virus, which when inoculated into mice caused hyperglycaemia and B cell necrosis with an inflammatory infiltrate. The virus was subsequently identified as having similarities to Coxsackie B4.

Menser, Forrest and Bransby (1978) reported a frequency of 40% for diabetes developing in patients with congenital rubella. In New York 21% of the congenital rubella population have islet cell antibodies and these are found in 50–80% of patients with altered carbohydrate metabolism. Insulin autoantibodies were found in 13% of the population compared with less than 1% of controls.

Should viruses be playing a part in the initiation of type 1 diabetes they could do so in a number of ways. Clearly the prime candidate role would be in instigating auto-immune phenomena which might result from their well demonstrated tropic effect. Altern-atively the tropic effect may be a sufficient explanation. Other suggestions are that certain viruses can inhibit proinsulin synthesis or insulin release; or that synthesis of other islet proteins might be affected, for example HLA antigens or interferons (Szopa *et al.*, 1993).

Chemicals

Chemicals that can be injected into animals, resulting in B cell destruction and diabetes, have been recognised for many years. The best known are alloxan and streptozotocin. In humans identification of destructive agents is more difficult due to the vast numbers of chemicals ingested daily. Traditionally animals are made diabetic by single-dose injection but it has been demonstrated that repeated subdiabetogenic doses can induce round cell infiltration of the islet and insulitis (Like and Rossini, 1976). Certain chemicals can cause massive B cell destruction in man when ingested for self-poisoning, of which the best known is a rodenticide available in the USA.

Of interest is the increased incidence of type 1 diabetes in groups which consume large quantities of smoked meat and fish (Helgason and Jonasson, 1981). More recently, prolonged breast feeding has seemed to protect against the development of diabetes or perhaps the introduction of cow's-milk protein leads to an increase in insulin-dependent diabetes (Dahl-Jorgensen, Joner and Hanssen, 1991). The risk of type 1 diabetes was decreased in children totally breast-fed for 2 or 3 months or, to put this another way, those children who were younger than 2 months or 3 months at the time when supplementary milk feeding was commenced had an increased risk of insulin-dependent diabetes (Virtanen *et al.*, 1992). Furthermore, there is an association of in-creased risk of insulin-dependent diabetes

and levels of cow's-milk antibodies such that high IgA antibodies are associated with in-creased risk (Virtanen *et al.*, 1994). This latter suggestion has led to a trial of avoidance of cow's-milk protein in first-degree relatives of insulin-dependent diabetics over the first 9 months of life in Finland, where incidence rates are high.

The synthesis of the genetic predisposition to diabetes and the environmental precipitat-ing agent remains tenuous. It has been argued that the genetic predisposition may influence the tendency to a viral infection on exposure, replication of the virus in the B cell or the efficacy with which an initial lesion is repaired. Environmental agents may lead to the pro-duction of antigens that stimulate an immune response against the islet itself or allow failure of regulation of the immune response or even lead to abnormal proliferation of lymphocytes.

IMMUNOLOGICAL FACTORS

For many years a link has been acknowledged between organ-specific endocrinopathies and diabetes. Diabetes occurs more commonly in association with thyroid disease, Addison's disease and pernicious anaemia. In the early 1970s antibodies to islet cells were detected in blood from diabetic patients with other auto-immune disorders (Bottazzo, Florin-Christensen and Doniach, 1974). While antibodies could be detected by indirect immunofluorescence in the blood of these patients, Lendrum, Walker and Gamble (1975) showed that they were particularly prevalent in blood from newly diagnosed type 1 diabetic patients. They were not specific for particular islet types but reacted with all cell types, yet not with islet hormones. Much work has gone into refining the detection of antibodies to the B cell and to fragments of the cell. Subgroups have been identified such as complement-fixing islet cell antibody, which some argue is more specific for B cell destruction.

Islet cell antibodies may be present for long periods before manifestation of overt diabetes. Following development and diagnosis of the disease the majority show a rapid decline in titre although 10–15% of patients may have persistent antibodies. In this latter group there is a female preponderance and many patients have evidence of other organ-specific antibodies, suggesting a specific subgroup of type 1 diabetes.

A puzzling feature with regard to islet cell antibodies has been their relative non-specificity. Appropriately named islet cell antibodies and not B-cell antibodies they possess the capacity to attack all cells of the islet yet the damage produced seems limited to the B cell. Bottazzo and his colleagues (1983) put forward the hypothesis of aberrant expression of class II antigens on endocrine cells as a prelude to damage. They (Bottazzo *et al.*, 1985) and others (Foulis, Farquharson and Hardman, 1987) confirmed that only the B cell showed aberrant expression of the DR antigens.

Insulin autoantibodies have also been reported in 40% of newly diagnosed insulin-dependent diabetes (Palmer *et al.* 1983).

Of more recent interest has been the identification of 64K autoantibodies circulating in more than 80% of newly diagnosed insulin-dependent patients. These appear to be targeted upon a 64K antigen in B cells. Baekkeskov *et al.* (1990) perceived a link between the rare but severe neurological disease stiff man syndrome, when antibodies to gamma-aminobutyric acid coexist with islet cell antibodies in most patients, and the 64K protein of insulin-dependent patients. They confirmed that the 64K antigen of islets was identical to the antigen for gamma-aminobutyric acid antibodies, i.e. the enzyme glutamic acid decarboxylase, found in high concentrations in B cells. There are two isoforms of GAD antibodies, the products of different genes. In the human islet GAD_{65} is predominantly expressed while in other species GAD_{67} is predominant in islets.

This is an area of intense investigation at present. A number of other islet autoantigens have been suggested, including insulin itself, proinsulin, gangliosides, heat shock protein 65, surface protein p69 and the ABBOS sequence.

Antigen–antibody complexes can also be detected in blood from newly or recently diagnosed diabetic patients. These immune complexes may react with cells that have surface receptors for complement fractions, damaging cells directly or interacting with specific T cell populations. Migration of leucocytes from type 1 patients is inhibited by islet fractions and a variety of other abnormalities have been found, including low-affinity E rosette-forming cells and decreased suppressor-T lymphocytes. Some abnormalities are found only in poorly controlled patients, suggesting that they are secondary to the metabolic abnormality.

PREDICTING INSULIN-DEPENDENT DIABETES

The above findings on the aetiology of type 1 diabetes have led to the firm conclusion that it is an autoimmune disease or more specifically that a particular environmental agent may cause B cell damage which, by interaction with a particular genetic make-up, leads to, or allows, a modified immune response. This immune response results in antibody formation, which can lead to further destruction of insulin secretory cells with an almost inevitable consequence of type 1 diabetes. Thus after the initial environmental insult the development of diabetes is an autoimmune process. A note of caution should be added to this, perhaps oversimplified, concept of progression since the antibody most intensively investigated, islet-cell antibody, shows deviation from this pattern. Islet-cell antibody is directed to all cells of the islet yet damage only occurs to the B cell, raising doubts as to its destructive role. In addition, injection of islet-cell antibodies into animals does not result

Table 1.5 Lifetime risk for the development of insulin-dependent diabetes (%)

General population	0.4
With DR_3/DR_4	2.4
With susceptible DR/DQ alleles	8.0
Identical twin of type 1 diabetic	36.0
Sibling	6.0
HLA identical	12.0
HLA non-identical	1.0
Offspring of a diabetic mother	1.3
Offspring of a diabetic father	6.0

in islet destruction and insulin-dependent diabetes.

Nevertheless, possibilities exist for intervention in this process and with this in mind prediction and prevention have become a priority. Prevention is discussed elsewhere in this volume (Chapter 13) but it is clear that prevention or even well designed trials of early intervention will depend upon an ability to predict those people at increased risk of developing insulin-dependent diabetes.

From the epidemiological data which are available it is apparent that clustering of cases of insulin-dependent diabetes occurs. Lifetime risk is set out in Table 1.5 for different groups of people.

The striking finding in Table 1.5 is that even in the group that is generally acknowledged as carrying a high risk the concordance for insulin-dependent diabetes is only about 1 in 3. Clearly, prediction of insulin-dependent diabetes from genetic markers will be limited. In view of this attention has turned to the use of immunological markers and to a much lesser extent metabolic markers. The best studied immunological marker is islet-cell antibodies.

Johnston *et al.* (1989) found that ten out of ten twins who developed diabetes had islet-cell antibodies, compared with seven of 19 who did not develop diabetes in 5 years of follow up. In prospective family studies the titre of islet cell antibodies has been found to correlate with the development of insulin-

dependent diabetes. All those with a titre > 80 JDF units followed for 7 years developed diabetes (Bonifacio *et al.*, 1990). At lower titres 14 of 16 family members who developed diabetes had islet-cell antibodies above the detection limit of 4 JDF units. Importantly, 4% of family members who did not progress to diabetes also had titres > 4 JDF units. In a 10-year study of nearly 5000 non-diabetic relatives of patients with insulin-dependent diabetes 27 of 40 who developed diabetes had pre-existing islet-cell antibodies (Riley *et al.*, 1990).

What of other potential immunological markers? Insulin autoantibodies do not appear to add significantly to the conclusions that can be drawn from the presence of islet-cell antibodies. Antibodies to the 64 kDa islet antigen may prove more specific but await further evaluation. Meanwhile the search continues for an autoantigen which can be specifically linked with the destructive process in the islet while metabolic markers are also being sought which can be used in the prediction of high risk individuals.

AETIOLOGY OF TYPE 2 DIABETES

The aetiology of type 1 diabetes is an area of clarity compared with that of type 2 diabetes. In part this is due to lack of knowledge of the pathogenic mechanism of type 2 diabetes and in particular the difficulty of dating the onset of the disease in a patient. There is a broad spectrum of presentation from asymptomatic individuals detected by routine medical examinations to apparently acutely ill patients with considerable metabolic abnormality who may even be in coma. The wide variety of presentation may lend support to the view that it is incorrect to consider type 2 diabetes as a homogeneous entity (McCarthy, Froguel and Hitman, 1994). In the original version of this book Malins discussed the aetiology of diabetes under one heading and it may be that after an equivalent time interval the discussion of aetiology of type 2 diabetes will be similarly out of date. At the moment, however, we are stuck with the label of type 2 diabetes, although the original suggestion by the classifiers that it should be 'not insulin-dependent' rather than 'non-insulin-dependent' may have considerable merit.

GENETIC FACTORS

Population studies

It is widely held that the prevalence of type 2 diabetes is of the order of 1–2% in Western cultures. Certain ethnic groups give higher figures than this – 5% in Indian subpopulations (Mather and Keen, 1985) – while some populations have extremely high prevalence rates. The well-investigated Pima Indians (Bennett and Knowler, 1980) and Nauruan islanders (Zimmet, 1982) yield a prevalence of 30%. Such high figures lend support to a genetic predisposition when taken with other evidence but the validity of extrapolation to other populations may be open to question. In some countries there is an impression of high prevalence rates approaching one-third to one-half of the population but confirmation is difficult due to absence of adequate population records.

Population studies have tended to concentrate upon ethnic groups where prevalence rates are high but extrapolation of findings is dubious. In Nauruan families there is a 40% prevalence of diabetes in the offspring of two diabetic parents while no diabetes occurs in the offspring of two non-diabetic parents. In islanders over the age of 60 the prevalence of diabetes is 83%. It is possible to detect genetic admixture in some individuals by HLA typing and in these people the prevalence over age 60 is only 17%.

In the Pima Indians of Arizona 50% over the age of 35 have non-insulin-dependent diabetes. Glucose tolerance in this population conforms to a bimodal distribution interpreted as a single gene determining diabetic status.

Twin studies

The strongest evidence of a genetic influence in the aetiology of diabetes comes from studies in identical twins (Barnett *et al.*, 1981). The concordance rate is of the order of 90% and approaches 100% when pairs are followed for 5–7 years. This contrasts with the 45–50% concordance rate for type 1 diabetes. It is of interest that with the late onset of the disease a number of pairs have lived apart in different environments for many years. This series of studies has been criticized on the grounds of differential ascertainment but it is supported by a USA survey of military records of monozygotic twins.

Family studies

Kobberling and Tillil (1982) have calculated that 38% of siblings of patients with non-insulin-dependent diabetes will become diabetic before the age of 80 years. In the South Indian population 580 offspring of 164 families where both parents had diabetes revealed 50% with a diabetes and a further 12% with impaired glucose tolerance (Viswanathan *et al.*, 1985). In islet-cell-antibody-negative patients with diabetes presenting before the age of 40, 89% of parents and 69% of siblings had diabetes or impaired glucose tolerance (O'Rahilly *et al.*, 1987).

Candidate genes

Despite the apparently strong genetic component to the aetiology of this type of diabetes there is only limited information on the likely genetic markers. Non-HLA chromosome 6 genetic markers such as glyoxylase, C2 complement and properdin factor B have proved disappointing, as has chlorpropamide–alcohol flushing.

The gene which encodes for the insulin receptor has also been a rather obvious target for investigation. Located on chromosome 19 it spans a region of 120 kb. Many restriction length fragment polymorphisms have been identified and studied in varied populations. Almost uniformly no association has been found between a specific allele and type 2 diabetes. The populations studied include caucasoids, Sikhs, American whites and blacks, and Japanese.

Glucose transporter genes have also been investigated. The glucose transporters that have been identified (Gould and Bell, 1990) share a similar basic structure but differ in tissue distribution. Glut 4, which is located in the mainly metabolic tissues of muscle and fat, has been studied because it could be linked with tissue insulin resistance. Early studies have not indicated any link between Glut 4 polymorphisms and non-insulin-dependent diabetes.

A number of other potential associations have been examined, including amylin and glucokinase. Associations with typically type 2 diabetes have not been found.

The HLA system instrumental in progress in the aetiology of type 1 diabetes has served type 2 diabetes less well. No strong associations emerge in caucasoid populations although weak associations with HLA-A$_2$ have been reported in South African blacks and Pima Indians, with HLA-BW$_{61}$ in Asian Indians in South Africa and Fiji, and with HLA-BW$_{22}$ in Polynesians.

ENVIRONMENTAL FACTORS

It is perhaps true to say that the commonly quoted environmental factors precipitating type 2 diabetes are so much part of man's everyday life that they reveal the paucity of our attempts at identification. Age, diet, obesity, exercise and stress are all suggested.

Age

One fact about diabetes which is never disputed is that it becomes more common as age increases, though there is a fall at the greatest ages in the incidence recorded in diabetic clinics (FitzGerald *et al.*, 1961). While it is conceivable that this deficit could be explained by a higher death-rate in the oldest diabetics compared with the general population it is more probable that the figures represent a failure to record aged patients because other diseases overshadow the diabetes and because such people are less mobile and less likely to be referred to a general hospital clinic. This view is supported by the findings in population surveys, which disclose a much greater proportion of unsuspected diabetes among those who are over 70 years of age. It is not unreasonable, therefore, to assume that the incidence of diabetes in relation to the population at risk rises steadily with age. The reason for this is not obvious beyond the general deterioration that age brings to every function. The manner in which glucose tolerance deteriorates with age has been remarked in many population surveys, and the finding of tests abnormal by agreed standards at that time in as many as 16% of the population over the age of 50 and 25% over the age of 70 in a survey in Birmingham (Report of a Working Party appointed by the College of General Practitioners, 1963) begins to suggest that the diagnosis of diabetes by such standards in old people is unrealistic. It is reminiscent of estimates made at one time of a prevalence of mental deficiency of nearly 50% in the British population.

Obesity

Many would consider this the strongest risk factor in the development of type 2 diabetes. It is impossible to sit in the clinic week by week and not be impressed by an apparent association. This view is endorsed by the Second Report of the WHO Expert Committee on Diabetes Mellitus (WHO, 1980), which put obesity top of the list of risk factors. Some degree of caution is necessary, since Pyke (1979) found the expression of diabetes in identical twins to be independent of obesity and it is clear that the influence of obesity does not explain high prevalence rates of diabetes in various ethnic groups in either their own or adopted countries. Population studies of the predictive nature of obesity for diabetes have yielded conflicting results while there is the overwhelming evidence that the majority of obese people, even morbidly obese, do not have diabetes.

More recently attention has been focussed upon a particular form of obesity, central obesity, which seems to correlate better with harmful consequences of obesity than body mass index.

Nevertheless there are important consequences of obesity upon insulin secretion and action, which support a relationship superseding the rather simpler explanations of earlier years. The simple explanation for the association between obesity and diabetes is that weight gain as a result of gluttony leads ultimately to exhaustion of the islets and thereby to diabetes. It is well known that glucose tolerance tests which have been diabetic can return to normal after weight has been shed. It has been reported that this result can be achieved in more than 90% of obese diabetics but in our experience the figure would more closely approximate 15%.

The thrifty genotype

There has been considerable interest in why the diabetic genotype has persisted in the population. Neel (1962) proposed the concept of a thrifty genotype to suggest that persistence of the gene must confer some specific survival advantage. This proposes that the genotype favours fat deposition in times of plenty which confers an advantage to be carried into times of limited food supply. Now that we are no longer in a hunter-gatherer society fat deposition does not carry the same benefits and indeed has become a liability. It is argued that the theory is manifest in the populations that endured hardship but have undergone rapid socio-

economic development, such as the Pima Indians and the Nauruan islanders. In these populations the prevalence of diabetes has risen dramatically with the 'benefits' of modern-day civilization.

Exercise

Exercise, or more strictly lack of exercise, has been considered as an environmental factor in precipitating non-insulin-dependent diabetes. Indirect support for this is given by the role of exercise as part of treatment of diabetes. More direct association is given by the societies which have recently experienced an explosion in incidence of non-insulin-dependent diabetes. In nearly all such groups there is an associated change in lifestyle from traditional to more sedentary. As part of this reduced physical activity takes its place but clearly other factors such as change in diet and obesity are difficult to divorce from exercise. Methods of quantifying habitual physical activity are imprecise while in epidemiological studies it may be difficult to discard the influence of disease-related inactivity. At present there is no firm evidence for a role of exercise lack in precipitating non-insulin-dependent diabetes.

Stress

The diabetologist is frequently asked to adjudicate on whether stress 'caused' diabetes. The situation is common when a road traffic accident or an industrial accident is followed by the detection of glycosuria or a raised blood glucose and diabetes is diagnosed. Lawyers, wishing to do the best for their clients, are anxious that a causal link should be established but their claims are given little support by the physician or the literature. While admitting the fact that diabetes may follow trauma it is usually considered today that the injury is not to be regarded as a primary cause but that it may bring to light previously undiagnosed diabetes. Other stressful events, particularly injury or illness, may unmask diabetes by way of the catabolic hormone responses and forced immobilization. Robinson and Fuller (1986) reported an association between the onset of insulin-dependent diabetes and preceding severe life events. Against any theory linking stress and non-insulin-dependent diabetes is the oft-quoted low prevalence during the two world wars.

Parity

Mosenthal and Bolduan (1933) noticed that the frequency with which diabetes was cited as a cause of death at ages over 45 was higher in married and widowed women than in single women. Initially this observation was attributed to an association with obesity while others thought that the excess of elderly women was related to previous childbearing. Pyke (1956) showed that the chances of developing diabetes for women were related to the number of children they had borne. He considered that this effect of parity could not be due merely to the greater obesity of multiparous women, which was not striking in those who had developed diabetes. The results from our own clinic (FitzGerald *et al.*, 1961) confirmed those of Pyke, showing that the incidence of diabetes increases with each increase in parity; compared with that in nulliparae it is about twice as common in women who have had three children and six times as common in those who have had six or more.

Big babies

That women with diabetes may bear very large babies was observed in the last century in spite of the rarity of pregnancy in the recognized diabetic at that time. Skipper (1933) seems to have been the first to suggest that this tendency might be present before the onset of the diabetes although others emphasized it and it became more widely

known with the demonstration that the mean birth weight of babies born to prediabetic women was significantly greater than that of a control series. Later reports are concerned with the incidence of babies weighing more than 4.5 kg (10 lb) in pre-diabetic and non-diabetic mothers. The figures vary widely, probably as a result of different methods of collecting and handling the data, from 31% to the 12.6% of our own patients. The tendency to give birth to large babies was present up to 60 years before the clinical diagnosis of diabetes and did not increase as the time of diagnosis approached. It is unlikely that fetal gigantism at this time is related to hyperglycaemia, for it is difficult to believe that the blood glucose is raised in pre-diabetic women 50 years before the clinical diagnosis.

Early nutrition

Hales *et al.* (1991) have argued that fetal and early-life nutrition are important determinants for the later development of impaired glucose tolerance and non-insulin-dependent diabetes. They assessed the degree of glucose tolerance in men in their 60s whose weights in early life were known. A clear relationship emerged between low birth weight and low weight at 12 months and abnormal glucose tolerance in later life. Body mass index at the time of testing was found to be an independent variable in that low body mass index seemed to protect against abnormal glucose tolerance even in men of low birth and 12-month weight. On the basis of these data it has been suggested that early, including *in utero*, nutritional factors that determine fetal and infant growth influence the size and vascularity of the adult pancreas. Combined in later life with obesity, inactivity or aging resulting in insulin resistance this could lead to the development of glucose intolerance.

REFERENCES

Baekkeskov, S., Aanstoot, H. J., Christgau, S. *et al.* (1990) Identification of the 64K autoantigen in insulin-dependent diabetes as the GABA-synthesising enzyme glutamic acid decarboxylase. *Nature*, **347**, 151–156.

Barnett, A. H., Eff, C. Leslie, R. D. G. and Pyke, D. A. (1981) Diabetes in identical twins. A study of 200 pairs. *Diabetologia*, **20**, 87–93.

Bennett, P. H. and Knowler, W. C. (1980) Increasing prevalence of diabetes in the Pima (American) Indians over a ten year period, in *Diabetes 1979*, (ed. W. K. Waldhausl), Excerpta Medica, Amsterdam, p. 507–511.

Bennett, S. T., Lucassen, A. M., Gough, S. C. L. *et al.* (1995) Susceptibility to human type 1 diabetes at IDDM2 is determined by tandem repeat variation at the insulin gene minisatellite locus. *Nat. Genet.*, **9**, 284–291.

Bertrams, J. and Baur M. P. (1984) Insulin-dependent diabetes mellitus, in *Histocompatibility Testing*, (eds E. D. Albert, M. P. Baur and W. R. Mayr), Springer-Verlag, Heidelberg, p. 348–358.

Bingley, P. J. and Gale, E. A. M. (1991) Lessons from family studies. *Clin. Endocrinol. Metab.*, **5**, 261–283.

Bonifacio, E., Bingley, P. J., Shattock, M. *et al.* (1990) Quantification of islet-cell antibodies and prediction of insulin-dependent diabetes. *Lancet*, **335**, 147–149.

Bottazzo, G. F., Florin-Christensen, A. and Doniach, D. (1974) Islet cell antibodies in diabetes mellitus with autoimmune polyendocrine deficiencies. *Lancet*, **ii**, 1279–1283.

Bottazzo, G. F., Pujol-Borrell, R., Hanafusa, T. and Feldmann, M. (1983) Role of aberrant HLA DR expression and antigen presentation in induction of endocrine autoimmunity. *Lancet*, **ii**, 1115–1118.

Bottazzo, G. F., Dean, B. M., McNally, J. M. *et al.* (1985) In situ characterization of autoimmune phenomena and expression of HLA molecules in the pancreas in diabetic insulitis. *N. Engl. J. Med.* **313**, 353–360.

Cammidge, P. J. (1934) Heredity as factor in aetiology of diabetes mellitus. *Lancet*, **i**, 393–395.

Dahl-Jorgensen, Joner, G. and Hanssen, K. F. (1991) Relationship between cows' milk consumption and incidence of IDDM in childhood. *Diabetes Care*, **14**, 1081–1083.

Davies, J. I., Kawaguchi, Y., Bennett, S. T. *et al.* (1994) A genome-wide search for human type 1 diabetes susceptibility genes. *Nature*, **371**, 130–136.

Degnbol, B. and Green, A. (1978) Diabetes mellitus among first- and second-degree relatives of early onset diabetics. *Ann. Hum. Genet. (Lond.)*, **42**, 25–34.

Diabetes Epidemiology Research International Group (1988) Geographic patterns of childhood insulin-dependent diabetes mellitus. *Diabetes*, **37**, 1113–1119.

FitzGerald, M. G., Malins, J. M., O'Sullivan, D. J. and Wall, M. (1961) The effect of sex and parity on the incidence of diabetes mellitus. *Q. J. Med.*, **30**, 57–70.

Foulis, A. K., Farquharson, M. A. and Hardman, R. (1987) Aberrant expression of class II major histocompatibility complex molecules by B cells and hyperexpression of class I major histocompatibility complex molecules by insulin containing islets in type 1 (insulin-dependent) diabetes mellitus. *Diabetologia*, **30**, 333–343.

Frisk, G., Friman, G., Tuvemo, T. *et al.* (1992) Coxsackie B virus IgM in children at onset of type 1 (insulin-dependent) diabetes mellitus: evidence for IgM induction by a recent or current infection. *Diabetologia*, **35**, 249–253.

Gamble, D. R. (1977) Viruses and diabetes: an overview with special reference to epidemiological studies, in *Diabetes*, (ed. J. S. Bajaj), Excerpta Medica, Amsterdam, p. 285–293.

Gamble, D. R. (1980) Relation of antecedent illness to development of diabetes in children. *Br. Med. J.*, **281**, 99–101.

Gamble, D. R. and Taylor, K. W. (1969) Seasonal incidence of diabetes mellitus. *Br. Med. J.*, **3**, 631–633.

Gamble, D. R., Kinsley, M. I., FitzGerald, M. G. *et al.* (1969) Viral antibodies in diabetes mellitus. *Br. Med. J.*, **3**, 627–630.

Gepts, W. and le Compte, P. M. (1981) The pancreatic islets in diabetes. *Am. J. Med.*, **70**, 105–115.

Gorsuch, A. N., Spencer, K. M., Lister, J. *et al.* (1981) Evidence for a long prediabetic period in type 1 (insulin-dependent) diabetes mellitus. *Lancet*, **ii**, 1363–1365.

Gould, G. W. and Bell, G. I. (1990) Facilitative glucose transporters: an expanding family. *Trends Biol. Sci.* **15**, 18–23.

Green, A., Gale, E. A. M. and Patterson, C. C. (1992) Incidence of childhood-onset insulin-dependent diabetes mellitus: the Eurodiab Ace study. *Lancet*, **339**, 905–909.

Gundersen, E. (1927) Is diabetes of infectious origin? *J. Infect. Dis.*, **41**, 197–202.

Hales, C. N., Barker, D. J. P., Clark, P. M. S. *et al.* (1991) Fetal and infant growth and impaired glucose tolerance at age 64. *Br. Med. J.*, **303**, 1019–1022.

Harris, H. (1950) Familial distribution of diabetes mellitus: study of relatives of 1241 diabetic propositi. *Ann. Eugen. Lond.*, **15**, 95–119.

Helgason, T. and Jonasson, M. R. (1981) Evidence for a food additive as a cause of ketosis-prone diabetes. *Lancet*, **2**, 716–720.

Johnston, C., Pyke, D. A., Cudworth, A. G. and Wolf, E. (1983) HLA-DR typing in identical twins with insulin-dependent diabetes: difference between concordant and discordant pairs. *Br. Med. J.*, **286**, 253–255.

Johnston, C., Millward, B. A., Hoskins, P. *et al.* (1989) Islet-cell antibodies as predictors of Type 1 (insulin-dependent diabetes). *Diabetologia*, **32**, 382–386.

Karvonen, M., Tuomilehto, J., Libman, I. and LaPorte, R. (1993) A review of the recent epidemiological data on the worldwide incidence of type 1 (insulin-dependent) diabetes. *Diabetologia*, **36**, 883–892.

Kilvert, A., FitzGerald, M. G., Wright, A. D. and Nattrass, M. (1986) Clinical characteristics and aetiological classification of insulin-dependent diabetes in the elderly. *Q. J. Med.* **60**, 865–872.

Kobberling, J. and Tillil, H. (1982) Empirical risk figures for first degree relatives of non-insulin-dependent diabetics, in *The Genetics of Diabetes Mellitus*, (eds J. Kobberling and R. B. Tattersall), Academic Press, London, p. 201–209.

Lendrum, R., Walker, G. and Gamble, D. R. (1975) Islet-cell antibodies in juvenile diabetes mellitus of recent onset. *Lancet*, **i**, 880–883.

Like, A. A. and Rossini, A. A. (1976) Streptozotocin-induced pancreatic insulitis: new model of diabetes mellitus. *Science*, **193**, 415–417.

McCarthy, M. I., Froguel, P. and Hitman, G. A. (1994) The genetics of non-insulin-dependent diabetes mellitus: tools and aims. *Diabetologia*, **37**, 959–968.

Mather, H. M. and Keen, H. (1985) The Southall diabetes survey: prevalence of known diabetes in Asians and Europeans. *Br. Med. J.*, **291**, 1081–1084.

Menser, M. A., Forrest, J. M. and Bransby, R. D. (1978) Rubella infection and diabetes mellitus. *Lancet*, **i**, 57–60.

Mosenthal, H. O. and Bolduan, C. (1933) Diabetes mellitus – problems of present day treatment. *Am. J. Med. Sci.*, **186**, 605–621.

National Diabetes Data Group (1979) Classification and diagnosis of diabetes mellitus and other causes of glucose intolerance. *Diabetes*, **28**, 1039–1057.

Neel, J. V. (1962) Diabetes mellitus: a 'thrifty' genotype rendered detrimental by 'progress'. *Am. J. Hum. Genet.*, **14**, 353–362.

Notkins, A. L. (1979) The causes of diabetes. *Sci. Am.*, **241**, 62–73.

Odugbesan, O., Fletcher, J., Mijovic, C. *et al.* (1987) The HLA-D associations of type 1 (insulin-dependent) diabetes in Punjabi Asians in the United Kingdom. *Diabetologia*, **30**, 618–621.

Olmos, P., A'Hern, P., Heaton, D. A. *et al.* (1988) The significance of the concordance rate for type 1 (insulin-dependent) diabetes in identical twins. *Diabetologia*, **31**, 747–750.

O'Rahilly, S., Spivey, R. S., Holman, R. R. *et al.* (1987) Type II diabetes of early onset: a distinct clinical and genetic syndrome. *Br. Med. J.*, **294**, 923–928.

Palmer, J., Asplin, C. M., Clemons, P. *et al.* (1983) Insulin antibodies in insulin-dependent diabetics before insulin treatment. *Science*, **222**, 1337–1339.

Platz, P., Jakobsen, B. K., Morling, N. *et al.* (1981) HLA-D and -DR antigens in genetic analysis of insulin dependent diabetes mellitus. *Diabetologia*, **21**, 108–115.

Pyke, D. A. (1956) Parity and incidence of diabetes. *Lancet*, **i**, 818–821.

Pyke, D. A. (1979) Diabetes: the genetic connections. *Diabetologia*, **17**, 333–343.

Report of a Working Party appointed by the College of General Practitioners (1963) Glucose tolerance and glycosuria in the general population. *Br. Med. J.*, **2**, 655–659.

Riley, W. J., Maclaren, N. K., Krischer, J. *et al.* (1990) A prospective study of the development of diabetes in relatives of patients with insulin-dependent diabetes. *N. Engl. J. Med.*, **323**, 1167–1172.

Robinson, N. and Fuller, J. H. (1986) Severe life events and their relationship to the aetiology of insulin-dependent (type 1) diabetes mellitus. *Ped. Adol. Endocrinol.*, **15**, 129–133.

Singal, D. P. and Blajchman, M. A. (1973) Histocompatibility (HL-A) antigens, lymphocytotoxic antibodies and tissue antibodies in patients with diabetes mellitus. *Diabetes*, **22**, 429–432.

Skipper, E. (1933) Diabetes mellitus and pregnancy. *Q. J. Med.*, **7**, 353–380.

Svejgaard, A., Jakobsen, B. K., Platz, P. *et al.* (1986) HLA associations in insulin-dependent diabetes: search for heterogeneity in different groups of patients from a homogeneous population. *Tissue Antigens* **28**, 237–244.

Szopa, T. M., Titchener, P. A., Portwood, N. D. and Taylor, K. W. (1993) Diabetes mellitus due to viruses – some recent developments. *Diabetologia*, **36**, 687–695.

Then-Bergh, H. (1938) Die Erbbiologie des Diabetes Mellitus. *Arch. Rass. Ges. Biol.*, **52**, 289.

Todd, J. A., Bell, J. I. and McDevitt, H. O. (1987) *HLA-DQ_B* gene contributes to susceptibility and resistance to insulin-dependent diabetes mellitus. *Nature*, **329**, 599–604.

Tuomilehto, J., Lounamaa, R., Tuomilehto-Wolf, E. *et al.* (1992) Epidemiology of childhood diabetes mellitus in Finland – background of a nationwide study of type 1 (insulin-dependent) diabetes mellitus. *Diabetologia*, **35**, 70–76.

Virtanen, S. M., Rasanen, L., Aro, A. *et al.* (1992) Feeding in infancy and the risk of type 1 diabetes mellitus in Finnish children. *Diabet. Med.* **9**, 815–819.

Virtanen, S. M., Saukkonen, T., Savilahti, E. *et al.* (1994) Diet, cow's milk protein antibodies and the risk of IDDM in Finnish children. *Diabetologia*, **37**, 381–387.

Viswanathan, M., Mohan, V., Snehalatha, C. and Ramachandran, A. (1985) High prevalence of type 2 (non-insulin-dependent) diabetes among the offspring of conjugal type 2 diabetic parents in India. *Diabetologia*, **28**, 907–910.

WHO (1980) WHO Expert Committee on Diabetes Mellitus, second report, *Technical Report Series 646*, World Health Organization, Geneva

WHO (1985) Diabetes mellitus. Report of a WHO Study Group, *Technical Report Series 727*, World Health Organization, Geneva.

Yoon, J. Y., Austin, M. Onodera, T. and Notkins, A. L. (1979) Isolation of a virus from the pancreas of a child with diabetic ketoacidosis. *N. Engl. J. Med.*, **300**, 1173–1179.

Zimmet, P. (1982) Type 2 (non-insulin-dependent) diabetes – an epidemiological overview. *Diabetologia*, **22**, 399–411.

The classification of diabetes based upon aetiology into type 1 and type 2 has important consequences for a consideration of pathogenesis. Clearly, if a particular type of diabetes originates in a set of specific inherited and environmental factors it follows logically that a type 2 diabetic can never become a type 1 patient nor *vice versa*.

It is clear that this dogmatic distinction based on aetiology cannot be carried into clinical presentation or course of the disease. The elderly patient presenting in diabetic ketoacidosis and subsequently well controlled by oral agents; the obese newly diagnosed patient with a short history of acute symptoms including significant weight loss; and many others at presentation, blur the distinction between insulin-dependent and non-insulin-dependent diabetes without regard to an aetiological classification. Furthermore, there may come a time in the course of type 2 diabetes when diet and oral agents fail and insulin is needed. The desire to maintain the aetiological separateness of the two types of diabetes has led to considerable verbal gymnastics to describe this person – the insulin-requiring non-insulin-dependent diabetic.

In part, the problem is created by the well entrenched interpretation of 'dependent', which continues to refer to a dependence upon insulin for avoidance of ketoacidosis. An insulin-requiring non-insulin-dependent diabetic patient is no less dependent upon insulin for the relief of symptoms, i.e. disease, yet such a definition is avoided.

Which of the two classifications, aetiological or clinical, is pertinent to pathogenesis? Logically it must be aetiology yet there is a certain pull towards clinical. Thus, while considering the pathogenesis of the two main types of diabetes separately, it is acknowledged that at the end of the spectrum, when type 2 diabetes becomes insulin-requiring, this may signal a progression in pathogenesis which, in expression, is similar to type 1 diabetes.

THE HISTOLOGY OF THE PANCREAS IN DIABETES (TABLE 2.1)

After the discovery that diabetes could be produced experimentally by removal of the pancreas the islets of Langerhans were extensively studied, in particular by Laguesse (1894) who first gave them that name and suggested their endocrine function. The changes in the islets in established diabetics were described by several writers and the appearance of the various abnormalities was generally agreed though the interpretation proved more difficult.

The lesions in the diabetic pancreas were fully discussed in the admirable monograph of Warren and LeCompte (1952) and may be classified as follows, the percentages in

Table 2.1 The histology of the diabetic pancreas

1. The pancreas	– reduced weight
	– lobular markings accentuated
	– fibrosis
	– fatty change
2. The islet	– hyalinization
	– arteriosclerosis
	– fibrosis
	– hypertrophy
3. The B cell	– vacuolization
	– fat deposits

brackets being the proportion of their 811 cases showing this abnormality.

1. Hyaline change (41%) was first described by Opie (1901) and like the other lesions recorded here may be seen with routine staining. The hyaline material is laid down in relation to the capillaries, usually between the lumina of the sinusoids and the B cells and sometimes obliterating the whole islet. The involvement of islets is patchy, some remaining normal when others are severely involved. The degree of hyalinization is not related to the severity of the diabetes (Bell, 1952), but this type of lesion is much more common in the elderly than in the young. Lacy (1964), using the electron microscope, found the hyaline to possess the ultrastructural features of amyloid and he considered it clearly distinct from the basement-membrane thickening of angiopathy.

   More recently, islet amyloid has been rediscovered in diabetic patients over the age of 40 (50–90%), in the spontaneously diabetic primate *Macaca nigra* and in a small number of normal people. Its occurrence in normal people continues to confuse the issue of whether it is specifically diabetes-related or more a feature of aging. The precursor of amyloid within the islet has been identified and termed diabetes-associated peptide (Cooper *et al.*, 1987) or islet amyloid polypeptide (Westermark *et al.*, 1987). The peptide has similarities to calcitonin gene-related peptide and, to a lesser extent, the A chain of insulin.

2. Fibrosis (23%) entails the formation of a fibrous capsule round the islet and the extension of fibroblasts into the interior. Although seen in children it is more often found in older subjects. The cause is not apparent, except when it occurs in association with obvious chronic pancreatitis.

3. Hydropic change (4%) was reported by Weichselbaum and Stangl (1902) and consists of a foamy and, later, vacuolated appearance of the B cells only. In experimental diabetes it is the earliest sign of strain or injury to the B cells and is reversible if the provocative agent is removed. It is seldom seen in man at autopsy and has to be carefully distinguished from those changes in the islets that normally occur after death.

   The hydropic appearance in many, if not all patients, has been shown to be due to infiltration with glycogen as occurs in many organs in diabetes and does not necessarily reflect an injurious insult.

4. Lymphocyte infiltration (1%) was recognized by Warren and Root (1925) and has been found most often in young patients with diabetes of acute onset. The affected islets are reduced in size and there is some loss of cells, those which remain being generally arranged in narrow cords. It seems that both the A and B cells are involved but the latter more severely. A variable degree of lymphocytic infiltration is seen in the damaged islets and slight fibrosis may be detected. Although originally suggested as being due to over-stimulation of the islets, it was thought by both LeCompte (1958) and Gepts (1965) to represent a response to viral infection or an immunological attack.

   Gepts (1965) examined the pancreases of 22 patients who were young and who died at presentation of diabetes. In 15 of them a chronic inflammatory cell infiltrate was found which affected a small proportion of the islets. The term 'insulitis' was used by both LeCompte (1958) and Gepts (1965) to describe these findings.

These changes are seen with routine staining, with which at least a third of all patients with diabetes show no abnormality at postmortem. Realization of this fact drew attention away from the pancreas as the centre of diabetic pathology at about the same time as the discoveries of Houssay and others offered an alternative field for study in the pituitary and adrenal glands. Some workers, too, were impressed by the outpouring of glucose from the liver and were almost ready to relegate insulin to a subsidiary position in the metabolic abnormality of diabetes (Soskin, 1948).

It remains true, however, that the only certain method of producing diabetes in man is by the destruction of the pancreas. At the most half of the cases of pituitary or adrenal oversecretion develop abnormal carbohydrate tolerance. It has been argued that the normal pancreas in man is able to resist all the stresses from other endocrine glands that are encountered clinically (sometimes quite different from the insults presented to the pancreas of the experimental animal) and that these stresses produce diabetes only in those with less than normal islet-cell endurance, whether inherited or acquired.

The introduction of new staining methods in the 1950s helped to bring the pancreas back to the centre of the picture. The Gros. Schultze silver stain was thought to differentiate A from B cells and by this method small islets and few B cells were found in 80% of diabetics. More consistent results were achieved with the stains introduced by Gomori. Using his chrome alum haematoxylin and phloxin stain MacLean and Ogilvie (1955) estimated the total weight of islet tissue and of A and B cells in 30 diabetics and 30 controls. They found the weight of these elements to be on average low in both growth-onset and maturity-onset diabetics, the mean weight of B cells in the growth-onset cases being most markedly reduced of all. Gepts (1957), in an extensive quantitative study of the islets, came to similar conclusions and found a reduction of B cells to be almost constant in the diabetic pancreas. Wrenshall, Bogoch and Ritchie (1952) found that the yield of insulin from the pancreas of growth-onset diabetics was very small, whereas that from maturity-onset diabetics was about half the normal, in general agreement with the histological work of MacLean and Ogilvie and of Gepts. The electron-microscopic studies of Lacy (1964)

produced nothing to conflict with these findings.

The importance of the pancreas in the pathogenesis of diabetes was restored by these findings. In experimental animals, diabetes, however produced, is associated with destruction of B cells and loss of their granules with an insignificant recovery of insulin from the pancreas at autopsy. In man, though there is a reduction of B cell activity, this is inconstant except that juvenile patients nearly always show a loss of B cell granules and have little or no insulin in the pancreas.

The possibility of arterial or arteriolar narrowing in the blood supply to the islets was indicated by Cecil (1909), who found evidence of it in 80% of cases who were mostly elderly. Its importance has been rejected by most writers and Warren and LeCompte (1952) rarely found severe arteriosclerosis in the diabetic pancreas. Moschcowitz (1951) noted a great excess of arteriosclerosis (not atherosclerosis) in the arteries of the pancreas in elderly diabetics and found hyalinization and fibrosis of the islets in about half these patients. While his attribution of the hyaline change to arteriosclerosis may not be sound the significance of local arterial disease as a contributory factor in the diabetes of the elderly remains to be assessed.

As with the search for aetiological factors, interpretation of the histological findings was confounded by the consideration of diabetes as a single disease. From our current standpoint of the two major types of diabetes with differing aetiology and pathogenesis, interpretation of the earlier histological studies becomes easier, although it must be constantly borne in mind that few of the early studies set out to examine a homogeneous diabetic population.

In type 1 diabetes the pancreas is often normal in size at diagnosis but microscopy reveals lymphocytic infiltration of the islets. Gepts (1965) found this insulitis in 16 of 23 (70%) young diabetic patients who died within 6 months of onset of the disease and

Foulis *et al.* (1986) observed it in 59 of 74 (80%) patients with recent-onset insulin-dependent diabetes. Infiltration of the islets does not occur in a uniform way and some may show B cell loss and fibrosis while others may be apparently normal.

In type 1 diabetes which is long-standing, islets of Langerhans are small, resulting from an almost total absence of B cells with a degree of fibrosis. Other secretory cells, A, D and PP cells are present in normal numbers.

Islet hyalinosis is rare in type 1 diabetes despite its original description by Opie (1901) in a 17-year-old diabetic.

In type 2 diabetes there is a reduction in B cell mass to about 50% of the normal although this is not a constant finding and there is considerable overlap with the non-diabetic pancreas. D cells and PP cells are normal in number but some reports suggest an increase in A cells. The most consistent finding is amyloid deposition, considered the commonest and most typical lesion of the pancreas in non-insulin-dependent diabetes. Fibrosis also occurs frequently, although the precise stimulus to the fibrosis remains unclear.

PATHOGENESIS OF TYPE 1 DIABETES

The pathogenesis of type 1 diabetes is, as yet, linked to the aetiology by a series of hypothetical steps (Figure 2.1).

In the BB rat, a spontaneously diabetic animal, hyperexpression of class I genes of the major histocompatibility complex (MHC) precedes insulitis (Walker *et al.*, 1988) while in the human pancreas islets may be found which hyperexpress class II antigens and class I. In the same pancreases some islets can be found which show only class I hyperexpression (Bottazzo *et al.*, 1983; Foulis, Farquharson and Hardman, 1987). A and D cells also express class I but only when adjacent to B cells, leading to the hypothesis of a B-cell secretory product causing hyperexpression. Foulis, Farquharson and Meager

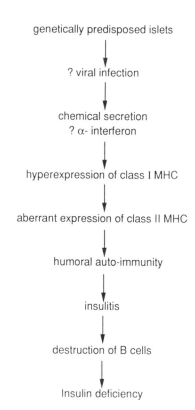

Fig. 2.1   A possible scenario whereby the aetiology of type 1 diabetes is linked to the pathogenesis.

(1987) identified alpha-interferon in islets with hyperexpression of class I but not in those islets devoid of hyperexpession. They suggested that this step precedes and indeed may prompt class II antigen expression, which is the crucial pathogenic step leading to insulitis and B cell destruction.

INSULIN

There is no doubt that in biochemical terms insulin deficiency is the crucial factor in the pathogenesis of insulin-dependent diabetes. It is difficult not to look at this hormone and marvel at its biochemical role. Insulin is well preserved through evolution, appearing in a number of primitive organisms.

In man the synthesis of insulin in the B cell of the islet of Langerhans of the pancreas has

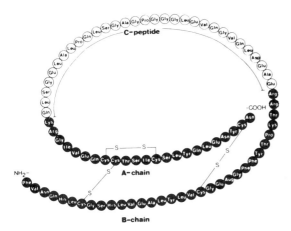

Fig. 2.2 The structure of human proinsulin.

cloning and sequencing can be carried out. To identify untranslated areas of genomic material other techniques have been used, including electron microscopy, digestion by restriction endonucleases and hybridization. It can now be stated with confidence that the human insulin gene is located on the short arm of chromosome 11 (Bell *et al.*, 1980; Owerbach *et al.*, 1981). It is 1355 base pairs long, made up of two introns and three exons (or coding regions). There is some species-specific allelic variation but in the main there is a remarkable similarity throughout nature. In the non-coding regions, particularly the 5'-flanking region, there is considerable within-species variation, the significance of which is uncertain.

been a subject of intense work in recent years. It is clear that there are a number of precursors of insulin within the cell. The first identified was proinsulin (Steiner *et al.*, 1967), which allowed explanation of the two-chain structure of insulin with the chains connected by disulphide bridges (Figure 2.2). Proinsulin has the A and B chain linked by an intervening peptide which has come to be known as connecting peptide (or C-peptide) and thus is a single polypeptide chain structure. In mature secretory granules connecting peptide is removed releasing equimolar quantities of insulin and C-peptide into the circulation.

Further examination of proinsulin has shown that it too is formed as a precursor (Chan, Keim and Steiner, 1976) with an additional 24 residue peptide chain and named preproinsulin. The peptide sequence of this compound has been elucidated partially by analysis of cloned rat preproinsulin mRNA and partly by degradative techniques. Preproinsulin mRNA has been characterized in material obtained from rat insulinoma and has a length of about 600 nucleotides. Characterization of mRNA formed the basis for studies of the insulin gene. mRNA may be used as the template for enzymic formation of complementary DNA. This can be inserted into bacterial plasmid DNA and synthesis,

METABOLIC EFFECTS OF INSULIN

Once it is released into the circulation the full range of the effects of insulin become apparent. These may be either positive, i.e. stimulatory, or negative, i.e. inhibitory of a metabolic process. It is important to acknowledge that in addition to effects produced by a rise in insulin concentration there are default actions. Thus, if metabolic activity is inhibited by a rise in insulin, a fall in insulin will release this inhibition. Similar considerations apply to stimulatory effects of a rise in concentration. These default or permissive actions of insulin are important in normal man for conservation of resources and survival through an antagonistic environment such as prolonged fasting. In excess, as in insulinopenia, they create major obstacles to the survival of the organism.

Hepatic effects of insulin

The liver has a crucial role in regulating blood glucose concentration. In the fasting state it is predominantly release of glucose by the liver which maintains fasting blood glucose. This is particularly important for brain and a number of other important tissues, in which

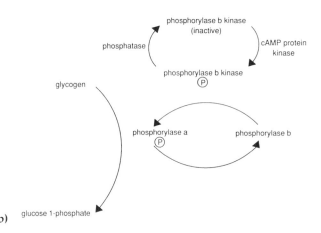

Fig. 2.3 (a) The synthesis of glycogen from glucose-1-phosphate. (b) The breakdown of glycogen to glucose-1-phosphate.

uptake of glucose is concentration-dependent and independent of insulin.

Any organ which is responsible for maintaining blood glucose levels during times of fasting or starvation would do well to avail itself of resources at times of plenty. In doing this the liver not only derives stores of glucose in the fed state but prevents entry of excessive amounts of glucose into the peripheral circulation.

After absorption of glucose from the small intestine approximately 60% is removed on first pass through the liver. Entry of glucose into the liver is independent of insulin, although conversion to glucose 6-phosphate by glucokinase is influenced by insulin. There is no obvious rapid modulation of enzyme activity by insulin, yet long-term insulin deficiency clearly reduces activity. Through glucose 6-phosphate a small amount of glucose enters hepatic glycolysis but the majority has storage as its fate.

Glucose assimilated during feeding is stored in the polymeric form as glycogen. Glycogen formation and deposition is through glucose 1-phosphate and regulated by glycogen synthase. The activation of this enzyme is through a phosphorylation/dephosphorylation cycle regulated by a cyclic-AMP-dependent protein kinase (Figure 2.3(a)). The process is inextricably linked with glycogenolysis regulated by phosphorylase. This enzyme is activated and deactivated through a phosphorylation/ dephosphorylation cascade. The active form of phosphorylase is the phosphorylated form while for glycogen synthase it is the dephosphorylated form. Phosphorylase is regulated by the same cyclic-AMP-dependent protein kinase (Figure 2.3(b)).

Glycogen synthase is activated by a rise in glucose concentration, although there is a lag with a fall in glucose 6-phosphate and UDP-glucose, suggesting that activation is somewhat more than simple substrate availability

(Hers, 1976). The lag period is due to inhibition of glycogen synthase phosphatase by active phosphorylase, and a decrease in the latter to < 10% of total phosphorylase is necessary for synthase activation. The net effect of this rather complex regulatory system is promotion of glycogen storage, and inhibition of glycogen breakdown, by insulin.

Gluconeogenesis is the hepatic pathway by which substrates released peripherally are recycled to glucose. Kidney also possesses the enzymes necessary for gluconeogenesis but under most conditions the liver is of prime importance. The main substrates for hepatic gluconeogenesis are lactate and pyruvate, amino acids, especially alanine, and glycerol. Regulation may occur by change in substrate supply to the liver, alteration in hepatic uptake of substrate and intrahepatic modulation.

The origin of the substrate is of interest. Lactate and pyruvate are derived from glucose while glycerol comes from triglyceride in the fat cell. The glycerol originates from glucose taken up by the fat cell and converted to alpha-glycerophosphate for esterification with fatty acids. While an amino acid in its own right, alanine also appears to function as a nitrogen transporter from the periphery to the liver. It is formed by transamination of pyruvate and thus the carbon skeleton is also derived from glucose (Chang and Goldberg, 1978).

Insulin is a potent regulator of peripheral production of these substrates. Glycerol release and alanine release are inhibited by insulin while lactate and pyruvate release from muscle is increased provided glucose is supplied to the peripheral tissues simultaneously with elevated insulin concentrations. Lactate is produced by muscle, skin and tissues which do not require insulin for glucose uptake, such as erythrocytes, brain and renal medulla. In these tissues hyperglycaemia and insulinopenia lead to increased lactate production. The splanchnic bed is also a potent producer of lactate immediately after a meal.

Uptake of substrate by the liver is altered

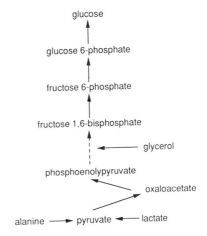

Fig. 2.4 Gluconeogenesis.

mainly by hormones other than insulin although insulin may increase fractional extraction of alanine while glucose appears to decrease extraction.

Within the liver a number of steps are targets for regulation. Of particular importance is the conversion of pyruvate, through which lactate and alanine flow, to phosphoenolpyruvate. This step involves formation of oxaloacetate from pyruvate by pyruvate carboxylase and phosphoenolpyruvate is then formed from oxaloacetate by phosphoenolpyruvate carboxykinase. A second regulatory step is at the fructose 6-phosphate/fructose 1,6-bisphosphate level and the final regulatory step at the glucose/glucose 6-phosphate stage (Figure 2.4).

Somewhat surprisingly there is little evidence of an effect of insulin upon gluconeogenesis within the liver. Insulin may antagonize the effects upon gluconeogenesis of other hormones but physiological rises in plasma insulin have only modest effects upon hepatic gluconeogenesis. Hyperglycaemia does have an inhibitory effect upon the conversion of both lactate and alanine into glucose (Shulman *et al.*, 1986).

The two processes of glycogenolysis and gluconeogenesis combine to give a hepatic glucose output which is inhibited by insulin, primarily through an effect upon glycogen breakdown, and reduced by glucose (Sacca, Hendler and Sherwin, 1978).

Hepatic glucose output is clearly raised in insulin-dependent diabetics although it is difficult to study them in a totally insulin-deficient state. Where this has been tried, particularly in diabetic ketoacidosis, there is wide variation between subjects and many have hepatic glucose production rates elevated in the face of a blood glucose of 20 mmol/l.

Lipogenesis

The liver also has a crucial role in fat synthesis. Dietary fat, plasma non-esterified fatty acids and *de novo* synthesis of fatty acids from glucose contribute to hepatic triglyceride synthesis and subsequent release. The starting block for synthesis of fatty acids within the liver is acetyl CoA derived from carbohydrate sources. Acetyl CoA is carboxylated to form malonyl CoA by the enzyme acetyl CoA carboxylase. Malonyl CoA undergoes repeated addition of acetyl CoA units until the required chain length is reached. In man the major product is palmitoyl CoA, from which other fatty acids are formed by saturation, desaturation and hydroxyl addition.

Acetyl CoA carboxylase rather than fatty acid synthetase appears to be the main site of regulation. Starvation and alloxan-induced diabetes in animals reduce fatty acid biosynthesis, which can be returned to normal by refeeding or insulin.

Peripheral effects

Effects upon carbohydrate metabolism

Certain tissues have an obligatory requirement for insulin to stimulate the bulk of their glucose uptake. These are muscle, which accounts for 85% of total body glucose uptake, and fat, which contributes a further 10%. Even in these tissues some glucose uptake is mediated by the prevailing glucose concentration while in another set of tissues – liver, brain and nervous tissue (including retina), renal medulla and erythrocyte – glucose uptake is independent of insulin.

Glucose uptake into tissues is mediated by a family of membrane proteins (Mueckler, 1990). These facilitative glucose transporters share the same basic structure but are specialized within certain tissues. Those identified that are of metabolic importance are listed in Table 2.2.

Glut 1 appears to be expressed in many tissues providing them with their basal glucose requirement. Glut 2 is predominantly a feature of tissues which release glucose as well as taking it up. At physiological glucose concentrations it displays pseudo-first-order kinetics, which is of value in allowing release of glucose. The muscle/adipocyte transporter, Glut 4, is the major transporter of the insulin-sensitive tissues.

Although there is evidence for an effect of insulin upon the translocation of Glut 4 from an intracellular location to the plasma membrane, the precise site of insulin regulation of

Table 2.2 The glucose transporter family

Name	Alternative name	Tissue location	Chromosome location
GLUT 1	Erythrocyte Hep G2 Brain	Fetal tissues, brain, kidney	1
GLUT 2	Liver	Liver, kidney, B cell	3
GLUT 3	Fetal muscle	Widely distributed	12
GLUT 4	Muscle/adipocyte	Skeletal and heart muscle, adipose tissue	17
GLUT 5	Small intestine	Small intestine	1

glucose uptake remains unclear. It is also true to say that while glycolysis is widely held to be stimulated by insulin this site too eludes description. Indeed it may be that glycolysis is stimulated simply by the availability within the cell of glucose following enhanced uptake, although there is evidence from substrate concentrations of an effect upon a key regulator of glycolysis, phosphofructokinase.

Zierler and Rabinowitz (1963) demonstrated a stimulatory effect of insulin upon forearm glucose uptake and a considerable amount of recent work using a variety of techniques has confirmed this effect. DeFronzo *et al.* (1983), using the hyperinsulinaemic glucose clamp, demonstrated a dose–response relationship for insulin upon glucose uptake.

A key step in glucose oxidation lies at the transition from glycolysis to the Krebs cycle (Figure 2.5). The conversion of pyruvate to acetyl CoA represents a loss to the organism of carbohydrate stores. In turn, the organism achieves a supply of substrate for energy production, or for fatty acid or cholesterol synthesis. Pyruvate dehydrogenase is an en-

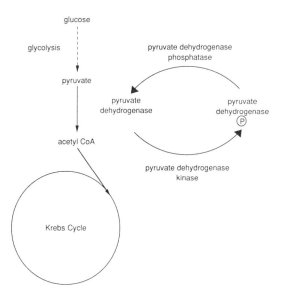

Fig. 2.5 The importance of the regulation of pyruvate conversion to acetyl CoA in the metabolism of glucose.

zyme complex regulated by phosphorylation/dephosphorylation. The balance between the phosphorylated enzyme (inactive) and dephosphorylated enzyme (active) is regulated through kinase and phosphatase enzymes. Regulation of the kinase is by ratios of acetyl CoA:CoA, NADH:NAD and ATP:ADP, with an increase in ratio activating the kinase and therefore inactivating pyruvate dehydrogenase (Pettit, Pelley and Reed, 1975). Insulin increases the proportion of active to inactive pyruvate dehydrogenase *in vitro* (Coore *et al.*, 1971) and the proportion is decreased in alloxan-diabetic rats. It is less clear *in vivo* whether this is a direct effect or mediated through metabolite changes, for example fatty acids and ketone bodies.

Effects upon protein metabolism

From early descriptions of diabetes mellitus it is apparent that tissue wasting was a readily observed feature of the disease. Protein synthesis from amino acids involves cellular uptake, activation and polymerization, which provides numerous sites for regulation. Insulin deficiency in laboratory animals results in a depression of protein synthesis that is corrected by insulin administration, which was ascribed to a reversal of restraint upon peptide chain initiation (Jefferson, 1980). Feeding, that is availability of amino acids, also stimulates protein synthesis (Rennie *et al.*, 1982), although this effect is somewhat offset by the effect of insulin in lowering circulating concentrations of amino acids. Insulin appears also to inhibit protein breakdown, with a 40% decrease in proteolytic rate in perfused rat liver following the addition of insulin (Mortimore and Mondon, 1970).

Effects upon fat metabolism

Adipose tissue stores energy reserves as triglycerides. Both deposition and breakdown of triglyceride are under hormonal control with insulin exerting a crucial influence.

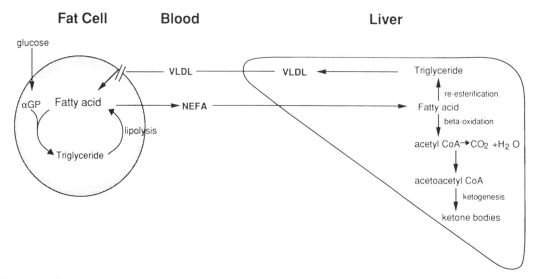

Fig. 2.6   The metabolism of triglyceride.

Triglyceride is synthesized within the fat cell from fatty acids and alpha-glycerophosphate (Figure 2.6). Fatty acids arrive at the fat cell as triglyceride, having been esterified in the liver. At the endothelial surface this triglyceride is degraded by lipoprotein lipase, releasing fatty aids which pass into the cell. The activity of this enzyme is a major determinant of fat storage and is increased by insulin. Deposition of triglyceride is also promoted by insulin through uptake of glucose into the adipocyte. Human adipocytes are deficient in alpha-glycerokinase, preventing reuse of glycerol in re-esterification, and *de novo* synthesis of alpha-glycerophosphate is from glucose.

Breakdown of triglyceride into fatty acids and glycerol is an important focus of action of insulin and other hormones. Since glycerol cannot be utilized in re-esterification it is released and taken up by the liver for utilization in gluconeogenesis. Some of the fatty acid is used in re-esterification and the remainder is released into the circulation. Breakdown of triglyceride is controlled by hormone-sensitive lipase, which is extremely sensitive to inhibition by insulin.

Non-esterified fatty acids pass to the liver,

where uptake is along a concentration gradient. Further breakdown is by beta-oxidation, which is intramitochondrial. Uptake into the mitochondrion involves creation of the fatty acyl CoA derivative, which is linked to carnitine by carnitine acyl transferase I on the outer mitochondrial membrane (Figure 2.7). Carnitine acyl transferase II, on the inner mitochondrial membrane, splits carnitine, leaving fatty acyl CoA within the mitochondrion. Here the fatty acids may undergo: complete beta-oxidation to acetyl CoA and via the Krebs cycle to CO_2 and water; partial oxidation to acetyl CoA followed by condensation to acetoactyl CoA and hence ketone bodies; or re-esterification within the liver and subsequent release of VLDL. The biochemistry of ketogenesis has aroused considerable interest in recent years (McGarry *et al.*, 1989).

The carnitine acyl transferases and the relationship of the fasting/fed liver have clarified the picture. It has been apparent for a number of years that fasting livers are primed for ketogenesis. The most likely explanation of this is through malonyl CoA, the first committed intermediate of fatty acid synthesis. High concentrations of malonyl CoA inhibit

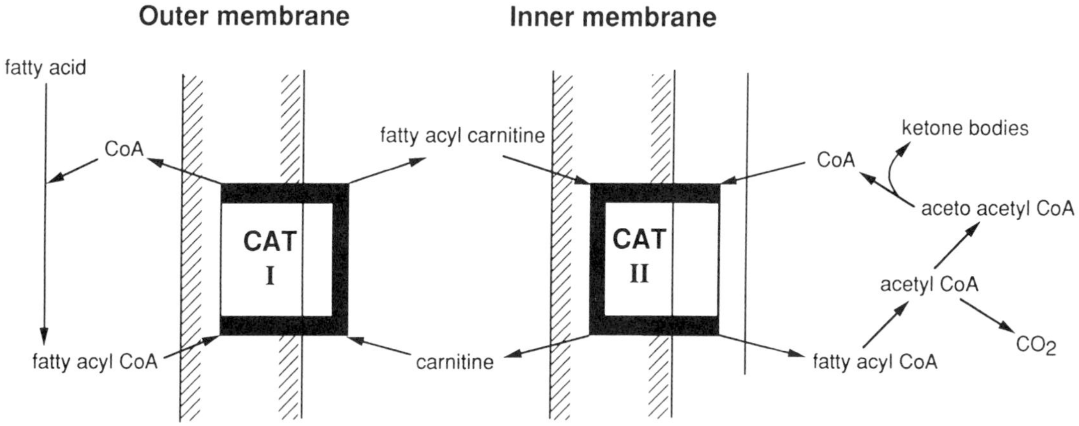

Outer membrane   **Inner membrane**

Fig. 2.7 The metabolism of fatty acids. Transport into the mitochondrion via the carnitine acyl transferase pathway and intramitochondrial fate.

ketogenesis while low concentrations allow ketogenesis. Glucagon, which increases keto-genesis, lowers malonyl CoA concentration.

While glucagon is clearly ketogenic it has proved most difficult to demonstrate a specific antiketogenic effect of insulin, although *in-vitro* evidence supports such an effect. Despite this, it remains unclear whether insulin determines ketogenic rates or whether the important factor is the insulin/glucagon ratio in portal blood.

CHANGES IN INSULIN-DEPENDENT DIABETES

The full-blown picture of total insulin deficiency is rarely seen. Even in diabetic keto-acidosis small amounts of insulin can be measured in plasma. The effects of inadequate insulin replacement, however, are similar to a degree of insulin deficiency. Blood glucose is raised due to overproduction by the liver and underutilization by the periphery. With the high circulating glucose concentration non-insulin-mediated glucose uptake is enhanced in both metabolically active tissues, which depend upon insulin stimulation of glucose uptake to meet most of their energy demands, and non-insulin-dependent tissues. Partial oxidation of glucose in these tissues

leads to enhanced release of lactate and pyruvate, which further drive gluconeogenesis to produce glucose.

Protein metabolism is affected, with enhanced proteolysis and inadequate synthesis.

Fat metabolism shows increased breakdown, with high non-esterified fatty acid levels promoting ketone body synthesis.

One point on the action of insulin which is underappreciated is the differential sensitivity of metabolic processes to insulin (Alberti and Nattrass, 1978). Lipolysis is exquisitely sensitive to inhibition by insulin, circulating levels of 10 mU/l having a demonstrable effect while stimulation of glucose uptake into muscle and adipose tissue requires five to ten times more; glucose output lies between these extremes.

PATHOGENESIS OF TYPE 2 DIABETES

THE ROLE OF INSULIN

Many gaps remain in our understanding of the actions of insulin and the consequences of insulin deficiency yet the pathogenesis of type 1 diabetes is infinitely clearer than the pathogenesis of type 2 diabetes. In type 2 diabetes difficulties arise from uncertainty over the homo- or heterogeneous nature of the disorder. Nowhere is this better illustrated than in the consideration of the obese diabetic. Is the pathogenesis of type 2 diabetes the same in obese patients as in the non-obese?

Non-obese diabetic patients may present difficulties in classification on clinical grounds and it is therefore not surprising that many of the studies of pathogenesis have used obese patients, where classification is on firmer ground. While this is sensible in terms of selecting a homogeneous group of patients it does complicate the issue, since obesity *per se* has effects upon insulin secretion and action.

Insulin action

Insulin action, or more specifically insulin resistance, is an important topic in non-insulin-dependent diabetes and is becoming more important in other forms of diabetes. The first step in any action of insulin is the binding to a specific receptor. There follows instigation and amplification of the signal via a second messenger to the metabolic action.

Insulin receptors

Insulin receptors are large glycoprotein components of tissue plasma membrane. By definition, and in common with other hormone receptors, they are specific and can be saturated in a reversible manner. There are four subunits: two alpha, linked by disulphide bridges, with two beta, linked to the alpha subunits by disulphide bridges (Figure 2.8) (Czech, Massague and Pilch, 1981). The alpha-subunits are extracellular and bind insulin on the cell surface while the beta-subunits traverse the plasma membrane and the intracellular domain contains a tyrosine-specific protein kinase. The insulin receptor gene has been cloned and is localized to chromosome 19 (Ullrich *et al.*, 1985).

Insulin binds to these receptors and causes aggregation within the membrane into pitted areas on the surface. Endocytosis results in

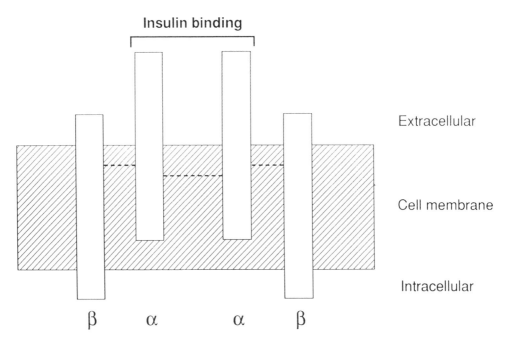

Fig. 2.8 Structure of the insulin receptor.

internalization of the hormone–receptor complex (Gorden *et al.*, 1980) and subsequently there is degradation of insulin and possibly receptor, with some recycling of receptors to the cell surface.

Using radiolabelled hormone, insulin binding to its receptor can be measured and techniques exist for determining receptor number on cells and affinity of insulin for its receptor. As in many aspects of insulin chemistry and biochemistry, the results present interpretative difficulties. Of these it is perhaps the shape of the binding curve which causes most difficulty, with uncertainty as to whether the curvilinear plot of bound versus bound/free (Scatchard plot) indicates two classes of receptor, high- and low-affinity, or whether it reflects one class of receptor where binding characteristics are modified by insulin occupation of adjacent receptors (negative cooperativity). The insulin receptor gene codes for the entire receptor (Ullrich *et al.*, 1985) so any suggestion of two types of receptor indicates post-translational modification.

Insulin second messenger

Elucidation of a clear picture of the mechanism of action of insulin has been elusive in the area of second messenger of hormone action. It has been even more frustrating since the mechanism of action of catecholamines and glucagon was clarified. Not for insulin the rather simple effect upon cyclic AMP, although there were many attempts to demonstrate that insulin acted through inhibition of the rise in cyclic AMP. The mechanism for insulin has proved considerably more difficult to elucidate and it is by no means completely worked out.

An important impetus was given with the discovery that a gene product resulted in phosphorylation of tyrosine residues in proteins. Furthermore, this tyrosyl kinase activity was expressed by human insulin receptors (Kasuga, Karlsson and Kahn, 1982).

Not only can exogenous proteins be phosphorylated by this tyrosine kinase activity but autophosphorylation of tyrosine residues within the insulin receptor also occurs. It has emerged that insulin binding to its receptor activates the tyrosine kinase immediately, which results in autophosphorylation of tyrosine residues in the receptor. Thus it appears that autophosphorylation or perhaps phosphorylation of other proteins in response to insulin binding to the insulin receptor is crucial for signal transmission. While some would argue that it is the autophosphorylation of the insulin receptor that results in a conformational change, which enables the intracellular effects of insulin, a number of other intracellular proteins have been identified which may be implicated. One of these is insulin receptor substrate 1 (IRS-1) and it is possible that phosphorylation of tyrosine residues on this, or similar, protein by the insulin receptor tyrosine kinase may be the initiator of intracellular insulin action.

The number of actions of insulin upon metabolism which are mediated through enzyme phosphorylation/dephosphorylation reactions suggests that autophosphorylation of the receptor or phosphorylation of another intracellular substrate would be a logical finding as the initiating event by which insulin exerts metabolic effects.

Regulation of insulin receptors

An important finding has been that insulin regulates its own receptor. Exposure of the receptor to high concentrations of insulin rapidly results in a decrease in receptor number. It is likely that this loss of receptors results from internalization rather than from destruction. Many tissues have been investigated for changes in insulin receptors and in general there is a consistency of response. In particular, the role of obesity and diabetes mellitus upon receptor number and affinity in metabolically active tissue has been a focus of study.

Briefly, some of the conditions altering receptor number or affinity are meals and activity, age, diet, sex hormones, particularly during the menstrual cycle, pregnancy and oral contraceptive use, and corticosteroid administration (Taylor, 1984).

Equally important has been the finding that maximal effects of insulin can be obtained when only 10–30% of receptors are occupied.

Hyperinsulinaemia

That some non-insulin-dependent diabetics have circulating insulin levels higher than normals has been obvious for a considerable time. Indeed the demonstration that obese patients were hyperinsulinaemic followed the development of methods for measuring insulin (Karam, Grodsky and Forsham, 1963). It is illuminating to look at the apparent levels of fasting plasma insulin in those early studies. Levels were grossly higher than would be expected or accepted today. Clearly the antibodies used in those early insulin radioimmunoassays left something to be desired.

Recently this area has been revisited, with the observation that non-insulin-dependent diabetics and patients with impaired glucose tolerance have elevated fasting proinsulin and split products of proinsulin. Indeed, when immunoradiometric assay for insulin, proinsulin, and split proinsulins is used rather than radioimmunoassay it becomes difficult to confirm that fasting hyperinsulinaemia is a feature of non-insulin-dependent diabetes. In contrast, a number of studies show elevated proinsulin concentrations, not only in patients with non-insulin-dependent diabetes or impaired glucose tolerance but also in subjects at high risk of developing the former (Haffner *et al.*, 1994).

Fasting hyperinsulinaemia was originally one of the main pointers suggesting insulin

resistance and it may be fortuitous that the correct conclusion of insulin resistance was arrived at from an erroneous observation. Nevertheless the conclusion that insulin resistance and hyperinsulinaemia are features of obesity, non-insulin-dependent diabetes and impaired glucose tolerance does not stand or fall by the assay used to measure fasting 'insulin'. It is clear that hyperinsulinaemia can be demonstrated in obesity and in non-insulin-dependent diabetes after oral glucose, test meals or in daily profiles. When accompanied by euglycaemia or hyperglycaemia this finding leads inevitably to the conclusion that insulin action is impaired, i.e. there is resistance to the action of insulin.

It should be said that interpretation of some studies of hyperinsulinaemia is fraught with difficulty. Two factors cause confusion: firstly, matching diabetic patients and controls for body weight has not always been an element in the design of studies. If obese non-insulin-dependent diabetics are matched with non-diabetic lean controls and given an oral glucose tolerance test the obese diabetics will have higher blood glucose and plasma insulin concentration than the lean non-diabetics, leading to the conclusion that they are insulin-resistant. If matched with appropriate obese non-diabetic controls, however, insulin responses in the diabetics are reduced, leading to the conclusion that there is also an element of insulin deficiency. The second confounding factor when comparing insulin responses in diabetics and non-diabetics is matching the groups for the stimulus to insulin secretion. This involves controlling for blood glucose concentration in the two groups and is a problem that is exceptionally difficult to solve.

Nevertheless the findings from a host of studies have firmly entrenched the idea that both obesity and non-insulin-dependent diabetes are states of insulin resistance. Recent techniques for studying insulin resistance support this view.

METHODS OF STUDYING INSULIN RESISTANCE

Studies of insulin action pre-date the development of radioimmunoassay for insulin. Himsworth (1936) was clear that diabetics fell into two groups – those that were insulin-sensitive and those that were insulin-resistant. The former were young and thin while the latter tended to be older and fatter. He studied the blood glucose response to simultaneous administration of glucose and insulin, showing wildly different responses in the two groups. Reaven, a great admirer of Himsworth, developed a technique of glucose and insulin infusion accompanied by adrenalin to inhibit endogenous insulin secretion and propranolol to block the metabolic effects of adrenalin. When the quadruple infusion was given to groups of patients such that similar insulin levels were achieved in the circulation, then the height of the blood glucose concentration in response to the fixed glucose infusion was a marker of the action of insulin to dispose of the glucose.

This technique was used extensively (Reaven, 1983) before being superseded by glucose clamping, which has several advantages, the main one being that it allows construction of dose–response curves. Simply put, an infusion of glucose maintains the starting blood glucose during infusions of insulin designed to produce logarithmically increasing circulating insulin concentrations of, say, 100, 1000 and 10 000 mU/l (Figure 2.9). The combination of insulin infusion to a circulating level of 100 mU/l with glucose infusion effectively blocks hepatic glucose output. Under these steady-state conditions the amount of glucose infused to maintain blood glucose concentration must equal the amount being taken up by peripheral tissues. Alternatively, during glucose and insulin infusion glucose turnover can be determined isotopically. Thus either a direct or indirect measure of peripheral glucose uptake is obtained and clearly the less uptake that can

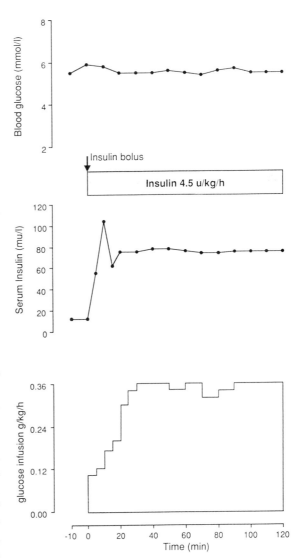

Fig. 2.9 An example of the technique of euglycaemic glucose clamping.

be obtained the greater the degree of insulin resistance (DeFronzo, Tobin and Andres, 1979).

Insulin sensitivity and insulin responsiveness

An important model of insulin resistance was promulgated by Kahn (1978). He proposed that the relationship of dose of hormone to effect could be more clearly understood if divided into two components. The first, insulin insensitivity, was where insulin in higher doses would eventually produce an effect up to and including a maximal biological action. The net result of insensitivity was therefore a right shift in a dose–response curve. The second component was when a maximal effect of insulin could not be achieved, no matter how high the dose of insulin, and this was called insulin unresponsiveness. Furthermore, it was argued that the correct interpretation of these abnormalities was that a pure right shift was due to a decrease in receptor number while unresponsiveness was due to a postreceptor defect in insulin action. The concept was worthy of a more thoughtful response than it received, although it has been widely and uncritically applied to results of glucose clamp experiments.

In obesity, be it in experimental animals or man, hyperinsulinaemia, insulin resistance and a reduced concentration of insulin receptors are well recognized features. In some patients a mild degree of insulin resistance accompanies a pure receptor defect but in the majority of people there is a postreceptor defect in insulin action. It is possible that there are differences between tissues, with muscle and adipocytes displaying an inability to obtain a maximal effect of insulin while in the liver there is a simple right shift of the dose–response curve.

It can be argued that, where the defective action is due to decreased insulin receptor concentration, this is a consequence of hyperinsulinaemia. In more severe forms, while a receptor defect is present, the predominance of a poor metabolic response may be due to hyperinsulinaemia or other causes. The alternative explanation, that hyperinsulinaemia arises as a consequence of defective action, has received less attention and investigation.

In diabetes the situation is more complex. Binding defects are well recognized in type 1

diabetes but are determined not only by the basic pathogenesis but by adequate or inadequate treatment. In non-insulin-dependent diabetes, patients who are not obese show decreased receptors and insulin resistance that is associated with decreased maximal action. In contrast, those with impaired glucose tolerance have only a receptor defect. It might be expected that the rapid developments in our understanding of specific hormone receptors and their abnormalities in particular disease states such as obesity and non-insulin-dependent diabetes would have contributed in a major way to understanding the pathogenesis of the disease. This has not been the end result, however, for while being of immense importance in the mechanism of how insulin works the clinical relevance has proved nebulous. Pure receptor defects are rare as a cause of insulin resistance. On the other hand, the inability of insulin to achieve a maximal effect is common in both diabetes and obesity.

CAUSES OF INSULIN RESISTANCE (TABLE 2.3)

CIRCULATING INSULIN ANTAGONISTS

Metabolites

It is possible that some circulating metabolites can cause insulin resistance, of which

Table 2.3   Circulating causes of insulin resistance

| Metabolites | Hormones | |
	Major	Minor
Non-esterified fatty acids	Catecholamines	Thyroxine
	Glucagon	ACTH
Ketone bodies	Cortisol	Vasopressin
Hydrogen ions	Growth hormone	Prolactin

'Pseudo-insulin resistance'
Familial hyperproinsulinaemia
Mutant insulin
Antibodies to exogenous insulin

the most important and interesting are non-esterified fatty acids and ketone bodies. These suggestions arise from the work of Randle and his colleagues and have been christened the Randle glucose–fatty-acid cycle (Randle *et al.*, 1963). *In vitro*, in a series of experiments in the perfused rat heart, it was observed that addition of fatty acids or ketone bodies to the perfusion media significantly reduced glucose oxidation by the heart. On the basis of these experiments it was suggested that a cycle existed whereby substrate supply of glucose for oxidation by muscle was promoted by insulin. When insulin concentrations fell fatty acids would be mobilized and be oxidized in the process, inhibiting glucose oxidation. Thus there is a glucose-sparing effect, and a feedback could be envisaged whereby the small rise in blood glucose from this would stimulate insulin secretion in the whole animal and a new equilibrium would be achieved.

It remains unclear whether in man *in vivo* this cycle is of importance. Some have argued that insulin regulation of fatty acid metabolism is the prime effect of insulin and that changes in glucose concentration are secondary to changes in fatty acid metabolism. While this is almost certainly an over-extrapolation of the data on which the cycle was based, there are many others who would not wish to disregard the cycle completely and have a sneaking affection for its importance.

Hormones

Perhaps of greater importance than intermediary metabolites in inducing insulin resistance is hormonal antagonism. The prime catabolic hormones, catecholamines, glucagon, cortisol, and growth hormone, are clearly capable of insulin antagonism to the degree where diabetes occurs. This finding is discussed elsewhere (Chapter 3). Other hormones – thyroxine, prolactin, ACTH and vasopressin – may have actions opposing insulin when

secreted in excess or when conditions allow. Yet other hormones may have differential effects upon the liver and the periphery, e.g. progesterone and oestrogens.

Pseudo-insulin resistance (see also Chapter 3)

There are some causes of 'apparent' or 'pseudo-insulin resistance' arising from circulating compounds. In familial hyperproinsulinaemia, or when a patient secretes a mutant insulin, the diagnosis is usually made when hyperglycaemia coexists with high circulating concentrations of 'insulin'. The insulin resistance is false, however, and indeed there is a normal response of blood glucose to exogenous insulin. Rather, the insulin is insulin measurable by radioimmunoassay, i.e. any product that is sufficiently similar to insulin to be identified as 'insulin' by the assay antibody, and not only the pure chemical, biologically active, human insulin. Similarly, pseudo-insulin resistance occurs when there are high titres of circulating antibodies to insulin, a problem less common with the purity of insulins today. Here, resistance to exogenous insulin occurs as the injected insulin is nullified by formation of antibody–antigen complexes. Once the antibodies are saturated the response to further insulin does not show resistance.

RARE SYNDROMES OF INSULIN RESISTANCE

True resistance occurs in some rare conditions which have diabetes as part of a syndrome. Perhaps the best investigated is the association of insulin receptor antibodies with acanthosis nigricans or ataxia telangiectasia. The majority of the very small number of cases reported have been North American black females with features of other immune disorders. Basal insulin was of the order of 100–1000 mU/l in the presence of abnormally elevated glucose levels but the striking feature is resistance to exogenous insulin. Doses of insulin used to treat their diabetes have ranged up to 24 000 units/day with one report of a patient given in excess of 150 000 units of insulin. Little effect is seen upon blood glucose but patients do not develop severe diabetic ketoacidosis. Two other syndromes of acanthosis nigricans and insulin resistance have been described. Type A, associated with virilization and hirsutism, has no circulating inhibitor but shows an abnormal receptor on fibroblast culture while Type C, of which there have been few patients, has the phenotype of Type A with no receptor defect and a probable postreceptor defect.

Some patients with lipoatrophic diabetes have insulin resistance with or without features of the above syndromes and there have been a couple of reports of patients with insulin resistance and leprechaunism.

None of these associations, rare syndromes, hormones, or metabolites explain the insulin resistance which is a feature of both non-insulin-dependent diabetes and obesity. Nor do they contribute to the understanding of the pathogenesis of the conditions.

INSULIN SECRETION IN NON-INSULIN-DEPENDENT DIABETES

The interpretation of insulin levels and responses in non-insulin-dependent diabetic patients is problematical. The major confounding feature is the difficulty, when comparing with normals, of matching blood glucose levels and hence stimuli to secretion. There is no satisfactory way of taking into account both glucose and insulin levels simultaneously and attempts to construct insulin/glucose or glucose/insulin ratios are virtually worthless. A second factor which must be taken into account is the reliance upon a single stimulus in the interest of investigative cleanliness. A glucose load may be the obvious choice but it is unclear how the response is influenced by a preceding period of hyperglycaemia. Protein or non-

glucose stimuli have been used in only a limited way to address this problem.

If, for the moment, discrepancies in blood glucose concentration are ignored, basal insulin levels in non-insulin-dependent diabetics are similar to age- and weight-matched non-diabetic subjects (Turner and Holman, 1976). It is pertinent to recognize, however, that the similarity is achieved in the face of different stimuli. The mechanism whereby this situation comes about is suggested to be as follows. As part of the aetiology and pathogenesis of the condition there is a small reduction in insulin secretion; consequently there is an increase in hepatic glucose production and hyperglycaemia follows. In turn this stimulates insulin secretion and a new equilibrium is reached. If attempts are made to match basal blood glucose levels it becomes apparent that the diabetics are insulinopenic, although neither glucose infusion of normals nor insulin infusion of diabetics is an ideal way to address this question.

If intravenous glucose is used as a stimulus to insulin secretion the normal response is biphasic (Figure 2.10) (Porte and Pupo, 1969). It is suggested that first-phase insulin release is from a readily releasable pool of synthesized insulin; second-phase insulin release is the slower release of newly synthesized

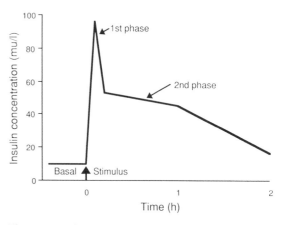

Fig. 2.10 The insulin response to an intravenous glucose stimulus.

insulin. In non-insulin-dependent diabetes first-phase insulin secretion is lost but second-phase may be normal or even exaggerated. Again, there is the problem of matching stimuli since inevitably inadequate first-phase insulin release results in hyperglycaemia, and thus a greater stimulus to second-phase secretion. This situation persists until the more severely hyperglycaemic stage of the disease is reached, when second-phase response becomes impaired or lost.

While the use of oral glucose is to be welcomed as a more physiological route of administration, if not a physiological substance which is given, it does make interpretation difficult. In essence, with this simple test, conclusions are being drawn which must take into account absorption, B cell secretion, hyperglycaemia, and insulin resistance. Small wonder that many studies are uninterpretable and many conclusions unwarranted. Having said that, the sheer volume of studies gives weight to the opinion that insulin responses are diminished in type 2 diabetes. There is greater controversy in the area of impaired glucose tolerance patients although it should not be assumed that these patients will develop frank diabetes. In similar fashion, the data from non-insulin-dependent diabetic patients does not take into account the natural history of the disease or at what stage in the evolution of his diabetes the patient is being studied. Similar conclusions of insulinopenia are apparent when non-glucose stimuli are used, provided other factors are taken into account.

Either reduced B cell mass or B cell dysfunction would explain the poor insulin responses in non-insulin-dependent diabetes. In animals more than 85% of islet tissue must be destroyed to give insulinopenic diabetes and it is likely therefore that both lesions coexist. Of interest is the increasing recognition that hyperglycaemia *per se* may impair insulin secretion. Animal studies show islet damage following prolonged exposure to hyperglycaemia which can be prevented by

treatment (Clarke *et al.*, 1982) and several studies show improved insulin response after correction of hyperglycaemia.

Other abnormalities of insulin secretion have been found in non-insulin-dependent diabetes, notably the loss of pulsatile insulin secretion (Lang *et al.*, 1981).

INSULIN RESISTANCE IN NON-INSULIN-DEPENDENT DIABETES

Decreased insulin action in diabetic patients was noted long ago by Himsworth (1949) but it is only in recent years that it has attracted an enormous amount of attention. More recent techniques for studying this problem – forearm perfusion, quadruple infusions of glucose, insulin, adrenalin and propranolol, and the euglycaemic clamp technique – produce similar results. It is clear that in established non-insulin-dependent diabetes there is insulin resistance. This insulin resistance is a result of both insulin insensitivity and insulin unresponsiveness. It is not clear whether both or either of these defects lies in hepatic glucose production, or peripheral glucose uptake which is insulin-mediated, or indeed whether the defect may lie in glucose-stimulated (insulin-independent) glucose uptake.

Hepatic glucose production in non-insulin-dependent diabetes is raised or inappropriately normal for the prevailing hyperglycaemia. Insulin suppresses hepatic glucose output but higher concentrations are needed in diabetics than in normals. Provided the insulin concentration is sufficiently high a maximal suppression can be achieved.

There is a weight of evidence indicating impaired peripheral glucose uptake in non-insulin-dependent diabetes. This impairment arises from a right shift in the dose–response curve with an inability to obtain maximal rates of uptake. In skeletal muscle both oxidative and non-oxidative pathways of glucose disposal are impaired (DeFronzo, Bonadonna and Ferrannini, 1992). With regard to non-oxidative pathways there is a general finding that the insulin effect on glycogen synthase in skeletal muscle of patients with non-insulin-dependent diabetes is reduced (Damsbo *et al.*, 1991).

Resistance in glucose-mediated glucose uptake is an interesting concept, relatively under-explored. Tissues that require basal glucose uptake are perhaps more important functionally than metabolically. Thus if there is resistance to glucose entry into brain or nervous tissue it is conceivable that the subsequent rise in blood glucose would be appropriate.

THE RELATIONSHIP OF INSULIN SECRETION AND INSULIN RESISTANCE

Without knowledge of the natural history of non-insulin-dependent diabetes it becomes difficult to assess the relationship between secretion and resistance. Some will agree that diminished secretion of insulin with low circulating levels leads to decreases in certain key enzyme activities, thus inducing insulin resistance. Others will argue that the development of insulin resistance imposes a strain upon the secretory mechanism of the B cell such that failure to increase secretion results in diabetes.

At present this debate cannot be resolved but mathematical models of secretion and resistance in non-insulin-dependent diabetic patients suggest that neither, on its own, can produce frank diabetes. What is needed for the development of non-insulin-dependent diabetes is a combination of both.

PREDICTING NON-INSULIN-DEPENDENT DIABETES

A number of studies have attempted to identify metabolic markers for the development of non-insulin-dependent diabetes. In general a group of patients at high risk of developing the condition are compared to a low-risk group. The former may include relatives of patients with non-insulin-dependent diabetes,

patients with impaired glucose tolerance, or racial groups with a high prevalence of the disease. The findings suggest that elevated insulin concentration or insulin resistance may predict subsequent development of the disease in subjects with normal glucose tolerance (Lillioja *et al.*, 1993). In contrast, and somewhat confusingly, lower post-glucose insulin concentrations also predict conversion to diabetes in patients with impaired glucose tolerance (Saad *et al.*, 1988).

Other abnormalities of insulin secretion, such as loss of pulsatile insulin secretion, which have been found in non-insulin-dependent diabetes, can also be found in relatives of patients with non-insulin-dependent diabetes (O'Rahilly, Turner and Matthews, 1988).

Metabolic defects have also been identified in subjects at increased risk of non-insulin-dependent diabetes. Non-oxidative glucose disposal may be reduced (Warram *et al.*, 1990) and there is abnormality of glycogen sythase activation (Vaag, Henriksen and Beck-Nielsen, 1992).

REFERENCES

Alberti, K. G. M. M. and Nattrass, M. (1978) Severe diabetic ketoacidosis. *Med. Clin. N. Am.*, **62**, 799–814.

Bell, E. T. (1952) Hyalinization of islets of Langerhans in diabetes mellitus. *Diabetes*, **1**, 341–344.

Bell, G. I., Swain, W. F., Pictet, R. L. *et al.* (1980) Sequence of the human insulin gene. *Nature*, **284**, 26–32.

Bottazzo, G. F., Pujol-Borrell, R., Hanafusa, T. and Feldmann, M. (1983) Role of aberrant HLA-DR expression and antigen presentation in induction of endocrine autoimmunity. *Lancet*, **ii**, 1115–1118.

Cecil, R. L. (1909) A study of the pathological anatomy of the pancreas in 90 cases of diabetes mellitus. *J. Exper. Med.*, **11**, 266–290.

Chan, S. J., Keim, P. and Steiner, D. F. (1976) Cell-free synthesis of rat preproinsulins: characterization and partial amino acid sequence determination. *Proc. Nat. Acad. Sci. USA*, **73**, 1964–1968.

Chang, T. W. and Goldberg, A. L. (1978) The

origin of alanine produced in skeletal muscle. *J. Biol. Chem.*, **253**, 3677–3684.

Clark, A., Brown, E., King, T. *et al.* (1982) Islet changes induced by hyperglycemia in rats: effect of insulin or chlorpropamide therapy. *Diabetes*, **31**, 319–325.

Cooper, G. J. S., Willis, A. C., Clark, A. *et al.* (1987) Purification and characterization of a peptide from amyloid-rich pancreases of type 2 diabetic patients. *Proc. Nat. Acad. Sci. USA*, **84**, 8628–8632.

Coore, H. G., Denton, R. M., Martin, B. R. and Randle, P. J. (1971) Regulation of adipose tissue pyruvate dehydrogenase by insulin and other hormones. *Biochem. J.*, **125**, 115–127.

Czech, M. P., Massague, J. and Pilch, P. F. (1981) The insulin receptor: structural features. *Trends Biochem. Sci.*, **6**, 222–225.

Damsbo, P., Vaag, A., Hother-Nielsen, O. and Beck-Nielsen, H. (1991) Reduced glycogen synthase activity in skeletal muscle from obese patients with and without type 2 (non-insulin dependent) diabetes mellitus. *Diabetologia*, **34**, 239–245.

DeFronzo, R. A., Bonadonna, R. C. and Ferrannini, E. (1992) Pathogenesis of NIDDM: a balanced overview. *Diabetes Care*, **15**, 318–368.

DeFronzo, R. A., Ferrannini, E., Hendler, R. *et al.* (1983) Regulation of splanchnic and peripheral glucose uptake by insulin and hyperglycemia in man. *Diabetes*, **32**, 35–45.

DeFronzo, R. A., Tobin, J. D. and Andres, R. (1979) Glucose clamp technique: a method for quantifying insulin secretion and resistance. *Am. J. Physiol.*, **237**, E214–E223.

Foulis, A. K., Farquharson, M. A. and Hardman, R. (1987) Aberrant expression of class II major histocompatibility complex molecules by B cells and hyperexpression of class I major histocompatibility complex molecules by insulin containing islets in type 1 (insulin-dependent) diabetes mellitus. *Diabetologia*, **30**, 333–343.

Foulis, A. K., Farquharson, M. A. and Meager, A. (1987) Immunoreactive alpha-interferon in insulin secreting beta cells in type 1 diabetes mellitus. *Lancet*, **ii**, 1423–1427.

Foulis, A. K., Liddle, C. N., Farquharson, M. A. *et al.* (1986) The histopathology of the pancreas in type 1 (insulin-dependent) diabetes mellitus: a 25-year review of deaths in patients under 20 years of age in the United Kingdom. *Diabetologia*, **29**, 267–274.

Gepts, W. (1957) Contribution a l'étude morpho-logique des ilots de Langerhans au cours du diabete. *Ann. Soc. Roy. Sci. Med. Nat. Brux.*, **10**, 5–108.

Gepts, W. (1965) Pathologic anatomy of the pancreas in juvenile diabetes mellitus. *Diabetes*, **14**, 619–633.

Gorden, P., Carpentier, J., Freychet, P. and Orci, L. (1980) Internalisation of polypeptide hormones: mechanism, intracellular localisation and significance. *Diabetologia*, **18**, 263–274.

Haffner, S. M., Bowsher, R. R., Mykkanen, L. *et al.* (1994) Proinsulin and specific insulin concentration in high- and low-risk populations for NIDDM. *Diabetes*, **43**, 1490–1493.

Hers, H. G. (1976) The control of glycogen metabolism in the liver. *Ann. Rev. Biochem.*, **45**, 167–189.

Himsworth, H. P. (1936) Diabetes mellitus; its differentiation into insulin-sensitive and insulin-insensitive types. *Lancet*, **i**, 127–130.

Himsworth, H. P. (1949) Syndrome of diabetes mellitus and its causes. *Lancet*, **i**, 465–472.

Jefferson, L. S. (1980) Role of insulin in the regulation of protein synthesis. *Diabetes*, **29**, 487–496.

Kahn, C. R. (1978) Insulin resistance, insulin insensitivity, and insulin unresponsiveness: a necessary distinction. *Metabolism*, **27 (suppl 2)**, 1893–1902.

Karam, J. H., Grodsky, G. M. and Forsham, P. H. (1963) Excessive insulin response to glucose in obese subjects as measured by immunochemical assay. *J. Am. Diet. Assoc.*, **12**, 197–204.

Kasuga, M., Karlsson, F. A. and Kahn, C. R. (1982) Insulin stimulates the phosphorylation of the 95,000 dalton subunit of its own receptor. *Science*, **215**, 185–187.

Lacy, P. E. (1964) Pancreatic beta cell. Colloquia on Endocrinology 15, The Aetiology of Diabetes Mellitus and its Complications. CIBA Foundation, Churchill, London, p. 78–85.

Laguesse, E. (1894) Sur quelques details de structure du pancreas humain. *C. R. Biol. Paris*, **1**, 667–669.

Lang, D. A., Matthews, D. R., Burnett, M. and Turner, R. C. (1981) Brief, irregular oscillation of basal plasma insulin and glucose concentration in diabetic man. *Diabetes*, **30**, 435–439.

LeCompte, P. M. (1958) Insulitis in early juvenile diabetes. *Arch. Pathol.*, **66**, 450–457.

Lillioja, S., Mott, D. M., Spraul, M. *et al.* (1993) Insulin resistance and insulin secretory dysfunction as precursors of non-insulin-dependent diabetes mellitus: prospective studies of Pima Indians. *N. Engl. J. Med.*, **329**, 1988–1992.

McGarry, J. D., Woeltje, K. F., Kuwajima, M. and Foster, D. W. (1989) Regulation of ketogenesis and the renaissance of carnitine palmitoyltransferase. *Diabetes/Metabol. Rev.* **5**, 271–284.

MacLean, N. and Ogilvie, R. F. (1955) Quantitative estimation of the pancreatic islet tissue in diabetic subjects. *Diabetes* **4**, 367–376.

Mortimore, G. E. and Mondon, C. E. (1970) Inhibition by insulin of valine turnover in liver. Evidence for a general control of proteolysis. *J. Biol. Chem.* **245**, 2375–2383.

Moschcowitz, E. (1951) The relation of hyperplastic arterio-sclerosis to diabetes mellitus. *Ann. Int. Med.*, **34**, 1137–1162.

Mueckler, M. (1990) Family of glucose transporter genes. *Diabetes*, **39**, 6–11.

Opie, E. L. (1901) The relation of diabetes mellitus to lesions of the pancreas. Hyaline degeneration of the islets of Langerhans. *J. Exp. Med.*, **5**, 397–428.

O'Rahilly, S., Turner, R. C. and Matthews, D. R. (1988) Impaired pulsatile secretion of insulin in relatives of patients with non-insulin-dependent diabetes. *N. Engl. J. Med.*, **318**, 1225–1230.

Owerbach, D., Bell, G. I., Rutter, W. J. *et al.* (1981) The insulin gene is located on the short arm of chromosome 11 in humans. *Diabetes*, **30**, 267–270.

Pettit, F. H., Pelley, J. W. and Reed, L. J. (1975) Regulation of pyruvate dehydrogenase kinase and phosphatase by acetyl CoA/CoA and NADH/NAD ratios. *Biochem. Biophys. Res. Comm.*, **65**, 575–582.

Porte, D. and Pupo, A. A. (1969) Insulin responses to glucose: evidence for a two pool system in man. *J. Clin. Invest.*, **48**, 2309–2319.

Randle, P. J., Garland, P. B., Hales, C. N. and Newsholme, E. A. (1963) The glucose fatty-acid cycle. Its role in insulin sensitivity and the metabolic disturbances of diabetes. *Lancet*, **i**, 785–789.

Reaven, G. M. (1983) Insulin resistance in non-insulin-dependent diabetes. Does it exist and can it be measured? *Am. J. Med.*, **74**, 3–17.

Rennie, M. J., Edwards, R. H. T., Halliday, D. *et al.* (1982) Muscle protein synthesis measured by stable isotope techniques in man: the effects of feeding and fasting. *Clin. Sci.*, **63**, 519–523.

Saad, M. F., Knowler, W. C., Pettit, D. J. *et al.* (1988) The natural history of impaired glucose intolerance in Pima Indians. *N. Engl. J. Med.*, **319**, 1500–1506.

Sacca, L., Hendler, R. and Sherwin, R. S. (1978) Hyperglycemia inhibits glucose production in man independent of changes in glucoregulatory hormones. *J. Clin. Endocrinol. Metab.*, **47**, 1160–1163.

Shulman, G. I., Lacy, W. W., Liljenquist, J. E. *et al.* (1986) Effect of glucose, independent of changes in insulin and glucagon secretion, on alanine metabolism in the conscious dog. *J. Clin. Invest.*, **65**, 496–505.

Soskin, S. (1948) *The Endocrines in Diabetes*, American Lecture Series 19, Charles C. Thomas, Springfield, IL.

Steiner, D. F., Cunningham, D., Spigelman, L. and Aten, B. (1967) Insulin biosynthesis: evidence for a precursor. *Science*, **157**, 697–700.

Taylor, R. (1984) Insulin receptor assays – clinical application and limitations. *Diabetic Med.*, **1**, 181–188.

Turner, R. C. and Holman, R. R. (1976) Insulin rather than glucose homeostasis in the pathophysiology of diabetes. *Lancet*, **i**, 1272–1274.

Ullrich, A., Bell, J. R., Chen, E. Y. *et al.* (1985) Human insulin receptor and its relationship to the tyrosine kinase family of oncogenes. *Nature*, **313**, 756–761.

Vaag, A., Henriksen, J. E. and Beck-Nielsen, H. (1992) Decreased insulin activation of glycogen synthase in skeletal muscles in young non-obese caucasian first-degree relatives of patients with non-insulin-dependent diabetes mellitus. *J. Clin. Invest.*, **89**, 782–788.

Walker, R., Bone, A. J., Dean, B. M. *et al.* (1988) Aberrant expression of class II MHC molecules on pancreatic B cells during development of insulin dependent diabetes; cause or consequence?, in *Frontiers in Diabetes Research*, (eds E. Shafrir and A. E. Renold), *Lessons from Animal Diabetes*, 2nd ed, Libbey, London, p. 185–189.

Warram, J. H., Martin, B. H., Krowlewski, A. S. *et al.* (1990) Slow glucose removal rate and hyperinsulinemia precede the development of type II diabetes in the offspring of diabetic patients. *Ann. Intern. Med.*, **1133**, 909–915.

Warren, S. and LeCompte, P. M. (1952) *The Pathology of Diabetes Mellitus*, 3rd edn, Lea & Febiger, Philadelphia, PA.

Warren, S. and Root, H. F. (1925) The pathology of diabetes, with special reference to pancreatic regeneration. *Am. J. Pathol.*, **1**, 415–429.

Weichselbaum, A. and Stangl, E. (1902) Weitere histologische Untersuchungen des Pankreas bei Diabetes Mellitus. *Wien. Klin. Wochenschr.*, **15**, 969–977.

Westermark, P., Wernstedt, C., Wilander, E. *et al.* (1987) Amyloid fibrils in human insulinoma and islets of Langerhans of the diabetic cat are derived from neuropeptide-like protein also present in normal islet cells. *Proc. Nat. Acad. Sci. USA*, **84**, 3881–3885.

Wrenshall, G. A., Bogoch, A. and Ritchie, R. C. (1952) Extractable insulin of pancreas. *Diabetes*, **1**, 87–105.

Zierler, K. L. and Rabinowitz, D. (1963) Roles of insulin and growth hormone, based on studies of forearm metabolism in man. *Medicine*, **42**, 385–402.

The term 'secondary diabetes' is a most unsatisfactory label to attach to the types of diabetes that do not fit comfortably into the insulin-dependent/non-insulin-dependent categories. After all, the two major types of diabetes are secondary in the sense that the metabolic disturbances are secondary to genetic and environmental factors. Nevertheless the term has a long tradition of use in the ares of diabetes resulting from disease of other organs and has been extended to include diabetes resulting from drugs and diabetes as either an accompaniment to or an integral part of specific syndromes.

PANCREATIC DISEASE

The literature of the association of diabetes with gross lesions of the pancreas is large and historically interesting. Cawley (1788) comes first but deserves little credit as he merely recorded a case of pancreatic lithiasis with diabetes, which he regarded as a disease of the kidneys, and it was Lancereaux (1877) who definitely associated diabetes with destruction of the pancreas. A case of pancreatic lithiasis described by Barron (1920), in which the relationship between islet cell damage and the appearance of diabetes was stressed, led Banting to the idea of extracting insulin from the pancreas after the acinar portion had been made to degenerate by ligation of the pancreatic duct – an inessential but important step in his experiments.

PANCREATITIS

Transitory hyperglycaemia and glycosuria are common during an attack of acute pancreatitis.

Occasionally the diabetes may persist but this is certainly infrequent. Warren and LeCompte (1952) pointed out that an inflammatory lesion sufficiently intense to destroy most of the islet tissue is usually severe enough to be fatal. Likewise, in chronic pancreatitis, diabetes only appears after the mass of the gland has been destroyed and the proportion of diabetics in a series of patients with chronic pancreatitis is a measure of the severity of the pancreatic insult.

In a large (551 cases) UK survey of acute pancreatitis 9% showed transient hyperglycaemia thought to indicate a severe attack yet none progressed to frank diabetes later, except where other predisposing factors were present, such as chronic pancreatitis, pre-existing diabetes or a family history of non-insulin-dependent diabetes (Trapnell, 1980).

In chronic pancreatitis James, Agnew and Bouchier (1974) found that 49 of 81 (60.5%) had an abnormal glucose tolerance test. Other reports suggest one-third with diabetes and one-third with impaired glucose tolerance. In this situation the severity of the glucose abnormality may reflect the severity of the underlying disease and there may be ready progression through impaired glucose tolerance to frank diabetes.

Clinically, chronic pancreatitis does not seem to be an important numerical cause of diabetes in Europe or North America. About one-third of young diabetic patients may show a low amylase output in the pancreozymin-secretin test while showing no clinical evidence of exocrine pancreatic disease. It is unclear whether this is related to the duration or severity of the diabetes. This finding has not been universally accepted and others have concluded that diabetes is not associated with abnormal exocrine secretion from the pancreas.

There is considerable geographic variation in diabetes secondary to chronic pancreatitis: 0.5% of diabetics at the Mayo clinic, but in Nigeria 8.6% of diabetics had chronic pancreatitis. In East Africa Kinnear (1963) found that 13% of all native patients presenting with diabetic symptoms had a calcified pancreas. Most of these patients were less than 20 years of age and they formed an easily recognizable group because they had steatorrhoea. This variation almost certainly results from different aetiologies. In the West, alcohol is the clearest underlying cause of chronic pancreatitis. Countries with a high prevalence include France, Italy and Portugal and most series record high alcohol intakes in their predominantly male population with chronic pancreatitis. In Asia and Africa, however, alcohol has not been implicated as a causative agent (see below). It has been suggested that this may be a degenerative condition occurring at a relatively young age. Factors implicated in its development are cassava, which is eaten in large amounts in Kerala in the south-west of India. A path can be traced from cassava to cyanide and an inability to detoxify the amounts generated. There is evidence that cyanide is hyperglycaemic.

Following the appearance of diabetes there is tremendous variation in insulin responses to oral glucose and subnormal, normal and supranormal responses are reported. Islet cell antibodies are not present and glucagon levels tend to be low. The histological change in the endocrine pancreas in chronic pancreatitis remains controversial. Some workers report islet preservation even when exocrine destruction is severe. When this occurs islet clustering may be seen. Others report decreases in the number of islets. Some islets show degeneration and round cell infiltration. With increasing hyalinization of fibrous tissue the islets are distorted into linear streaks.

Within the islet it is unclear whether normal A:B cell ratios persist. Immunocytochemistry suggests normal numbers of D cells, a slight increase in PP cells, B cells reduced to 60% of controls and A cells increased, sometimes to equal the total number of B cells (Kloppel *et al.*, 1978).

CARCINOMA OF THE PANCREAS

Warren and LeCompte (1952) and others have pointed out that this somewhat uncommon neoplasm is found with much greater frequency than expected at autopsy among unselected diabetic patients and our own comparative study of diabetic mortality confirms this, the incidence of carcinoma as a whole being normal in the diabetic.

A large proportion of patients with carcinoma of the pancreas have a diabetic type of glucose tolerance test. Murphy and Smith (1963), in a review of 245 unselected patients with this growth subjected to operation at the Lahey Clinic between 1955 and 1961, found 91 (37.4%) with abnormal glucose tolerance at the time of laparotomy. A total of 25 of the patients had developed clinical diabetes which needed insulin or oral treatment.

Clinically the association is important because diabetes may precede the obvious features of the pancreatic growth by several months, occasionally more than a year. Characteristically the patient presents with glycosuria, having been to the doctor complaining of loss of weight and malaise but not thirst. The diabetes is usually mild and the weight loss seems to be more rapid and considerable than one would expect. Restriction of diet and, if necessary, oral treatment quickly controls the diabetes but the weight continues to fall and the patient feels no better. After a few months abdominal pain or backache makes it obvious that all is not well and if obstructive jaundice supervenes the diagnosis becomes obvious. As a corollary the finding of glycosuria and abnormal glucose tolerance in a patient with obstructive jaundice suggests a diagnosis of pancreatic carcinoma. The diagnosis of diabetes is worth making since it may be quite severe and need treatment.

A mysterious feature of the diabetes associated with carcinoma of the pancreas is that islet cell destruction from involvement by the growth or associated pancreatitis is not often extensive and a considerable part of the gland may appear normal on routine examination. Further histological studies of biopsy material at the time of operation would be helpful.

TOTAL PANCREATECTOMY

Complete pancreatectomy leads inevitably to diabetes which has to be treated with insulin to maintain life and which does not respond to sulphonylurea drugs. Withdrawal of insulin leads rapidly to symptoms of diabetes and usually ketosis, although cases have been described when patients did not become ketosed after 3 days without it despite well marked hyperglycaemia and thirst. The daily requirement of insulin is usually small, though there is a single record of insulin resistance in which the diabetes was not controlled by 180 units daily. Commonly the dose is 10–20 units, seldom more than 40 units and certainly less than the average for insulin-dependent diabetes arising spontaneously. The reason for this is uncertain. Loss of humoral agents such as glucagon is probably not sufficient to explain the low requirement, but nutritional defect resulting from the removal of the exocrine secretions of the pancreas is more likely to be important. Similarly, irregular intestinal absorption accounts for the occasionally unstable character of the diabetes.

HAEMOCHROMATOSIS

The first description of an association of diabetes with haemochromatosis was given by Trousseau in 1865. His observations were extended by Troisier, who in 1871 reported diabetes, hepatic cirrhosis and pigmentation while the term bronze diabetes was introduced in 1886. Sheldon (1935) was the first to propose that primary haemochromatosis was an inherited metabolic abnormality, when describing five families.

Early theories that diabetes results from infiltration of the pancreas by iron have gone largely unchallenged. The iron content of the pancreas is increased 50–100 times in idiopathic haemochromatosis and as a result there is extensive pancreatic fibrosis. The pigment, which may be so marked as to colour the pancreas reddish-brown or deep brown, is deposited in acinar and ductal tissues. The islets also show pigmentation in 80% of cases. The end result is a reduction in number or complete absence in 62% and fibrosis in 25% of the reported cases collected by Sheldon (1935). The involvement is not uniform: the islets being involved to a variable extent but the B cells are selectively affected, the A cells remaining quantitatively normal.

The incidence of diabetes in any series of patients with haemochromatosis depends upon the stage at which the diagnosis is made. In earlier times, when diabetes was almost a cardinal feature, it was naturally higher, being present in 78% of Sheldon's patients, but later series reported only 42%. Usually the diagnosis of diabetes is made before that of haemochromatosis although a greater awareness of the genetics of idiopathic haemochromatosis and identification of relatives at risk will alter this picture. Singh *et al.* (1992) screened 400 caucasian diabetic patients and found two probable heterozygotes and two probable homozygotes, giving a prevalence of the homozygote of 4.9 per 1000. This figure is lower than other studies and is the same as in the general population.

The diabetes of haemochromatosis cannot be distinguished from other types of diabetes. A male predominance, younger age of onset or insulin responses to oral glucose do not help to distinguish a specific type of diabetes. Most patients end up being treated with insulin although early reports of significant insulin resistance are not borne out in clinical practice. There have been suggestions that the diabetes improves significantly with chelation therapy, which is tacitly accepted as being due to an effect upon the pancreas. It would seem more likely that any initial improvement is due to an improvement in liver function (Cutler, 1989). I tend toward the opinion that diabetes does not improve significantly with depletion of iron stores, i.e. there is no decisive change in the need for insulin. Any effect upon insulin dosage is usually lost in a striving to improve diabetic control.

Haemochromatosis should be borne in mind in diabetic clinic practice. It is, of course, an exceptionally rare cause of diabetes, occurring in less than 1% of diabetic patients (O'Brien *et al.*, 1990). Bronze diabetes is not always an appropriate label. The pigmentation, especially if it is metallic rather than melanotic, may escape detection but a suspicious colour of the skin in association with enlargement of the liver calls for investigation. Estimation of the serum iron and iron binding capacity, with calculation of the percentage saturation, is a most useful screening procedure although serum ferritin measurement is a more specific assessment of iron stores. Liver biopsy may be confirmatory but often seems to cloud the issue. Except in a total abstainer the question always seems to arise of whether the haemochromatosis observed truly represents haemochromatosis or may be from alcohol-induced cirrhosis. Absorption of radioactive iron from the gut is abnormal but is a test rarely needed for diagnosis.

MALNUTRITION-RELATED DIABETES

The reclassification of diabetes by the World Health Organization (WHO, 1985) recognized malnutrition-related diabetes as an important cause of diabetes worldwide. The syndrome has a variety of other names, including J-type diabetes, Z-type diabetes, tropical diabetes, tropical calcific pancreatitis, fibrocalculous diabetes and protein-deficient diabetes. These names reflect clinical and biochemical variation in the disease, with malnutrition proposed as the unifying theme. Currently accepted nomenclature (WHO, 1985) is that there are two major subtypes of malnutrition-related diabetes: fibrocalculous pancreatic diabetes (also known as tropical calcific pancreatitis) and protein-deficient pancreatic diabetes.

Hugh-Jones (1955) first reported difficulty in classifying some Jamaican diabetics. Of 215 Jamaican patients 13 were neither insulin-dependent nor non-insulin-dependent. The patients were characterized by young age of onset, lack of ketosis, absence of obesity and a degree of insulin resistance. He coined the term 'J-type' (Jamaican-type) to describe this group. Tulloch and MacIntosh (1961) added a further 11 cases to this series from the University College Hospital of the West Indies, reporting 3–8 years of observation. In addition to the characteristics previously reported, normal liver histology was found, and only one of seven patients had pancreatic calcification. Similar cases of diabetes have been reported around the world from Malaya, Indonesia, Fiji and many countries in Africa. Zuidema (1955), in Indonesia, described patients with pancreatic calcification and fibrosis and a history of malnutrition or malnutrition at presentation. He called this type of diabetes 'Z-type'.

The prevalence of malnutrition-related diabetes around the world varies somewhat with different criteria being used. In Jamaica it is around 7% of diabetics, in Nigeria 50% of diabetics under the age of 20, in Indonesia 80% of diabetics and in India 23%. Problems of definition in India are compounded by an increased frequency of MODY.

As with most syndromes there has been a clear overdiagnosis of the rarity. It is a strange affliction of the physician that rarities are prized and characteristics of patients may be remoulded to fit a rare syndrome. Clearly many patients labelled malnutrition-related

Table 3.1 Protein-deficient pancreatic diabetes

1. Blood glucose > 11.1 mmol/l (200 mg/dl)
2. Onset before the age of 30 years
3. History of childhood malnutrition
   or
   Poor socioeconomic status
4. Body mass index < 19 kg/m^2
5. Insulin requirement > 60 units/day or greater than 1.5 u/kg
6. Absence of ketosis on insulin withdrawal

Table 3.2 Fibrocalculous pancreatic diabetes

1. Blood glucose > 11.1 mmol/l (200 mg/dl)
2. Onset before the age of 30
3. History of childhood malnutrition
   or
   Poor socioeconomic status
4. Body mass index < 19 mg/m^2
5. Insulin requirement > 60 units/day
   or greater than 1.5 u/kg
6. Absence of ketosis on insulin withdrawal
7. Chronic pancreatitis as evidenced by
   (a) pancreatic calculi
   or
   (b) history of recurrent abdominal pain since childhood
   and/or steatorrhoea
   and/or abnormal pancreatic morphology
   and/or abnormal exocrine pancreatic function test
8. Absence of gallstones, alcoholism or primary hyperparathyroidism

diabetes have been type 1 or more commonly type 2 diabetic patients with minor variation from the norm at presentation. Nevertheless, there remain two main groups of diabetic patients that lie uneasily in the predominantly Western classification of type 1 and type 2 diabetes. These are malnutrition-related diabetes without evidence of exocrine pancreatic disease (protein-deficient pancreatic diabetes) and tropical pancreatic diabetes with features of exocrine pancreatic disease (fibrocalculous pancreatic diabetes). The criteria for protein-deficient pancreatic diabetes (Table 3.1) have been attacked by a number of writers as being too non-specific in a tropical population. Malnutrition is common when poverty abounds, high insulin requirements may reflect the immunogenicity of the insulin preparations available, body mass index may be less abnormal than at first sight taking into account the distribution of BMI in the whole population, and ketosis resistance may not be a consistent finding. There is a lack of aetiological and diagnostic features of this condition, which leaves a considerable doubt as to whether it is a distinct entity or perhaps a slowly evolving insulin-dependent diabetes.

Fibrocalculous pancreatic diabetes is better defined as a separate entity. Similar criteria apply as to pancreatic diabetes, although many workers in the field have argued that young age and underweight are of only minor importance. The cardinal feature is a history of chronic pancreatitis. Evidence of this is accepted if there are pancreatic calculi. Where

these are not obvious a history of recurrent abdominal pain from an early age, steatorrhoea, an abnormal pancreatic CT scan or ERCP, or abnormal pancreatic exocrine function test may make the diagnosis in the absence of other causes of chronic pancreatitis (Table 3.2) (Mohan *et al.*, 1985).

The clinical presentation is often with severe diabetes, marked hyperglycaemia and dehydration in an emaciated patient. Patients are underweight yet by definition ketosis is absent. The response to oral hypoglycaemic agents is poor and doses of insulin > 60–80 units/day are required to control the blood glucose. Even following insulin withdrawal ketosis does not occur. Quite why this should be so is unclear and a number of explanations have been put forward. There may be sufficient residual B cell secretion to inhibit hepatic ketogenesis; damage to the A cells may result in the loss of the ketogenic effect of glucagon; or there may be hepatic carnitine deficiency. Alternatively, at the fat cell subcutaneous fat loss may lead to a poor supply of NEFA to the liver for ketogenesis, or the action of catecholamines upon lipolysis may be impaired, which would also result in impaired delivery of NEFA to the liver. Experimental evidence suggests that the answer lies at the level of adipose tissue lipolysis (Yajnik *et al.*, 1992)

As befits a syndrome with many names a large number of aetiological factors have been implicated. Kambo *et al.* (1985) reported an association in fibrocalculous pancreatic diabetes with the hypervariable 5′ flanking region of the insulin gene, although this was also found in type 2 diabetes. They suggested this genetic predisposition to diabetes with an additional environmental stimulus of pancreatitis. Environmental agents have been largely favoured as aetiological factors, particularly malnutrition, with or without cassava consumption. Other factors include herbal remedies and alcohol. Protein calorie malnutrition in experimental animals results in damage to both the exocrine and endocrine pancreas and is therefore a prime candidate in aetiology, yet there is the nagging doubt that this exists in many parts of the world where malnutrition-related diabetes is unrecorded.

Cassava intake is high in many areas where this type of diabetes occurs. Cassava contains linamarin, a glycoside that on hydrolysis releases hydrocyanic acid. This is normally inactivated by conjugation with the sulphhydryl groups of the amino acids methionine, cystine and cysteine, which are deficient in protein calorie malnutrition. In Kerala, malnutrition-related diabetes is endemic and cassava is the main staple food yet there are areas, such as Madras, where the syndrome is common yet the intake of cassava is low. Currently the link remains non-proven.

DRUGS (TABLE 3.3)

Hyperglycaemia as a result of drug administration for either therapeutic or experimental reasons may come about in a number of ways. In experiments where non-diabetic animals are made diabetic this is usually

Table 3.3 Therapeutic agents with diabetogenic side effects

Drugs affecting the cardiovascular system
1. Diuretics
   Benzothiadiazines especially diazoxide, loop diuretics
2. Antihypertensive agents
   Propranolol, atenolol, metoprolol, nifedipine

Drugs affecting the respiratory system
1. Beta-agonists
   Salbutamol, ritodrine, terbutaline
2. Beta-stimulants
   Theophylline, caffeine
3. Expectorants
   Benylin®

Anti-infective agents
1. Antituberculous
   Rifampicin, isoniazid
2. Antibacterial
   Nalidixic acid
3. Antiprotozoal
   Pentamidine

Drugs acting upon the gastrointestinal system
Cimetidine

Drugs acting upon the central nervous system
Phenytoin, chlordiazepoxide, morphine, lithium

Hormonal preparations
Glucocorticoids, growth hormone, glucagon, somatostatin, adrenalin, noradrenalin, anabolic steroids, oral contraceptives

Other drugs
Aspirin, L-asparaginase, cyclosporin A

brought about by destruction of the B cells. Except when treating an insulinoma this is rarely an aim in clinical practice. A multitude of other drugs, however, are able to produce hyperglycaemia through a number of different mechanisms. From first principles it could be argued that hyperglycaemia would result not only from B cell destruction but also if insulin secretion was impaired, insulin resistance induced, a combination of these two, or as a result of a direct effect upon metabolic pathways.

It should be acknowledged that the terminology used in describing the interrelationship of drug administration and hyperglycaemia may be erroneous or misleading. It is difficult to state with certainty that a drug causes hyperglycaemia or diabetes. This remains true even when a demonstrable effect upon insulin secretion or glucose metabolism is observed. One can always point to a host of patients who take a specific drug yet do not develop diabetes. For this reason, clinically the appearance of diabetes after the use of a particular drug has been assumed to be an indication of a diabetic predisposition unmasked by the drug.

BENZOTHIADIAZINES

Hyperglycaemia after taking benzothiadiazines was noted in man by Goldner, Zarowitz and Akgun (1960). The phenomenon was especially striking in the case of the antihypertensive agent diazoxide when it was submitted for clinical trial (Dollery, Pentecost and Samaan, 1962) to the extent that it has probably had as much subsequent use in the treatment of non-diabetic hyperglycaemia as it has as an antihypertensive agent.

The mechanism by which these drugs alter carbohydrate tolerance is unclear. The principal mechanism is probably direct inhibition of insulin release but it has been found that they can cause pancreatitis in mice, increase hepatic output of glucose in dogs, and that adrenergic hormones may be involved. Hyperglycaemia is accompanied by increased hepatic glycogenolysis, a beta-adrenergic effect, with a rise in serum lactate and pyruvate. It has been observed that tolbutamide and other sulphonylureas, as well as insulin, suppress the effect even in alloxanized mice. This has led to the suggestion that there may be some competitive antagonism at the level of the sulphonylurea receptor, either through competition for binding to the receptor or upon the effect upon the potassium channel.

In man the plasma insulin levels in response to secretogogues are reduced. This is likely to be due to potassium depletion, which impairs insulin secretion and is an effect of benzothiadiazines (Carlsen *et al.*, 1990). There is no evidence to support the view that it is a simple unmasking of undiagnosed diabetes or a diabetic predisposition, judging from the incidence of family history, although this has been suggested. Hyperglycaemia appears within a variable time from a few days to many months after starting treatment and is usually of moderate degree. It may subside rapidly when the drug is withdrawn and reappear equally rapidly if it is given again. In some instances the diabetes does not seem to be reversible. The response to a sulphonylurea is excellent and complete in most cases. A worsening of established diabetes has the same characteristics as that which appears *de novo*.

The frequency of this phenomenon is hard to gauge in ordinary clinic practice. Hypertension and diabetes are both common in the general population and patients with either are in well screened populations. It would not be surprising that hypertension appeared more common in the diabetic population and *vice versa*, purely from the viewpoint that diabetics are more likely to have their blood pressure measured while hypertensive patients are more likely to have their urine tested. In fact we know that there is a genuine and real increase in the association of non-insulin-dependent diabetes and hypertension. It is certain also from detailed clinical studies that the effect is a real one. In the treatment of mild hypertension (Medical Research Council Working Party, 1981) hyperglycaemia was found to be four to six times as common in the thiazide group as in the placebo group although a rather high dose of thiazide was used.

The use of thiazide diuretics in the treatment of hypertension has declined in recent years partly due to more potent agents with fewer side effects, particularly hyperglycaemia, but also due to the realization that an equivalent antihypertensive effect can be obtained with fewer side effects through using a lower dose. As diuretic treatment, thiazides have largely been replaced by the loop diuretics such as frusemide and bumetamide. These are chemically distinct but also contain a halogenated sulphamoylbenzene ring, which occurs also in thiazide diuretics. Without doubt they have less of a diabetogenic action.

ANTIHYPERTENSIVE AGENTS

Other antihypertensive agents have been reported to alter glucose homoeostasis. The most important of these are the beta-blocker group of drugs. A number of studies have shown that propranolol can result in glucose intolerance in previously non-diabetic patients, although the effect is small and of doubtful clinical significance. In a comparative study in patients with non-insulin-dependent diabetes Wright *et al.* (1979) found that both propranolol and the more specific beta$_1$-antagonist metoprolol increased postprandial blood glucose concentrations by approximately 1 mmol/l (18 mg/dl) compared with placebo. The mechanism whereby beta-blockers cause glucose intolerance is unclear. Despite higher glucose concentrations Wright *et al.* (1979) found unchanged insulin concentrations presenting interpretative difficulties – does this indicate insulin resistance or why did not the higher glucose stimulate an increase in insulin secretion?

Calcium-channel-blocking drugs seem to be metabolically neutral, with little evidence to support an effect upon either glucose or insulin. There are occasional reports of overdosage producing hyperglycaemia with or without an acidosis in non-diabetic patients.

ADRENERGIC BETA-AGONISTS

Adrenergic beta$_2$-agonists are widely used in the treatment of bronchial asthma but it is their use in premature labour that has led to

reports of effects upon glucose homoeostasis. Salbutamol, terbutaline and ritodrine have all been shown to raise blood glucose, increase blood lactate and induce hypokalaemia. A metabolic acidosis may accompany these abnormalities. The mechanism is unclear although the raised glucose is accompanied by raised circulating insulin.

CORTICOSTEROIDS

Corticosteroid preparations are potent precipitators of overt diabetes and cause loss of control in established diabetic patients when given in large doses. This remains an under-acknowledged fact which can lead to an ignoring of the hyperglycaemia and metabolic upset of ill patients. Clearly any treatable aspect of an ill patient should not be missed through ignorance.

Hyperglycaemia in response to corticosteroid therapy is associated with hyperinsulinaemia. Despite this hyperinsulinaemia hepatic glucose output is raised and peripheral glucose disposal is impaired. *In vitro* steroids alter the dose–response curve for the effect of insulin upon glucose uptake into cells and glucose oxidation.

The pathogenic mechanism is discussed in more detail below under endocrine disease. It is also part of the stress response, i.e. the precipitation of diabetes by trauma or illness, and as such is of importance in the development of ketoacidosis.

The frequency with which corticosteroids produce diabetes will depend primarily upon the dose rather than the steroid. There is nothing to suggest that any particular steroid is less inclined to have diabetes as one of its side effects than the next. High doses of a specific steroid are more likely to result in diabetes and the majority of studies have focussed upon the use of high-dose steroids. In these studies about 20% of patients develop diabetes.

OTHER DRUGS

The only other major groups of drugs which have attracted particular interest are the oral contraceptive preparations and the immuno-suppressive agents. The former are more of historical interest while the latter are a problem for the future.

Clear-cut effects upon glucose tolerance can be observed during the use of oral contraceptive preparations (provided a large enough patient sample is taken) but much of the literature refers to earlier preparations with a high oestrogen content and the problem seems less apparent with low-dose-oestrogen preparations. Even with low-dose-oestrogen combined preparations, and also with progestagen-only preparations, metabolic effects are demonstrable although sufficiently subtle to allow us the opinion that a young diabetic woman should not be advised against taking an oral contraceptive preparation solely on the grounds of the effect upon control of her diabetes.

Of more pressing interest is the development of diabetes or impaired glucose tolerance in post-transplant patients receiving immunosuppressive agents. It is clear that this effect is not due solely to concomitant administration of corticosteroids, since it persists after discontinuing steroids (Krentz *et al.*, 1993). The abnormality is not associated with insulinopenia and may be attributable to insulin resistance with or without a subtotal impairment of insulin secretion.

Many other drugs affect glucose tolerance (Table 3.3) but the clinical impact is small. The effect is of more interest to clinical pharmacologists and the pharmaceutical industry than to the doctor in the clinic, who will be rightly sceptical of claims that specific agents are better than the rivals in the treatment of diabetic patients. Few people would deny patients the benefit of lithium or rifampicin because of a marginal effect upon a glucose tolerance test.

Drugs which fall into this category include nifedipine, cimetidine and salbutamol. All have been reported as causative agents in precipitating the infrequent case of keto-acidosis or non-ketotic diabetic coma. Central nervous system agents such as phenothiazines and benzodiazepines also exhibit effects upon glucose metabolism, as does phenytoin, which is used occasionally in the treatment of islet cell tumours. Lithium may also alter carbohydrate metabolism.

ENDOCRINE DISEASE

CUSHING'S SYNDROME

Oversecretion of corticosteroids has long had an association with diabetes. Lukens, Flippin and Thigpen (1937) reported glycosuria in 44% of 55 proven cases while others quote 90% with abnormal glucose tolerance test and 15% with frank diabetes (Plotz, Knowlton and Ragan, 1952). Corticosteroids are potent antagonists of insulin with effects upon carbohydrate, protein and fat metabolism.

In normal man administration of a synthetic ACTH-like peptide for 2–3 days results in an increase in fasting blood glucose of about 2 mmol/l (36 mg/dl) (Johnston *et al.*, 1979). More prolonged corticosteroid excess is associated with glucose intolerance but fasting blood glucose returns to normal. This pattern is found in Cushing's syndrome (Johnston *et al.*, 1980a). The increase in blood glucose is due to stimulation of hepatic gluconeogenesis by corticosteroids through an effect upon key enzymes such as phosphoenol-pyruvate carboxykinase. Supply of gluconeogenic precursors is also increased (Johnston *et al.*, 1979). Cortisol also inhibits glucose-dependent and insulin-stimulated glucose uptake into muscle and adipose tissue.

In normal man these effects are counteracted by a rise in circulatory insulin concentrations. This compensatory rise in insulin also nullifies any ketogenic effect of cortisol in normal man. In insulin deficiency, however, ketone body concentrations are elevated by cortisol excess (Schade, Eaton and Standefer, 1977). In Cushing's syndrome levels of ketone bodies and non-esterified fatty acids are normal. Alanine, the major gluconeogenic amino acid, is increased by cortisol.

It is tempting to conclude that the metabolic effects of corticosteroids can be overcome where sufficient insulin secretory reserve exists to maintain hyperinsulinism. This cannot be the true explanation in a disease where approximately two-thirds of patients show abnormalities of glucose tolerance.

The suggestion that abnormal glucose tolerance and hyperinsulinism precede a degree of insulin deficiency and frank diabetes seems somehow too logical and compartmentalized.

Special mention should be made of the association of diabetes with the ectopic ACTH syndrome. At presentation the diabetes looks to be undoubtedly insulin-dependent, with the history of weight loss. Weakness may also be a dominant feature in the presentation, due more to hypokalaemia than diabetes *per se*. Palmar pigmentation and pigmentation at other sites is usually obvious. Sadly, the course of the disease is rarely lengthy and insulin is required for all too short a time.

ACROMEGALY

Studies of the incidence of glucose tolerance abnormalities in acromegaly give a variable incidence both of glycosuria and diabetes ranging from 17–38%. Where the glucose tolerance test has been employed systematically the higher figure is more appropriate. While it is surprising that diabetes is not more common after long-standing excess of growth hormone, acromegaly is probably the most common cause of diabetes as a secondary disturbance following another disease.

The diabetes of acromegaly is usually biochemically mild. Pharmacological amounts of growth hormone given to normal man impairs glucose tolerance within 1–2 hours. In insulin-deficient man a hyperglycaemic effect is readily apparent (Schade, Eaton and Peake, 1978), which results from increased hepatic glucose output and decreased peripheral glucose uptake. Where insulin secretory reserve exists hyperinsulinaemia results. Growth hormone also has a lipolytic effect and raises ketone body concentrations even before an increase in non-esterified fatty acids is apparent (Gerich *et al.*, 1976).

As with cortisol excess similar stages in the progression to frank diabetes have been postulated, from normal glucose tolerance with hyperinsulinaemia, though impaired glucose tolerance despite hyperinsulinaemia to diabetes with insulin deficiency. Only 5–10% of acromegalic patients fall into the frank diabetes category and it cannot be concluded either that the stages denote the natural history of acromegaly or that those in the final category have coexisting acromegaly and 'idiopathic' diabetes.

PHAEOCHROMOCYTOMA

Chromaffin tumours are rare (about 1 per 100 000 adults) but occasionally come to light in the investigation of patients with high blood pressure. Among cases of phaeochromocytoma frank diabetes was present in 10% and abnormal glucose tolerance in a further 9% (Graham, 1951); certainly a higher incidence than that of diabetes in the age-group involved. These tumours secrete either mainly adrenalin or mainly noradrenalin.

Catecholamines are potent inducers of insulin resistance, while the alpha-adrenergic effect of adrenalin is well recognized to inhibit insulin secretion. A prime metabolic effect of catecholamines is to increase hepatic glucose output. This is achieved by both stimulation of glycogen breakdown and an increase in hepatic gluconeogenesis. These effects are mediated through changes in cyclic 3',5'-AMP. In the periphery, catecholamines are potent lipolytic agents through increased activity of hormone-sensitive lipase. Glycerol is taken up by the liver for gluconeogenesis and non-esterified fatty acids are also extracted from the blood by the liver. Whether catecholamines divert fatty acids into ketone bodies within the liver remains unresolved.

Fasting blood glucose tends to be normal in patients with phaeochromocytoma although the response to oral glucose is impaired. Alpha-adrenergic blockade may restore glucose tolerance to normal, as may resection of the tumour, although normal glucose tolerance is not always guaranteed by restoration of normal insulin secretion.

PRIMARY HYPERALDOSTERONISM

First described by Conn and Louis (1956), primary hyperaldosteronism is associated with glucose intolerance in about 50% of cases. The biochemical disorder is mild and it would seem unlikely to be due to the rather weak glucocorticoid effect of this potent mineralocorticoid. Interestingly glucose intolerance in hypokalaemic hepatic cirrhosis associated with secondary aldosteronism also occurs. In both primary and secondary hyperaldosteronism glucose intolerance may be corrected by repletion of total body potassium stores. The glucose intolerance of Conn's syndrome is also corrected by removal of the adenoma.

PANCREATIC ENDOCRINE TUMOURS

Glucagonoma

Although McGavran *et al.* (1966) described a glucagon secreting pancreatic A-cell carcinoma in 1966 it was not until the early 1970s that many cases were identified and reported. Mallinson *et al.* (1974) described the clinical syndrome associated with a glucagon-secreting tumour composed of necrolytic migratory erythema, weight loss, normochromic normocytic anaemia, stomatitis, glucose intolerance and markedly elevated levels of circulating glucagon.

The effect of the massive elevations in glucagon upon glucose tolerance is perhaps easier to understand than the other clinical features produced. Glucagon has potent metabolic effects, increasing glycogen breakdown and gluconeogenesis and promoting ketogenesis. An interesting sequel to the acute effect of glucagon upon hepatic glucose output is that with prolonged exposure hepatic glucose output returns to normal.

Unlike other catabolic hormones it has proved difficult to identify an effect of glucagon upon lipolysis in man. The effect upon ketogenesis is therefore independent of an effect upon fatty acid availability and is truly intrahepatic. Whether regulation is by glucagon concentration or the portal insulin to glucagon ratio has been fiercely debated.

Glucose intolerance in the glucagonoma syndrome varies in reports from mild to uncontrollable. Since the majority of tumours are malignant complete resection is rarely possible and glucose intolerance persists.

Somatostatinoma

Tumours of the D cells of the islets of Langerhans have been reported in recent years. Initially the diagnosis was coincidental in patients having cholecystectomy but subsequent reports have confirmed gallstones as a true association. Other commonly associated features are dyspepsia, diarrhoea and weight loss. Somatostatin is a potent inhibitor of insulin secretion and glucagon secretion and it is therefore not surprising that diabetes is associated with somatostatinoma. Interestingly, although the diabetes is associated with hypoinsulinaemia it does not appear to be ketosis-prone. As with the glucagonoma syndrome, the majority of somatostatinomas are malignant (Christensen, 1986).

THYROID DISEASE

Glucose intolerance in hyperthyroidism undoubtedly occurs but probably not to the prevalence of more than 50% reported by some. Usually the intolerance is mild with a normal fasting blood glucose. The potential for glucose intolerance induced by thyroid hormones is great. They alter gastric emptying and glucose absorption, increase insulin turnover and induce sympathetic overactivity.

PROLACTINOMAS

Early reports that prolactin was diabetogenic were probably a result of contamination of the preparation with traces of growth hormone. Nevertheless there are reports of impaired glucose tolerance with hyperinsulinaemia in patients with prolactin-secreting adenomas where growth hormone levels were normal. Johnston *et al.* (1980b) found normal glucose tolerance with an exaggerated insulin response during metabolic rhythms in nine hyperprolactinaemic females. Blood glycerol and ketone bodies were lower in their patients although other reports suggest that non-esterified fatty acids are increased.

CARCINOID SYNDROME

Glucose tolerance is impaired in patients with the carcinoid syndrome when serotonin levels are high. This appears to be due to inhibition of insulin secretion by serotonin (Feldman *et al.*, 1975). Fasting glucose and insulin is normal, with a reduced insulin response to glucose stimuli.

SYNDROMES OF DIABETES

DIDMOAD

The DIDMOAD syndrome of diabetes insipidus, diabetes mellitus, optic atrophy and deafness is an uncommon syndrome. Wolfram and Wagener (1938) noted diabetes mellitus associated with optic atrophy in a family and De Lawter (1949) added to this diabetes insipidus. Deafness with optic atrophy and diabetes mellitus was described by Shaw and Duncan (1958) and the full syndrome by Ikkos *et al.* (1970).

The diabetes mellitus is typically insulin-dependent and shows a tendency to the development of ketoacidosis. The insidious onset of diabetes insipidus may be difficult to recognize, thirst and polyuria being ascribed to poor diabetic control. When optic atrophy is present with diabetes mellitus this may alert the physician to the possibility of the DIDMOAD syndrome and for this reason diagnosis of optic atrophy usually precedes that of diabetes insipidus. The recognition of diabetes insipidus is of importance since it may lead to dilatation of the urinary tract (Page, Asmal and Edwards, 1975). Deafness often passes unnoticed without objective testing. The association of diabetes mellitus and optic atrophy seems commoner than the full syndrome. Indeed it seems that optic atrophy may be commoner in the diabetic population than the normal population, although such associations are difficult to prove or disprove. Few normal populations have their eyes screened as intensively as the diabetic population. It is unclear whether the association is partial penetrance of the full-blown syndrome or whether the other defects would eventually develop in these patients.

Other abnormalities have been noted in the syndrome, although rarely, including ataxia and psychiatric disorder, cardiomyopathy, sideroblastic anaemia and thrombocytopenia. Hypogonadism is also reported but where studies of hypothalamo-pituitary function have been performed there has been no evidence of endocrine abnormality other than diabetes mellitus and insipidus.

A number of authors have argued for a single recessive gene to explain the familial nature of the DIDMOAD syndrome. There is considerable variation in manifestation, however, which has led to alternative explanations being sought. Bundey *et al.* (1992) described abnormal mitochondria, both morphological and biochemically, in a patient with DIDMOAD and a number of patients have been described with a mutation in the mitochondrial DNA. Not all patients labelled

DIDMOAD have abnormalities of maternally inherited mitochondrial DNA and as with other 'types' of diabetes there seems scope for heterogeneity.

The natural history of the syndrome reveals early onset of diabetes mellitus, in most cases before the age of 10 years, and blindness from optic atrophy by early adult life. Sudden death is reported and I would support the view that this is commoner than in type 1 diabetes.

MATERNALLY INHERITED DIABETES AND DEAFNESS

For many years it has been apparent that there is a maternal effect in the inheritance of diabetes. Thus, for example, if a person is diagnosed below the age of 25 years with diabetes and a parent has the disease also it is twice as likely to be the mother as the father. This raises the possibility that mitochondrial DNA may play a part in the transmission, since only maternal mitochondrial DNA is passed to the next generation. Paternal mitochondrial DNA is carried in the tail of the sperm and is therefore not transmitted at fertilization.

Mitochondrial DNA is a circular molecule of 16 569 base pairs and each mitochondrion carries two to ten copies. Its main function is to code for some mitochondrial proteins and especially subunits of the respiratory chain and transfer RNAs. A number of groups have reported families with maternal transmission of predominantly non-insulin-dependent diabetes associated with a sensorineural deafness (van den Ouweland *et al.*, 1992). These patients have a point mutation in their mitochondrial DNA at position 3243 in the mitochondrial tRNA$^{LEU(UUR)}$ gene. This same mutation is responsible for the MELAS syndrome of myopathy, encephalopathy, lactic acidosis and stroke-like episodes in which a defect in insulin secretion has also been identified (Suzuki *et al.*, 1994).

MATURITY-ONSET DIABETES OF THE YOUNG (MODY)

In contrast to the DIDMOAD syndrome, maturity-onset diabetes of the young (MODY) is a less well demarcated syndrome. The heterogeneous nature of non-insulin-dependent diabetes ensures this. As originally described (Fajans and Conn, 1960) MODY described a syndrome of biochemically mild, possibly asymptomatic diabetes affecting children, adolescents or young adults. The strong familial segregation of this type of diabetes was recognized soon after the original description and much later attention was drawn to the long natural history which led to only minimal diabetic complications.

In this form MODY was readily recognizable in a few families in most diabetic clinics but two failings of human nature have led to subsequent clouding of the syndrome.

The first is the desire to attach a diagnostic label to a patient. There is little doubt in the minds of most diabetologists that both insulin-dependent and non-insulin-dependent diabetes can present in atypical ways. This is especially true if one goes looking for diabetes, as is done in familial studies. I have no doubt that many studies reporting patients with MODY are simply recording the early diagnosis of non-insulin-dependent diabetes. Prevalence rates for MODY of around 5% of non-insulin-dependent diabetes have been reported from Germany and India, while the figure rises to 10% of black Americans and South African Indians, and 18.5% of Indians around Madras (Fajans, 1990).

Secondly, with the urge to redefine and classify, confusion has arisen with the change in oral glucose load in an oral glucose tolerance test – up from 50 g in many countries, down from 100 g in the USA, and the revision of the diagnostic criteria of an oral glucose tolerance test (WHO, 1985). With this latter point goes the introduction of the new category of impaired glucose tolerance. Many patients described as having MODY require a glucose tolerance test for diagnosis, and classification as diabetic by old criteria may not find support in the new criteria. These confounding factors bias the natural history of the syndrome. Thus, if the group which is followed includes substantial numbers with impaired glucose tolerance we might conclude that few patients develop specific diabetic complications. On the other hand, if our group contains substantial numbers who are truly non-insulin-dependent diabetics diagnosed early, then prolonged follow-up might lead to the conclusion that these MODY patents are as prone to diabetic complications as their fellow non-insulin-dependent diabetics! At present, with such an ill-defined phenotype I can see no way of resolving these problems without a specific genetic marker for the syndrome.

Autosomal dominant inheritance, while a possible marker, is rarely of help without sufficient relatives available for study. HLA antigens, mutant insulins and linkage with the insulin gene, insulin receptor gene, and erythrocyte HepG2 glucose transporter locus have not clarified the situation nor has the chlorpropamide alcohol flush phenomenon. More recently Froguel *et al.* (1992) and Hattersley *et al.* (1992) have reported an association between MODY and mutations of the glucokinase gene. It is clear however that when a glucokinase mutation is present genetic heterogeneity exists and that not all families labelled MODY have glucokinase mutations. Vaxillaire *et al.* (1994) have sought, without success, linkage of MODY with other markers such as fatty-acid-binding protein 2, glucagon-like peptide-1 receptor and phosphoenolpyruvate carboxykinase.

These statements, of course, demand the qualification that they are based upon studies in correctly identified MODY patients. Young age at onset of non-insulin-dependent diabetes is clearly insufficient and is only strengthened slightly by adding a strong family history.

This leaves us in the difficult position of wondering whether there is a true syndrome of MODY. My feeling is that it does indeed exist but I would be in favour of diagnosing it only if:

- there was a strong family history; **and**
- the biochemical disorder was mild, probably requiring a glucose tolerance test for diagnosis at least in some members of the family (a severe biochemical abnormality would preclude the diagnosis); **and**
- normoglycaemia was obtainable by diet only or by a small dose of a sulphonylurea.

Patients who do not fulfil these criteria may be regarded as 'pending a diagnostic label' until the future course of their disease clarifies the category.

LIPOATROPHIC DIABETES

Lawrence (1946) is credited with the first detailed description of lipoatrophic diabetes, although earlier cases were reported. The features are total absence of all normal fat depots, diabetes with insulin resistance, hepatomegaly with increased fat storage progressing to fibrosis and cirrhosis, hyperlipidaemia with eruptive xanthomata, and a raised metabolic rate (Table 3.4).

The clinical appearance is striking and has been described as cadaveric. The total absence of subcutaneous fat highlights the anatomy of muscles and veins, giving an appearance of muscular hypertrophy. Biochemically, hyperglycaemia is rarely accompanied by mild ketonaemia and never by ketoacidosis. Massive insulin resistance is documented: Law-

Table 3.4 Features of lipoatrophic diabetes

1. Total lipoatrophy involving all normal fat depots
2. Hepatomegaly with increased lipid storage and progressive fibrosis
3. Diabetes with insulin resistance but no tendency to ketosis on insulin withdrawal
4. Raised basal metabolic rate without hyperthyroidism
5. Hyperlipidaemia with cutaneous xanthoma

rence's patient required more than 2000 units per day. Portal cirrhosis has been reported from autopsies. The hyperlipaemia is mainly due to triglyceride elevation, occasionally cholesterol also, and may be found in relatives. Some patients have received antithyroid treatment because of the raised metabolic rate but there is no evidence of thyrotoxicosis and the response to thyroidectomy has been that of a normal patient.

It is unclear whether two forms of the syndrome exist – congenital and acquired. Clearly, a congenital form occurs, from the many reports in which parental consanguinity and familial occurrence are common. These children also manifest growth disorders, with prepubertal acceleration that tapers off at puberty. Other patients present in later life, although rarely after the age of 30 when onset of lipoatrophy may precede or be simultaneous with onset of diabetes. These cases tend not to be familial.

Partial lipoatrophy

In some patients the lipoatrophy is partial, affecting mainly the face and trunk or even specific areas of the upper body. Onset may follow a severe infection and associated immune disease may be present.

Leprechaunism

It is likely that leprechaunism is a severe form of lipoatrophic diabetes. The absence of subcutaneous fat combined with lanugo hair on the face, low-set ears, wide eyes and thick hair give the appearance of the leprechaun of Irish mythology. Whereas the leprechaun is a benign elf, the disease is far from benign. Insulin resistance of the postbinding type is readily apparent.

MENDENHALL SYNDROME

Mendenhall (1950) described a syndrome of short stature with pineal hyperplasia, phallic enlargement, facial dysmorphism, premature dentition and acanthosis nigricans. Insulin-resistant diabetes presents in the first decade and death in ketoacidosis in the second decade. Doses of insulin of thousands of units are without effect and hypophysectomy has been tried with scant success, while some patients show a partial response to IGF-1.

GENETIC SYNDROMES AND DIABETES

Since diabetes is a relatively common disease it has been associated with many genetic syndromes. It is commoner than would be anticipated in Down's syndrome, Turner's syndrome and Klinefelter's syndrome.

Diabetes accompanying Down's syndrome may require insulin or may be controlled with oral agents or diet. When associated with primary hypothyroidism the diabetes tends to be insulin-dependent. In Turner's syndrome 60% of young adults have diabetes, which is usually non-insulin-dependent. Diabetes is less common in Klinefelter's syndrome, when abnormal insulin binding to the receptor has been observed.

Other syndromes associated with diabetes include: the Prader–Willi syndrome of hypotonia, obesity, mental retardation and hypogonadotrophic hypogonadism; the Lawrence–Moon–Biedl syndrome of mental retardation, hypogonadotrophic hypogonadism, retinitis pigmentosa and digital abnormalities; and Alstrom's syndrome of obesity, retinitis pigmentosa and deafness. All three of these syndromes are generally associated with non-insulin-dependent diabetes.

Occasional patients with these syndromes are seen in the diabetic clinic but the reader is more likely to encounter the association with neurological disease in the form of dystrophia myotonica, Huntingdon's chorea or Friedreich's ataxia. In the first two the diabetes is usually non-insulin-dependent while Friedreich's ataxia may be associated with insulin-dependent diabetes.

Table 3.5 Syndromes of insulin resistance and acanthosis nigricans

Type	Abnormality	Sex/age	Cardinal features	Associated features
Type A	Abnormal insulin receptor – genetic	Female 10–30 years	Glucose intolerance Insulin resistance Acanthosis nigricans Virilization	Ovarian dysfunction Polycystic ovaries Accelerated growth Acral hypertrophy Muscle cramps
Type B	Anti-insulin-receptor antibodies	Female:male 2:1 30–50 years	Glucose intolerance Insulin resistance Acanthosis nigricans Virilization	Polycystic ovaries Systemic lupus erythematosus Sjögren's syndrome
Type C	Postreceptor abnormality	Female 10–30 years	As Type A	As Type A
Rabson–Mendenhall syndrome	Postreceptor abnormality	Female < 20 years	Glucose intolerance (severe) Acanthosis nigricans Virilization	Pineal hyperplasia Dystrophic nails and teeth
Ataxia–telangiectasia	Anti-insulin-receptor antibodies	< 20 years	Glucose intolerance Insulin resistance Cerebellar ataxia Widespread telangiectasia Acanthosis nigricans	Thymic dysplasia Immune deficiencies

SYNDROMES OF PSEUDO-INSULIN RESISTANCE

Insulin is measured by radioimmunoassay and the assay is only as good as the antibody. Even antibodies with good specificity may show cross reaction with C-peptide or, more commonly, proinsulin. Apparent insulin resistance can then be found when euglycaemia or hyperglycaemia are accompanied by high concentrations of RIA-insulin. Recently it has become clear that proinsulin is measured in the majority of radioimmunoassays for insulin.

In familial hyperproinsulinaemia the cause of the massive rise in RIA insulin is proinsulin. A number of mutant human insulins are also described. In both conditions the response of blood glucose to exogenous insulin is normal. Individuals who secrete a mutant insulin also produce human insulin and have been found to be heterozygotes. Differences in clearance of the two insulins, however, lead to a greater relative proportion of the mutant insulin in the circulation. Glucose intolerance or diabetes is not an invariable accompaniment and it is perhaps surprising that it occurs at all, with 50% of the secreted insulin being normal human. Peripheral insulin resistance has been invoked to explain the development of hyperglycaemia but the answer may lie in differences in receptor affinity with blocking by mutant insulin. As would be expected, the mutant insulins sequenced all have replacement of an amino acid at or near the active site of insulin. The two phenylalanines at B24 (Insulin Los Angeles) and B25 (Insulin Chicago) are typical in this respect although the mutant insulin A3 (Insulin Wakayama) is less typical. The active site feature of the two insulins may be misleading since it is clear that the properties of insulin may be modified dramatically by substitutions elsewhere in the molecule.

SYNDROMES OF INSULIN RESISTANCE AND ACANTHOSIS NIGRICANS (TABLE 3.5)

A number of syndromes in which insulin resistance is associated with acanthosis nigricans have been reported. Type A is mainly a syndrome of females in which the features are diabetes or glucose intolerance, severe insulin resistance, acanthosis nigricans and excessive androgen secretion. There is a variable degree of virilization, with polycystic ovaries, amenorrhoea and moderate elevations in testosterone levels. Age of onset is usually younger than 30 years.

The insulin resistance is impressive, with little effect of doses of insulin in excess of 1000 or even 10 000 units, and lies at the receptor level. Abnormal insulin binding to its receptor or defective autophosphorylation have been demonstrated which are not associated with circulating antibodies. Although some mutations of the insulin receptor have been found these do not explain the majority of patients or families with the condition (Moller *et al.*, 1994).

The type B syndrome has an onset after the age of 30 and is associated with other immunological disease. Antinuclear and anti-DNA antibodies may be present, associated with clinical features of systemic lupus erythematosus. The majority of patients (80%) have acanthosis nigricans and all have IgG antibodies directed at the insulin receptor. Occasional variants of both syndromes have been reported. Where the type A syndrome has normal receptors and a postbinding defect the phrase 'Type C' has been coined.

The Rabson–Mendenhall syndrome includes pineal hyperplasia and nail and teeth dystrophia with the type A syndrome.

REFERENCES

Barron, M. (1920) The relation of the islets of Langerhans to diabetes with special reference to cases of pancreatic lithiasis. *Surg. Gynec. Obstet.*, **31**, 437–448.

Bundey, S., Poulton, K., Whitwell, H. *et al.* (1992)

Mitochondrial abnormalities in the DIDMOAD syndrome. *J. Inher. Metabol. Dis.*, **15**, 315–319.

Carlsen, J. E., Kober, L., Torp-Pedersen, C. and Johansen, P. (1990) Relation between dose of bendrofluazide, antihypertensive effect and adverse biochemical effects. *Br. Med. J.*, **300**, 975–978.

Cawley, T. (1788) A singular case of diabetes, consisting entirely in the quality of the urine; with an enquiry into the different theories of that disease. *Lond. Med. J.*, **9**, 296–308.

Christensen, S. E. (1986) Somatostatinoma, in *Recent Advances in Diabetes 2*, (ed. M. Nattrass), Churchill Livingstone, Edinburgh, p. 61–70.

Conn, J. W. and Louis, L. H. (1956) Primary aldosteronism, a new clinical entity. *Ann. Intern. Med.*, **44**, 1–15.

Cutler, P. (1989) Deferoxamine therapy in high-ferritin diabetes. *Diabetes*, **38**, 1207–1210.

De Lawter, D. E. (1949) *Med. Ann. DC*, **18**, 198.

Dollery, C. T., Pentecost, B. L. and Samaan, N. A. (1962) Drug-induced diabetes. *Lancet*, **ii**, 735–737.

Fajans, S. S. (1990) Scope and heterogeneous nature of MODY. *Diabetes Care*, **13**, 49–64.

Fajans, S. S. and Conn, J. W. (1960) Tolbutamide-induced improvement in carbohydrate tolerance of young people with mild diabetes. *Diabetes*, **9**, 83–88.

Feldman, J. M., Plonk, J. W., Bivens, C. H. and Lebovitz, H. E. (1975) Glucose intolerance in the carcinoid syndrome. *Diabetes*, **24**, 664–671.

Froguel, P., Vaxillaire, M., Sun, F. *et al.* (1992) Close linkage of glucokinase locus on chromosome 7p to early-onset non-insulin-dependent diabetes mellitus. *Nature*, **356**, 162–164.

Gerich, J. E., Lorenzi, M., Bier, D. M. *et al.* (1976) Effects of physiologic levels of glucagon and growth hormone on human carbohydrate and lipid metabolism. *J. Clin. Invest.*, **57**, 875–884.

Goldner, M. G., Zarowitz, H. and Akgun, S. (1960) Hyperglycemia and glycosuria due to thiazide derivatives administered in diabetes mellitus. *N. Engl. J. Med.*, **262**, 403–405.

Graham, J. B. (1951) Pheochromocytoma and hypertension: an analysis of 207 cases. *Surg. Gynecol. Obstet.*, **92**(suppl), 105–121.

Hattersley, A. T., Turner, R. C., Permutt, M. A. *et al.* (1992) Linkage of type 2 diabetes to the glucokinase gene. *Lancet*, **339**, 1307–1310.

Hugh-Jones, P. (1955) Diabetes in Jamaica. *Lancet*, **ii**, 891–897.

Ikkos, D. G., Fraser, G. R., Matsouki-Gavra, E. and Petrochilos, M. (1970) Association of juvenile diabetes mellitus, primary optic atrophy, and perceptive hearing loss in three sibs, with additional idiopathic diabetes insipidus in one case. *Acta Endocrinol.*, **65**, 95–102.

James, O., Agnew, J. E. and Bouchier, I. A. D. (1974) Chronic pancreatitis in England: a changing picture? *Br. Med. J.*, **ii**, 34–38.

Johnston, D. G., Postle, A., Barnes, A. J. and Alberti, K. G. M. M. (1979) The role of cortisol in direction of substrate flow, in *Lipoprotein Metabolism and Endocrine Regulation*, (eds L. Hessel and H. M. J. Krans), Elsevier, Brussels, p. 117–134.

Johnston, D. G., Alberti, K. G. M. M., Nattrass, M. *et al.* (1980a) Hormonal and metabolic rhythms in Cushing's syndrome. *Metabolism*, **29**, 1046–1052.

Johnston, D. G., Alberti, K. G. M. M., Nattrass, M. *et al.* (1980b) Hyperinsulinaemia in hyperprolactinaemic women. *Clin. Endocrinol.*, **13**, 361–368.

Kambo, P. K., Hitman, G. A., Mohan, V. *et al.* (1985) The genetic predisposition to fibrocalculous pancreatic diabetes. *Diabetologia*, **32**, 45–51.

Kinnear, T. W. G. (1963) The pattern of diabetes mellitus in a Nigerian teaching hospital. *E. Afr. Med. J.*, **40**, 288–294.

Kloppel, G., Bommer, G., Commandeur, G. and Heitz, P. (1978) The endocrine pancreas in chronic pancreatitis. Immunocytochemical and ultrastructural studies. *Virchows Arch. Pathol. Anat.*, **377**, 157–174.

Krentz, A. J., Dousset, B., Mayer, D. *et al.* (1993) Metabolic effects of cyclosporin A and FK 506 in liver transplant patients. *Diabetes*, **42**, 1753–1759.

Lancereaux, E. (1877) Notes et reflections apropos de deux cas de diabete sucré avec alteration du pancreas. *Bull. Acad. Med. Paris*, **6**, 1215.

Lawrence, R. D. (1946) Lipodystrophy and hepatomegaly with diabetes lipaemia and other metabolic disturbances. *Lancet*, **i**, 724–731.

Lukens, F. D. W., Flippin, H. F. and Thigpen, F. M. (1937) Adrenal cortical adenoma with absence of the opposite adrenal. Report of a case with operation and autopsy. *Am. J. Med. Sci.*, **193**, 812–820.

Mallinson, C. N., Bloom, S. R., Warin, A. P. *et al.* (1974) A glucagonoma syndrome. *Lancet*, **ii**, 1–5.

McGavran, M. H., Unger, R. H., Recant, L. *et al.* (1966) A glucagon-secreting alpha-cell carcinoma of the pancreas. *N. Engl. J. Med.*, **274**, 1408–1413.

Medical Research Council Working Party (1981)

Adverse reactions to bendrofluazide and propanalol for the treatment of mild hypertension. *Lancet*, **ii**, 539–543.

Mendenhall, E. N. (1950) Tumor of the pineal body with high insulin resistance. *J. Indiana Med. Assoc.*, **43**, 32–36.

Mohan, V., Mohan, R., Susheela, L. *et al.* (1985) Tropical pancreatic diabetes in South India: heterogeneity in clinical and biochemical profile. *Diabetologia*, **28**, 229–232.

Moller, D. E., Cohen, O., Yamaguchi, Y. *et al.* (1994) Prevalence of mutations in the insulin receptor gene in subjects with features of the Type A syndrome of insulin resistance. *Diabetes*, **43**, 247–255.

Murphy, R. and Smith, F. G. (1963) Abnormal carbohydrate metabolism in pancreatic carcinoma. *Med. Clin. N. Am.*, **47**, 397–405.

O'Brien, T., Barrett, B., Murray, D. M. *et al.* (1990) Usefulness of biochemical screening of diabetic patients for hemochromatosis. *Diabetes Care*, **13**, 532–534.

Ouweland, J. M. W. van den, Lemkes, H. H. P. J., Ruitenbeek, W. *et al.* (1992) Mutation in mitochondrial tRNA$^{LEU (UUR)}$ gene in a large pedigree with maternally transmitted type II diabetes mellitus and deafness. *Nature Genet.*, **1**, 368–371.

Page, M. McB., Asmal, A. C. and Edwards, C. R. W. (1975) Recessive inheritance of diabetes: the syndrome of diabetes insipidus, diabetes mellitus, optic atrophy and deafness. *Q. J. Med.*, **45**, 505–520.

Plotz, C. M., Knowlton, A. I. and Ragan, C. (1952) The natural history of Cushing's syndrome. *Am. J. Med.*, **13**, 597–614.

Schade, D. S., Eaton, R. P. and Standefer, J. (1977) Glucocorticoid regulation of plasma ketone body concentration in insulin-deficient man. *J. Clin. Endocrinol. Metab.*, **44**, 1069–1079.

Schade, D. S., Eaton, R. P. and Peake G. T. (1978) The regulation of plasma ketone body concentration by counter-regulatory hormones in man. II Effects of growth hormone in diabetic man. *Diabetes*, **27**, 916–924.

Shaw, D. A. and Duncan, L. J. P. (1958) Optic atrophy and nerve deafness in diabetes mellitus. *J. Neurol. Neurosurg. Psychiat.*, **21**, 47–49.

Sheldon, J. H. (1935) *Haemochromatosis*, Oxford University Press, Oxford.

Singh, B. M., Grunewald, R. A., Press, M. *et al.* (1992) Prevalence of haemochromatosis amongst patients with diabetes mellitus. *Diabetic Med.*, **9**, 730–731.

Suzuki, S., Hinokio, Y., Hirai, S. *et al.* (1994) Pancreatic beta-cell secretory defect associated with mitochondrial point mutation of the tRNA$^{LEU(UUR)}$ gene: a study in seven families with mitochondrial encephalopathy, lactic acidosis and stroke-like episodes (MELAS). *Diabetologia*, **37**, 818–825.

Trapnell, J. E. (1980) Patterns of pancreatitis in Great Britain – with special reference to diabetes, in *Secondary Diabetes: The Spectrum of the Diabetic Syndromes*, (eds S. Podolsky and M. Vishwanathan), Raven Press, New York, p. 77–88.

Tulloch, J. A. and MacIntosh, D. (1961) 'J'-type diabetes. *Lancet*, **ii**, 119–121.

Vaxillaire, M., Vionnet, N., Vigouroux, C. *et al.* (1994) Search for a third susceptibility gene for maturity-onset diabetes of the young. *Diabetes*, **43**, 389–395.

Warren, S. and LeCompte, P. M. (1952) *The Pathology of Diabetes Mellitus*, 3rd edn, Lea & Febiger, Philadelphia, PA.

Wolfram, D. J. and Wagener (1938) Diabetes mellitus and simple optic atrophy among siblings: report of four cases. *Proc. Mayo Clin.*, **13**, 715–718.

WHO (1985) Diabetes mellitus. Report of a WHO Study Group, *Technical Report Series 727*, World Health Organization, Geneva.

Wright, A. D., Barber, S. G., Kendall, M. J. and Poole, P. H. (1979) Beta-adrenoceptor-blocking drugs and blood sugar control in diabetes mellitus. *Br. Med. J.*, **i**, 159–161.

Yajnik, C. S., Shelgikar, K. M., Naik, S. S. *et al.* (1992) The ketosis-resistance in fibro-calculous-pancreatic diabetes. *Diab. Res. Clin. Pract.*, **15**, 149–156.

Zuidema, P. J. (1955) Calcification and cirrhosis of the pancreas in patients with deficient nutrition. *Accum. Med. Geogr. Trop.*, **7**, 229–251.

THE HISTORY

The history of diabetic symptoms is of the greatest importance and an accurate appreciation of their severity far exceeds an estimation of the blood glucose as a means of assessing the need for treatment. Having said this I must admit that it is far from easy. Abnormal thirst and fatigue are not always recognized and intelligent patients may deny them although their relatives give a convincing account of their onset and degree. Moreover, the consultant is usually presented with a patient in whom glycosuria has already been found and who is ready to admit symptoms which may have been discussed for some days before the visit.

The urgency of the symptoms in the worst cases is obvious enough. Generally speaking an acute onset of thirst and polyuria indicates severe diabetes likely to need insulin. Sometimes this onset can be defined to within a few hours but in my experience such a catastrophe is rarely related to any shock or trauma. Much more frequent is a story of gradual weight loss and perhaps occasional pruritus vulvae over a period of many months, culminating in the subacute onset of thirst and polyuria.

SYMPTOMS

Analysis of the presenting symptoms was made by Beaser (1948) but this was based on an examination of case records not intended for the purpose. Table 4.1 shows the presenting complaint in 547 consecutive patients some years ago. There is no reason to think that in recent years these have been modified.

Those who were diagnosed on admission to hospital are excluded. It is, in many in-

Table 4.1 Presenting symptoms in 547 consecutive patients with diabetes (% in brackets)

Age	0–39	40–59	60+
Males/females	28/27	98/108	100/186
Thirst	34 (62)	46 (22)	61 (22)
Wasting	8 (14)	19 (9)	14 (5)
Fatigue	2 (4)	18 (9)	22 (8)
Pruritus vulvae	–/5 (20)	–/41 (38)	–/57 (31)
Balanitis	0/–	2 (2)/–	6 (6)/–
Sepsis	1 (2)	14 (7)	19 (6)
Visual	0	12 (6)	29 (10)
Other	0	9 (4)	16 (5)
None	5 (9)	45 (22)	62 (22)

stances, very difficult to decide what symptom was decisive in causing the patient to seek advice. Pruritus vulvae is the most definite presentation of all and fatigue the least. Under the category 'no symptoms' are included those who were picked up at routine examinations, and a certain number with lesions that were not sufficiently frequent to be analysed separately are grouped under 'other'.

THIRST AND POLYURIA

This, the classical presentation of diabetes, is always a prominent feature of severe diabetes and the fluid intake may be as high as 15 pints or 9 litres a day. Occasionally, the thirst is of such intensity that the patient must have a drink while sitting in the clinic waiting area. It may reasonably be attributed to loss of water from osmotic diuresis. The ability of the renal tubules to reabsorb glucose is exceeded when the blood glucose rises and the glucose, of necessity, takes with it an excess of water in the urine. Polyuria begets thirst, and not the converse, as nearly every patient believes.

Clinically the situation is not clear-cut. For one thing there is a wide variation in the normal habit of drinking. Those who normally drink little and do not pass much urine are easily impressed by moderate polyuria, while those who are accustomed to a large intake and may have a big bladder capacity are slow to notice an increased volume. It is certainly striking that some patients with constant hyperglycaemia (above 15 mmol/l; 270 mg/dl) deny thirst and have no obvious excess of fluid intake. In general, however, quantitative studies show that the amount of fluid consumed and excreted is related to the weight of glucose lost in the urine. Patients with thirst, even those with severe diabetes and mild ketonuria, may be relieved at once by drastic restriction of carbohydrate in the diet. In the insulin-dependent patient this effect is short-lived.

There is evidently some variation in the response of the body to hyperglycaemia for there are patients who notice polyuria and dryness of the mouth within an hour of a moderate rise in blood glucose such as follows a meal. Others may sustain an equivalent or greater rise without any subjective symptoms. In insulin withdrawal experiments a rise in blood glucose of 10 mmol/l (180 mg/dl) may not provoke thirst. The onset of thirst seems to bear greater relation to a decline in body weight from dehydration (Milles, Baylis and Wright, 1981). It is not apparent whether this difference is determined by renal factors or others concerned with urinary excretion such as vasopressin.

EXCESSIVE APPETITE AND POLYPHAGIA

Polyphagia is mentioned in most accounts of the leading symptoms of diabetes but in my experience it is uncommon even on direct questioning. The appetite is usually normal, sometimes impaired when thirst is urgent. Rare also is a craving for sweet things.

Excessive hunger could be explained as a result of the inability of the tissues to use glucose and the loss of fuel in the urine, an explanation which reveals much of our ignorance of appetite regulation.

LOSS OF WEIGHT

Loss of weight in the diabetic may be attributed to the mobilization of fat stores and breakdown of protein. In addition, there may be considerable calorie loss in the urine, often exceeding 100 g of glucose in a day.

As a manifestation, if not a symptom, of diabetes, wasting would seem to be the most common. That may be because observation of weight is rather more objective than that of other symptoms and a number of our patients have kept records of their weight for over 20 years when they first attended the clinic. Table 4.1 indicates that loss of weight is not prominent as a presenting symptom. In the young it is overshadowed by thirst and in middle age it is welcomed by those who have been trying in vain to reduce by dieting. These middle-aged patients often recall a grossly excessive weight 5–10 years before the diagnosis which has gradually declined without any attempt to eat less. Whether this period represents the initial stage of diabetes is uncertain.

FATIGUE

Tiredness, a weariness of the flesh, is not easy to identify in the diabetic history. It is often rejected as a symptom by the patient, who attributes it to advancing age, worry or overwork, all of which appear to be equally inevitable in the British population. A tendency to drop off to sleep too easily is common and especially noticeable when watching television. Fatigue is probably a common manifestation in all but the mildest diabetes, but does seem to be absent in some patients with severe diabetes, perhaps those who replace their losses of fuel and fluid by hearty eating and drinking. Inefficient utilization of glucose or electrolyte losses could explain the muscular weakness which is the basis of fatigue.

PRURITUS VULVAE

Although properly a complication, pruritus vulvae is so commonly a feature in the history of diabetes that it wins a place as a leading symptom. Table 4.1 shows that it was the presenting complaint in 103 out of 321 women and it was mentioned by a further 106 when they were questioned directly so that it is a symptom in two-thirds of all women who develop diabetes. Though predominantly a complaint of the stout and middle-aged it is not rare in girls and young women with diabetes.

In the great majority diabetic pruritus is associated with definite and visible vulvitis, so that a normal appearance of the vulva in a diabetic woman with pruritus leads one to seek for other causes for the itching. The vulvitis is most obvious on the labia, which are reddened and swollen, while there is often an extension to the skin of the thighs, perineum and perianal areas. Vaginal discharge is not a feature. Older writers attributed the vulvitis to fungal growth in the saccharine urine but the discovery that *Monilia* was often found on the vulva in patients who seemed normal led to the belief that some other mechanism was responsible, perhaps merely the irritant effect of glucose in the urine. Hesseltine and Campbell (1938) showed that glucose as powder or solution applied to the normal vulva produced no symptoms and were convinced that diabetic vulvitis is a mycosis and rarely, if ever, an irritation from products in the urine. They considered that glucose favours the development of the mycosis and that glycosuria is the underlying cause. Clinically, glycosuria is always abundant in diabetic vulvitis and the lesion clears rapidly when the urine is rendered sugar-free, so that local treatment is seldom required. If the symptoms are not relieved in this way it is necessary to look for other lesions such as *Trichomonas* infection.

BALANITIS

Inflammation and pruritus of the prepuce and glans penis, though relatively uncommon compared with vulvitis in women, is evidently more frequent than many doctors realize, to judge from the number of men who are referred to a surgeon for circumcision or to a venereologist without the urine being tested. It is usually the leading symptom, but others are elicited on questioning. Circumcised men are very rarely affected. Phimosis, with considerable swelling of the prepuce, maintains infection which is often monilial, and reddening round the urethral orifice is characteristic. Glycosuria is always abundant and when it is abolished the balanitis quickly resolves. Obviously it is necessary, but not always easy, to stay the hand of the surgeon who wishes to carry out circumcision, which may prove unnecessary in the end.

OTHER SYMPTOMS OF DIABETES

Abnormalities of taste

A sweet taste in the mouth is an uncommon symptom of untreated diabetes. More often a sensation of 'stickiness' with no precise taste is described. This may be experienced by insulin-treated patients as soon as the blood glucose rises to abnormal levels and is a useful warning to them that all is not well. Diabetics are said to show a slight but significant rise of the taste threshold for dextrose (Schelling *et al.*, 1965), correlated with the blood glucose level (Le Floch *et al.*, 1989).

White marks on clothing

A white crystalline deposit on trousers and shoes from splashes of urine is commonly noticed by men and may be the presenting symptom. It is relatively common and indicates glycosuria of such a degree that it can be regarded as pathognomonic of diabetes as distinct from other causes of glycosuria. It is associated with heavy glycosuria and is interesting because some of the men who report it have noticed the deposit for years before the diagnosis, a point in support of the belief that diabetes may exist for a long time in a symptomless form.

One of our patients from the Black Country near Birmingham saw white marks on his shoes and knew what this meant. He put himself on a diet without consulting a doctor and controlled his treatment by an ingenious method. He kept an old shoe on to which he passed urine and then allowed it to dry in the back-yard. If a white deposit appeared he intensified the diet, if not he was encouraged to eat a little more.

The symptom is not quite unknown in women, for those who have a little stress incontinence occasionally report that their underclothes are stiff.

The report of an unusual deposit in the chamber-pot is still mentioned but rarely now that this diagnostically useful article is falling into desuetude.

Visual symptoms

A change in refraction, usually in the direction of myopia, may outweigh other complaints at the time of diagnosis and is an indication of significant diabetes. More commonly the onset is delayed until after treatment has been started. Lens opacities, if truly diabetic rather than senile cataract, are a feature of severe diabetes which will need insulin treatment.

Impotence

Impotence may be an early manifestation and is usually attributed to neuropathy. The diabetes may be comparatively mild, in which case the outlook for improvement is poor. When the classical symptoms are urgent the impotence may be part of a general loss of strength and may disappear when they are abolished.

Amenorrhoea

Amenorrhoea may occur in severe diabetes but is overshadowed by other symptoms. It may recur in phases of poor insulin control and is three times commoner in the diabetic woman compared with non-diabetic women (Kjaer *et al.*, 1992).

Infections

Infections, especially in the skin, or the failure of wounds to heal may be the first indication of the presence of diabetes. The association is now well known and urine tests are commonly carried out in such cases. If a glucose tolerance test then shows a very slight abnormality its relation to the infection is doubtful. Probably, infection related to diabetes is a manifestation of definite and persistent hyperglycaemia.

PHYSICAL SIGNS

There are no characteristic features in the examination of the untreated diabetic. The picture of really severe diabetes, most often seen in the young, is unlike that of other wasting diseases. The severe wasting is accompanied by obvious signs of considerable dehydration. In such patients acetone can usually be detected on the breath.

Sometimes complications are present at the time of the initial examination. The most important and valuable from the point of view of diagnosis is retinopathy, which is found in about 10% of our newly discovered patients. The physical examination at diagnosis may reveal abnormality in the nervous system; vibration sense may be impaired or ankle jerks may be absent. Undoubtedly, a transient or temporary impairment of nerve conduction can occur in the presence of prolonged hyperglycaemia and the finding may not indicate a true diabetic peripheral neuropathy. Only the course after treatment of the hyperglycaemia clarifies the issue.

METHODS OF PRESENTATION

From our experience over the years we have gained some indication of the manner in which diabetes is discovered in the population. Table 4.2 shows the reason for testing the urine and hence reference to the diabetic clinic in 1678 consecutive newly diagnosed patients. The importance of testing the urine of any patient whose symptoms do not suggest diabetes is underlined by the large number of people with confirmed diabetes in this category and it will be seen that routine examinations contribute a significant proportion of the confirmed cases.

Table 4.3 indicates who first suspected diabetes and tested the urine in 3176 consecutive patients with proven diabetes seen at our clinic. There is no indication that the relative distribution of the various categories has changed significantly since these data were collected.

The general practitioner, in the UK, is still the most likely person to suspect the diagnosis.

The patients with glycosuria discovered in general hospitals were mostly found by routine testing of the urine during an un-

Table 4.2 Reason for testing urine (1678 consecutive patients)

	Diabetes confirmed	Diabetes not confirmed
Diabetic symptoms	774	85
Routine with symptoms (not diabetic)	363	194
Routine without symptoms	99	163
Total	1236	442

Table 4.3 Suspicion of diabetes (testing for glycosuria) in 3176 confirmed cases (% in brackets)

General practitioner	2070 (65.2)
General hospitals	508 (16.0)
Eye hospitals (including opticians)	165 (5.2)
Women's hospitals	73 (2.3)
Maternity hospitals	35 (1.1)
Employer's medical department	109 (3.4)
Regional medical officer	42 (1.3)
Insurance examination	50 (1.6)
Patient or relative	77 (2.4)
Miscellaneous	47 (1.5)
Total	3176 (100)

related illness, but persistent infection makes an important contribution to this group.

The majority of referrals from eye hospitals were patients with senile cataract, but retinopathy was not uncommon and a few attended because of a change in refraction.

It is still common for patients to be referred to a women's hospital with pruritus vulvae without the urine being tested and this is the main reason for the comparatively large number in this category.

Employer's medical examinations are comparatively frequent now that large firms have a medical department. Routine tests are carried out on entry to the firm's payroll and when employees report sick at the works surgery.

The Regional Medical Officer examines a sample of patients who have claimed sickness benefit for more than 2–3 weeks and it is not surprising that his routine urine examination sometimes discloses diabetes. These patients are referred back to the general practitioner, who commonly confirms the finding of glycosuria and sends them to the diabetic clinic. The figure given here may be an understatement, although efforts were made to elicit tactfully from each patient the manner in which glycosuria was first found.

Insurance examinations contribute fewer cases than might be expected. There may be a significant deficiency here, because a medical examination for the purposes of a life insurance proposal is not always performed unless the sum involved exceeds a certain figure. Thus higher income groups, perhaps more likely to be private patients, will probably make up much of the population to be examined.

Urine testing by patients or their relatives may be expected to increase as public knowledge of diabetes and its symptoms is extended and as rapid blood glucose measurement finds its way into chemists' shops, hospital open days and charity fetes (Singh *et al.*, 1994).

THE CLINICAL DIAGNOSIS OF DIABETES

The evidence for the diagnosis of diabetes in 1871 consecutive patients is shown in Table 4.4. It appears that a clinical diagnosis can be made with the help of a single blood glucose estimation in the great majority of patients. It is, in fact, virtually unknown in our clinic for such a diagnosis to need revision, always provided that diagnostic criteria are kept constant. Occasionally a doubt arises because the blood glucose is found to be repeatedly normal after the first attendance, but a glucose tolerance test then confirms the original diagnosis. The only non-diabetic patients attending the diabetic clinic are the few in whom the diagnosis was based on stricter criteria that preceded current diagnostic levels.

Great care is needed in the use of a single blood glucose. A careful and dispassionate history usually enables one to make a provisional diagnosis and the blood glucose, preferably taken after a substantial meal, is related to it. A specimen of urine at the same time is a useful check and any gross discrep-

ancy between the findings in blood and urine calls for repetition of the tests.

TYPES OF CLINICAL DIABETES

There have been many attempts to classify diabetic patients by their age, physique, response to insulin or the supposed site of the lesion responsible for their diabetes. Anyone looking at the serried ranks of a diabetic clinic would quickly perceive a predominance of elderly overweight patients, indeed the distinction of *diabete gras* from *diabete maigre* was made over a century ago by Bouchardat (1875) and others. As the stout patients are usually middle-aged at the time of diagnosis they were often said to have 'maturity-onset diabetes' while those who are thin and need insulin at diagnosis are usually young so that this type of diabetes was called 'juvenile'. Recognition that some elderly patients need insulin at diagnosis and a few youngsters do not has led to replacement of this imperfect classification. In the newer imperfect classification juvenile diabetes is termed 'insulin-dependent' and maturity-onset diabetes is renamed 'non-insulin-dependent' diabetes.

Divisions of diabetes by clinical type are convenient but it must be recognized that there are exceptions which are by no means rare. Mild diabetes occurs in children, although with the exception of the specific syndrome of maturity-onset diabetes of young people it is unlikely to remain mild. Diabetes over the age of 80 is more often severe than mild. It is necessary always to see diabetes as a dynamic process which can only be designated mild or severe at the time of the description. It is galling to see a letter one has written about a patient 10 years previously with the description of mild diabetes as the patient now comes with retinopathy and foot ulceration. In general the disease becomes more severe with the passage of time but the reverse process may occur. Mild diabetes may rather acutely deteriorate under stress.

Table 4.4 Evidence for the diagnosis of diabetes in 1871 patients (% in brackets)

Raised blood glucose	1666	(89.0)
Abnormal glucose tolerance test	197	(10.5)
Ketosis	8	(0.4)

This is an important point. It is all too common to find that a patient has been pigeon-holed as having slight diabetes so that the possibility of it becoming very significant is forgotten when some other acute illness arises. I have seen elderly patients suffer needlessly from diabetic symptoms because it had been decided that their diabetes must be mild in view of their age.

STARTING TREATMENT (TABLE 4.5)

It cannot be stressed too often that diabetes must be diagnosed before any treatment is instigated. Even in the age of rapid, simple blood glucose measurement patients are still seen where treatment was started after the finding of glycosuria. The diagnosis must be confirmed by blood glucose measurement. The ramifications of being labelled diabetic – for life insurance, driving, employment – are of such importance that surety of diagnosis is demanded.

The question then arises of what treatment should be started. To answer this a number of factors are taken into account, weighted, and a choice made.

Despite the withdrawal of the terms 'juvenile-onset' and 'maturity-onset' diabetes, age still figures near the top of this list. Relative youth increases the probability of insulin-dependence while middle-age to elderly points towards non-insulin-dependent diabetes.

The history is important but, far from one symptom pointing specifically to treatment, rather it is the acute nature of the symptoms

Table 4.5 Factors taken into account in the choice of treatment for a newly diagnosed diabetic patient

- Age
- Acute history
- Weight loss
- Ketonuria
- Family history
- Degree of obesity
- Potential for dietary modifications

that suggest a need for insulin. From the history it is weight loss which has most importance. Weight loss points towards a loss of protein stores and of fat in addition to the disordered glucose metabolism. It is clear that fat breakdown is prevented by insulin in a concentration which is an order of magnitude less than the concentration needed to facilitate glucose uptake into tissues. Thus loss of fat stores is likely to indicate a marked reduction in insulin secretion and hence insulin-dependence.

Ketonuria is a sequel to this. Ketone bodies are from fat breakdown and again suggest marked insulinopenia.

Where there is a family history of diabetes some attention may be paid to the type of diabetes in the sibling or parent, but this is of less importance.

Thus, an acute history including weight loss and with ketonuria present suggests a need for insulin treatment. Older patients, with no weight loss or ketonuria are likely to respond to diet.

The potential for dietary modification is always assessed either informally, i.e. by the degree of overweight or obesity of the patient, or more formally by a dietary history. Patients above their ideal body weight can have their diets modified to eat less. Where the patient is not overweight a dietary history can reveal the extent to which dietary modifications can or cannot be made.

These guidelines work well in practice but do not deal with 100% of newly diagnosed diabetics. Occasionally patients of 150% ideal body weight are seen to present with weight loss and ketonuria. Here choice of treatment may be difficult and we often adopt the policy that initial treatment with insulin is a safe option. After treatment with insulin for 2–3 months it is often clear whether diet and tablets or insulin is really needed. The guidelines are similarly inadequate in the thin elderly patient who has insulin-dependent diabetes and nowhere are their limitations more exposed than in the comparatively rare instance of maturity-onset diabetes in young people (MODY).

INITIAL TREATMENT WITH DIET

It is clear that some patients who do not require insulin can be treated solely by diet. This presupposes a willingness to attempt to follow a diet and a persistence in this approach when symptoms have been relieved and forgotten. Sadly, the doctor's hopes and expectations are not often matched by the patient's resolve. On the other hand it is possible to see a marked reduction in hyperglycaemia and glycosuria with the minimal of dietary modification. The avoidance of refined sugars where a high intake existed previously may often be sufficient in the normal-weight patient, while in the obese patient persuasion to eat less may be sufficient to produce a dramatic improvement.

In the obese patient improved control may precede a major change in body weight but when followed by a significant improvement in body weight the benefits may be apparent for years. It is often difficult to know, in this dietary controlled phase, when repeated blood glucose measurements are in the normal range and when the patient's weight may be 10–20% less than at presentation, whether diabetes is still present or whether normality has returned, albeit only temporarily. It is a brave man who argues for a return of complete normality to the patient. In our own clinic the only patients who show persistently normal blood glucoses for year after year have probably not got diabetes and were diagnosed before the advent of the revised diagnostic criteria. We have not felt brave enough to tell them that, after 15 years of 'diabetes' by older diagnostic criteria they are no longer diabetic, not through any efforts on their or their doctor's part, but by dint of a redefinition made by experts in the field.

INITIAL TREATMENT WITH TABLETS

Standard texts invariably advocate that where insulin is not thought necessary at diagnosis diet should always be tried as first-line treatment and oral agents only introduced when diet alone is inadequate. Physicians seeing large numbers of newly diagnosed diabetic patients do not follow this advice rigidly. The symptomatic underweight patient may be given diet and sulphonylurea together as immediate treatment, as may the normal-weight patient where initial inquiry reveals little prospect of substantial dietary modification. Clearly, however, the use of either a sulphonylurea or a biguanide as initial treatment in an overweight patient cannot be justified and merely indicates an inability to give adequate dietary advice.

SUBSEQUENT PROGRESSION

There is no doubt that some patients with diabetes progress slowly if at all. Patients in this category tend to escape from follow-up and it is difficult to estimate their number in relation to those who deteriorate. The latter are frequently forced on our attention when they return to the clinic with diabetic symptoms having defaulted for several years. There does seem to be a tendency for an initially slight biochemical abnormality to become worse, either gradually or in a stepwise fashion as a result of stresses or infections.

No doubt some patients, after the initial shock of learning that they are diabetic, diet carefully but later grow careless so that the diabetes seems to deteriorate. Others maintain control without difficulty until an infection, an accident or a pregnancy causes a return of glycosuria and hyperglycaemia, which may remit as the stress subsides but may initiate a new phase of more severe diabetes. Many a patient passes through the stages of successful diet, sulphonylurea, sulphonylurea with biguanide, and eventually insulin, the whole sequence taking 10 or more years. In the majority it often seems inevitable that deterioration will occur. When control worsens it is simple to blame a lack of dietary compliance, although the worsening of diabetes may play a role too often ignored by the physician. There appears an inevitable progression from diet to tablets to insulin. On the whole, and although it is far from proven, I am of the opinion that diabetes worsens with time.

INITIAL TREATMENT WITH INSULIN

It is impossible to forecast the response of a patient to insulin and the daily dose required to establish control varies from 10 to 100 or more units. Treatment is always initiated with a lower rather than a higher dose. Once control is achieved there is a tendency for the requirement to drop somewhat, even apart from the phenomenon of remission, and to settle at an average of 20–60 units daily. There follows a stable period in which good biochemical control can often be maintained throughout the day with rare hypoglycaemia. After about 18 months, and perhaps in relation to an infection, there is a sudden change for the worse and a stormy period with instability and increased insulin requirement leads to a phase of less satisfactory control, in which hypoglycaemia is difficult to avoid. The control of diabetes by insulin is affected by a number of intercurrent factors. Infection, trauma, immobilization, weight gain, pregnancy (usually) and unhappiness aggravate the diabetes. Physical exercise, weight loss and happiness make it better. Striking examples of the alternating effect of immobilization from depression and activity from hypomania can be seen in the insulin charts of our manic-depressive patients. The beneficial effect of exercise depends on an adequate supply of insulin and if this is lacking it may lead to an increase rather than a fall in blood glucose. Weight loss usually lowers the insulin dose significantly and this is notable in patients who waste from malignant disease. In the terminal stage of tuberculosis it was common for the insulin requirement to fall almost to zero. A similar change is the rule in advanced renal failure, but in this instance many factors are probably involved.

REFERENCES

Beaser, S. B. (1948) The clinical characteristics of early diabetes mellitus. *N. Engl. J. Med.*, **239**, 765–769.

Bouchardat, A. (1875) *De la glycosurie ou diabete sucré*, vol 2, Germer-Baillière, Paris.

Hesseltine, H. C. and Campbell, L. K. (1938) Diabetic or mycotic vulvovaginitis. *Am. J. Obstet. Gynecol.*, **35**, 272–283.

Kjaer, K., Hagen, C., Sando, S. H. and Eshoj, O. (1992) Epidemiology of menarche and menstrual disturbances in an unselected group of women with insulin-dependent diabetes mellitus compared to controls. *J. Clin. Endocrinol. Metab.*, **75**, 524–529.

Le Floch, J. P. Le Lievre, G. L., Sandoun, J. *et al.* (1989) Taste impairment and related factors in type 1 diabetes mellitus. *Diabetes Care*, **12**, 173–178.

Milles, J. J., Baylis, P. H. and Wright, A. D. (1981) Plasma vasopressin during insulin withdrawal in insulin-dependent diabetes. *Diabetologia*, **20**, 607–611.

Schelling, J. L., Tetreault, L., Lascagna, L. and Davis, M. (1965) Abnormal taste threshold in diabetes. *Lancet*, i, 508–512.

Singh, B. M., Prescott, J. J. W., Guy, R. *et al.* (1994) Effect of advertising on awareness of symptoms of diabetes among the general public: the British Diabetic Association study. *Br. Med. J.*, **308**, 632–636.

DEFINITION

Diabetes mellitus is usually defined as a chronic disorder of carbohydrate metabolism characterized by hyperglycaemia and glycosuria. A persistently raised blood glucose concentration can only be due to diabetes mellitus. A brief rise, not exceeding 1 hour, may occur as a response to carbohydrate feeding or during an oral glucose tolerance test to levels considered abnormal yet not denoting diabetes. This pattern has been called a lag storage curve, although the name is not entirely appropriate. Hyperglycaemia lasting several weeks sometimes follows trauma, burns or other acute stress. The condition has been called pseudo-diabetes because glucose tolerance later becomes normal. Again the title is not helpful since some patients may require insulin during the hyperglycaemic phase and the term pseudo-diabetes tempts the unwary into ignoring the metabolic abnormality. In addition the eventual outcome of such cases has proved difficult to record but there are many suggestions of an increased incidence of diabetes in later life in groups of such patients.

The mildest forms of diabetes, in which hyperglycaemia may be only occasional or even entirely absent, are defined by the glucose tolerance test. The distinction of normal from abnormal tests is made by reference to arbitrary standards of normality.

In recent years many of the diagnostic levels have been revised to take into account epidemiological evidence relating particularly to the development of microvascular complications. With the exception of certain well defined populations we do not know with certainty whether normal and abnormal may be distinguished by such criteria or whether there is a smooth gradation from the most normal to the most abnormal. Other fields of medicine have provided similar debate, for example hypertension. These debates, on blood pressure or blood glucose, are not without consequence since bimodality adds weight to the importance of genetic factors in aetiology while a smooth change from normal to abnormal lends support to the role of environmental factors in pathogenesis.

Perhaps too much time and energy is spent on the argument over trivial abnormalities of the glucose tolerance test. In the majority of patients with diabetes mellitus the diagnosis is clear-cut. Concentration upon the glucose tolerance test has misled many of our colleagues, relatively inexperienced in diabetes, into thinking that diabetes must be diagnosed in this way, thus wasting laboratory time and subjecting a patient to needless investigations. Nevertheless, without clear standards of normality and abnormality the definition of diabetes mellitus will inevitably lack precision.

In an attempt to improve on the definition some writers are prepared to add that hyperglycaemia and glycosuria depend on a deficiency of insulin, resulting from either insufficient supply or diminished effectiveness. This concept is supported by early work using simultaneous administration of glucose and insulin to diabetic patients (Himsworth, 1936; Himsworth and Kerr, 1939) and by a wealth of recent work utilizing a variety of techniques of investigation (Chapter 2).

The implication of insulin in defining diabetes mellitus adds further to our original definition in view of the wide-ranging effects upon metabolism. Thus we arrive at the position of Marble (1971) who defined diabetes as 'a chronic disorder of metabolism, not only carbohydrate but protein and fat'. These considerations are not superfluous to a definition of diabetes when faced with a child who is growing slowly or a diabetic with ketoacidosis.

Concentration upon a definition of diabetes mellitus based entirely upon metabolism must be incomplete. In addition to the biochemical disorder there is the development of a clinical syndrome. Microvascular disease, neuropathy, macrovascular disease and a wealth of other changes in, for example, platelets and lipids form as much a part of the disease of diabetes as do the more acute biochemical changes. In some of these the link between a chronic biochemical abnormality and the development of histological and clinical changes is becoming clear and has formed the basis for the long-running debate on diabetic control and the development of complications. In others, notably macrovascular disease, the link is more tenuous and until further evidence becomes available the clinical consequences should be included in any definition of diabetes mellitus.

The purist, therefore, will want included in any definition a chronic disorder of metabolism, particularly carbohydrate, protein and fat, and the development of a clinical syndrome of disease characterized by microangiopathy, neuropathy and macrovascular disease.

PREVALENCE

It is uncertain whether the prevalence of diabetes has fluctuated through the ages. Hippocrates makes no mention of it and the only convincing description in classical literature is that of Aretaeus the Cappodocian (second century AD). The often quoted Papyrus Ebers merely refers to polyuria while the *Ayur Veda* of Susruta, a Hindu manuscript of the sixth century AD may have been in great part a copy of Greek medicine transmitted through Arab sources (Saundby, 1891). It clearly describes the urine of diabetes as sweet and the disease is given the name *madhumeha*, or 'honey urine.' Weakness and thirst are mentioned as symptoms, carbuncles and phthisis as complications (Frank, 1957).

This knowledge persists in a Cingalese treatise of the 15th century, but no mention of it appears in European writings until two centuries later, when Thomas Willis (1621–1675) wrote of 'the diabetes or pissing evil' and described the urine as 'wonderfully sweet as if it were imbued with honey or sugar'. He thought the disease had been rare among the ancients but continued: 'in our age given to good fellowship and guzzling down chiefly of unallayed wine we meet with examples and instances enough, I may say daily of this disease'.

From that time diabetes was familiar to physicians, but we cannot guess how common it was until the recording of death-rates in the 19th century gives us some indication. Trousseau (1870) told his students that they would seldom see a diabetic patient in the hospital wards but emphasized that the disease was much more common than was generally supposed. In 1875 Bouchardat wrote that one was sure to find glycosuria in one of 20 men from the professional and commercial classes between the age of 40 and 60. By 1880 the mortality rate from diabetes in Paris was recorded as 9.6 per 100 000, in London it was 5.9 and in England as a whole 5.8. An estimate of the death-rate in the USA for this year was 2.8 per 100 000.

There was a general belief that diabetes was very common in India and Ceylon at this time, though the Cingalese considered it disgraceful and concealed its existence as long as they could, looking upon it as a punishment for ill-gotten wealth. The editor of the *Indian Medical Gazette* in 1871 stated that among the upper and middle class of natives from

Calcutta almost every family had lost one or more of its members from diabetes. In 1907 Bose reckoned that nearly 10% of the well-to-do class of Bengali gentlemen suffered from diabetes and Chakravarti attributed 10% of the total mortality in Calcutta to the disease.

Mortality statistics for diabetes indicate the trend of prevalence over considerable periods of time but are of little value in calculating the number of cases in the population because diabetes is commonly not mentioned on death certificates or may be excluded from the causes of death by methods of registration.

PRESENTATION OF PATIENTS WITH DIABETES

I have often thought that a good question for medical students' final examinations, where such relics of the past still exist, would be on the multitudinous ways in which a diabetic can present. The majority are diagnosed on the basis of classical symptoms and/or signs, glycosuria and hyperglycaemia. Many others are diagnosed following what is euphemistically termed 'routine' urine or blood testing. Sometimes the label is correct as, for example, in insurance or works medical examinations. At other times it is inappropriately used. When a patient attends the genitourinary clinic with balanitis or pruritus vulvae, or the eye department with cataract, testing blood or urine is not a routine test. Glycosuria is sought because of the association with diabetes of the presenting condition. What to one person is a high index of suspicion is, to another, an unthinking 'routine' urine test. Certainly, the number of diabetic patients in whom diabetes is suspected because of a positive urine test in medical or surgical clinics, casualty departments and on-ward testing testifies to the usefulness of the test.

It is unclear whether the screening of urine for sugar is being replaced by immediate blood glucose measurement with reagent strips. It seems likely that as some of the functions of the clinical chemistry laboratory move nearer the bedside this will occur. What is clear is the continuing and erroneous view that glycosuria warrants a fasting blood glucose measurement or that this should be done even when a postprandial blood glucose is unequivocally raised. While there are valid reasons for measuring fasting blood glucose these do not include diagnosis unless equivocal values are obtained from random or postprandial samples.

It is important that some concept of what is being measured is held by anyone called upon to interpret the findings of glucose in urine or measurement of blood glucose.

MEASUREMENT OF GLUCOSE IN URINE

> **Falstaff**: Sirrah, you giant, what says the doctor to my water?
>
> **Page**: He said, sir, the water itself was a good healthy water; but, for the party that owed it, he might have more diseases than he knew for.
>
> Shakespeare, *Henry IV Part II*: 1;2.

Young, healthy subjects consistently excrete a small quantity of glucose averaging 72 mg/day but rarely exceeding 200 mg/day (Froesch and Renold, 1956). A similar observation was made by Fine (1965), who found that glycosuria exceeding 15 mg/dl increased with advancing age and was more prevalent in men than women. This agrees with the results of random blood sugar estimations in surveys for diabetes, which show the same increase with age, but is hardly in accord with the common observation that the renal threshold for glucose is higher in the elderly. The increase of glycosuria with age probably truly represents the increasing prevalence of hyperglycaemia over the age of 50 years.

In clinical practice significant glycosuria is present when the urine contains 100 mg/dl or more of glucose. It is an anomaly of practice that, despite adopting SI units for blood glucose measurement, millimoles per litre has rarely been accepted for quantification of glycosuria.

There are many quick and easy reagent strip methods for measuring urine glucose, testifying to both their usefulness and the potential for remuneration of pharmaceutical companies. Early urine testing depended upon Benedict's test (Benedict, 1911). A solution of sodium bicarbonate, sodium nitrate and copper sulphate gave a colourful reaction after the addition of glucose and boiling. Clinitest was a convenient tablet form of this test much used by diabetic patients to assess control. When the tablet was added to five drops of urine plus ten drops of water, boiling occurred with colour development over 15 seconds. Up to 2% (2 g/dl) glycosuria could be detected in this way or, by adjustment of the proportions of urine and water, up to 5% (5 g/dl). The test worked well, although it was a little cumbersome to perform, but occasional problems resulted from the hygroscopic property of the tablets. The test has been superseded by other tests for urine sugar or glucose. There was much interest in the fact that Clinitest measured reducing substances in urine rather than glucose specifically. This led to false positives, which were of little consequence, although the ability to detect other reducing sugars was of interest in paediatric practice.

GLUCOSE OXIDASE METHODS

These tests, which are specific for glucose, depend upon the oxidation of glucose to gluconic acid by enzyme impregnated into a reagent strip. Absorbent indicator papers are impregnated with glucose oxidase and a compound which can be oxidized by hydrogen peroxide to give a colour. The strip also contains the enzyme necessary for this, peroxidase. Clinistix was best regarded as a qualitative test and had the drawback that it was too sensitive. Quantities as small as 0.01% of glucose were detected, which included those normal subjects excreting up to

0.1% glucose. Partly for this reason but mainly for the poor quantification, it was a test inappropriate for monitoring diabetic control. The newer range of urine tests are based on the same principle.

USE OF URINE TESTS

Specimens of urine should be tested for sugar within a few hours of collection. For the detection of diabetes it is best to have a specimen passed 1–2 hours after a substantial carbohydrate meal. If this is negative the diagnosis is unlikely but not excluded, especially when the patient is elderly and may have a high renal threshold. The quantity of glycosuria is of some diagnostic value. The greater it is the stronger the probability that diabetes is present. In the Birmingham Survey (Report of a Working Party Appointed by the College of General Practitioners, 1962) 92.6% of those who were found to have definite diabetes passed 1% or more of glucose in the urine 1–2 hours after taking 50 g of glucose by mouth.

BLOOD GLUCOSE MEASUREMENT

It should not be necessary to stress that glycosuria does not diagnose diabetes. It merely gives weight to the suggestion derived from the symptoms and signs or establishes the hypothesis from an unexpected finding. Blood glucose measurement is always necessary to make the diagnosis.

Capillary or venous samples may be used but the nature of the sample should always be stated. Arterio-venous differences that are negligible in the fasting state may be up to 4 mol/l (72 mg/dl) one hour after the ingestion of glucose. The average difference is about 1.5 mmol/l (27 mg/dl), but a sensible rule of thumb is to take a difference of 10% higher in capillary blood, which more loosely approximates arterial blood, than venous blood. The choice of method depends very largely upon the laboratory facilities available. Capillary samples require expert technique to extract a small volume. Venous samples require little skill and a larger volume can be divided for other assays. When whole blood is left at room temperature for 3 hours, half the glucose is converted to lactate by enzymes of glycolysis within the erythrocyte. This loss is prevented by sodium fluoride which, when mixed with potassium oxalate, prevents clotting.

Glucose can be assayed in whole blood or plasma. Serum is not advisable because the inevitable delay while the clot retracts allows glucose metabolism. Intracellular glucose cannot be measured because of rapid metabolism and including ruptured red cells in the assay achieves the effect of diluting plasma glucose. Thus plasma glucose is 14% higher than blood glucose, although again a reasonable working figure is 10%.

The much-used enzyme strips which are discussed below require capillary blood. There has been a lack of specificity in acknowledging what is measured. A membrane surrounds the reagent pad, which does not allow red cells to reach the reagent. Even if they do there is no guarantee of red cell rupture and it seems correct to acknowledge that plasma glucose is being measured.

Much has been written on measuring blood glucose (Burrin and Price, 1985). Older methods, such as those of Hagedorn and Jensen or Folin and Wu, measured reducing substances. Other methods more suited to adaptation for autoanalysers, such as Somogyi-Nelson and Hoffmann's method, measured glucose or glucose plus other sugars. There is little excuse nowadays for using anything other than a glucose-specific method and for referring to blood glucose rather than blood sugar. Glucose oxidase or hexokinase methods are appropriate.

Reagent sticks such as Dextrostix, BM 1–44 stix or other similar productions are glucose oxidase sticks with peroxidase and chromagen also impregnated in the reagent pad. They are extremely convenient but whether they should be used alone to diagnose diabetes is debatable (Price, Burrin and Nattrass, 1988). Under the supervision of the laboratory, with adequate quality control and the test carried out by trained staff, there would seem to be little objection. In the family practitioner's surgery with only occasional tests being performed an answer which is read by eye cannot be considered satisfactory as a means of diagnosis. Diabetes is a disease with major consequences for work, driving and insurance, among others, and a single strip-reading by a little-practised physician or nurse seems rather flimsy evidence upon which to base this important diagnosis.

'RANDOM' BLOOD GLUCOSE MEASUREMENT

Blood is collected by venepuncture or finger stab into fluoride/oxalate tubes. It is sensible to get into the habit of noting the last mealtime. Blood glucose concentration varies during a day within relatively narrow limits although nearly everyone underestimates these limits (Figure 5.1). In our studies of blood glucose measured by hexokinase method at half-hourly intervals during the day we found that for normal subjects the 95th centile 1 hour after the evening meal was 9.8 mmol/l (176 mg/dl). Most estimates put the range at 3–7 mmol/l (54–126 mg/dl). Although our patients were relatively young others have accepted values up to 10 mmol/l (180 mg/dl) in older people (Alberti, Dornhorst and Rowe, 1975).

FASTING BLOOD GLUCOSE MEASUREMENT

There is less normal variation in fasting blood glucose concentration and it is less important whether blood is taken from a vein or from capillaries. There is an interesting seasonal variation and a tendency for fasting blood glucose to rise with age (Figure 5.2).

For diagnosis a single blood glucose can be taken in the fasting state or 1–2 hours after a meal. Practical considerations to some extent dictate the choice, usually depending on the

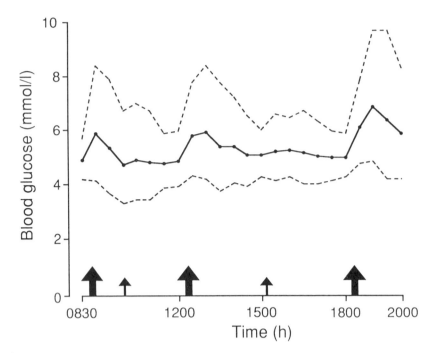

Fig. 5.1 Blood glucose concentration over 12 hours in 23 normal subjects. Mean at each time point is shown (●━━●) with 5th and 95th centile (– – – –). Large arrows indicate meals and small arrow snacks.

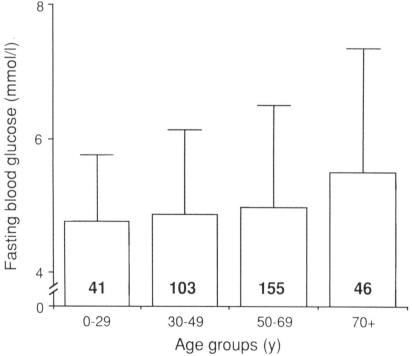

Fig. 5.2 Fasting capillary blood glucose (mean + 2 s.d.) by age group.

distance the patient has to travel to the doctor or hospital. For random blood glucose I am unhappy about calling abnormal anything less than the quoted vales for diagnosis for 2 hours after a glucose load. In practice anything upward of 8 mmol/l (144 mg/dl) increases suspicion but the diagnosis will need confirmation. Occasionally much higher values can be found which do not signify diabetes, but these occur almost exclusively in patients who have had partial or total gastrectomy.

When using single blood glucose estimations for diagnosis one must remember that no laboratory is infallible. Technical errors in measurement do occur from time to time and specimens may be wrongly labelled or wrongly identified. With fasting samples there is only the word of the patient that the fact has been observed. In a doubtful case further evidence should be sought.

THE DIAGNOSIS OF DIABETES

The correct diagnosis of diabetes is a matter of importance in both a positive and a negative sense. It is as wrong to neglect the minor but significant symptoms of early diabetes as it is to inflict needless restrictions and the fears of complications on those who are only under suspicion. Coma, blindness and gangrene are consequences well-known wherever the illness is discussed by patients, and fear of diabetes is widespread – with some justification, it must be admitted.

In most cases referred to a hospital clinic the diagnosis is beyond reasonable doubt by the time the history and physical examination are complete. The diagnosis is suggested in these patients by a previous finding of glycosuria or hyperglycaemia.

Before the test the possibility of diabetes may be far from obvious. Symptoms may be absent, vague or bizarre, or may be overshadowed by those of an accompanying illness. It is not difficult to make a case for a routine test for glucose in every clinical examination.

The importance of the diagnosis is such that with an equivocal result or when doubt exists a glucose tolerance test should be performed. It is often forgotten that to demonstrate normality is a justifiable reason for a glucose tolerance test. Once the suspicion is placed in a patient's mind that diabetes is a possibility reassurance of normality is often gratefully received.

The minor abnormalities of glucose tolerance that are discussed later in this chapter present a problem which must be considered individually in each case with due attention to age, body weight and personality of the patient. It is as well to remember that in the borderline groups there is no test which clearly distinguishes normality from nonnormality despite numerous efforts to provide enhanced diagnostic tests.

THE PROBLEM OF DIAGNOSING DIABETES

The first question which must be addressed is whether our common usage of 'disease' and 'non-normality' as synonyms should be accepted as such. No one would dispute the importance of identifying disease and attempting to bring relief. The dis-ease brought by symptoms of acute diabetes – excessive thirst and urination, balanitis and pruritus, and lethargy – not always appreciated until relieved, are worthy of treatment. Similarly, the long-term disabling complications are an avoidable consequence.

It might be concluded that the population who develop acute symptoms or are at risk of complications can be safely thought to have diabetes. They will be unified by a degree of hyperglycaemia which identifies them as being at risk. Yet is is clear that a proportion of patients run little risk of either symptoms or complications. I refer to the milder degrees

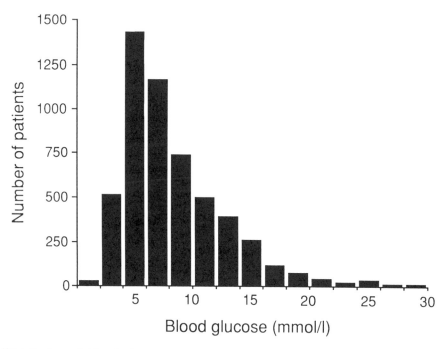

Fig. 5.3 Distribution of blood glucose concentration in a hospital population (inpatients and out-patients). Results from 4900 measurements are shown.

of carbohydrate disturbance rather than the established clear-cut diabetic without complications. Most of the latter group will develop acute symptoms if treatment is withdrawn.

It has to be faced that hyperglycaemia requires definition and can only be a term relative to normoglycaemia. Our reliance upon statistics in this situation raises the second problem and may be misleading. Blood glucose concentration, either fasting or postprandial, does not follow the gaussian distribution beloved of statisticians and clinical chemists fond of compiling reference ranges. Yet, importantly, neither does it break into two distinct populations, the normal and the diabetic. Rather there is a skew to the right (Figure 5.3).

Given this, we can still define a normal population and state with confidence a range for fasting or postprandial blood glucose concentration which will include 90–95% of normal subjects. Subjects lying to the right of a calculated upper limit of normal may then be normal, not normal or diabetic. We can say with some confidence that the farther to the right, i.e. the higher the blood glucose concentration, the greater the likelihood of the patient having diabetes. What cannot be done except in a totally arbitrary way is to derive a blood glucose value one side of which is normal and the other side of which is diabetic. This is well acknowledged among physicians treating diabetes yet the temptation to lay down diagnostic criteria is irresistible. Every august body in diabetes has spoken authoritatively on the subject of diagnosing diabetes in recent years and there is no doubt that some revision of criteria had become necessary (WHO, 1980, 1985; National Diabetes Data Group, 1979).

'OLD' DIAGNOSTIC CRITERIA

The diagnostic criteria for diabetes produced by the secretaries of the British Diabetic Association in 1964 (FitzGerald and Keen, 1964) laid down values for a glucose tolerance test which were aimed at dividing the population into normal and diabetic. A fasting capillary blood glucose of 6.1 mmol/l (110 mg/dl) with a value 2 hours after 50 g glucose of 6.7 mmol/l (120 mg/dl) marked the limit of normality. If these values seem somewhat arbitary numerals it is because they derive from the pre-SI-unit days of 110 and 120 mg/dl.

At the same time as these criteria were in use other diagnostic tests were employed. Oral glucose could be given in 100 g amounts as in the USA; glucose could be given intravenously for diagnosis; and other provocative tests were being used in an attempt to identify people regarded as pre-diabetic, or potential diabetics. In addition, proposals for giving a weight-related dose of glucose have always attracted supporters capable of arguing endlessly on a dose per kilogram or a dose per metre squared!

One aim of a redefinition of criteria was therefore to introduce a consensus view and achieve some standardization of the procedure, particularly the stimulus to be used, and interpretation. A masterful compromise of a dose of glucose of 75 g was chosen by both the World Health Organization (WHO, 1980) and the National Diabetes Data Group (1979), thus devaluing at a stroke previous work on diabetes which had used 50 g and 100 g diagnostic tests.

THE RATIONALE FOR NEW DIAGNOSTIC CRITERIA

When it came to deciding on diagnostic values during a glucose tolerance test a more rational approach prevailed. The awareness of previous values as too tight was supported by a number of studies.

Firstly, there are a number of populations around the world who have been much investigated because of their high prevalence of diabetes. The groups themselves tend to be small but give meaningful results because of the high prevalence (30–50%). They include the Pima Indians of Arizona (Bennett *et al.*, 1976), Nauru Micronesians (Zimmet and Whitehouse, 1978) and Western Samoan Polynesians (Zimmet, 1979). The high prevalence is a consequence of bimodality in the distribution of blood glucose levels. Thus the diabetic population can be distinguished from the normal population, although a small degree of overlap of necessity occurs. The 2-hour post-glucose value which distinguishes normal from diabetic in these populations is around 10–11 mmol/l (180–200 mg/dl) and this has influenced the revised diagnostic criteria.

Secondly, and still with these quaint populations, retinopathy due to diabetes is confined to the diabetic mode, as is proteinuria and renal failure from diabetes. Similarly, in the Bedford survey (Jarrett and Keen, 1976) it was reported that diabetic retinopathy that developed subsequently was mainly, although not exclusively, in those subjects with a 2-hour plasma glucose greater than 11.1 mmol/l (200 mg/dl). Consistent results were reported also from the Whitehall Survey (Jarrett and Al Sayegh, 1978). Thus support is given to the idea that the diagnosis and the disease can be equated above a 2-hour value for plasma glucose of 11.1 mmol/l (200 mg/dl).

A corollary of the loosening of the diagnostic criteria was that a small group of patients was identified, previously labelled as having borderline or pre-diabetes, who were not entirely normal on glucose tolerance testing yet did not qualify for the diagnosis of diabetes. These patients were placed in a new diagnostic category called 'impaired glucose tolerance'. The justification for a separate category distinct from normality was twofold: firstly, this group has an increased risk of progression to diabetes and secondly, they display a risk for cardiovascular disease which is intermediate between the normal and the diabetic population (Mykkanen *et al.*, 1993).

'NEW' DIAGNOSTIC CRITERIA

There have been many attempts to set out clearly the more recent diagnostic criteria. Interpretation of the recommendations was not helped by the publication in quick succession of two reports from the World Health Organization, especially as there were subtle but significant differences between the two. In the succeeding paragraphs are set out the diagnostic criteria of the 1980 and the 1985 report, which presumably superseded the 1980 report. The diagnostic levels of glucose were not the same in the two reports mainly because of the policy adopted in the 1980 report of rounding values to the nearest millimole per litre.

When a glucose tolerance test is not necessary diagnosis is relatively simple.

Diagnosing diabetes:

1. When symptoms of diabetes are present a single random venous plasma glucose value of 11 mmol/l (200 mg/dl) or more or fasting of 8 mmol/l (140 mg/dl) or more are diagnostic of diabetes (WHO, 1980).
2. In the absence of symptoms an additional abnormal blood glucose result is needed to confirm the clinical diagnosis (WHO, 1980).
3. When symptoms of diabetes are present or even if they are trivial or absent a single random venous plasma glucose value greater than 11.1 mmol/l (200 mg/dl) establishes the diagnosis (WHO, 1985).
4. For the asymptomatic patient, if the glucose value obtained is just in the diagnostic range, at least one additional test result with a value in the diabetic range is de-

sirable to confirm the clinical diagnosis (WHO, 1985).

'Diagnosing' normality:

1. Random venous plasma values below 8 mmol/l (140 mg/dl) and fasting below 6 mmol/l (100 mg/dl) exclude the diagnosis of diabetes (WHO, 1980).
2. A random venous plasma glucose value below 5.5 mmol/l (100 mg/dl) makes the diagnosis of diabetes unlikely (WHO, 1985).

It is rather pointless to criticize in detail these diagnostic recommendations. Backed by expert might, most national diabetic associations have accepted the criteria. Some early criticism led to attempted clarification in the second WHO report which probably only served to confuse. Loose definition such as 'if the glucose value obtained is **just in** the diagnostic range' was most unhelpful, but probably the greatest defect was not to be clear about what constituted normality in the second report. After all, it could be argued that, if normality could not be defined, how was abnormality to be defined?

Two points which are advised are not adhered to in our clinic. Firstly, taking symptoms into account to help classify patients is probably useless. Some with marked hyperglycaemia may have negligible symptoms while normal subjects often have diabetic symptoms. Their value as a discriminant function is probably so low as to be unworthy of study.

Secondly, we regularly contravene the WHO recommendations by basing the diagnosis upon one blood glucose measurement even in the absence of symptoms. This is a result of working on the shop floor rather than in an ivory tower.

In the main the diagnosis of diabetes does not present great problems. Hyperglycaemia is the detectable hallmark. Only when results are 'equivocal' does interpretation of the diagnostic criteria occasionally present problems. When this occurs a good helping of common sense is preferred to a rigid line-by-line knowledge of the WHO reports.

Although the instructions are relatively straightforward, care must still be exercised in applying them. Many patients are capable of fasting for short or even long periods before their appearance in the clinic and it is all too easy to imagine that a postprandial value is normal until it is revealed that it is an abnormal 'fasting' value. If in doubt, either because the blood glucose levels are inter-mediate or because there is a high clinical index of suspicion, the situation can be labelled equivocal. This label should never be the fallback of the indecisive but a specific tag with a particular consequent action. Then a glucose tolerance test becomes necessary.

ORAL GLUCOSE TOLERANCE TEST

In an ideal world we would look at the patho-genesis of diabetes and devise a suitable dynamic diagnostic test. Undersecretion of a hormone by an endocrine gland is best diagnosed by a stimulation test. The oral glucose tolerance test derives from the time when both major types of diabetes were held to be faults in insulin secretion either near total or some minor degree of impairment. While near total loss of insulin secretion occurs in insulin-dependent diabetes it is rarely necessary to conduct a glucose toler-ance test to diagnose this type of diabetes. Non-insulin-dependent diabetes has its origins in diminished insulin secretion and insulin resistance. It is fortuitous that the oral glu-cose tolerance test takes both into account, albeit imperfectly, with insulin secretion indirectly assessed in the early stages and peripheral glucose disposal in the later stages (Reaven *et al.*, 1993). Of course the test is not independent of the rate of intestinal absorp-tion of glucose, although this is rarely a confounding factor.

It is remarkable that the test has survived as the standard investigation of the doubtful case of diabetes. So far it continues to survive despite the help of people who would like to aim at a mathematical expression of results or computer modelling. Although the curves are not highly reproducible the intrapatient variation is not usually a source of confusion except where values lie close to diagnostic cut-off levels. Normal curves on repetition are still normal and definitely abnormal curves are definitely abnormal in the great majority of cases, and perhaps too much is made of minor degrees of abnormality, which on repeti-tion move between diagnostic categories.

Technique (Table 5.1)

An adequately nourished patient needs no special dietary preparation. Conn (1940) showed that a severely restricted (20 g) carbo-hydrate intake for 5 days before a test would produce a diabetic curve in subjects who had given a normal curve on a full diet. Others have shown that as little as 50 g carbohydrate daily is sufficient to overcome this effect and those who have restricted their diet more severely can be restored to normal by an intake of 150 g daily for 4 days before the test. An undernourished patient should take no less than this.

After a fast of 12 hours the first samples of blood and urine are collected and 75 g glu-cose given in 250 ml water. Subsequent blood

Table 5.1 Procedure for an oral glucose tolerance test

1. Ensure preceding diet of > 150 g carbohydrate for 3 days prior to test
2. Fast patient for 10–14 hours before test
3. After blood for fasting glucose is withdrawn give 75 g anhydrous glucose in 300 ml (flavoured) water drunk over 5 minutes
4. Patient should sit quietly and not smoke
5. Second blood sample at 2 hours
6. Urine samples should be collected at 0 and 2 hours for detection of renal glycosuria with a normal OGTT

samples are withdrawn at 1 and 2 hours along with urine specimens. The practice of taking half-hourly samples for 2 hours has little meaning now that diagnosis is based on fasting and 2-hour values, whereas the 1-hour value may be useful confirmation if either fasting or 2-hour values are equivocal.

During the test the patient should sit quietly. Lying alters glucose absorption while exercise will clearly lower blood glucose. It is often stated that smoking is not allowed, although there is little evidence from blood glucose measurements to support such a ban (Walsh *et al.*, 1977). Nevertheless, it makes the job of the venepuncturist more pleasant.

Reporting of results should include the type of specimen analysed, blood or plasma, venous or capillary. It has been confirmed that 75 g anhydrous glucose should be given and if hydrolysates of starch are used this should be equivalent to 75 g anhydrous glucose. In children the dose is 1.75 g glucose per kilogram body weight up to a maximum of 75 g.

Diagnostic criteria

Diagnosis from a glucose tolerance test is based upon results fasting and 2 hours after a 75 g glucose load (or 1.75 g/kg body weight in children to a maximum of 75 g). Diagnostic criteria from the 1985 report are set out in Table 5.2. Briefly, a fasting venous plasma glucose equal to or greater than 7.8 mmol/l (140 mg/dl) is diagnostic of diabetes. A fasting value less than 7.8 mmol/l (140 mg/dl) can occur either in normals or in people with impaired glucose tolerance. For 2-hour values, less than 7.8 mmol/l (140 mg/dl) is normal, 7.8–11.1 mmol/l (140–200 mg/dl) the category of impaired glucose tolerance and 11.1 mmol/l (200 mg/dl) or greater diagnostic of diabetes. Sadly, as an example of the confusion which can and has been generated, the figure of 11.1 mmol/l (200 mg/dl) appears in both the definition of impaired glucose tolerance and diabetes mellitus!

A handsome measure of common sense is necessary when applying the criteria. Other than for the 2-hour value the criteria (WHO, 1985) do not indicate what is to be regarded as normal beyond the rather bland statement that a random venous plasma glucose below 5.5 mmol/l (100 mg/dl) makes diabetes unlikely!

Furthermore, only a minor knowledge of mathematics is necessary to conclude that if the fasting value can be classified at two levels and the 2-hour value at three levels (WHO, 1985) the number of combinations is six. Worse, since the 1980 report was clearer about what might be considered normal, both fasting and 2-hour values can be classified at three levels, resulting in nine possible combinations. The reports could have been clearer in detailing the interpretation of, say, a normal fasting value with a 2-hour value indicative of impaired glucose tolerance.

Table 5.2   Intepretation of the oral glucose tolerance test (values in millimoles per litre; milligrams per decilitre in brackets)

	Venous whole blood	Capillary whole blood	Venous plasma	Capillary plasma
Diabetes				
Fasting	⩾ 6.7 (120)	⩾ 6.7 (120)	⩾ 7.8 (140)	⩾ 7.8 (140)
2-hour	⩾ 10.0 (180)	⩾ 11.1 (200)	⩾ 11.1 (200)	⩾ 12.2 (220)
Impaired glucose tolerance				
Fasting	< 6.7 (120)	< 6.7 (120)	< 7.8 (140)	< 7.8 (140)
2-hour	6.7–10.0 (120–180)	7.8–11.1 (140–200)	7.8–11.1 (140–200)	8.9–12.2 (160–220)

Interpretation

Many factors modify a glucose tolerance test result. Analytical considerations are considered above. Others, such as the seasonal variation which occurs, are also extrinsic to the patient. Of this group, the diurnal variation is much studied but is of little relevance since glucose tolerance tests are not performed in the evening. Factors within the patient are of most importance although their effects are variable.

Age

In survey studies which include random glucose tolerance tests an age effect is always apparent (Report of a Working Party Appointed by the College of General Practitioners, 1962). Since diagnostic criteria are not age-related there is an increase of 'abnormal' tests in the elderly. Even if we include only those patients defined as normal by a 75 g

oral glucose tolerance test and current criteria the trend is still present (Figure 5.4) although removing abnormal fasting and 2-hour values leaves the focus on the intervening times.

This could be regarded as a normal accompaniment of aging in the same way that a moderate increase in blood pressure with age has been considered normal. From the practical point of view the difficulty lies, in each instance, in distinguishing between a mild harmless aberration and an abnormality that may lead to serious complications. It is small comfort to a man who is in congestive heart failure as a result of hypertension or crippled by diabetic neuropathy to be told that he is merely at the upper end of the distribution scale for blood pressure or blood glucose.

This difficulty – of distinguishing true abnormality that is diabetes from an artefactual abnormality because of rigid diagnostic criteria – is encountered with other factors that modify glucose tolerance.

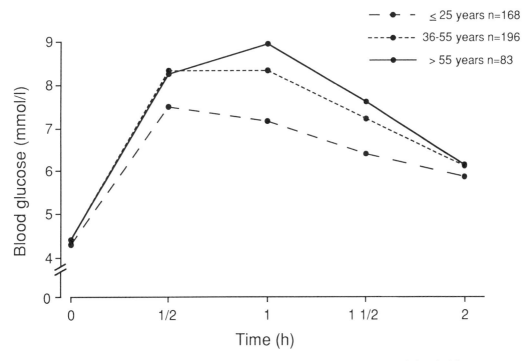

Fig. 5.4 Results from oral glucose tolerance tests in non-diabetic subjects subdivided by age group.

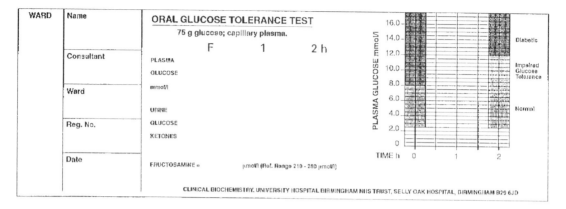

Fig. 5.5   A conventional method of expressing the results of a glucose tolerance test.

Body weight

The relationship of blood glucose with body weight has been interpreted as an increase of diabetes with obesity. This view has to be correct since diagnostic criteria pay no attention to body weight. If obese patients with diabetes and impaired glucose tolerance are excluded is there a detectable effect of obesity upon glucose tolerance? I am struck by the normality of glucose tolerance tests in many massively obese patients we have studied.

Drugs

If anything the situation is even more confusing when the effect of drugs upon glucose tolerance is considered. The most profound effects are found with thiazide diuretics and corticosteroids. Do they make pre-existing diabetes more likely to be detected? Do they unmask diabetes in patients with a tendency? or do they convert a normal person into a diabetic or into a normal person with a temporary abnormality of glucose tolerance due to administration of a particular drug? The answers do not exist to these simple questions yet they are surely more important than the pseudo-accuracy of the diagnostic criteria obtained by quoting one decimal place of blood glucose values. My own view in all these situations is that it cannot be

predicted when an abnormality is not pathological, nor when it is temporary, and since the consequences of diabetes are so important the assumption should be that diabetes exists and should be treated.

Recording results

It is by no means easy for the busy physician to carry these diagnostic values in the memory. Fortunately, the laboratory can help as ours has done by producing a graphical or tabular representation as an *aide-memoire* in the clinic (Figure 5.5). This also serves to remind the physician whether we measure glucose in blood or plasma, and is it capillary or venous blood?

Classification

Whenever glucose tolerance tests are performed distinct patterns emerge. Most patients can be classified as diabetic or having impaired glucose tolerance while some may be inferred as being normal on the criteria in Table 5.2. As always, it is the minor degrees of abnormality that are most difficult. The apparent precision denoted by the less than or equals to sign has to be ridiculous and indeed, it elicited criticism. The numerical values of the 1980 report were, after all, rounded after conversion from milligrams

Table 5.3 Diagnostic categories for results from venous plasma samples during an oral glucose tolerance test (Source: the figures are taken from WHO, 1985 – see text)

Fasting blood glucose	2-hour blood glucose		
	A < 7.8	B 7.8–11.1	C ≥ 11.1
1. < 5.5	Normal		
2. 5.5–< 7.8		Impaired glucose tolerance	
3. ≥ 7.8			Diabetic

Table 5.4 Difficulties in classifying the oral glucose tolerance test in 699 patients (Source: diagnostic levels for venous plasma glucose are taken from WHO, 1985)

Fasting blood glucose	2-hour blood glucose		
	< 7.8	7.8–11.1	≥ 11.1
< 5.5	306 (44%)	97 (14%)	39 (6%)
5.5–< 7.8	24 (3%)	48 (7%)	69 (10%)
≥ 7.8	3 (0.4%)	10 (1.4%)	103 (15%)

per decilitre. This criticism was acknowledged in the revised report of 1985 – the response of the expert committee was to alter the numerical values to more 'accurate' figures. In theory it is possible for a patient to have been diabetic in 1978, normal in 1982 and diabetic again in 1987 simply through changes in the numerical criteria for diagnosis.

Unclassified or unclassifiable results are found commonly. Clearly, if diagnosis is based on two values, fasting and 2-hour, and each of these results is classifiable on three levels, as was suggested in the 1980 report, or two levels, as suggested in the 1985 report, there are nine or six possible combinations (Table 5.3). If we extrapolate from the suggestion in the 1985 report that a venous plasma glucose of less than 5.5 mmol/l (100 mg/dl) makes diabetes unlikely to the conclusion that a fasting value of less than 5.5 mmol/l (100 mg/dl) excludes the diagnosis, then both reports give nine categories, as defined in Table 5.3. Of the combinations in the table, it is clear that 1A is normal, 2B impaired glucose tolerance and 3C diabetes. The remainder do not classify comfortably, although this conclusion can be influenced by the individual reading of the diagnostic criteria. Thus some may regard 1B as impaired glucose tolerance, 2C as diabetes and 3B as diabetes.

In a selected population referred for oral glucose tolerance tests we found that only 66% of results from 699 patients fell into the clear-cut diagnostic categories (Table 5.4).

Of course, it can be argued that such a referred population, including as it does ill patients and those who take medication which interferes with glucose metabolism, might be expected to produce some confusing results. Yet this is the very population in whom unequivocal diagnosis can present problems and who are most likely to be referred for glucose tolerance tests.

Alternative results

The commonest aberrant result, the detection of which is a good reason for requesting a glucose tolerance test, is that of renal glycosuria. The blood glucose values are all within the normal range but glycosuria is found in one or more of the urine collections (Figure 5.6).

Renal glycosuria was first recognized by Klemperer (1896), who observed that glycosuria could occur without hyperglycaemia. He referred to renal diabetes, but this title has been understandably rejected by those who regard this condition as entirely benign. The use of the term should be restricted to glycosuria with normal blood glucose levels and normal glucose tolerance. In the Birmingham survey we adopted this definition and found renal glycosuria to be uncommon but by no means rare, having a prevalence of 3 per 1000. It was strikingly more common in men than in women in spite of the inclusion of six pregnant women in the tested population, and was not seen over the age of 70,

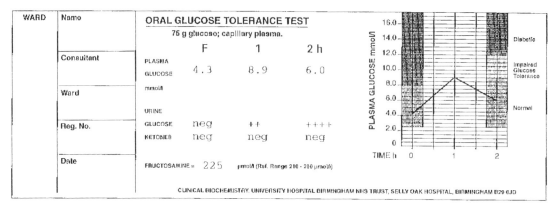

Fig. 5.6   A typical example of results from a patient showing renal glycosuria.

perhaps as a result of diminished glomerular filtration rates with advancing years.

In pregnancy renal glycosuria is certainly common and a frequency of between 5% and 35% in all pregnancies has been reported. Flynn, Harper and De Mayo (1953) found glycosuria in 24% of antenatal attendances, two-thirds of the patients showing glycosuria at some time during pregnancy, although lactosuria was considerably more frequent even in the third month of pregnancy. The renal glycosuria of pregnancy disappears rapidly after delivery and is not found 1 week later.

There have been several reports of families with a high incidence of renal glycosuria but only in a minority of cases is there a known familial incidence. The familial form is considered to be a congenital abnormality in otherwise healthy subjects, inherited as a dominant mendelian trait and detected most often in the second decade.

Renal glycosuria seems to be due to inadequate resorption of glucose in the renal tubules. Renal blood flow and glomerular filtration are normal but tubular resorption is diminished when the blood glucose is not raised. The mechanism of the defect in the proximal renal tubule has not been identified. Decreased phosphorylase has been suggested, as phlorizin is believed to produce glycosuria

by inhibition of this enzyme, and there is some evidence for hormonal control of tubular function (Bland, 1948), which may be disturbed in pregnancy.

Renal glycosuria is symptomless except under conditions of starvation or ketosis, when dehydration may occur. Pruritus vulvae is occasionally encountered, especially in renal glycosuria of pregnancy. It is generally agreed that the renal defect is not progressive. Most writers who have followed their cases for 10 years or more have concluded that there is no undue incidence of diabetes.

McLean (1922) coined the phrase 'lag storage' to describe glucose tolerance curves which were normal yet had an apparently elevated value up to 1 hour after glucose ingestion. There is a rapid and excessive rise in blood glucose following oral ingestion of glucose to values exceeding 10 mmol/L (180 mg/dl). It is therefore not the curve which lags but, it was suggested, the storage of glucose. Galactose tolerance curves in subjects who show the lag-storage effect have the same shape as that produced by glucose. There are no figures for the prevalence of this type of result using the new diagnostic criteria.

It is a common sequel to gastrectomy but may occur also in cases of peptic ulcer which have not been subjected to operation. The high peak may be followed at 2–3 hours from the start of the test by an exaggerated fall in the blood glucose, presumably as a result of excessive insulin output. True hypoglycaemia symptoms are uncommon. More often, complaints during the test are atypical and not necessarily related to the nadir in blood glucose levels.

OTHER DIAGNOSTIC TESTS

Many other forms of the glucose tolerance test have been used over the years.

THE INTRAVENOUS GLUCOSE TOLERANCE TEST

This test was introduced in the hope of achieving a precise measurement of carbohydrate tolerance. Following the injection of glucose intravenously there is an immediate rise in blood glucose followed by a fall which, in the first 15 minutes, is mainly due to diffusion through the extracellular fluid, the osmotic dilution of the blood with water being trivial. After 15 minutes blood glucose is reduced by entry into the tissues and to a much lesser extent by urinary excretion. The plasma immunoreactive insulin rises, reaching a maximum 60 seconds after the end of a rapid glucose infusion. Samols and Marks (1965) proposed that the change in plasma insulin was the main reason for the disappearance of injected glucose. It is established that plasma immunoreactive insulin rises less in the intravenous than in the oral test and it may be that the difference is due to glucagon secretion which is provoked by orally administered glucose and can in its turn stimulate further insulin secretion (Samols, Marri and Marks, 1965).

After preparation as for the oral test, 25 g of glucose in a 50% solution are injected over a period of 3 minutes. Blood samples are collected every 10 minutes for 1 hour and the blood glucose is plotted semilogarithmically against time. The fall in blood glucose forms a straight line from which the disappearance rate of glucose can be calculated.

Those who have devoted much time to this test argue that it should replace the oral test because it takes less time, avoids the gastrointestinal tract and produces a result which can be stated as a single figure (Lundbaek, 1962). There is good evidence that it is of special value in the presence of abnormal function or motility of the stomach, as in pregnancy. However, there is a certain risk of venous thrombosis from the glucose injection if given by unpractised hands and in most centres long experience with the oral test make it easier to manage and interpret. In addition, it is a fallacy to suppose that a glucose tolerance test can be used to make a sharp distinction between the diabetic and the non-diabetic and this fallacy is somewhat encouraged by the use of tolerance indices.

The remainder of alternative procedures for glucose tolerance testing are mentioned briefly for historical reasons. None contributes to present-day diagnosis of diabetes.

The Exton–Rose test gave 50 g glucose after a fasting blood specimen with a second 50 g half an hour later. In normal subjects the fasting and half-hour levels were normal and the 1-hour value not more than about 0.5 mmol/l (9 mg/dl) higher than the half-hour. In diabetics the increase was more than 1.5 mmol/l (27 mg/dl).

The sodium–tolbutamide test used intravenous injection of tolbutamide to lower blood glucose. While normal subjects reach a nadir 20–40 minutes after injection the fall is detectably more gradual in diabetics.

The cortisone glucose tolerance test used two doses of cortisone acetate before a glucose tolerance test. Numerical values were laid down to differentiate normal from the potential diabetic. The prednisone–glycosuria test depended upon an increase in glycosuria in response to prednisone. Subjects with a pre-diabetic background showed a higher rate than normals.

GLYCATED PROTEINS IN DIAGNOSIS

The measurement of glycated protein concentrations might be expected to replace the glucose tolerance test as a diagnostic marker for diabetes. The usefulness of glycated proteins lies in the post-translational glycation being dependent upon prevailing blood glucose concentration. Thus they give an integrated estimate of blood glucose concentration over the life of the protein.

Glycated haemoglobin has been studied most extensively, with fructosamine the more recent focus of attention. Several workers have shown that only 20–60% of patients with an abnormal glucose tolerance test have elevated HbA_{1c}, depending upon the criteria for abnormality (Dods and Bolmey, 1979; Dix *et al.*, 1979; Little *et al.*, 1988).

We (Albutt, Nattrass and Northam, 1985) compared the oral glucose tolerance and glycated haemoglobin measurement in 535 patients having the glucose tolerance test for diagnostic purposes. In a number of patients the oral glucose tolerance test was unclassifiable by WHO (1980) criteria but if these patients were excluded the remaining results are shown in Table 5.5.

The sensitivity of glycated haemoglobin in detecting diabetes was 81% and the specificity 96%. The predictive value of a positive test for the diagnosis of diabetes was therefore 83%. Since publication of these data we have extended our observations to compare the usefulness of other glycated proteins in diagnosis. In 164 patients undergoing an oral glucose tolerance test glycated haemoglobin, fructosamine and glycated albumin were measured. The assessment of these results is given in Table 5.6.

Correcting serum fructosamine values for the level of serum albumin as advocated by some actually worsened the results. These

Table 5.5   Comparison of glycated haemoglobin levels and oral glucose tolerance test in the diagnosis of diabetes – WHO, 1980 diagnostic criteria (Source: adapted from Albutt *et al.*, 1985)

Normal	
Fasting blood glucose < 5.5 mmol/l and	
2-hour blood glucose < 8.0 mmol/l	
Number of patients	260
Mean glycated haemoglobin	6.91%
Standard deviation	0.95%
Number of patients with glycated haemoglobin > 9.0%	7
Impaired glucose tolerance	
Fasting blood glucose 5.5–6.9 mmol/l and	
2-hour blood glucose 8.0–10.9 mmol/l	
Number of patients	28
Mean glycated haemoglobin	7.87%
Standard deviation	1.31%
Number of patients with glycated haemoglobin > 9.0%	5
Diabetic	
Fasting blood glucose ≥ 7.0 mmol/l and	
2-hour blood glucose ≥ 11.0 mmol/l	
Number of patients	70
Mean glycated haemoglobin	11.01%
Standard deviation	2.27%
Number of patients with glycated haemoglobin > 9.0%	57

Table 5.6 Glycated proteins and the oral glucose tolerance test in the diagnosis of diabetes; reference ranges were calculated as the 2.5–97.5th centile from all patients classified as normal glucose tolerance

OGTT diagnosis	No. of patients (%) with glycated protein level above upper limit of reference range		
	Glycated Hb	Fructosamine	Glycated albumin
Normal ($n = 46$)	0	0	0
Impaired glucose tolerance ($n = 20$)	3 (15)	1 (15)	6 (30)
Diabetic ($n = 33$)	24 (73)	25 (76)	29 (88)

figures show the assays in their best light, since if the difficult to classify glucose tolerance test results are included there is a deterioration, particularly in the sensitivity of the test. For example, if patients are included who have a fasting blood glucose of 5.5–6.9 mmol/l (100–125 mg/dl) and a 2-hour value of > 11.1 mmol/l (200 mg/dl) only three of 28 patients had an elevated glycated haemoglobin level.

It was perhaps naive to expect a perfect relationship between the level of glycated protein and the glucose tolerance test, especially since the latter is a definition of diabetes rather than a detection of a well limited disease. Currently there seems little reason to change our earlier conclusion that a raised glycated protein is useful for confirming the diagnosis of diabetes but that glycated haemoglobin (for example) is within the reference range in approximately one in three diabetics where diagnosis is by oral glucose tolerance test and in a majority (83%) of patients with impaired glucose tolerance (Table 5.7).

Table 5.7 Percentage sensitivity, specificity and predictive value of a positive test for glycated proteins in detecting diabetes

	Glycated Hb	Fructosamine	Glycated albumin
Sensitivity	73	76	88
Specificity	95	99	91
Predictive value	89	96	83

GLYCOSURIA

The use of specific glucose oxidase test strips for urine has largely removed the false positive glucosuria result seen with tests detecting reducing substances. These findings were of interest mainly in children. While glucose is the commonest reducing sugar in the urine, lactose, fructose, galactose and pentose all give positive results. Lactosuria is commonly found in the urine of newborn babies in amounts related to the quantity of lactose in the feeds. It also occurs about twice as often as glucose in pregnancy and is found in 94% of pregnant women at some stage (Flynn, Harper and De Mayo, 1953). In the puerperium lactosuria is often abundant and at this time the renal glycosuria of pregnancy rapidly disappears.

Essential fructosuria is a very rare familial condition due to defective phosphorylation of fructose to fructose-1-phosphate. The ingestion of large quantities of fructose, especially when liver function is impaired, may cause fructosuria. After taking 100 gm fructose about 10% of normal subjects will pass some fructose in the urine.

Galactosuria is an important means of early recognition of the harmful inborn error of metabolism galactosaemia. The deficiency of the enzyme UDP galactose-1-phosphate transferase results in failure to thrive from a few days after birth, followed by hepatosplenomegaly, jaundice, ascites and cataract. Mental retardation results unless milk is withdrawn from the diet.

Pentosuria, by contrast, is a benign congenital error of metabolism. The pentose excreted is L-xylulose. Transient pentosuria may follow the eating of large quantities of fruit, particularly cherries, plums and grapes. It has also been reported after morphine, salicylates and cortisone, which may be due to enzyme induction of glucoronic acid pathways.

In addition to false-positive glycosuria from other sugars, certain drugs are capable of confusing the result. The best known is the reducing agent ascorbic acid.

Enzyme test strips are more costly than the older Clinitest method but less prone to false-positive results. Since the latter are rarely a source of confusion convenience is a more appropriate argument in their favour. It may well be impossible to persuade users to adopt the term glucosuria.

REFERENCES

Alberti, K. G. M. M., Dornhorst, A. and Rowe, A. S. (1975) Metabolic rhythms in old age. *Biochem. Soc. Trans.*, **3**, 132–133.

Albutt, E. C., Nattrass, M. and Northam, B. E. (1985) Glucose tolerance test and glycosylated haemoglobin measurement for diagnosis of diabetes mellitus – an assessment of the criteria of the WHO Expert Committee on diabetes mellitus 1980. *Ann. Clin. Biochem.*, **22**, 67–73.

Benedict, S. R. (1911) The detection and estimation of glucose in urine. *J. A. M. A.*, **57**, 1193–1194.

Bennett, P. H., Rushforth, N. B., Miller, M. and LeCompte, P. M. (1976) Epidemiologic studies of diabetes in the Pima Indians. *Rec. Prog. Hormone Res.*, **32**, 333–371.

Bland, J. H. (1948) Renal glycosuria: a review of the literature and a report of four cases. *Ann. Intern. Med.*, **29**, 461–468.

Bose, R. K. C. (1907) Discussion on diabetes in the Tropics. *Br Med. J.*, **2**, 1051–1064.

Bouchardat, A. (1875) *De la glycosurie ou diabete sucré*, vol II, Germer-Baillière, Paris.

Burrin, J. M. and Price, C. P. (1985) Measurement of blood glucose. *Ann. Clin. Biochem.*, **22**, 327–342.

Conn, J. W. (1940) Interpretation of the glucose tolerance test. The necessity of a standard preparatory diet. *Am. J. Med. Sci.*, **199**, 555–564.

Dix, D., Cohen, P., Kingsley, S., *et al.* (1979) Glycohemoglobin and glucose tolerance tests compared as indicators of borderline diabetes. *Clin. Chem.*, **25**, 877–879.

Dods, R. F. and Bolmey, C. (1979) Glycosylated hemoglobin assay and oral glucose tolerance test compared for detection of diabetes mellitus. *Clin. Chem.*, **25**, 764–768.

Fine, J. (1965) Glucose content of normal urine. *Br. Med. J.*, **1**, 1209–1214.

FitzGerald, M. G. and Keen, H. (1964) Diagnostic classification of diabetes. *Br. Med. J.*, **1**, 1568.

Flynn, F. V., Harper, C. and De Mayo, P. (1953) Lactosuria and glycosuria in pregnancy and the puerperium. *Lancet*, **ii**, 698–704.

Frank, I. L. (1957) Diabetes mellitus in the texts of old Hindu medicine. *Am. J. Gastroenterol.*, **237**, 76–95.

Froesch, E. R. and Renold, A. E. (1956) Specific enzymatic determination of glucose in blood and urine using glucose oxidase. *Diabetes*, **5**, 1–6.

Himsworth, H. P. (1936) Diabetes mellitus. Its differentiation into insulin-sensitive and insulin-insensitive types. *Lancet*, **i**, 127–130.

Himsworth, H. P. and Kerr, R. B. (1939) Insulin-sensitive and insulin-insensitive types of diabetes mellitus. *Clin. Sci.*, **4**, 119–152.

Jarrett, R. J. and Al Sayegh, H. (1978) Impaired glucose tolerance: defining those at risk of diabetic complications. *Diabetologia*, **15**, 243.

Jarrett, R. J. and Keen, H. (1976) Hyperglycaemia and diabetes mellitus. *Lancet*, **ii**, 1009–1012.

Klemperer, G. (1896) Ueber regulatorische glycosurie und renal diabetes. *Berl. Klin. Woschenschr.*, **33**, 571.

Little, R. R., England, J. D., Wiedmeyer, H. M. *et al.* (1988) Relationship of glycosylated hemoglobin to oral glucose tolerance. Implications for diabetes screening. *Diabetes*, **37**, 60–64.

Lundbaek, K. (1962) Intravenous glucose tolerance as a tool in definition and diagnosis of diabetes mellitus. *Br. Med. J.*, **i**, 1507–1513.

McLean, H. (1922) *Modern Methods in the Diagnosis and Treatment of Glycosuria and Diabetes*, 3rd edn, Constable, London.

Marble, A. (1971) Current concepts in diabetes, in *Joslin's Diabetes Mellitus*, (eds A. Marble, P. White, R. F. Bradley and L. P. Krall), Lea & Febiger, Philadelphia, PA.

Mykkanen, L., Kuusisto, J. Pyorala, K. and Laakso, M. (1993) Cardiovascular disease risk factors as predictors of Type 2 (non-insulin-dependent) diabetes mellitus in elderly subjects. *Diabetologia*, **36**, 553–559.

National Diabetes Data Group (1979) Classification and diagnosis of diabetes mellitus and other causes of glucose intolerance. *Diabetes*, **28**, 1039–1057.

Price, C. P., Burrin, J. M., and Nattrass, M. (1988) Extra-laboratory blood glucose measurement: a policy statement. *Diabetic Med.*, **5**, 705–709.

Report of a Working Party Appointed by the College of General Practitioners (1962) A diabetes survey. *Br. Med. J.*, **i**, 1497–1503.

Reaven, G. M., Brand, R. J., Chen, Y-D. I. *et al.* (1993) Insulin resistance and insulin secretion are determinants of oral glucose tolerance in normal individuals. *Diabetes*, **42**, 1324–1332.

Samols, E. and Marks, V. (1965) Interpretation of the intravenous glucose test. *Lancet*, **i**, 462–463.

Samols, E., Marri, G. and Marks, V. (1965) Promotion of insulin secretion by glucagon. *Lancet*, **ii**, 415–416.

Saundby, R. (1891) *Lectures on Diabetes*, John Wright, Bristol.

Trousseau, A. (1870) *Lectures on Clinical Medicine* (translated from the edition of 1868), New Sydenham Society, London.

Walsh, C. H., Wright, A. D., Allbutt, E. and Pollock, A. (1977) The effect of cigarette smoking on blood sugar, serum insulin and non-esterified fatty acids in diabetic and non-diabetic subjects. *Diabetologia*, **13**, 491–494.

WHO (1980) WHO Expert Committee on Diabetes Mellitus, second report, *Technical Report Series 646*, World Health Organization, Geneva.

WHO (1985) Diabetes mellitus. Report of a WHO Study Group *Technical Report Series 727*, World Health Organization, Geneva.

Zimmet, P. (1979) Epidemiology of diabetes and its macrovascular manifestations in Pacific populations: the medical effects of social progress. *Diabetes Care*, **2**, 144–153.

Zimmet, P. and Whitehouse, S. (1978) Bimodality of fasting and two-hour glucose tolerance distributions in a micronesian population. *Diabetes*, **27**, 793–800.

AIMS OF TREATMENT

The short-term aim of diabetic treatment is to achieve for the patient, as far as possible, a state in which health is taken for granted and seldom obtrudes into consciousness. Obviously this is not too difficult when a minor modification to diet, usually some form of restriction, is all that is needed, but in the severe insulin-dependent patient it can never be fully achieved for there must be always at least some regard for the timing and quantity of meals. For this reason the initial period of education in diet and insulin administration is vital for it gives the patient a chance to take command of the diabetes so that the daily time-table becomes second nature. A failure to get down to this training is responsible for many poor results and avoidable complications.

The aims of treatment are summarized in Table 6.1. It is the fifth on this list, the avoidance of diabetic complications which gives greatest impetus to our efforts to achieve good control. It is pertinent, therefore, to review the evidence which indicates whether good diabetic control can influence the development of complications.

Table 6.1 Aims of treatment

1. The elimination of diabetic symptoms
2. The avoidance of side effects of treatment, notably hypoglycaemia
3. A normal life in society
4. The maintenance of good health for a reasonable span
5. The amelioration of complications

DOES GOOD CONTROL INFLUENCE THE DEVELOPMENT OF COMPLICATIONS?

In the assessment of the impact of diabetic control upon complications some definition of terms is necessary. The development and extent of complications may be theoretically influenced in a number of ways.

PRIMARY PREVENTION

Complications of diabetes would not occur if diabetes itself was prevented. To date there is no evidence that this can be achieved. It should be noted that in many publications the term 'primary prevention' is used erroneously to refer to the prevention of complications in a diabetic patient; that is secondary prevention.

SECONDARY PREVENTION

This refers to the situation where diabetes is manifest yet complications can be prevented by some aspect of management. As with primary prevention there is no evidence that this can be regarded as a realistic goal.

The case for such a hypothesis is non-proven. It is difficult to design studies to test the hypothesis. In insulin-dependent patients, where diagnosis and duration approximately coincide, any study would have to last beyond 10 years for a reasonable number of patients to develop complications. During this time many aspects of management would be likely to change making the study of one variable, e.g. blood glucose, open to confounding influences. In addition, for such a study to show secondary prevention it would have to carry on long after the 10 years for it to become clear that complications were being prevented rather than simply that the onset of complications was being delayed by the intervention.

In non-insulin-dependent patients the confounding factor is the time from onset to diagnosis, never known with certainty, and therefore the unknown of how far complications may have progressed subclinically before treatment is instigated.

DELAY IN PROGRESSION

To most people this is what is meant by control influencing complications – that good control delays perhaps the onset, and certainly the progression, of diabetic complications. The evidence for this is examined below.

REVERSIBILITY OF DIABETIC COMPLICATIONS

Whether established diabetic complications are reversible depends, to an extent, on definition. Long-term diabetic complications, such as neuropathy and retinopathy, are not reversed by improvements in blood glucose control. Indeed, I know of no evidence in support of the reversibility of long-term complications. At diagnosis of diabetes, however, slowing of nerve conduction times may be observed which improve with treatment of the hyperglycaemia. Is this an example of reversibility of diabetic complications? or is it that the state of the nerves at diagnosis does not constitute a true diabetic neuropathy? I am inclined to the latter view in exactly the same way as I would not consider blurred vision at diagnosis as a 'diabetic complication'.

GOOD DIABETIC CONTROL DOES DELAY THE PROGRESSION OF LONG-TERM COMPLICATIONS!

The evidence in support of this statement accrues from three distinct types of study:

retrospective clinical studies, intervention studies in diabetic animals and prospective clinical studies in man.

RETROSPECTIVE STUDIES IN MAN

Firstly, the retrospective study of diabetic care. Many such studies have been performed with a similar generalized pattern. Usually a physician in charge of a diabetic clinic who is either about to retire or has just retired reviews the medical records of a cohort of patients for whom he or she has cared. The patients may be divided into two groups, patients with or without complications. More ambitious classifications may even be attempted according to severity of complications or time from diagnosis of diabetes to detection of complications. The notes of each patient are then reviewed with the object of making a qualitative or semi-quantitative judgement of their degree of control.

Such studies are grossly flawed. In reality the central question posed by the physician is 'has my time in the clinic been well worth while?' In other words . . . all the time and effort which has gone into attempting to improve diabetic control in these patients . . . has it saved some of them from developing complications or resulted in a lesser severity of complications in those who achieved the goal of better control? . . . or was it all a waste of time? It would be a remarkable physician who was prepared for the results to show that the working life had been of little benefit.

More practical objections also exist. Anyone familiar with a busy diabetic clinic will agree on the difficulties of assessing long-term control before the introduction of glycated protein measurements. Most studies have adopted an approach based on a semi-quantitative assessment of control from repeated blood glucoses or even urine glucose measurements over the years. An accurate measure is probably impossible and the best that can be hoped for is a crude index which is arbitrarily defined as poor, moderate or good control.

Nevertheless the number of studies along these lines which have made it into the literature are legion and we should all be grateful to the distinguished American diabetologist Harvey Knowles (1964). He collated more than 300 of these studies and in a critical indictment concluded that most contained insufficient data for any conclusions. Of those containing sufficient data for analysis a relationship between the degree of control and the development (or severity) of complications was apparent in 50 studies; a relationship did not appear to exist in 25; and in a further 10 studies the data did not support either conclusion.

A further large retrospective study was published by Pirart (1978). In 4400 diabetic patients he found a clear relationship between diabetic control and the severity of retinopathy, nephropathy and neuropathy. This study has attracted considerable attention because of its size but it shares the drawbacks of earlier studies. The title of a prospective study is misleading. A prospective study of control and the development of complications has an *a priori* requirement for two levels of control throughout the study period and it is mandatory that patients are allocated randomly to one of the two levels. In other words the patient, at incorporation into the study, must have an equal chance of being assigned to good control or poor control. Without this randomization it is the patient and not the investigator who decides which group they end up in and we can never dismiss the concept of easy and difficult diabetes. In other words, patients predisposed to severe complications may have a type of diabetes which is difficult to control and a similar case could be made for a benign variant of diabetes. Pirart's study falls down in this crucial area and epitomizes the deficiencies of the retrospective study.

ANIMAL STUDIES

A second area which has contributed to the debate is studies of the development of complications in small animals. It is clear that animals made diabetic by alloxan or streptozotocin will develop tissue changes with time. There has been debate over the specificity of the ultrastructural change in comparison with the change in human diabetics (Siperstein *et al.*, 1977) but most workers now accept the similarities. Restoration of normal metabolism by insulin or, more convincingly, by islet cell transplantation leads to regression of tissue changes (Fox *et al.*, 1977; Slater *et al.*, 1978; Mauer *et al.*, 1974).

Despite the vast amount of animal work in diabetes, however, there is always a lingering doubt over its extrapolation to humans. Whether this is always justified can be debated but alloxan- or streptozotocin-induced diabetes may not be a terribly good model for a disease such as insulin-dependent diabetes or non-insulin-dependent diabetes, where there is a major genetic influence in the aetiology of the human condition.

PROSPECTIVE STUDIES

We might conclude that only prospective human studies will answer the question. There have been few attempts, although an increase is noted in recent years.

In the extensively investigated group of patients from the Pima Indian tribes of Arizona the percentage developing nephropathy as evidenced by proteinuria was twice as high in the group with 2-hour OGTT blood glucose in the range 11.1–16.6 mmol/l (200–300 mg/dl) compared with those in whom it was 7.8–8.9 mmol/l (140–160 mg/dl) (Kamenetzky *et al.*, 1974). Similarly, Jarrett and Keen (1976) found a relationship between 2-hour blood sugar levels and the presence and development of retinopathy. These studies are often quoted as evidence of a relationship between hyperglycaemia and complications and while they may have some predictive value they should not be confused with studies of long-term control of diabetes.

True prospective studies have been hampered by the belief that it is ethically unacceptable to allocate patents to a group where diabetic control is deliberately designated poor. The argument is made that since some people believe that good control has long-term beneficial effects anything less than a striving for this would be immoral. To exclude other influences, however, this prerequisite is mandatory. Tchobroutsky and his colleagues (Job *et al.*, 1976; Tchobroutsky, 1978), with typical French flair, circumvented these objections. They designated a poorly controlled group based on standard therapy and a well-controlled group of intensive therapy and this has become the template for prospective studies. The former group received a single daily injection of insulin, which was an accepted way of treating diabetes in their clinic at that time, and the latter twice or thrice daily insulin. Patients had to agree to participate before any allocation to a group was made. They observed that the mean yearly increase in the number of microaneurysms and the mean fasting blood glucose concentration were lower in the multiple injection group. Despite the random allocation to one or other group some shifting of patients between groups occurred, which was extensively criticized at the time the results were presented. The practical details of a study such as this are enormous and the outcome moderately convincing even if not totally sufficient to dispel all doubt in the debate.

Since the studies of Tchobroutsky and his colleagues others have attempted similar prospective trials, often utilizing newer methods of insulin delivery. There is a certain consistent view to emerge from the findings of these studies (Hanssen *et al.*, 1992; Dahl-Jorgensen *et al.*, 1994).

Continuous subcutaneous insulin infusion (CSII) to improve metabolic control delayed the progression of diabetic retinopathy (Dahl-

Jorgensen *et al.*, 1986; Reichard *et al.*, 1988) as did pancreas transplantation (Lawson *et al.*, 1982). With CSII there was a paradoxical and usually transient worsening of the retinal change in the early phase of treatment (Lauritzen, Frost-Larsen and Deckert, 1983; Dahl-Jorgensen *et al.*, 1986) and, in a exception to the overall picture of a beneficial effect, no evidence of a delaying effect could be found for the progression of retinopathy from the preproliferative to the proliferative stage.

There are conflicting data on the progression of established diabetic nephropathy with improved glycaemic control (Bending *et al.*, 1986) although it is clear that once creatinine levels are increased there is no effect of improving control (Viberti *et al.*, 1983). At the earlier stage of microalbuminuria evidence suggests that good control delays the progression from normal albumin excretion to microalbuminuria (Dahl-Jorgensen *et al.*, 1986; Reichard *et al.*, 1988) and may reduce the rate of microalbumin excretion (Viberti *et al.*, 1979).

The influence of control upon neuropathy is more difficult to assess. Impaired conduction times early in the disease may not represent true diabetic neuropathy while at the other end of the spectrum nerves that are terminally damaged will not be capable of recovery. Holman *et al.* (1983) found an improvement in vibration sensory threshold with 2 years of intensified management, but pancreas transplant did not result in any improvement in the late stage of distal polyneuropathy (Solders *et al.*, 1987). In the Oslo study 8 years of strict glycaemic control retarded the deterioration of motor and sensory nerve conduction velocities (Amthor *et al.*, 1994).

The question posed by these findings is of importance and is referred to above. If control and complications are related, is the effect upon development, progression or reversibility? Studies to date have concentrated upon delaying progression. Even with more sophisticated insulin delivery systems and better ways of assessing control the concept of good control until the development of complications is probably too difficult. As regards reversibility, it has not been shown to date that this is an achievable goal (Schiffrin, 1986).

A further point of concern is that, while studies have examined the impact of control upon microvascular complications and neuropathy, there is no suggestion that control of blood glucose can prevent, delay or reverse macrovascular disease (Nielsen and Ditzel, 1985; Knuiman *et al.*, 1986). This has caused some worry in the light of the argument for an association of hyperinsulinaemia and atheroma. Improving control in insulin-dependent diabetic patients carries with it the assumption that higher insulin doses will be necessary to achieve this goal. Higher doses of insulin, given into the peripheral circulation, must inevitably lead to higher circulating insulin concentrations. In turn, if there is any truth in the hyperinsulinaemia/atheroma hypothesis, this could lead to an increased risk of macrovascular disease. To put the argument crudely, improving control may save sight but not lives and indeed may truncate life! Even leaving aside the lack of support for the hypothesis, which has been lurking in the shadows of diabetes for more than 20 years with little in the way of further sightings, the argument is flawed at the outset. It is by no means certain that the only way to ensure an improvement in control would be by increasing the dose of insulin. Attention to diet, exercise, alterations in insulin sensitivity by these or other means could all improve control without an increase in insulin requirement.

The Diabetic Control and Complications Trial

The Diabetic Control and Complications Trial (DCCT) was initiated in the US in 1982 by the US National Institute of Diabetes, and Digestive and Kidney Disorders to examine the relationship of control and complications. Specifically the study was designed to answer two questions:

• Would intensive therapy for insulin-dependent diabetes prevent the development of diabetic retinopathy in patients without retinopathy at recruitment?
• Would intensive therapy for insulin-dependent diabetes delay the progress of retinopathy in patients with a mild degree of retinopathy at recruitment?

The first patients were enrolled in 1983 and the study expanded to a full-scale trial in 1985. Data collection was completed in 1993.

The main results were reported in a series of publications beginning in 1993 (Diabetes Control and Complications Trial Research Group, 1993).

In 29 centres, 1441 patients with insulin-dependent diabetes were recruited between 1983 and 1989. They were aged between 13 and 39 years, C-peptide deficient, and without hypertension, hypercholesterolaemia, severe diabetic complications or major medical condition. About half of them (726) had diabetes of 1–5 years duration, no retinopathy and normal urinary albumin excretion (< 40 mg/day) at recruitment. The remainder (715) had diabetes of 1–15 years duration, mild retinopathy and a urinary albumin excretion of < 200 mg/day. Patients were randomized to receive either intensive or conventional treatment.

Intensive treatment was by insulin administration three or four times daily, by subcutaneous injection or by continuous subcutaneous insulin administration with hospitalization for initiation of treatment. The doses of insulin were adjusted in response to the results of home blood glucose monitoring four times daily and a weekly 3 a.m. blood glucose measurement. Intensive education and support were also given with monthly clinic visits and at least weekly (sometimes daily) telephone contact with a health-care provider.

Conventional treatment was by once- or twice-daily insulin, daily blood or urine tests and 3-monthly review in the clinic.

The aims of treatment were different between groups. In the intensive group the aims were to maintain: preprandial blood glucose levels of 3.9–6.7 mmol/l (70–120 mg/dl); postprandial < 10 mmol/l (180 mg/dl); 3 a.m. blood glucose > 3.6 mmol/l (65 mg/dl); and HbA_{1c} measured monthly < 6.05%. In the conventional group an aim was to keep patients free of symptoms. The HbA_{1c} result was only made known if it was > 13.1%.

The main outcome was development of clinically significant diabetic retinopathy or progression of retinopathy as judged by fundal photography against a standard scale. Other complications and hypoglycaemic episodes were also monitored.

Mean HbA_{1c} fell in the intensive treatment group by about 2% but was unchanged in the conventional group. This separation was maintained for the duration of the trial. Mean blood glucose difference between the groups was of the order of 2.8 mmol/l (50 mg/dl). Follow-up was for a mean of 6.5 years with a range from 3–9 years. In what was a quite remarkable achievement for this type of study 99% completed the study!

In the group without retinopathy at entry the incidence curves for the development of retinopathy were similar up to 3 years. Thereafter the curves separated and from 5 years onwards the cumulative incidence was approximately 50% less in the intensive treatment group. Over a mean of 6 years of follow-up retinopathy developed in 6.6% of the intensively treated group and 24.1% of the conventionally treated group. Intensive therapy achieved a risk reduction of 76%. In the group with retinopathy at entry the figures were 21.2% (intensive) and 40.6% (conventional). The risk reduction for progression was 54%. Intensive treatment also halved the risk of developing proliferative retinopathy and of receiving photocoagulation. With regard to other outcomes intensive treatment reduced the risk of progression to, or of, microalbuminuria by 34% and 45% respectively, and clinical neuropathy by 69% and 57%.

There was no increase in cardiovascular events in the intensive treatment groups and if anything the trend was towards a reduction. Similarly, there was no difference in treatment groups for quality of life, cognitive function or emotional assessments.

The major difference in side effects was in hypoglycaemic episodes. Intensive treatment increased hypoglycaemic episodes threefold (Diabetes Control and Complications Trial Research Group, 1991).

Weight gain was a problem in the intensive treatment group. At 5 years patients in this group had gained a mean of 4.6 kg more than patients receiving conventional treatment.

These conclusive findings should bring to an end the uncertainty over the role of diabetic control in the development of complications. An important message is that any improvement of diabetic control leads to beneficial effects in reducing complications. Conversely, the risk of severe hypoglycaemia increased continuously with lower glycated haemoglobin levels.

The legacy of this quite magnificent study is how best to apply the results to everyday clinical management (Santiago, 1993). It is self-evident that with a 99% follow-up rate over this length of time the patients were highly motivated. The majority (96%) were caucasian. On average they had spent 14 years in education and the intelligence quotient in both groups averaged 113. Over the period of the study 633 physicians were involved! All conspire to make the prospect of translating the results into the diabetic clinic a daunting prospect.

CRITERIA OF DIABETIC CONTROL

The hallmark of diabetes is an elevated blood glucose concentration. Controlling diabetes therefore means lowering the degree of hyperglycaemia. The degree to which success is achieved in this aim can be measured by blood glucose profiles or surrogate measures. Recent years have seen a major advance in assessment of control with the development of assays for glycated proteins. These estimations can give an overall assessment of diabetic control in the preceding weeks before the blood sample is drawn. Other measurements sometimes used as secondary measures of long-term control, such as lipoproteins, are of some value, although changes in them may be inconsistent and affected by factors other than diabetes.

In the past some have advocated 'clinical' rather than 'chemical' control, suggesting that hyperglycaemia and glycosuria can be ignored if the patient is free from the symptoms of diabetes. The objection to this point of view is a simple one. It is manifestly impossible to judge from what the patient says whether the symptoms of diabetes are present or not. Sometimes the symptoms are not recognized, sometimes they are deliberately concealed, but the story is unreliable in just those cases in which it is of the greatest importance. Unfortunately loss of weight, which is at least a measurable manifestation, is a rather late indication of poor control and is no substitute for a record of blood and/or urine tests. Often the patient who tests blood or urine regularly and is accustomed to a good result at the start of each day is put on the alert by finding hyperglycaemia or considerable glycosuria two or three mornings running. This leads to the correction of errors in diet or an early visit to the doctor before things have got out of hand. Conversely a patient who fails to test may drift imperceptibly into a state of grossly uncontrolled diabetes with damaging infection or acute neuropathy as a consequence.

Clearly a purely 'clinical' assessment of control is wholly unsatisfactory in this day and age except in a very few patients in whom other problems outweigh any thought of controlling the diabetes. For the majority of patients the production and maintenance of normoglycaemia should be the aim and our standard of good control. In the case of treatment with diet alone or oral drugs it is reasonable to expect a normal blood glucose at any time of the day and to think of an increase or change of treatment if the patient persistently fails to achieve it. When insulin is used some relaxation of the standard is usually necessary because we know from experience that attempting to obtain and maintain euglycaemia throughout the day is excessively difficult and carries a risk of hypoglycaemia.

Obviously there are difficulties in applying such a standard; not least the difficulty of assessment which results from the impossibility of obtaining blood samples at all hours of the day and night; but also of maintaining preprandial and postprandial normoglycaemia with current insulin regimens. In a young patient in apparently good health it is perfectly possible to record a blood glucose of 4 mmol/l (72 mg/dl) a few minutes before the midday meal and another of 15 mmol/l (270 mg/dl) one hour after it. Which of these represents the state of diabetic control?

Difficulties in applying this standard universally among the patient population and the well-nigh impossible task of achieving it in certain groups of patients have led many authorities to devise alternative standards of control. Marble (1964) set the following criteria:

1. During treatment of non-insulin-dependent patients with diet or oral hypoglycaemic agents:
   (a) good control – no glycosuria; the majority of blood glucose values no more than 6.1 mmol/l (110 mg/dl) before meals.
   (b) fair control – glycosuria in 24 hours should not exceed 5% of the total carbohydrate intake; the majority of blood glucose values no more than 7.2 mmol/l (130 mg/dl) before meals;

Table 6.2 Targets for metabolic control

	Good	Acceptable	Poor
Fasting blood glucose			
(mmol/l)	4.4–6.7	< 7.8	> 7.8
(mg/dl)	80–120	< 140	> 140
Postprandial blood glucose			
(mmol/l)	4.4–8.9	< 10.0	> 10.0
(mg/dl)	80–160	< 180	> 180
Glycosylated proteins	< mean + 2 s.d.	< mean + 4 s.d.	> mean + 4 s.d.
Urine glucose (%)	0	< 0.5	> 0.5
Total cholesterol			
(mmol/l)	< 5.2	< 6.5	> 6.5
(mg/dl)	< 200	< 250	> 250
Fasting triglycerides			
(mmol/l)	< 1.7	< 2.2	> 2.2
(mg/dl)	< 150	< 200	> 200
HDL-cholesterol			
(mmol/l)	> 1.1	> 0.9	< 0.9
(mg/dl)	> 40	> 35	< 35

urine free from ketone bodies; serum cholesterol below 6.5 mmol/l (250 mg/dl).

2. During treatment of insulin-dependent patients with insulin therapy:
   (a) good control – glycosuria in 24 hours should not exceed 5% of the total carbohydrate intake; no ketonuria; the majority of blood glucose values no more than 7.2 mmol/l (130 mg/dl) before a meal (3 hours or more after the last meal); serum cholesterol below 6.5 mmol/l (250 mg/dl);
   (b) fair control – glycosuria in 24 hours not exceeding 10% of the total carbohydrate intake; blood glucose level no more than 8.3 mmol/l (150 mg/dl) before meals.

Some standard such as this is implied by the terms 'good' or 'fair' in most publications that refer to control. It must be emphasized that over a long period this judgement is no more than an estimate and often a very inaccurate one.

A recent attempt to define standards of diabetic control has come from Alberti and Gries (1988) writing on behalf of the European non-insulin-dependent diabetes mellitus policy group. They set targets for biochemical monitoring, although with the proviso that they should be individualized according to the specific objectives of treatment in a particular patient. It should be stressed that these targets are for patients with non-insulin-dependent diabetes (Table 6.2).

THE DIABETIC CLINIC

The common nature of diabetes mellitus in the general population and the consequences of long-term complications, demoralizing for the patient and costly for the nation, demand some attempt at organizing care within a structured format. Except where payment for service directly is involved, either by the patient or an insurer, the format that has evolved in the UK has traditionally centred around the hospital diabetic clinic.

Before the discovery of insulin there was little to offer a patient with diabetes except advice on dieting. This was in the province of general medicine and specialists in diabetes were few. When insulin was made available the situation was immediately transformed. Diabetics could be maintained in fair health by rather elaborate treatment. The numbers attending hospital for advice and supervision mounted rapidly and the outpatient physicians were unwilling or unable to give up the considerable time involved. As a result diabetic clinics were set up, primarily, I suspect, in order to get rid of these unwanted patients rather than to provide them with expert care. In some instances the clinic was under the care of a consultant physician but in some, a specialist in a limited but not necessarily related field, such as venereology, was put in charge and in a few the future care was carried out by a biochemist with no medical degree. All things considered diabetic clinics in Britain were highly successful in providing a necessary service often only grudgingly recognized by the hospital.

The clinic at King's College Hospital, London, under the forceful leadership of Dr R. D. Lawrence, was a striking example, and the widespread adoption of his eminently sensible methods of treatment was all to the good. In some ways it is unfortunate that diabetes does not fit easily into any specialty and has never been at home with other disorders of metabolism or with endocrinology. The main reason is the size of the diabetic problem, which is apt to oust all other work unless the intake of patients is strictly controlled; no easy matter. As a result the clinic is apt to become large and unwieldy, comparatively junior assistants have to be employed to get through the work and the way is open for those critics who claim that diabetes is just a result of empire building. Most of the work, they add, could be carried out by the general practitioner.

As to this point, most physicians who run diabetic clinics would be glad to know of any satisfactory method by which patients could be returned to the care of their own doctor. At present it seems that it would require a far stronger liaison between hospital and practitioner than time permits.

Table 6.3 The objectives of a diabetic clinic

1. The creation of a skilled team, including physicians, nurses, health visitors, medical social workers, dieticians and chiropodists
2. The education of the patients
3. The education of those who have to look after diabetics; general practitioners, district nurses
4. The care of diabetic patients in other major illness and with complications requiring hospital care, e.g. gangrene
5. Research into special aspects of diabetes
6. The provision of material for research by other specialists, e.g. renal disease
7. Therapeutic trials

The justification for diabetic clinics lies in the objectives listed in Table 6.3.

This list leaves out the controversial routine supervision of diabetic patients, but with or without this activity it could be argued that a good diabetic clinic achieves more for the health of the people than any other department in a general hospital.

Unfortunately the laudable and theoretical aims of a diabetic clinic tend to be swamped by the routine supervision of diabetic control and in many centres the hospital diabetic clinic is firmly ensconced in an era of stagnation. The aims and justification of the traditional diabetic clinic are no longer tenable without revision, given the advances which have occurred in diabetic management. Some 30 years ago treatment of diabetic retinopathy was limited and ineffective and the detection of retinopathy was an intellectual exercise on the part of the doctor. With effective treatment has come the requirement for regular screening of eyes in a systematic way, early detection of retinopathy, and referral and treatment at the appropriate stage.

Management of end-stage renal disease in the diabetic was also minimal, with the approach that little could influence the rate of downward progression. Today diabetic patients benefit from dialysis and transplantation, as do their non-diabetic counterparts, and the detection of microalbuminuria and the management of hypertension have consequently increased in importance.

The one basic belief of the traditional diabetic clinic was that control of blood glucose made a difference to the development of complications and the clinic was organized with assessing and improving control as a major, if not the only aim. The special skill of the doctor in the diabetic clinic lay in the manipulation of therapy, in particular the titration of insulin dose to improve control. This urgency regarding the improvement of control has not been diminished by more recent evidence confirming the role of metabolic control in the rate of progression of diabetic complications. The case is almost watertight and it is widely and loudly publicized. As a result it is pushed to the forefront as the *raison d'être* of the diabetic clinic. Patients sense the importance from the publicity, other health professionals see it as the main aim of education, and junior medical staff in the clinic, faced with the most recent glycosylated protein, clinic blood glucose measurement or books of blood or urine tests, focus upon control, altering therapy in a minor way and seeking early review of the patient to see if improvement results. The early review reinforces the patients' view of control and increases the workload of the clinic to a point where other goals are diminished.

Throughout this cycle we cannot display sufficient honesty to admit that obtaining and maintaining normoglycaemia is a sheer impossibility in the majority of patients who depend upon insulin, yet we set the unattainable goal. It is only when directly questioned by the frustrated patient that we admit the limitations of present-day insulin regimens. It is not in our nature, however, to set lower goals and while this illogical situation exists there will always be too much work for all but the most recently established clinic.

The diabetic clinic has become the site for dietitians dispensing diets which few patients follow, nurses educating by dispensation of knowledge that few comply with, and doctors manipulating doses with marginal and temporary effect upon control. All conspire in the unquestioned belief that attendance at the diabetic clinic is important in the degree of control achieved.

The response of some to this critique of the traditional diabetic clinic has been to discard it. Others have sustained a more rational approach. It is laudable that time has been made to think of alternatives, for many were so busy doing the work they had no time to stand back and question the achievement. Whether suggested alternatives really meet the requirements may be questioned. Our response has been to work within the clinic format, setting time aside specifically for particular functions. Annual review for the detection of complications; management of patients with diabetic complications; diagnosis; all have time set aside for them in our clinic and these times are fiercely guarded. The scheme is still in its infancy but appears to work well, to the benefit of the patient. The main difficulty was in finding time to think of our aims and design a new approach. While the final result would not be applicable to every clinic the approach – of sitting down and asking what are we trying to achieve – is mandatory for every clinic prepared to face the challenge of diabetic patient management rather than blood glucose management.

MANAGEMENT OF THE DIABETIC PATIENT

Anton Chekhov was once asked by an actor at a rehearsal of *The Seagull* how his part should be played, and after a long pause replied 'as well as possible'. The same answer might serve for the question of how diabetes should be managed. There is no formula. Technically correct treatment can be offset by the defects of rigid and unimaginative care of the individual. Conversely, inadequate treatment can be compensated to a great extent by wise and perceptive management.

Nevertheless a good deal may be achieved by organization at every level. A certain routine in the continuing care of the patient is desirable and need not make it impersonal. A brief interview which makes no attempt to penetrate their reticence allows careless or fearful patients to escape without revealing their true situation and gives support to the desire to put off the day of reckoning; it confirms the intelligent and experienced diabetic in the belief that a visit to the doctor or the clinic is a waste of time and that she would do better to look after his/her diabetes by him/herself. The patient may be right in thinking so but s/he suffers from one severe handicap – s/he has experience of treating only one patient and that is not a guide to every aspect of diabetes management. The following routine is relevant to specialist and non-specialist alike, since it assumes no special knowledge of diabetes on the part of the doctor.

FIRST VISIT

Diagnosis of diabetes is the most important part of the first attendance in a previously undiagnosed patient. The history records the presence or absence of thirst, polyuria, wasting and fatigue, together with any other presenting symptoms such as pruritus vulvae, balanitis or neuritic pain. A family history of diabetes may be elicited and in women the obstetric history, with birth weights, is often interesting.

At the beginning of the examination weight and height are measured and at least one pupil is dilated. We have done this as a routine in thousands of new patients without mishap and unless the pupil is dilated it is commonly impossible to observe details of the retina. The physical examination pays special attention to the visual acuities, blood pressure, and the state of the feet, notably the foot pulses and skin sensation. Enlargement of the liver may arouse suspicion of haemochromatosis. At the end of the examination

the pupil will be sufficiently dilated for a full examination of the retina. If retinopathy is observed both pupils must be dilated to assess the extent.

Once the suspicion of diabetes is aroused the urine or blood is tested. A positive urine result indicates a significant (more than 0.1%) glycosuria which demands investigation. Tests for acetone and protein are carried out. Blood glucose is measured using any one of the rapid methods available which provides an immediate result. A result of over 11.1 mmol/l (200 mg/dl) in conjunction with a typical history is confirmatory evidence sufficient for treatment to be started.

It is debatable whether any investigations other than blood glucose estimation and urine testing need to be done at this stage. Of course, if clinically indicated a chest X-ray, ECG, full blood count and biochemical profile may be helpful. It is surprising how often these baseline results are helpful in the future but I doubt that doing them solely for a baseline is a justifiable reason.

The first visit ends with initiation of treatment (Chapter 4). This should include the dietary advice, a prescription of oral agents or insulin where appropriate and an initial educational package.

SUBSEQUENT VISITS

At each attendance the patient is asked to bring one or more samples of urine, labelled with the time in each case. It is usually wise to collect a further sample at the hospital or surgery and this can be correlated with a blood sample taken about the same time.

The weight is then recorded. At the interview the symptoms of diabetes are specifically asked for whether the patient complains of them or not. A home record of blood or urine tests is often a helpful focus for discussion. In insulin-taking patients it is most important to probe for possible hypoglycaemic attacks because patients are so often reticent about them. In addition the technical problems of insulin injection can be mentioned. Occasionally it is helpful if the means whereby insulin is administered is produced to confirm that it is in sound condition. It is much easier to talk about diet problems if the details have been recorded at the first attendance.

ANNUAL REVIEW

In recent years it has become fashionable to insist that each diabetic patient should have an examination annually. Quite where this dictum has originated from is unclear. Nevertheless the call for an annual review has been taken up by patients' groups and there is some pressure from the consumer to participate in this. The physical examination follows the lines outlined above for the first attendance – visual acuity and dilatation of the pupils; examination of the lower limbs for peripheral pulses, reflexes and vibration sense, and inspection of the feet for overall standard of care; not forgetting the measurement of blood pressure. Some degree of biochemically annual review can also be undertaken at this time, including measurement of cholesterol and triglycerides, creatinine and microalbuminuria.

There is no doubt that this annual examination reveals defective aspects of management at times. Elderly patients are identified who have been battling on cutting their own toe/ nails despite impaired vision and loss of manual dexterity. Also, the first detection of diabetic retinopathy is always of importance. It is not always clear, however, what action should be taken with some of the other findings. Absent reflexes or foot pulses alert the doctor and patient to the need for greater foot care but not necessarily conduction studies or arteriography. Junior doctors who are perfectly competent to detect the abnormalities do not always have the breadth of clinical experience to interpret the findings in the light of required action or inaction.

RECORDS

One of my teachers used to divide doctors into two groups – those who made notes and bad doctors. There may be exceptions but anyone who has to make his/her way through the records of a diabetic patient, extending perhaps over 20 or 30 years, will be inclined to agree. One cannot but admire the capacity of some doctors to carry so much information about so many patients in their heads without a single note committed to paper, but one cannot commend it. None of us can be available on every occasion to perform a feat of memory and none of us is immortal.

The documents used at the Diabetic Clinic of the Birmingham General Hospital are illustrated in Figures 6.1 and 6.2. The record of first attendance is sufficiently simple to be completed with ease at the time of the examination. It is not so easy to devise a method of adding the notes of subsequent attendances in such a way that they produce a coherent account of the diabetic odyssey. The sheets (Figure 6.2) ensure that every visit is entered and in the right order.

This provides a graphic record of weight, blood glucose and insulin dosage, which can be very valuable when making a rapid assessment of the trends over an extended period. Our continuing record, and I suspect that similar charts can be found around the world, concentrate upon urinanalysis, weight and blood glucose concentration. Urinalysis remains a valuable guide both to treatment and to developing nephropathy. Time and again the development of intermittent proteinuria followed by constant proteinuria can be observed, prompting alterations in approach.

Weight, presented graphically, is a most useful guide to treatment. Gain in weight with poor control often indicates poor dietary adherence while poor control with weight loss is likely to be the development of insulin deficiency. Of course, other reasons for these observations may be present, such as congestive cardiac failure or a neoplasm, but

HMR4b/WRG 4003

DIABETIC   CLINIC

RACE

FAMILY HISTORY

PREVIOUS ILLNESSES

ONSET

SYMPTOMS

THIRST

POLYURIA

WASTING

PRURITUS

FATIGUE

PRESENT CONDITION

EYES

OFFSPRING

STILL BIRTHS
LIVE BIRTHS
BIRTH WEIGHTS

DRUGS

MAXIMUM WEIGHT

GLYCOSURIA DISCOVERED

Fig. 6.1 Patient record sheet for a first attendance at the diabetic clinic (as used at the General Hospital, Birmingham, UK).

University Hospital Birmingham

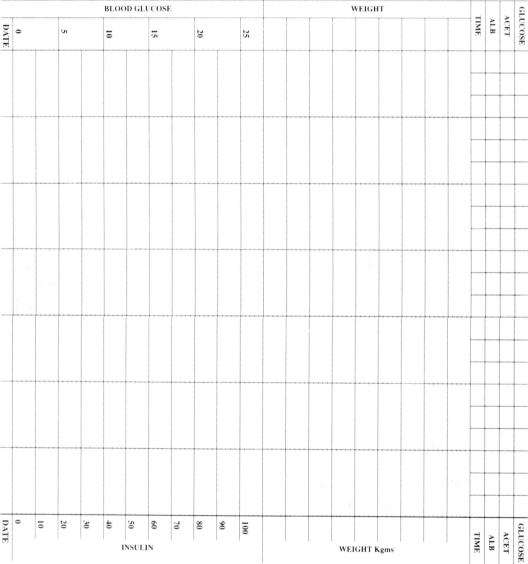

Fig. 6.2　Follow-up record of attendance in the diabetic clinic.

these do not detract from the usefulness of weight measurement. I would exhort those doctors intending to establish, or in the process of establishing, diabetic clinics to incorporate a graph of weight.

Our record sheets have not adapted well to developments in diabetic care. The focus of the subsequent visits section remains firmly lodged in diabetic control and yet we have not introduced a graphical record of glycated protein results. Nor have we achieved any means of a formal recording of the findings on annual review. These continue to be written in longhand.

A further point worthy of mention is the release of clinic records to other departments or hospitals. With a central storage of records there is little that can be done to supervise this procedure and the clinic doctor must accept the inevitability of missing patient notes. Even in our own clinic, where records of diabetic patients are kept separately, we cannot deny our colleagues the use of the full notes. We can ensure that photocopies are made of the diabetic clinic record for release, allowing us to retain the original, which may gain several entries before the full set of notes returns. Any expense of materials or personnel is surely justified when weighed against the uselessness of a patient visit without records and the justifiable anger of the patient with this situation.

BIOCHEMICAL ASSESSMENT IN CLINIC

Blood glucose measurement

A major question mark lies over the value of random blood glucose measurement in the clinic. It is quite clear that the result is influenced by a number of factors, few of which escape the notice of the patient.

Obviously the time of the last meal is important and for an afternoon clinic a patient may well omit lunch, a fact that is rarely volunteered but which can be elicited by a direct question; results in our clinic show

an unusual improvement in one quarter of patients with the Muslim festival of Ramadan; the number of patients who only remember to take their tablets for the 2–3 days before a clinic appointment can only be guessed at; and there can be no doubt from our 12-hour studies that the time of the clinic influences the results obtained, an afternoon clinic producing better blood glucose readings than a morning one.

The alternative to a random or postprandial blood glucose measurement in clinic is to measure fasting blood glucose. This has considerable advantage for non-insulin-dependent diabetic patients, where there is reproducibility from day to day (Holman and Turner, 1977). My prejudice against asking patients to attend fasting undoubtedly stems from working in a big city. The thought of 100 diabetic patients criss-crossing the city by public transport or private car while fasting is not one that is instantly appealing.

Despite these limitations on its value we cannot bring ourselves to dispense totally with clinic blood glucose measurement and there are clear-cut uses for the data, but as an assessment of overall control it leaves a lot to be desired. Fortunately, other methods of assessment have evolved. A number of methods have been described that allow the patient to take a blood sample at home for subsequent measurement in the hospital laboratory. A drop of capillary blood from a finger prick can be placed on filter paper and dried (Burrin *et al.*, 1981) or drawn into a special container with diluent (Holman *et al.*, 1985). This useful technique does allow fasting blood glucose to be estimated without the anxieties outlined above.

Home blood glucose monitoring

More useful is the technique of home blood glucose monitoring. Independently Tattersall and colleagues (Walford *et al.*, 1978) in Nottingham and Sonksen, Judd and Lowy (1978) in London described the usefulness of this procedure as an aid to diabetic management. Perhaps for the first time they indicated that not only the super-intelligent patient had a valuable contribution to make to management. Since then measurement of blood glucose, at home or work or play, by visually read strips or by the use of a meter has largely replaced home urine testing. Its success depends not only upon increased education and interest of the patient but upon a confidence to participate actively in therapy decisions. Without this latter the results are little more valuable than the endless books of urine tests that patients accumulated. Potentially, however, it can provide reassurance and confidence to make changes in insulin dose.

Patients should be instructed to measure at particular times of the day and record the results. Some enthusiasts suggest 11 times per day, including samples in the middle of the night. Others will recommend an occasional test, perhaps when there seems something awry. There has to be a sensible balance between these two viewpoints. Four times per day before meals and bed, on two days per week – a working day and a leisure day – provides about as much information as can be assimilated at review. The patient must be provided with sufficient information to allow logical alteration of insulin dose and encouraged to use this information, often on a try-it-and-see basis.

Glycated proteins

The chemistry of glycated proteins is discussed elsewhere in this volume. Although several applications of their use have been suggested the monitoring of diabetic control is the only area where a definite role exists for measurement.

Synthesis of proteins or glycoproteins is under enzymatic control in the majority of instances in the human body. Reducing sugars such as glucose will react non-enzymatically, that is, post-translational.

Haemoglobin A_{1c}, a post-translation modification of HbA_0 was noted to be raised in the blood of diabetic patients by Rahbar (1968). In subsequent studies it was shown that biosynthesis is slow, takes place over the life of the red cell and, importantly, the amount synthesized is dependent upon the prevailing degree of glycaemia. When this is taken in the light of the life of the erythrocyte as 120 days, the level of HbA_{1c} becomes an indirect marker of the level of glycaemia integrated over the life-span of red cells. Thus it reflects glycaemic control over the 6 weeks before the sample is taken. Normal levels are of the order of 5–9%, depending upon methodology, and in particular whether a labile fraction is removed before analysis and whether HbA_{1c} is specifically measured or total HbA_1, which also contains HbA_{1a} and HbA_{1b}. Falsely low levels can be obtained, the commonest being due to a predominance of young erythrocytes as in haemolytic anaemia. Presumably because they have been exposed to glucose for a lesser time, young erythrocytes contain less HbA_{1c} than older red cells. Patients with haemoglobinopathies and persistent HbF also give abnormal values. Levels of glycated haemoglobin show a good correlation with other measures of control and have provided a useful adjunct to monitoring therapy.

Measurement of other glycated proteins have also contributed, particularly serum fructosamine. Fructosamine is not a single protein entity but is rather a name for a cumulative protein, one of the main constituents being albumin. It (or they) is glycated in a similar way to haemoglobin but reflects glycaemia in the 2 weeks preceding blood sampling. It has to be more useful, therefore, in pregnancy, when the 6-week measure is too slow to indicate that change is necessary. It is distinctly less useful in conditions where albumin turnover is increased. The major time for this to occur in the diabetic population is when the patient has proteinuria.

Of course, while glycated proteins can indicate how well or how badly a patient is doing they do not give any indication on how to improve control. For this the day-by-day pattern of blood glucose measurement is necessary.

Studies of glycated haemoglobin concentrations in various clinics have confirmed the poor control of most insulin-dependent diabetic patients. Since it is an integrated measure of control glycated proteins are less open to manipulation of either clinic blood glucose or home blood glucose results. In the latter instance big discrepancies have been noted between patients' own recording of their results and readings retained in a memory recorder. The psychology of this situation, deliberate misrecording of results or deliberate manipulation of behaviour to ensure a good blood glucose reading in the clinic, has been underinvestigated. It is tempting to say that it is hardly worth detecting since even discovery is unlikely to change behaviour. Yet these patents will still adopt the attitudes of 'the doctor knows best' and will accept advice even to the extent of insulin treatment.

REFERENCES

Alberti, K. G. M. M. and Gries, F. A. (1988) Management of non-insulin-dependent diabetes mellitus in Europe: a consensus view. *Diabetic Med.*, **5**, 275–281.

Amthor, K. F., Dahl-Jorgensen, K., Berg, T. J. *et al.* (1994) The effect of 8 years of strict glycaemic control on peripheral nerve function in IDDM patients: the Oslo study. *Diabetologia*, **37**, 579–584.

Bending, J. J., Viberti, G. C., Watkins, P. J. and Keen, H. (1986) Intermittent clinical proteinuria and renal function in diabetes: evolution and the effect of glycaemic control. *Br. Med. J.*, **292**, 83–86.

Burrin, J. M., Worth, R., Laws, S. and Alberti, K. G. M. M. (1981) Simple filter paper method for home monitoring of blood glucose, lactate, and 3-hydroxybutyrate. *Ann. Clin. Biochem.*, **18**, 243–247.

Dahl-Jorgensen, K., Brinchmann-Hansen, O., Hanssen, K. F. *et al.* (1986) Effect of near-normoglycaemia for two years on progression of early diabetic retinopathy, nephropathy, and neuropathy: the Oslo study. *Br. Med. J.*, **293**, 1195–1199.

Dahl-Jorgensen, K., Brinchmann-Hansen, O., Bangstad, H. J. and Hanssen, K. F. (1994) Blood glucose control and microvascular complications – what do we do now? *Diabetologia*, **37**, 1172–1177.

Diabetes Control and Complications Trial Research Group (1991) Epidemiology of severe hypoglycemia in the Diabetes Control and Complications Trial. *Am. J. Med.*, **90**, 450–459.

Diabetes Control and Complications Trial Research Group (1993) The effect of intensive treatment of diabetes on the development and progression of long-term complications in insulin-dependent diabetes mellitus. *N. Engl. J. Med.*, **329**, 977–986.

Fox, C. J., Darby, S. C., Ireland, J. T. and Sonksen, P. H. (1977) Blood glucose control and glomerular capillary basement membrane thickening in experimental diabetes. *Br. Med. J.*, **2**, 605–607.

Hanssen, K. F., Bangstad, H. J., Brinchmann-Hansen, O. and Dahl-Jorgensen, K. (1992) Blood glucose control and diabetic microvascular complications: long-term effects of near-normoglycaemia. *Diabetic Med.*, **9**, 697–705.

Holman, R. R. and Turner, R. C. (1977) Diabetes: The quest for basal normoglycaemia. *Lancet*, **i**, 469–474.

Holman, R. R., Dornan, T. L., Mayon-White, V. *et al.* (1983) Prevention of deterioration of renal and sensory-nerve function by more intensive management of insulin-dependent diabetic patients. *Lancet*, **i**, 204–208.

Holman, R. R., Rees, S. G., Moore, J. C. *et al.* (1985) Patient-orientated metered capillary blood collection. *Ann. Clin. Biochem.*, **22**, 141–143.

Jarrett, R. J. and Keen, H. (1976) Hyperglycaemia and diabetes mellitus. *Lancet*, **ii**, 1009–1012.

Job, D., Eschwege, E., Guyot-Argenton, C. *et al.* (1976) Effect of multiple daily insulin injections on the course of diabetic retinopathy. *Diabetes*, **25**, 463–469.

Kamenetzky, S. A., Bennett, P. H., Dippe, S. E. *et al.* (1974) A clinical and histologic study of diabetic nephropathy in the Pima Indians. *Diabetes*, **23**, 61–68.

Knowles, H. C. (1964) The problem of the relation of the control of diabetes to the development of vascular disease. *Trans. Am. Clin. Climatol. Assoc.*, **76**, 142–147.

Knuiman, M. W., Welborn, T. A., McCann, V. J. *et al.* (1986) Prevalence of diabetic complications in relation to risk factors. *Diabetes*, **35**, 1332–1339.

Lauritzen, T., Frost-Larsen, H. W. and Deckert, T. (1983) Effect of 1-year of near-normal blood glucose levels on retinopathy in insulin-dependent diabetics. *Lancet*, **i**, 200–204.

Lawson, P. M., Champion, M. C., Canny, C. *et al.* (1982) Continuous subcutaneous insulin infusion (CSII) does not prevent progression of proliferative and preproliferative retinopathy. *Br. J. Opthalmol.*, **66**, 762–766.

Marble, A. (1964) *Diabetes Mellitus*, American Diabetes Association, New York.

Mauer, S. M., Sutherland, D. E. R., Steffes, M. W. *et al.* (1974) Pancreatic islet transplantation. Effects on the glomerular lesions of experimental diabetes in the rat. *Diabetes*, **23**, 748–753.

Nielsen, N. V. and Ditzel, J. (1985) Prevalence of macro- and microvascular disease as related to glycosylated hemoglobin in Type I and II diabetic subjects. An epidemiologic study in Denmark. *Horm. Metab. Res.*, **17**(suppl), 19–23.

Pirart, J. (1978) Diabetes mellitus and its degenerative complications: a prospective study of 4400 patients observed between 1947 and 1973. *Diabetes Care*, **1**, 168–188; 252–263.

Rahbar, S. (1968) An abnormal hemoglobin in the red cells of diabetics. *Clin. Chem. Acta*, **22**, 296–298.

Reichard, P., Britz, A., Cars, I. *et al.* (1988) The Stockholm diabetes intervention study (SDIS): 18 months results. *Acta Med. Scand.*, **224**, 115–122.

Santiago, J. V. (1993) Lessons from the Diabetes Control and Complications Trial. *Diabetes*, **42**, 1549–1554.

Schiffrin, A. (1986) Reversibilty of diabetic complications, in *Recent Advances in Diabetes* 2, (ed. M. Nattrass), Churchill Livingstone, Edinburgh, p. 195–208.

Siperstein, M. D., Foster, D. W., Knowles, H. C. *et al.* (1977) Control of blood glucose and diabetic vascular disease. *N. Engl. J. Med.*, **296**, 1060–1063.

Slater, D. N., Mangnall, Y., Smythe, A. *et al.* (1978) Neonatal islet cell transplantation in the diabetic rat: effect on the renal complications. *J. Pathol.*, **124**, 117–124.

Solders, G., Wilczek, H., Gunnarsson, R. *et al.* (1987) Effects of combined pancreatic and renal transplantation on diabetic neuropathy: a two-year follow-up study. *Lancet*, **ii**, 1232–1235.

Sonksen, P. H., Judd, S. L. and Lowy, C. (1978) Home monitoring of blood-glucose. *Lancet*, **i**, 729–732.

Tchobroutsky, G. (1978) Relation of diabetic control to development of microvascular complications. *Diabetologia*, **15**, 143–152.

Viberti, G. C., Bilous, R. W., Mackintosh, D. *et al.* (1983) Long-term correction of hyperglycaemia and progression of renal failure in insulin dependent diabetes. *Br. Med. J.*, **286**, 598–602.

Viberti, G. C., Pickup, J. C., Jarrett, R. J. and Keen, H. (1979) Effect of control of blood glucose on urinary excretion of albumin and B2-microglobulin in insulin-dependent diabetes. *N. Engl. J. Med.*, **300**, 638–641.

Walford, S., Gale, E. A. M., Allison, S. P. and Tattersall, R. B. (1978) Self-monitoring of blood glucose. *Lancet*, **i**, 732–735.

Stolen waters are sweet and bread eaten in secret is pleasant

Proverbs 9:17

It seems strange that early writers did not discover the effect of carbohydrate restriction on the symptoms of diabetes, for we see often enough patients, even the young, with acute symptoms who are dramatically relieved of these by the exclusion of sugar and bread from their diet. Some of the herbs advocated, for instance by Avicenna (980–1037), may have produced such disturbances of digestion as to promote undernutrition. Thomas Willis (1621–1675) gave a diet of milk and barley water boiled with bread and may have achieved a reduction in calories which could have helped his patients and foreshadowed the later undernutrition cures. Thomas Sydenham (1624–1689) said: 'let the patient eat food easy of digestion such as veal, mutton and the like and abstain from all sorts of fruits and garden stuff' (Saundby, 1891), not bad advice but as vague as the instructions often given verbally to patients today.

John Rollo (1797) may be regarded as the pioneer of modern dietary treatment in that his regime was definite and based on scientific principles, albeit his theory of the nature of diabetes was totally wrong. Rollo's instructions were as follows:

Breakfast, 1½ pints of milk and ½ pint of lime water, mixed together; bread and butter. For noon, plain blood puddings, made of blood and suet only. Dinner, game, or old meats, which have been long kept; and as far as the stomach may bear, fat and rancid old meats, as pork, to eat in moderation. Supper, the same as breakfast.

The strenuous and unpleasant character of the treatment accounts for the failure of Rollo's method to survive, but restriction of carbohydrate was a feature of most diets about this time and the principles were revived in an entirely acceptable form by Appollinaire Bouchardat (1875), who eliminated the unpleasant features such as rancid fat and concentrated rather on the value of eating little, especially carbohydrate ('manger le moins possible'). The effect of the privations of the siege of Paris in 1870 on his patients confirmed his views. He tried to fit the diet to the individual patient and was the first to emphasize the value of exercise.

The special feature added by Cantani (1870) was extreme austerity of management. Patients were segregated under lock and key and allowed only lean meat and some fat with water and dilute alcohol. Fast days were enforced if necessary to eliminate glycosuria and the treatment lasted up to 9 months. As far as we know Cantani had a large and lucrative practice and it seems there will always be a following for those who offer nothing but mortification of the flesh at considerable pecuniary cost. To this day patients pay large fees for the privilege of submitting to a meagre (and very cheap) dietetic rule under strict discipline.

The practice of undernutrition was carried to the extreme limit by Allen (1914), who was able to extend the life expectancy of diabetic children from 1.3 to 2.9 years by restricting calories severely and reducing carbohydrate to 30 g or in some cases even as low as 5 g per day. The patients were often so weak that they could not get out of bed but they did live longer and a few survived until insulin rescued them.

Since the introduction of insulin there has been a gradual relaxation of diet restriction but, as in the past, advocates have not been lacking for every permutation of the proportions of protein, carbohydrate and fat. Some problems have remained constant, particularly how to persuade the overweight or frankly obese patient to lose weight. This problem can be placed high in a list of concepts guaranteed to unify the opinions of diabetic physicians. Few disagree on the difficulties of achieving this aim in all but a scant number of patients.

It would not be true to say that such unity is lacking on the appropriateness or otherwise of the latest revolution in dietary content. Rather there has been a grudging acceptance of the changes in diet by doctor and patient alike. The two changes in diabetes which have served to confuse both doctors and patients are the biochemical redefinition of diabetes and the radical change in dietary advice. With the first, some patients considered diabetic by old diagnostic criteria for 20 years were suddenly decreed non-diabetic. Surprisingly few lost faith with a medical profession which had so misled them and many continue to make the annual pilgrimage to the diabetic clinic, resisting all attempts at reassurance. Similarly, patients advised on the wisdom of carbohydrate restriction for 20–30 years with periodic exhortation to follow the diet somehow had to adjust to the startling news that restriction was out and indeed a high carbohydrate diet was to be eaten. That so many accepted this reversal of thought testifies to the stoicism of the diabetic patient. As to the musings of expert committees, the judgement of the patient is likely to be more generous than the comment of peers.

THE DIETARY NEEDS OF THE DIABETIC

ENERGY

The difficulty in determining the calorific needs of the diabetic patient is compounded by the wide variation within the population as a whole. Nevertheless energy expenditure calculations, taking into account age, sex and a broad category of physical activity (e.g. light or heavy) have been performed and the results are available to all (Lean and James, 1986). More traditional approaches include taking a dietary history and then calculating energy requirements on the basis of the information obtained. Whichever method is used calculation of the energy content of the diet should be the first step in the dietary prescription. Only when this is decided can the relative proportions of the dietary constituents be applied and the actual amounts calculated.

CARBOHYDRATE

A certain amount of carbohydrate is essential as an energy source, for in its absence protein is used for this purpose. Diets containing 100 g of carbohydrate or more are fully adequate to prevent protein loss and the excessive metabolism of fat that occurs in carbohydrate starvation. While small amounts of carbohydrate exert a protein-sparing effect in non-diabetic individuals the intake of a diabetic patient must always be considered in the light of urinary losses. Glycosuria of 20–50 g/l severely affects the net figure for carbohydrate intake.

PROTEIN

There is no reason for the diabetic diet to contain more or less than the normal adequate ration of protein. The recommended daily intake for adult males is 50–60 gm/day and for females 40–50 gm/day (HMSO, 1990). The National Advisory Committee on Nutrition Education (1983) considered that protein should form not less than 11% of the energy allowance of the diet of adults or 14% for nursing mothers, infants and adolescents.

FAT

Fat is essential in the diet only as a source of fat-soluble vitamins, most of which can be obtained from other sources, and to supply essential fatty acids. Far richer as an energy source than carbohydrate and protein, it confers a major advantage of a decreased bulk as energy supply. With this in mind 30–60 g fat per day could be considered appropriate for a daily calorie intake of 1350–2700 cal. In practice it is more likely to be found that an intake of 1350–2700 calories contains 50–105 g fat.

INTER-RELATIONSHIP OF MACRONUTRIENTS

In the whole animal

It is a generalization but one which holds some truth that the daily intake of protein in the developed world is guided mainly by the financial status of the eater. The source of protein for most people is meat, bread, eggs, fish and milk and not all of these have a benefit of concentrate without bulk. With protein intake in the average diet relatively static at about 15% of daily calorie intake there remains great scope for manipulation of carbohydrate and fat intake. To a larger extent the recent revision of dietary advice for diabetics resulted from the predictable realization that if protein was dictated by finance, and advice was given to restrict carbohydrate, then the daily calorie intake would inevitably be made up by fat. Gram for gram, of course, this is likely to produce unwanted adiposity but worse consequences have been argued. High fat intake must be ill-advised, it is forcefully suggested, in a disease where atherosclerosis remains the major cause of mortality.

Many doctors would happily accept this vague suggestion of pathogenesis if it could be delivered with rather less fervour. Few issues cause more fervent appeals, advice or dogmatic approaches. Would that these were replaced by more moderate advice based on some scientific principle.

At the cellular level

While it may be convenient to compartmentalise dietary constituents into carbohydrates, protein, and fat, once absorbed the body is less discriminating. Monosaccharides may on reaching the liver be stored as glycogen, or be used through acetyl CoA to produce fatty acids or cholesterol. Both within the liver and at the adipocyte fatty acids are esterified with glycerol derivatives, produced exclusively in the metabolism of glucose, to produce triglycerides.

Triglyceride and hence fatty acids are less efficient at branching into other pathways. Carbohydrate or more strictly glucose cannot be synthesized from fatty acids because oxidation of fatty acids results in acetyl CoA, which feeds into the Krebs cycle after the reversible steps of glycolysis. Glycerol, as a product of lipolysis, is transported to the liver and contributes to glucose or glycogen production through gluconeogenesis.

As for proteins, the majority of amino acids are capable of interconversion into non-nitrogen-containing carboxylic acids, which supply energy through metabolism in carbohydrate pathways. The major gluconeogenic acid, alanine, is known to derive its carbon skeleton from pyruvate, accepting nitrogen from other amino acids.

The 'separateness' of dietary intake is indeed a myth once digested and nothing illustrates this more than the centrality of acetyl CoA. Formed from carbohydrate metabolism and fat breakdown, and metabolized to fatty acids, cholesterol and in the Krebs cycle, its widespread role has important ramifications for our approach to diet treatment. For example, surely attempts to reduce cholesterol in the diet in order to lower blood cholesterol must be doomed while its source within the body is a compound as ubiquitous as acetyl CoA.

FAT AND VASCULAR DISEASE

A casual link between dietary fat and atherogenesis remains to be established. Nevertheless, the concept underpins recent thinking on the composition of the diabetic diet. In fairness, it is not the sole consideration and the awareness that high carbohydrate diets, far from worsening diabetic control, may actually improve blood glucose levels is at least responsible for equal impetus.

Apart from the prevention of obesity the only reason for modifying the intake of fat is to alter the pattern of plasma lipids in the hope of preventing or delaying the onset of atheroma (Steiner, 1989). This goal is particularly attractive in diabetes because the incidence of coronary disease is known to be abnormally high in both male and female diabetics. There is also ample evidence that the plasma lipids are abnormal in the uncontrolled diabetic. The milky appearance of the plasma in uncontrolled diabetes has been known at least since the 18th century, when it was said that it resembled common cheese whey.

The precise role of circulating lipids in the aetiology of vascular disease in normal subjects or diabetic patients is still uncertain. There is some observational evidence that in the non-diabetic population cholesterol is a risk factor for atheromatous disease but agreement on the role of triglycerides is more difficult to come by. The subfractionation of plasma lipids has clarified the situation somewhat but the majority of information favouring causality remains epidemiological (Jarrett, Keen and Chakrabarti, 1982) In the general population, countries with a high incidence of ischaemic heart disease have a mean plasma cholesterol level of the population higher than that in countries with little ischaemic heart disease, and this difference is found before the clinical evidence of heart disease appears. At the level of the individual rather than the population, patients with familial hypercholesterolaemia are about three times more prone to ischaemic heart disease than normal subjects.

In Japan the mortality from ischaemic heart disease is of the order of one-eighth of Western developed countries for otherwise comparable diabetic populations. Similar observations have emanated from other parts of the world, including South Africa and Central America. It is clear that where there is a low incidence of ischaemic heart disease there coexists an intake of diets high in carbohydrate and low in saturated fat.

As poorly controlled diabetes is associated with lipid abnormalities and ischaemic heart disease is much more common in diabetics than non-diabetics the assumption is often made that a derangement of blood lipids is responsible for the excess mortality and morbidity. This view may be challenged. It is not entirely clear that lipid abnormalities are more common in the diabetic population than in the general population. Indeed the recent suggestions from our lipidologist colleagues is that diabetic patients have qualitatively different lipids rather than that there is any quantitative change either in numbers with abnormal lipids or in the degree of abnormality in the individual patient. Furthermore many, perhaps the majority, of diabetics at no time in their diabetic lives have a raised plasma cholesterol.

TYPES OF DIET

THE RESTRICTED CARBOHYDRATE DIET

Now mainly of historical interest, the low carbohydrate diet went unchallenged for half a century. Before insulin the Allen diet of severe carbohydrate restriction prolonged life. When insulin became available there was a cautious increase in carbohydrate. In the early days of insulin low carbohydrate diets allowed the use of relatively small doses of insulin, which initially had economic implications. In 1923 in England, 100 units of insulin cost £1.25, although the cost rapidly fell and by 1927 it was 20p.

While restriction of amount of carbohydrate in the diabetic diet has all but been replaced, two facets of restriction remain.

Firstly, there continues a restriction upon day-to-day variability in quantity of carbohydrate intake. Some constancy of amount both overall during the day and throughout the day continues to be advised. This is no longer so severe that it is given in the form of 'portions' or 'rations' but similar amounts at broadly similar times of day is still a hallmark of dietetic advice. This approach may not last much longer. There has never been a great deal of point in advising non-insulin-dependent patients in this manner. Provided the carbohydrate intake is spread somewhat throughout the day there is little necessity for dinner always to contain 60 g carbohydrate. For the insulin-taking patient the 'ration' system performed a useful function alongside rigid insulin regimens. With once-daily insulin injections constancy of distribution of carbohydrate throughout the day could aid avoidance of hyper- or hypoglycaemia. The penalty incurred by such a regimen was lack of variability in amount and in timing, although one of the main purposes of the exchange system was to allow variation in content. The advent of more flexible insulin regimens, particularly those using three- or four-times-daily insulin with at least three doses of rapid-acting insulin should see the total demise of a constant-amount regimen. Varying insulin dose before a meal will allow freedom in amount of carbohydrate and it is likely that the ration system will continue only as a rough guide to amount of carbohydrate being eaten, thus giving some indication of insulin dose, rather than a day-to-day constant.

Secondly, there remains a tendency to restrict refined carbohydrate. Indeed many authors have drawn attention to the dangers of a high carbohydrate diet should the patient interpret this as freedom to increase refined carbohydrate intake. Reaven (1980) warns of the dangers of equating high carbohydrate intake with an increased Danish pastry intake! Those interested in dietary theory and practice continue to debate the pros and cons of refined carbohydrate. Does it really result in a deterioration in blood glucose control if taken in excess? in moderation? or as an occasional treat? There remains considerable confusion in the literature but instinctively there is a feeling that a can of refined sugar in solution ought to produce a swing in blood glucose concentration as a consequence of rapid absorption. In the light of this debate it is hardly surprising that the pronouncements on sugars in the diet of the diabetic have been a compromise. The Diabetes and Nutrition Study Group of the European Association for the Study of Diabetes (1988) suggested that the total intake of added sucrose in the diet be limited to 30 g per day. For some peculiar reason the Nutrition Subcommittee of the British Diabetic Association's Professional Advisory Committee (1990) found this amount excessive and advocated 25 g!

THE RESTRICTED CALORIE DIET

This is the most commonly advised diet in treating diabetes. Patients presenting with non-insulin-dependent diabetes who are overweight or obese may require little else in the way of treatment. Other non-insulin-dependent diabetics run the risk of excessive weight gain on sulphonylurea therapy, while patients with either insulin-dependent or non-insulin-dependent diabetes run the risk of developing obesity with insulin treatment.

It should not be a difficult diet to advise. The exhortation to eat less takes little time to get across yet, judging by our own clinic, there is plenty of scope for failure. Sound practical advice on decreasing fat intake can easily falter when set against a lifetime's eating habits. One of our patients in his 70s, although accepting the potential benefits of grilling meat as opposed to frying it, still cannot resist pouring the fat from the grill pan over the cooked meat! In similar fashion advice may founder upon cultural habits. Who can resist the joys of Indian cooking, ignoring the amount of oil used in frying nearly every constituent of the meal?

The scope of the problem is enormous, not only in the diabetic population but in the general population of the Western world. It has been established that at any one time 65% of the female population of the UK and 30% of men are trying to lose weight. Perhaps the most difficult thing to get across is the slowness of attainable weight reduction. Sensible goals are necessary and few people can manage more than 1 kg (2 lb) per week for a month and 0.5 kg (1 lb) per week after that. Instant cures are much more attractive, testifying to the success of very low calorie diets, slimming clubs and a seemingly endless list of periodicals devoted to those wishing to lose weight. Success rates are hard to come by in the literature and are often so biased by patient selection and dropouts that any findings have little meaning.

THE DIABETIC DIET

Evolution

After the privations of the Allen era there was a gradual increase in the amount of carbohydrate allowed in the diet of the diabetic. Initially the increase was only to less than 200 g per day but by the 1930s levels up to 400 g per day were being allowed and indeed encouraged. It was claimed that on this intake the patient felt more normal without any serious problem of control by insulin. Rabinowitch (1935) was a forceful advocate of a high carbohydrate intake, up to 400 g, with fat not exceeding 50 g so that the total calorie

intake was kept in the region of 2000. Previous work had shown no adverse effect of the high carbohydrate intake upon control and further claims that ketosis and tuberculosis were less frequent with a reduction to normal of blood cholesterol followed (Rabinowitch, 1935). Only with his claim that gangrene 'is disappearing' did optimism prove excessive. Others had difficulty in substantiating the metabolic benefits of the diet, leaving the unanswered question of whether the value lay in restricted fat or restricted calories.

After the elegant studies of Himsworth, the high carbohydrate diet seemed to fall into limbo. This was surprising when Himsworth's findings are examined. Using glucose tolerance tests with or without insulin administration he studied insulin sensitivity. Diabetics – and at that time there was no particular distinction between types of diabetes – fell into two main categories: those who were sensitive to insulin and those who were not. In response to dietary manipulation, sensitivity to insulin could be enhanced. Thus the plasma glucose response of normal subjects improved when dietary carbohydrate was increased. Furthermore, there was a parallel improvement in insulin sensitivity (Himsworth, 1935).

The debate was revived by Brunzell *et al.* (1971). They showed lower fasting blood glucose, insulin and improved glucose tolerance in normal persons and those with 'mild' diabetes when the carbohydrate content of the diet was increased from 45% to 85%. In view of the oft-quoted nature of this paper it is appropriate to point out that the definition of diabetes was by criteria in use in 1971 and at least half of the diabetic patients would not be labelled diabetic by revised criteria. Indeed, none of the diabetics had a fasting plasma glucose diagnostic of diabetes. Similar results were obtained by other groups who studied chemical diabetes.

Rather more convincing than these studies are the succession published which showed no change in diabetic control on a comparison of low- and high-carbohydrate diets

(Patel *et al.*, 1969; Weinsier *et al.*, 1974). Lest it be thought that a proven case exists, it should be declared that there are also studies showing deterioration in glucose control with high carbohydrate feeding in normal subjects, chemical diabetics and untreated non-insulin-dependent diabetics (Reaven and Olefsky, 1974; Brunzell *et al.*, 1974). As with many aspects of diabetes, support or argument with a particular view can be found in the literature and results may be determined by who is treated, chemical diabetics, non-insulin-dependent diabetics or insulin-dependent diabetics, and with what. Many high carbohydrate studies have used liquid-formula feeds, others basic diets and yet others differing forms of carbohydrate.

The studies of the Oxford group (Simpson *et al.*, 1979) clarified the issue somewhat. They treated 11 insulin-dependent diabetics with low-carbohydrate (40%) and with high-carbohydrate diets (60%). There was a significant reduction in insulin dose, basal and postprandial glucose, although not in glycosylated haemoglobin or diurnal area under the glucose curve. Thus some improvement in control was noted but, perhaps as importantly, no deterioration occurred with the high-carbohydrate diet.

What is carbohydrate?

Reaven's view of the Danish pastry diet has been alluded to above. Dietary carbohydrate has both chemical structural features and form which have gained in importance in recent years. The process of digestion of carbohydrate has been known for many years and instinctively it is held that a monosaccharide must be absorbed more readily than an oligosaccharide, which requires hydrolysis before absorption. Part of the restricted nature of the low-carbohydrate diet was the exclusion of the disaccharide sucrose and other simple sugars. Even these views may be challenged, with studies showing that isolated starch preparations have rates of

absorption and glycaemic effect similar to glucose and greater than that of sucrose (Thompson, Hayford and Danney, 1978).

Rather than the chemical structure being of importance it is clear that the features, i.e. the way in which carbohydrate is presented for digestion, are important. Apple juice, stewed apple and whole apple display different absorption patterns when equal carbohydrate loads are given. Perhaps this is due to the remaining fibrous content of the food. Before considering dietary fibre, however, it should be emphasized that equivalent amounts of natural carbohydrates do not produce superimposable patterns of glycaemia. This concept has been refined further in recent years, with attempts to construct a 'glycaemic index'. This index compares the glycaemic excursion after ingestion of a named carbohydrate and compares it with the glycaemic excursion after an equivalent amount of the monosaccharide glucose. Thus numerical values can be ascribed to potatoes, rice, bread, etc. which give a comparative indication of glycaemic consequence. The concept is useful to the research worker but how many of our patients would be able to cope with the mountain of information generated remains questionable. At least the information is there, however, if it is sought by the patient.

There is still some relevance in the observations re absorption of starch versus monosaccharides. The latter are freely available on the corner of every street for consumption to promote energy, an image, or simply to quench thirst. With the exception of fast foods, dishing out solitary potatoes or jam-filled doughnuts, starch is rarely provided in this way. Generally, and even with boiled potatoes, the starch is presented in a fibre-containing food where the presentation may be of value. Naturally occurring fibrous fibre such as cereal fibre may affect absorption of carbohydrate. Miranda and Horwitz (1978) fed diets equal in carbohydrate but with different levels of fibre and found postprandial glucose values to be significantly reduced. Other studies have been less clear – the majority producing similar results – but with less certainty as to the reason for the improvement. There is a tendency to fail to separate high carbohydrate and high fibre in diets which have been tested. It then becomes difficult to ascribe improvement to one or the other (Kiehm, Anderson and Ward, 1976). Further confusion has been added by failure to categorize fibre.

Support for the view that dietary fibre increases improved diabetic control can be found in an impressive array of studies which have used a gelatinous fibre. These fibres, particularly guar and pectin, are unusual sources of fibre in the Western diet and, with the exception of small amounts of pectin in marmalade, nearly always need to be supplied as a dietary supplement. Significant reductions in postprandial glucose using guar added to meals has been shown in both non-insulin-dependent and insulin-dependent diabetics (Jenkins *et al.*, 1976, 1978). Unfortunately, and underappreciated, there is no support for the view that the findings with respect to guar and pectin can be transferred to fibrous fibres. Perhaps the enthusiasm for increasing fibrous fibre intake in diabetic patients owes as much to middle-class concepts of healthy eating and bowel movements as to scientific fact.

Summary

With all the reservations outlined above and after due consideration of the findings of many studies it has been recommended that:

- there is no reason to restrict carbohydrate in the diabetic diet and indeed an increase to 50% may have a beneficial effect upon control;
- some restriction of mono- or disaccharides should persist wherever possible, except as treatment for hypoglycaemia or when illness necessitates this type of intake;

- the use of foods rich in fibre should be encouraged.

Fat

There is some evidence to support the view that carbohydrate restriction in the diet of diabetics led to a consequent increase in fat intake. Birkbeck, Truswell and Thomas (1976), in a study of fat intake in a paediatric clinic, found that 44% calories were supplied by fat in the diabetic children's diets while Dorchy, Mozin and Loeb (1981) found 43% of calories from fat in adult diabetics.

Evidence that dietary fat and the development of atherosclerosis are linked is controversial and there is little sign that a reduction in dietary fat would reduce atherosclerotic disease. Epidemiological studies from Japan are often quoted and in other populations a fall in cardiovascular morbidity has coincided with alterations in eating habits. How can dietary fat relate to known risk factors for macrovascular disease? The major risk factor appears to be total cholesterol levels, with an inverse relationship between the subfraction HDL cholesterol and cardiovascular risk. A raised serum triglyceride level is not widely held to confer primary risk for the development of coronary artery disease. Dietary restriction of cholesterol, short of a strict vegetarian diet, is probably not feasible. Cholesterol is widely available from animal sources and the ready availability of acetyl CoA for cholesterol synthesis within the body does not suggest that dietary restriction could modify levels significantly. Nevertheless, there is a relationship between diabetic control and cholesterol, HDL cholesterol and triglycerides; diabetic patients may have higher cholesterol levels than non-diabetics; and diabetes is well recognized as a cause of hypertriglyceridaemia. The obvious goal in order to effect lowering of these two lipids is improvement in diabetic control to normoglycaemia or near-normoglycaemia. Where this is not possible, perhaps still in the majority of insulin-dependent patients and a substantial proportion of non-insulin-dependent patients, then an attack on a second front, that is directly at lipids, may be indicated. The front line of this attack tends to be dietary fat restriction.

Not all suggestions on altering fat intake are so poorly supported. Polyunsaturated fats can reduce cholesterol levels and thrombogenesis (Siess *et al.* 1980) yet it is only circumstantial evidence that places a figure of half the fat intake as polyunsaturates.

Summary

In the hope of reducing arterial disease it is recommended:

- that not more than 35% of total calories be derived from fat; and
- that this reduction in fat intake should be achieved primarily by reducing cooking and spreading fat, dairy products, and meat and meat products;
- for palatability and practicability about 50% of the remaining fat should be in the polyunsaturated form.

Other measures

These considerations can be described as the primary goals of the diabetic diet – high carbohydrate, low fat, increased fibre and a greater proportion of polyunsaturated fats. A number of other recommendations for the diabetic diet are in existence which are, in importance, far behind these goals. These secondary recommendations involve tampering with the diet and since radical restructuring is not necessary they are perhaps easier to implement.

Sweetening agents

Many people cannot adjust their lifetime habit by suddenly denying themselves sugar in tea, coffee or drinks. For them there are a number of sweeteners that can be substituted. Other sugars or sugar alcohols, fructose, xylitol and sorbitol have been extensively used. Fructose and xylitol are as sweet as sucrose but, since they enter glycolysis at the triosephosphate level the effect upon blood glucose is less. Entry to glycolysis at this level is also a drawback, since they can be metabolised to lactate, giving a substantial rise in this compound under certain circumstances. Sorbitol is less sweet than sucrose, less well absorbed and produces osmotic diarrhoea in susceptible individuals or if taken in excess. These compounds are carbohydrates and thus count in energy intake. Probably their major use is as bulking agents in commercial manufacture, a role usually fulfilled by sucrose, as most food labels testify.

Saccharin and cyclamates are non-nutritive sweeteners with quite long careers. More recently both have been linked with cancer. A number of weighty committees, including the American Diabetes Association and the American Dietetic Association, have considered the evidence on saccharin and bladder cancer (Smith, 1978). Conclusions were, as always with committees, guarded, assessing the evidence as neither supporting nor refuting the hypothesis of a link or suggesting a low risk of carcinogenesis in man. A summary of the views would be that these synthetic sweeteners should be discouraged.

Fortunately in the late 1970s a new generation of artificial sweeteners was born. For many years a non-metabolisable, naturally occurring compound was sought, with D-glucose a favourite for some time. It did not have to be non-metabolisable, however, if it was other than carbohydrate. The di-amino acid L-aspartate-L-phenylalanine methyl ester or aspartame was identified as fitting this pattern. Although weight-for-weight isocaloric with sucrose, it was 180 times sweeter allowing the use of minute quantities. It has the added advantage of no unpleasant aftertaste!

Alcohol

It would have been too much to expect alcohol to escape the scrutiny of committees asked to make recommendations. Alcohol is an easy target and the opportunity to hit it overwhelmingly attractive. In view of these temptations the Nutrition Subcommittee of the British Diabetic Association (Connor and Marks, 1985) exercised laudable restraint, simply pointing out that alcohol was energy and as such should be counted in the diet. They also drew attention to the high alcohol content and cost of beers brewed for diabetics. Many diabetics do want to know about alcohol intake and the majority of dieticians would regard advice as to non-sugar-containing mixers, dry wines and light-beers as a minimum of advice to be offered.

THE MAIN CONSIDERATION – CALORIE RESTRICTION

Only a few of our diabetic patients can ignore the overwhelming consideration of calorie restriction. The majority, be they overweight or obese non-insulin-dependent diabetics or patients on insulin attempting to avoid excessive weight gain, will consider some restriction of calories as a necessary evil. For the non-insulin-dependent diabetic, restriction of calorie intake may be sufficient to control their diabetes. When allied with weight loss towards an ideal body weight, normoglycaemia may be achieved for years. Whether this represents a cure for diabetes or a temporary remission can be debated. Perhaps more appropriately, it should be regarded as adequate treatment.

A fact which is often lost sight of is the beneficial effect on blood glucose of calorie restriction occurring before weight loss. Newly diagnosed patients who eat a restricted intake show improvements in blood glucose with diminution of glycosuria after approximately 1 week, whereas appreciable weight loss takes longer. Although of little consequence,

since the two go hand in hand, for clarity we should acknowledge that the primary aim of this treatment is to restrict intake and the secondary aim is reduction in body weight.

That is not to decry the value of weight reduction. There is a body of substantial evidence that weight reduction lowers blood glucose levels and numerous possible mechanisms for this improvement can be demonstrated. Glucose-stimulated insulin secretion is improved, as is suppressibility of glucagon by glucose (Savage *et al.*, 1979). Insulin sensitivity is improved (Hale *et al.*, 1988). In some of these long-term studies, however, there are poor correlations between weight loss and blood glucose levels (Streja, Boyko and Rabkin, 1981).

For the insulin-dependent diabetic patient, avoidance of weight gain is a primary aim. It remains unclear whether peripheral administration of insulin furthers weight gain, as is suggested by the depressed fatty acid and glycerol levels seen during normoglycaemia attained in this way (Nosadini *et al.*, 1982). If fat breakdown is inhibited by high peripheral insulin levels obtained in a drive for appropriate hepatic insulinization then it seems inevitable that maintenance of an ideal body weight presents problems. Regardless of how convincing this argument is, most would agree that once overweight, a weight-reducing diet presents special problems to a patient taking insulin. Since the population at large finds such difficulty in shedding weight the additional burden of insulin injections and cries for normoglycaemia must put this goal beyond all but a tiny few of patients on insulin. Avoidance of excessive weight gain must be the key. In terms of treating most people the calorie-restricted diet must be the most useful in the therapeutic armamentarium. Of course there are certain practical considerations which cannot be ignored, yet the message for most patients can be kept simple. The concept of input and output to maintain/reduce/increase body weight is relatively easy to get across, although time and careful explanation is necessary in response to the 'I eat like a bird' riposte often heard from the obese patient. What seems sadly lacking is any useful practical advice on cutting down intake. Realistic goals must be set. A person eating 3000 calories per day is unlikely to reduce intake to 800 calories per day for more than 1–2 days before reverting to the previous intake. Weight loss on 2000 calories per day will be slow but at least a realistic aim.

What of the wide discrepancy that can occur in otherwise identical individuals in energy intake? There are many studies which propose this as a real finding. Widdowson (1936) studied the diets of 63 healthy Englishmen, most of them leading moderately active lives. The mean calorie intake was 3067, but the range was 1772–4955. A teacher aged 28 was slightly overweight and consumed 1772 calories, while an electrician aged 29 was not overweight on 4955 calories. In general there was no significant correlation between energy intake and body weight. For many years it has been known that metabolic rates of individuals in the basal state differ markedly. As important is the adaptive response to a reduced energy intake which lowers resting energy output (Apfelbaum, Bostsarron and Lucatis, 1971). What has not been confirmed is any difference in basal metabolic rates between obese people and lean people. In general the suggestion is that BMR is **increased** in obese people, although there are appreciable differences from individual to individual (Halliday *et al.*, 1979) and the expression of a numerical value presents problems.

In looking at this problem from a different angle, the ability of an individual to dissipate excess energy may be important. Many studies vividly demonstrate that major changes in energy intake can be accepted with the consequence of only minor changes in body weight. The general nature of these findings is well known. Perhaps too well known! Nearly all people eat (and drink) more than

they admit to, yet there is a tendency to believe the cries of the obese 'on a starvation diet'. This raises a major practical question. If energy intakes may vary widely to maintain a particular degree of obesity, how are realistic goals to be set for a reduction in intake? Dietitians seem to feel they have the answer to this one by taking a dietary history and individualizing advice. Much time is spent in this battle of wits with the patient who, it must be said, nearly always wins. The dietitian estimates the patient's intake from a verbal account of intake and generally ignores (a) that it is likely to be a gross underestimate; (b) that it is an account of the 2 days before the hospital visit and after the finding of glycosuria; (c) that it is deliberately misleading. Calculating the imaginary calorific intake and reducing it to what is a totally unrealistic figure begins the spiral of non-compliance and dietary failure. An alternative approach is to use a nomogram for potential intake (Lean and James, 1986).

Within this framework of calorie restriction it is recommended that the high-carbohydrate/low-fat diet be advised, although whether this gives the diet a greater or lesser chance of success is not known. In as much as this type of diet, particularly by a reduction in fat, may allow a greater decrease in calorific intake than in real intake it is sensible advice.

TIMING

Some degree of consistency of timing as well as composition is important in insulin-dependent diabetics. The fact that many patients on once-daily or twice-daily insulin regimens can display laxity in timing is due to the difficulties of controlling blood glucose with insulin. Attempts to improve control yet allow freedom form the basis for regimens using multiple injections. Non-insulin-dependent patients, other than those treated with insulin, need not be so rigorous although certain rules should still be observed. Although sulphonylureas do not produce acute elevations in insulin when used chronically, there is still a risk of hypoglycaemia if meals are missed. Patients on diets may find it easier to lose weight if smaller meals are eaten three times per day rather than a single large meal, although there is no direct evidence to support this view.

PRACTICAL CONSIDERATIONS

The two-pronged aim of the diet in the treatment of diabetes is firstly to produce a correct body weight and secondly to control blood glucose, i.e. to strive for normoglycaemia without allowing hypoglycaemia. The first decision, therefore, is on the number of calories. This should take into account previous intake, type of work, whether manual or sedentary, and exercise other than work. Following this assessment either isocaloric, if the patient is of normal body weight, or restricted in calories should be prescribed. From the total calories the number of grams of carbohydrate to give 50–60% of calories can be readily calculated; approximately 15–20% of calories will be allowed as protein and the remainder allowed as fat. Minerals and vitamins will almost always be adequate on such a diet unless less than 1000 calories is eaten for any length of time. The diet must be simple enough for the understanding of the individual patient, cheap enough for the patient's income and acceptable to the palate. Some degree of individualization of the diet for each patient is therefore necessary, taking into account the mode of life, social habits and recognizing the wide variation in normal feeding customs. Mealtimes are often a social occasion with details developed over many years. The task of changing these deeply rooted customs should not be underestimated. Similarly, the urge to be strict with patients in their 70s should be avoided.

It should go without saying that the diet should have a reasonable chance of success. In the case of weight reduction it is often possible to reduce the intake of calories painlessly but this is largely because there is a recognizable objective and a tangible and welcome result is achieved. A lifelong diet with no other object than that of avoiding complications is another matter, especially in the milder cases where overeating brings no immediate retribution. It is true that a proportion of patients will follow with surprising accuracy a diet that violates all their previous habits. Some even make dieting their principal hobby in life. We must cater for these willing dieters with adequate and detailed advice. It is probably a mistake to discourage those who carry diet to obsessional lengths; the obsession is part of their personality and will only be transferred to some other and often less desirable object. These receptive patients take much time and, on the whole, repay it, but it is easy to overlook the large group of those who cannot or will not understand any but the simplest instructions. There should be no illusions about the success of indoctrination in dieting.

COMPLIANCE

There is ample evidence that patients do not and will not follow their prescribed diet. This view is too judgemental of human fallibility. Perhaps it would be as appropriate to state the case as 'there is ample evidence that the diets prescribed for diabetic patients do not lead to compliance'. Whatever the reason, the gulf between prescribed advice and the intake by patients remains wide. Tunbridge (1953) carried out a survey of 94 patients attending the clinic at Leeds General Infirmary, a department adequately staffed with doctors and dietitians. The accuracy of the diet was satisfactory in 16, moderately satisfactory in 44 and hopeless in 34. In a recent study from the same clinic food records were used to estimate intake in 92 diabetic patients. Only three patients were achieving the recommended > 50% energy intake as carbohydrate; four took < 30% of their calories as fat;

one patient ate < 10% saturated fat (Close *et al.*, 1991).

The state of the art was elegantly summed up by the late Kelly West (West, 1973) with the catchy and appropriate title 'Diet therapy of diabetes: an analysis of failure'. He documented how rarely diabetic patients understand and comply with the diet prescribed. Apart from a feeling that the physician was to blame he was concerned at the apparent waste of resources which were being ploughed into counselling fat non-insulin-dependent diabetics.

Studies of diet are notoriously difficult to perform. Both recall of a day's intake and dietary diaries are open to omission or manipulation. While this casts doubt upon actual figures for patients who do or don't follow their diet, it is unlikely that real figures would be better. There is always a risk of bias improving figures from reality, although there seems little reason for deliberately deceiving an interviewer that a diet is not being followed when it is. Some measure of compliance can be obtained by seeing the effectiveness, for example, the effect upon body weight or upon blood glucose control. Here, of course, the bias will be towards favourable reporting. Few people will have the courage to publish results showing poorly controlled diabetics getting fatter and fatter. But at least good results give the lesson of what can be done.

The UK prospective diabetes study has reported early results for dietary treatment (UKPDS, 1983). The allocation of dietitian time in this study is considerable and the first 12-month results on 286 patients have been reported (UKPDS, 1983). With initial advice 30% of patients were satisfactory on diet treatment alone. The difference between the median percentage ideal body weight at 12 months versus recruitment was 10%.

Similar results have been obtained in Belfast by Hadden and his colleagues (Hadden *et al.*, 1975; Wilson *et al.*, 1980), who report a fall in mean weight from 81 kg at diagnosis to 71.3 kg by 12 months and maintenance of this low at 3 years (70.8 kg). After grading their impression of dietary adherence it was concluded that weight loss and blood glucose control was better in those whose following of their diet was good or fair. Interestingly, their approach to dietary advice is described by the authors as didactic. Simplicity of instruction, forward planning and assessment were the hallmarks of their approach. After all, if patients will not follow simple advice why should they listen to more complex advice?

Just how representative of the general diabetic population these study groups are cannot be assessed. Nor can we derive which patients respond and which do not. Currently all patients get advice and a good deal of head-banging goes on cajoling, exhorting or attempting to persuade patients to diet – included among these are no-hopers who utilize valued resources. What proportion of patients they are we do not know. Some attend, disappear from the clinic, then return with not a kilogram difference to show at any stage. Will patients comply with newer diets? The omens are not good. Horrocks, Blackmore and Wright (1987) from our clinic reported results of analysis of diet in 65 patients with non-insulin-dependent diabetes. After 3 years only 14% patients took 50% of calories as carbohydrate and fibre content was doubled rather than increased three- to four-fold as originally advised.

DIETARY ADJUNCTS

GELATINOUS FIBRES

In recent years a number of adjuncts to diet have appeared. The most publicized is guar and its derivatives and it is referred to above. Guar is a preparation of the Indian cluster bean. As a gelatinous fibre it can slow absorption of glucose, leading to smoother glucose profiles. To do this it must be intrinsically mixed with the food, which presents a major problem. Experiments with guar have used it in a distinctly unpalatable form and attempts to mix it with soups or bread have had only limited success.

Although affecting absorption, guar does not produce a malabsorption syndrome yet gastrointestinal side effects can be unpleasant. Of these, abdominal fullness is unpleasant while excessive flatus with cramps is both unpleasant and embarrassing. Commercial preparations of guar are considered less potent in producing these side effects but this probably depends on the quantity rather than any minor qualitative differences. Small quantities, for example 10 g with breakfast, did not reduce postprandial rise in glucose significantly when compared with an identical meal without guar (Williams, James and Evans, 1980). It is now clear that a large amount of the fibre is required to alter absorption of glucose and interest in this approach has dwindled (Nuttall, 1993).

ALPHA-GLUCOSIDASE INHIBITORS

It might seem perverse to include this class of drugs in a chapter dedicated to diet. Nevertheless the end product of treatment is modification of absorption of nutrients by non-absorbable drugs. To that extent their inclusion here is justifiable.

Alpha-glucosidase inhibitors present an alternative approach to gelatinous fibres in interfering in the processes of digestion and absorption. They inhibit digestion of complex carbohydrates through enzyme inhibition leading to delayed absorption of the mono-saccharide.

The alpha-glucoside hydrolase inhibitor acarbose diminished postprandial rise in blood glucose in insulin-dependent diabetics (Walton *et al.*, 1979), while in a similar study insulin requirement decreased by 36%. In non-insulin-dependent patients glucose tolerance was improved (Sachse and Willms, 1979). In normal people addition of acarbose to a sucrose load decreases absorption of the sucrose by 40% and fermentation by colonic

bacteria results in flatulence. This is a common side effect in studies and evidence that it lessens with continuing use is anecdotal. Jenkins *et al.* (1979) combined guar and acarbose in a study of non-diabetic men. An additive effect upon blood glucose was found, reducing the mean postprandial rise to 0.6 mmol/l. Again, flatulence and a laxative effect were noted, although these were not worse than either agent alone.

In the past couple of years there has been a resurgence of interest in acarbose and its use in the treatment of non-insulin-dependent diabetes and a number of studies have shown a degree of improvement in diabetic control of the order of 0.4–0.9% in haemoglobin A_{1c} (Chiasson *et al.*, 1994).

REFERENCES

Allen, F. M. (1914) Studies concerning diabetes. *J.A.M.A.*, **63**, 939–943.
Apfelbaum, M., Bostsarron, J. and Lucatis, D. (1971) Effect of calorie restriction and excessive calorie intake on calorie expenditure. *Am. J. Clin. Nutr.*, **24**, 1405.
Birkbeck, J. A., Truswell, A. S. and Thomas, B. J. (1976) Current practice in dietary management of diabetic children. *Arch. Dis. Childhood*, **51**, 467–470.
Bouchardat, A. (1875) *De la glycosurie ou diabete sucré*, vol II, Germer-Baillière, Paris.
Brunzell, J. D., Lerner, R. L., Hazzard, W. R. *et al.* (1971) Improved glucose tolerance with high carbohydrate feeding in mild diabetes. *N. Engl. J. Med.*, **284**, 521–524.
Brunzell, J. D., Lerner, R. L., Porte, D. and Bierman, E. L. (1974) Effect of a fat free, high carbohydrate diet on diabetic subjects with fasting hyperglycemia. *Diabetes*, **23**, 138–142.
Cantani, A. (1870) *Cura del diabete mellito*, Morgagni, Naples.
Chiasson, J. L., Josse, R. G., Hunt, J. A. *et al.* (1994) The efficacy of acarbose in the treatment of patients with non-insulin-dependent diabetes mellitus. *Ann. Intern. Med.*, **121**, 928–935.
Close, E. J., Wiles, R. G., Lockton, J. A. *et al.* (1991) Diabetic diets and nutritional recommendations: what happens in real life? *Diabetic Med.* **9**, 181–188.

Connor, H. and Marks, V. (1985) Alcohol and diabetes. *Diabetic Med.* **2**, 413–416.

Diabetes and Nutrition Study Group of the European Association for the Study of Diabetes (1988) Nutritional recommendations for individuals with diabetes mellitus. *Diab. Nutr. Metab.*, **1**, 145–149.

Dorchy, H., Mozin, M. J. and Loeb, H. (1981) Unmeasured diet versus exchange diet in diabetics. *Am. J. Clin. Nutr.*, **34**, 964–965.

Hadden, D. R., Montgomery, D. A. D., Skelly, R. J. *et al.* (1975) Maturity onset diabetes mellitus: response to intensive dietary management. *Br. Med. J.*, **3**, 276–280.

Hale, P. J., Singh, B. M., Crase, J. *et al.* (1988) Following weight loss in massively obese patients correction of the insulin resistance of fat metabolism is delayed relative to the improvement in carbohydrate metabolism. *Metabolism*, **37**, 411–417.

Halliday, D., Hesp, R., Stalley, S. F. *et al.* (1979) Resting metabolic rate, weight, surface area, and body composition in obese women. *Int. J. Obesity.* **3**, 1.

Himsworth, H. P. (1935) The dietetic factor determining the glucose tolerance and sensitivity to insulin of healthy men. *Clin. Sci.*, **2**, 67–94.

HMSO (1990) *Dietary reference values for food energy and nutrients for the United Kingdom.* Her Majesty's Stationery Office, London.

Horrocks, H. M., Blackmore, R. and Wright, A. D. (1987) A long-term follow-up of dietary advice in maturity onset diabetes. The experience of one centre in the UK prospective study. *Diabetic Med.* **4**, 241–244.

Jarrett, R. J., Keen, H. and Chakrabarti, R. (1982) Diabetes, hyperglycaemia and arterial disease, in Complications of diabetes, 2nd edn, (eds H. Keen and J. Jarrett), Edward Arnold, London, pp. 179–203.

Jenkins, D. J. A., Goff, D. V., Leeds, A. R. *et al.* (1976) Unabsorbable carbohydrates and diabetes: decreased post-prandial hyperglycaemia. *Lancet*, **ii**, 172–174.

Jenkins, D. J. A., Taylor, R. H., Nineham, R. *et al.* (1979) Combined use of guar and acarbose in reduction of postprandial glycaemia. *Lancet*, **ii**, 924–927.

Jenkins, D. J. A., Wolever, T. M. S., Nineham, R. *et al.* (1978) Guar crispbread in the diabetic diet. *Br. Med. J.*, **2**, 1744–1746.

Kiehm, T. G., Anderson, J. W. and Ward, K. (1976) Beneficial effects of a high carbohydrate high-fibre diet on hyperglycemic diabetic men. *Am. J. Clin. Nutr.*, **29**, 895–899.

Lean, M. E. J. and James, W. P. T. (1986) Prescription of diabetic diets in the 1980s. *Lancet*, **i**, 723–725.

Miranda, P. M., Horwitz, D. L. (1978) High-fiber diets in the treatment of diabetes mellitus. *Ann. Intern. Med.*, **88**, 482–486.

National Advisory Committee on Nutrition Education (1983) Proposals for nutritional guidelines for health education in Britain, Health Education Council, London.

Nosadini, R., Noy, G. A., Nattrass, M. *et al.* (1982) The metabolic and hormonal response to acute normoglycaemia in Type I (insulin dependent) diabetes. *Diabetologia*, **23**, 220–228.

Nutrition Subcommittee of the British Diabetic Association's Professional Advisory Committee (1990) Sucrose and fructose in the diabetic diet. *Diabetic Med.*, **7**, 764–769.

Nuttall, F. Q. (1993) Dietary fiber in the management of diabetes. *Diabetes*, **42**, 503–508.

Patel, J. C., Metha, A. B., Dhirawani, M. K. *et al.* (1969) High carbohydrate diet in the treatment of diabetes mellitus. *Diabetologia*, **5**, 243–247.

Rabinowitch, I. M. (1935) Arteriosclerosis in diabetes. I. Relationship between plasma cholesterol and arteriosclerosis. II. Effects of the high CHO, low calorie diet. *Ann. Intern. Med.*, **8**, 1436–1474.

Reaven, G. M. (1980) How high the carbohydrate? *Diabetologia*, **19**, 409–413.

Reaven, G. M. and Olefsky, J. M. (1974) Increased plasma glucose and insulin responses to high-carbohydrate feeding in normal subjects. *J. Clin. Endocrinol. Metab.*, **38**, 151–154.

Rollo, J. (1797) *An Account of Two Cases of the Diabetes Mellitus; to Which are Added a General View of the Disease and Its Appropriate Treatment.* T. Dilly at the Poultry, London.

Sachse, G. and Willms, B. (1979) Effect of the alpha-glucosidase-inhibitor BAY-g-5421 on blood glucose control of sulphonylurea-treated and insulin-treated diabetics. *Diabetologia*, **17**, 287–290.

Saundby, R. (1891) *Lectures on Diabetes*, John Wright, Bristol.

Savage, P. J., Bennion, L. J., Flock, E. *et al.* (1979) Diet-induced improvement of abnormalities in insulin and glucagon secretion and in insulin receptor binding in diabetes mellitus. *J. Clin. Endocrinol. Metab.*, **48**, 999–1007.

Siess, W., Roth, P., Scherer, B. *et al.* (1980) Platelet-membrane fatty acids, platelet aggregation, and thromboxane formation during a mackerel diet. *Lancet*, **i**, 441–444.

Simpson, R. W., Mann, J. I., Eaton, J. *et al.* (1979) High-carbohydrate diets and insulin-dependent diabetics. *Br. Med. J.*, **ii**, 523–525.

Smith, R. J. (1978) NAS saccharin report sweetens FDA position, but not by much. *Science*, **202**, 852–853.

Steiner, G. (1989) From an excess of fat, diabetics die. *J.A.M.A.*, **262**, 398–399.

Streja, D., Boyko, E. and Rabkin, S. W. (1981) Nutrition therapy in non-insulin dependent diabetes mellitus. *Diabetes Care*, **4**, 81–84.

Thompson, R. G., Hayford, J. T. and Danney, M. M. (1978) Glucose and insulin responses to diet. Effect of variations in source and amount of carbohydrate. *Diabetes*, **27**, 1020–1026.

Tunbridge, R. E. (1953) Socio medical aspects of diabetes mellitus. *Lancet*, **ii**, 893–899.

UKPDS (1983) UK Prospective Study of therapies of maturity-onset diabetes 1. Effect of diet, sulphonylurea, insulin or biguanide therapy on fasting plasma glucose and body weight over 1 year. *Diabetologia*, **24**, 404–411.

Walton, R. J., Sherif, I. T., Noy, G. A. and Alberti, K. G. M. M. (1979) Improved metabolic profiles in insulin-treated diabetic patients given an alpha-glucosidehydrolase inhibitor. *Br. Med. J.*, **1**, 220–221.

Weinsier, R. I., Seeman, A., Herrera, M. G. *et al.* (1974) High- and low-carbohydrate diets in diabetes mellitus. *Ann. Intern. Med.*, **80**, 332–341.

West, K. M. (1973) Diet therapy of diabetes: an analysis of failure. *Ann. Intern. Med.*, **79**, 425–434.

Widdowson, E. M. (1936) A study of English diets by the individual method. *J. Hyg. Camb.*, **36**, 269–292.

Williams, D. R. R., James, W. P. T. and Evans, I. E. (1980) Dietary fibre supplementation of a 'normal' breakfast administered to diabetics. *Diabetologia*, **18**, 379–383.

Wilson, E. A., Hadden, D. R., Merrett, J. D. *et al.* (1980) Dietary management of maturity-onset diabetes. *Br. Med. J.*, **280**, 1367–1369.

The search for natural remedies for diabetes has been as persistent as in most chronic ailments. Few countries are without a traditional remedy and in the treatment of diabetes the effect may be real enough if the remedy is accompanied by a sparse diet or is sufficiently nauseating to reduce the intake of food. The periwinkle, *Vinca rosea*, enjoys a widespread reputation in the treatment of diabetes in the West Indies but no effect has been demonstrated. Throughout India the root bark of *Ficus religiosa* has been used as a remedy for diabetes and together with garlic and the common onion (*Allium caper*) appears to have some blood-glucose-lowering effect. More striking is the hypoglycaemic action of the unripe nut of *Blighia sapida*, the *ackee* in Jamaica or *isim* in Nigeria. This is due to hypoglycins, biologically active polypeptides which cause a marked fall in the concentration of liver glycogen and a profound drop in blood glucose (Hassall, Reyle and Feng, 1954).

Naive attitudes to natural cures of diabetes (and to other aspects of diabetic treatment as well) are by no means confined to so-called developing countries. Acetylsalicylic acid was used in the pre-insulin era and work has confirmed the anti-diabetic effect of large doses of aspirin. The basis for this effect, generally thought to be through inhibition of gluconeogenesis, is not fully explained and under some circumstances salicylates can cause a rise in blood glucose in normal subjects. Toxic side effects and weak antidiabetic activity make their use impractical.

Watanabe (1918) found guanidine to have hypoglycaemic properties but, together with a number of early derivates, it was found to have severe neurotoxic side effects. In 1926 Synthalin A (decamethylenediguanidine) and later Synthalin B (dodecamethylenediguanidine) were introduced as oral antidiabetic agents by Frank (Frank, Nothmann and Wagner, 1928). Perhaps the synthalins appeared at an inopportune time, for the results could not stand comparison with those of insulin, which had just revolutionized the treatment of diabetes. Synthalin was effective only in the mild or moderately severe diabetes of adult life. Moreover it caused anorexia, vomiting and a bad taste in the mouth. Worse still, a number of cases of acute yellow atrophy of the liver occurred for which the drug was held responsible and its use was discontinued soon after 1930, on what seems now to be rather inadequate evidence. Interest in the synthalins was revived by the introduction of the chemically related diguanides by Ungar, Freedman and Shapiro (1957) and Pomeranze, Fujiy and Mouratoff (1957).

The hypoglycaemic action of several sulphonamide compounds was reported in 1930 by Ruiz, Silva and Libenson, but not systematically studied until Janbon *et al.* (1942) observed severe hypoglycaemia in patients with typhoid fever who were being treated with a thiodiazol derivative of sulphonamide. The mechanism of the hypoglycaemic action of this substance, p-aminobenzene sulphamido isopropylthiodiazol, was studied in a series of experiments by Loubatières (1944) which would have been remarkable at any time but were especially so in the France of 1942–1946. Loubatières (1957) stressed the possible therapeutic application of his early work but almost 10 years passed before Franke and Fuchs (1955) reported the use of carbutamide, a

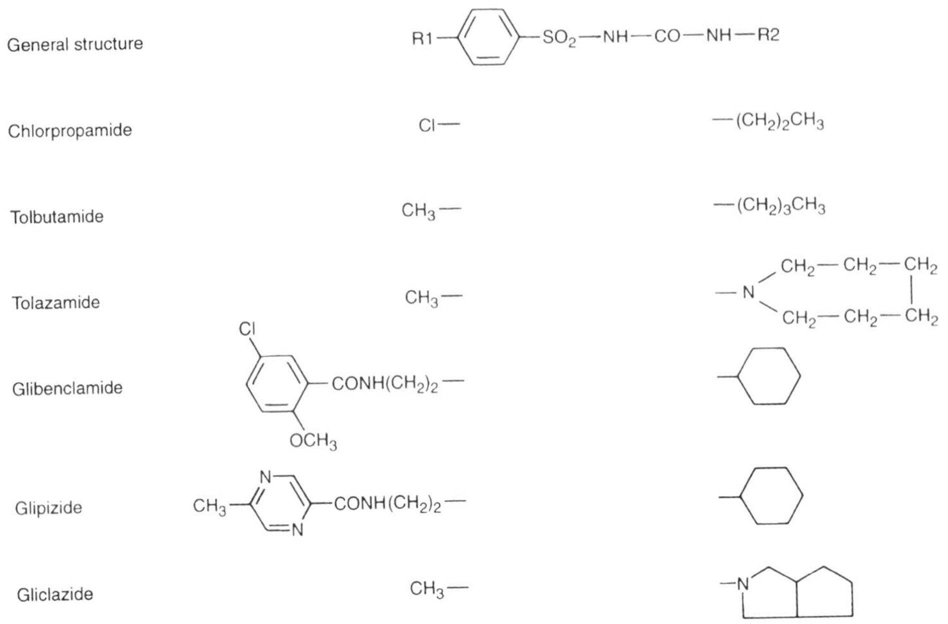

General structure   R1 —⟨benzene⟩— SO₂—NH—CO—NH—R2

Chlorpropamide   Cl—   —(CH₂)₂CH₃

Tolbutamide   CH₃—   —(CH₂)₃CH₃

Tolazamide   CH₃—   —N(CH₂—CH₂—CH₂ / CH₂—CH₂—CH₂)

Glibenclamide   (Cl, OCH₃ substituted benzene)—CONH(CH₂)₂—   ⟨cyclohexyl⟩

Glipizide   CH₃—(pyrazine)—CONH(CH₂)₂—   ⟨cyclohexyl⟩

Gliclazide   CH₃—   —N(bicyclic ring)

Fig. 8.1 Comparative structure of some sulphonylureas.

sulphonylurea compound, and found that it could be successfully substituted for insulin in a number of middle-aged and elderly diabetics. This drug, and a later introduction, methexamide, were subsequently withdrawn owing to toxic side effects but the closely related tolbutamide, chlorpropamide and acetohexamide were extensively employed and represented the most significant advance in diabetic treatment since the introduction of insulin.

SULPHONYLUREAS

PHARMACOLOGY

The active part of the sulphonylureas is a sulphonyl group linked to a ureide. The prosthetic radicals round this essential core determine the side reactions of the various compounds and their pathways of metabolism. There are many sulphonylureas on the market, a testament to their usefulness and income-generating properties. They are listed in Figure 8.1, which illustrates their structural differences.

CLASSIFICATION

The drugs can be grouped according to two classifications. The commoner is based in history, with chlorpropamide and tolbutamide labelled as first-generation sulphonylureas and the remainder as second-generation drugs. Apart from the chronological division, this classification also serves to separate sulphonylureas by potency, with the more recent drugs displaying greater potency per unit weight. This is a distinction which has little relevance clinically.

A better classification of the drugs is into short-acting, such as tolbutamide and glipizide, and long-acting, for example chlorpropamide and glibenclamide. This distinction is relevant clinically, as described below. Confusion may arise from pharmaceutical companies loudly proclaiming the half-life of a drug. While this may suggest that a particular drug is short-acting, when treating patients we are rarely concerned with the drug half-life (i.e. the pharmocokinetic property) but pay considerable attention to the length of half-life of the hypoglycaemic effect – the pharmacodynamic property. In addition to the half-life of the pure chemical this will necessitate consideration of its pathways of metabolism, hypoglycaemic activity or otherwise of its metabolites, and method of excretion. These are major influences, even disregarding the extent to which individual patients may modify these concerns.

Another grouping of the drugs, used only in special situations, is into those which are liver-metabolized and those metabolized or excreted unchanged in the urine. The argument is that the former may be used in patients with kidney disease and the latter in patients with hepatic disease. It ignores the question of whether sulphonylureas should be used in the presence of significant hepatic or renal disease.

MODE OF ACTION

Attempts to explain mode of action of sulphonylureas have provoked an immense amount of work and posed important questions. Present uncertainties reflect our basic ignorance about the pathogenesis of non-insulin-dependent diabetes. Since both insulin resistance and diminished insulin secretion have their advocates for the pathogenesis it is no surprise that this is paralleled in beliefs abut the mechanism of action of sulphonylureas. Both a decrease in insulin resistance and enhancement of insulin secretion are proposed as the major mode of action. While the former explanation is relatively recent, the latter was originally found in the early work of Loubatières (1957). He set out that the blood-glucose-lowering effect was caused by direct stimulation of the insulin-secreting cells of the pancreas. Indeed, in these early studies a substantial body of evidence was accumulated that the effect of sulphonylureas

was upon the pancreas directly. It could be clearly demonstrated that there was a decrease in islet B-cell granulation and a decrease in the insulin content of the pancreas; infusion into the pancreatic artery of dogs produced a greater fall in blood glucose than injection into peripheral vessels; and while they were not effective in the depancreatectomized animal, perfusion of the isolated pancreas with a sulphonylurea liberated insulin.

In clinical trials of sulphonylureas one major feature serves to confound this particular explanation of the mechanism of action. With all sulphonylureas there is a lowering of blood glucose concentration following the introduction of treatment, which is associated with an enhanced insulin response. With prolonged treatment, however, the improvement in blood glucose is maintained but insulin concentrations return to pretreatment levels. A typical example from Feldman and Lebovitz (1971) is shown in Figure 8.2. They carried out oral glucose tolerance tests in non-insulin-dependent diabetic patients before treatment and at 2 and 6 months after glibenclamide was introduced. The improvement in blood glucose after 2 months is maintained at 6 months, despite a return of insulin response to pretreatment levels.

This long-term effect has been labelled the extrapancreatic mechanism of action. Explanations for it have included altered hepatic extraction of insulin, increases in the number of insulin receptors on cell membranes, and enhancement of postreceptor pathways of glucose metabolism. Conclusive proof has proved elusive, in part because of difficulties of divorcing effects of increased insulin from effects of lower blood glucose upon these events. Nor does the suggestion of a mechanism of action through an extrapancreatic effect deter supporters of the insulin secretion hypothesis, for it is justifiable to consider the insulin responses of 0 and 6 months intrinsically linked to the glucose response. At 6 months similar insulin levels are obtained for

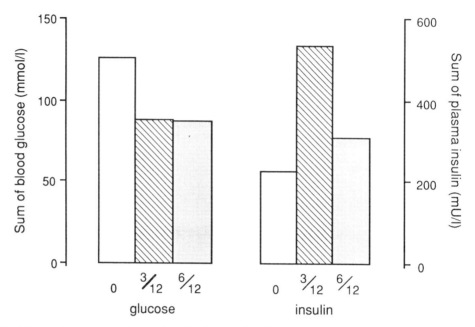

Fig. 8.2 Blood glucose and plasma insulin during the glucose tolerance test in non-insulin-dependent diabetic patients before and at 3 and 6 months after starting glibenclamide. (Source: adapted from Feldman and Lebovitz, 1971.)

a markedly reduced glucose stimulus, which can be interpreted as an enhancement of secretion.

Support for both hypotheses may be found in the extensive literature on sulphonylureas. In the promotion of insulin secretion the drug binds to receptors on the B cell surface membrane and inhibits potassium efflux from the cell through inhibition of the ATP-sensitive potassium channel (Sturgess *et al.*, 1985). The end result of this is depolarisation of the B cell. Sulphonylureas can also enhance insulin sensitivity in liver and peripheral tissues (Greenfield *et al.*, 1982; Simonson *et al.*, 1984; Jeng *et al.*, 1991). Both hepatic glucose production and peripheral metabolic clearance of glucose display increased sensitivity to insulin with chronic sulphonylurea treatment. Somewhat unresolved in these findings is the effect upon insulin secretion and insulin sensitivity of a reduction in circulating glucose with treatment, i.e. the effect of

correcting glucotoxicity. Hypocaloric diets without sulphonylurea administration will similarly improve secretion and sensitivity. It is unlikely that clearer views will emerge until the relative contributions of insulin resistance and decreased secretion to the pathogenesis of non-insulin-dependent diabetes are determined.

THERAPEUTIC USE

The sulphonylureas have been used on an enormous scale for nearly 40 years and their merits and defects are now well understood. The German workers who pioneered the clinical trials pointed out that the prospects of successful treatment increased with age, being good when the disease started over the age of 40; that they were better when the duration of diabetes was less than 5 years or if previous insulin treatment had been used for less than 2 years; and that the previous insulin dose should not have exceeded 28 units.

In the early days of sulphonylurea treatment these drugs were used in every new patient except those considered to have diabetes mild enough to be controlled by diet alone or severe enough to need insulin at once. It soon became apparent that those patients who were considered to have total diabetes with loss of beta-cell function did not respond. Notably, there was no effect in those who had suffered total pancreatectomy.

Later experience has confirmed the early generalizations and it is accepted that the sulphonylureas should never be used in children or adolescent diabetics and are best avoided in the obese, who should be treated by dietary restriction. As there are exceptions to most rules in diabetes it is tempting to use the method of trial and error, for the only certain means of identifying response is by use of the drug, but there are some patients in whom the attempt to control the diabetes by sulphonylureas should never be made and some in whom the prospect of success for any length of time is so slender that the attempt is not worthwhile.

Those who are obese but cannot or will not lose weight by dieting – a considerable group in any diabetic population – present a problem. It is all very well to deliver a homily at each visit in the knowledge that it will be ignored and that hyperglycaemia will continue. The patient continues to suffer from pruritus vulvae or other diabetic symptoms and is exposed to the risk of acute neuropathy and perhaps accelerated vascular disease. Is it enough to say that the patient deserved to suffer because of a lack of willpower? I believe that there is a case for the use of sulphonylurea drugs in obese subjects whose diabetes is uncontrolled, but they should be given only after a determined, but realistic, effort to achieve weight reduction by dieting has failed. As with all diabetic patients their efficacy can not be guaranteed,

and indeed, they are unlikely to prove wholly successful in the face of continued dietary anarchy.

CONTRAINDICATIONS

Sulphonylureas should not be used alone in patients who cannot secrete insulin. The largest group of patients are those with insulin-dependent diabetes but the occasional patient who has had a total pancreatectomy should not be overlooked. Insulin dependence is, however, a clinical definition and at times cannot be made with certainty. Even the presentation of a patient with diabetic keto-acidosis, the hallmark of insulin dependence, may not preclude satisfactory control of the diabetes with a sulphonylurea after the acute illness. This is particularly true in the elderly (Kilvert *et al.*, 1984) but the statement should not be generalized to the typical presentation of a teenager with insulin-dependence. Senile or demented patients who cannot be relied upon to take tablets or meals regularly should not be prescribed sulphonylureas. The enhanced supervision and care which comes from daily insulin administration by the nurse or a member of the family is to be encouraged. In addition, the outside agencies which may supply meals are well aware of the dangers of an insulin-taking patient failing to get their meal, while being less aware of the importance of the tablet-taking diabetic having a meal provided.

The other situation, already alluded to, that causes hesitancy in the prescription of a sulphonylurea is when coexisting hepatic or renal disease is present.

The use of sulphonylureas in pregnancy is a special case. Tolbutamide has been reported to have teratogenic effects in rats and mice, but the dosage was very high. When pregnant rabbits were given amounts which were smaller, although still much in excess of those normally used in man, congenital defects were not observed. Recorded experience of the treatment of pregnant women with sulphonylureas has on the whole been reassuring.

Nevertheless, there are grounds for doubting the wisdom of sulphonylurea use in the pregnant diabetic. Sulphonylureas cross the placenta and would be expected to stimulate fetal insulin secretion. Since hyperinsulinism of the fetus may result in excessive fetal weight and neonatal hypoglycaemia, it would seem inappropriate to expose the fetus to such risks. Stowers and Sutherland (1975) reported good results in gestational diabetics using only a small dose of chlorpropamide but were probably the last group in the UK to pursue this policy. Currently, insulin is advocated in all pregnant diabetic patients except the occasional situation where dietary modification is sufficient.

INDICATIONS

To summarize the indications for use: patients should have a high probability of having non-insulin-dependent diabetes; should be below or at ideal body weight or, at the very least, non-obese; and should have had a trial of dietary restriction alone. In practice, this final consideration is not followed rigidly. Dietary treatment depends for its success on a preceding diet which lends itself to modification and a patient who is not underweight. Most of us see little harm in using a sulphonylurea as an adjunct to simple dietary advice in elderly or underweight patients from diagnosis, which is a view that purists may challenge.

Beyond diagnosis the indications for sulphonylureas become less clear. When dietary advice fails a number of factors contribute. Inappropriate advice may have been given, there may be an initial surge of enthusiasm followed by relapse, or there may be failure from the outset from lack of inclination, motivation or just plain stubbornness. The most difficult group of patients is that of obese non-insulin-dependent diabetics inadequately controlled by diet. These patients are assumed to have hyperinsulinism and a

reluctance to introduce sulphonylureas stems from the desire to avoid accentuating hyperinsulinism and the consequence of weight gain. A biguanide might be a more logical choice in this situation although, in my opinion, the blood-glucose-lowering effect cannot match that of the sulphonylureas. The two other choices are diet, which is referred to above, and insulin, yet this will similarly enhance circulating insulin and lead to weight gain. There is no simple answer to this dilemma. Logical choice depends upon careful weighing of the potential risks of being obese versus hyperglycaemia.

METHOD OF USE

In practice the use of sulphonylureas is greatly simplified by two considerations. Firstly, and grossly underappreciated, there is only a limited dose–effect relationship, and secondly, the chemical response is rapid.

Schemes for dosage are made easy by the fact that there is an optimum level, which is fairly constant for each drug. This dose does not approach the maximum recommended dose and increasing the dose above this optimum does not increase the magnitude or duration of the hypoglycaemic effect. In view of this, instigation of treatment should always be at the lowest recommended dose. The continued use of these drugs is only justified if symptoms are relieved, glycosuria abolished and the blood glucose after a meal does not exceed 10 mmol/l (180 mg/dl). Partial responses to sulphonylureas can and do occur and it is tempting to persist or increase the dose. The end result of these courses of action should always be viewed in the light of the criteria outlined above. Case histories in diabetic clinics are littered with patients in whom a poor or moderate response to sulphonylureas has been allowed for years. Assuming dietary restriction is satisfactory, a less than complete response is an indication for the addition of a biguanide or a transfer to insulin. It is depressing to look back through the clinic record of a patient on sulphonylureas and wonder why insulin was not started 5 years ago.

It is nearly always possible to identify a successful response within a week and certainly within a month of treatment. As a rule a positive response is immediate and complete as soon as an adequate blood level is achieved. Interestingly, a poor response to the acute phase of sulphonylurea treatment is never rescued by a good response once extrapancreatic mechanisms of action can be invoked.

PROPHYLACTIC USE

Following his own observation that sulphonylureas may cause regeneration of the B cells in alloxan diabetic animals Loubatières (1960) suggested that the drugs could have prophylactic value in arresting the development of clinical diabetes in potential, latent or subclinical cases. Tolbutamide has not been shown to have a beneficial effect in delaying the progression of borderline diabetes to clinical diabetes, although the daily dose which has been used has been on the low side. The position has been complicated by the redefinition of diabetes whereby impaired glucose tolerance becomes a category between normal and clinical diabetes. Only 5–10% of these patients will progress to overt diabetes and, at present, these patients cannot be predicted.

TRANSFER FROM INSULIN

When oral therapy was introduced it was feared that many hours would have to be spent dissuading patients on insulin from trying to achieve control of their diabetes with oral drugs. In the event such demands were comparatively few and many of them half-hearted. A grumbling minority can be found in any clinic, with some requests justified as patients started on insulin to cover surgery or similar situation remind

their doctors to review the reason for starting insulin. For the remaining patients it is clear that the initiative for a transfer from insulin should not come from the doctor unless there is a real problem – hypoglycaemia or some social difficulty in insulin administration – which makes oral treatment safer. There may be a case for maintaining insulin treatment in the old and disabled because it ensures a daily visit by a responsible person. Oral drugs may be prescribed easily and forgotten just as easily by a forgetful or wayward patient. Patients who wish to transfer from insulin can be told that the experiment is not worth making:

- if there is a history of diabetic ketoacidosis at any time;
- in the non-obese patient when the blood glucose record displays wildly fluctuating values and glycated protein measurement confirms poor control despite a determined attempt to alter the insulin dose in order to improve control.

Even these criteria have their exceptions. There are case reports of elderly patients who, despite an episode of ketoacidosis, can be satisfactorily controlled on oral agents. In our own clinic we have seen this in recent years (Kilvert *et al.*, 1984).

It is worthy of emphasis once more that the insulin dosage is only a general indication of the need for insulin and that some very severe diabetics require less than 20 units per day. Conversely some markedly obese patients may require large amounts of insulin, well in excess of 40 units, at times in excess of 100 units, yet clearly they are not insulin-dependent in the sense of being ketosis-prone. In any doubtful case the transfer from insulin to tablets should take place under strict clinic control, with daily observation for the first week. A short-acting sulphonylurea should be chosen because of its rapid effect but any sulphonylurea may be used. There is no evidence of a long-term suppressive effect of insulin upon B cell secretion akin to that of corticosteroids upon ACTH and cortisol secretion. It follows then that a normal therapeutic dose of sulphonylurea should be used and not the maximum recommended dose, which may cause hypoglycaemia in a responsive patient.

Are there cases which can be described as being other than doubtful? Rarely can a response be reliably predicted but a well controlled patient who has no glycosuria and blood glucose concentrations < 10 mmol/l (180 mg/dl) with normal levels of glycated protein and with a daily dose of < 40 units of insulin per day suggests a good chance of success.

COMBINED THERAPY – INSULIN AND SULPHONYLUREA

The use of sulphonylurea drugs in patients who have to take insulin has been claimed to improve control and well-being. Recently, there has been a resurgence of interest in this type of combination therapy. The rationale is different depending upon whether insulin-dependent diabetic patients or non-insulin-dependent patients are to be treated.

Any beneficial effect of a sulphonylurea in insulin-dependent patients would depend upon a significant extrapancreatic effect of the drug. At the most it might be expected to reduce insulin requirement somewhat. Whether this is a laudable aim is in the eye of the beholder, but justification relies on a series of claims without solid ground. For example, if it is believed that hyperinsulinism is an aetiological factor in atherosclerosis it could be argued that a drug that allowed reduction of insulin dose was a beneficial adjunct to insulin. On the other hand, the total daily dose of insulin varies so widely from patient to patient that this argument may have little relevance. I am of the mind that complicating therapeutic regimens simply to reduce a daily dose of insulin, without a concomitant improvement in control, is an unworthy end in itself.

In non-insulin-dependent diabetic patients the theoretical considerations may be more plausible. If the action of sulphonylureas is to increase sensitivity of the B cells to secretory stimuli then insulin can be given to provide a baseline supplement while sulphonylureas help in controlling postprandial swings. This focusses upon a relatively small group of patients in defining this role. They must not be totally or almost totally insulin-dependent but must have significant residual secretion. In turn this would seem to argue the case that combination therapy should be used earlier in the natural history of the disease. An analogous situation occurs in obese patients poorly controlled on oral agents and requiring insulin. It has to be remembered that, even though poorly controlled, the obese patient may be producing vast quantities of insulin from the pancreas, albeit inadequate amounts. If the sulphonylurea is discontinued at this stage daily insulin dose will have to replace this amount before increasing the dose will improve control. This could be 100 units or more. This logical approach has a certain attraction and I suspect we will hear more along this line. Clinical reports show decreased insulin dosage, less hyperinsulinaemia, less weight gain (Yki-Jarvinen *et al.*, 1992; Chow *et al.*, 1995), but earlier claims of smoother control of blood glucose and greater well-being are not entirely convincing. Periods of close observation and of enhanced interest on the part of the physician have a significant effect upon diabetic control apart from any revision of the type of treatment. Most authorities have not found combined treatment useful in practice and will need firm evidence of benefit before assimilating it into their therapeutic armamentarium.

FAILURE TO RESPOND TO SULPHONYLUREA THERAPY

A small proportion of patients, who seem in all ways suitable, fail unexpectedly to respond to sulphonylurea treatment from the start. This primary failure, which may be defined as that which occurs within 3–6 months of beginning treatment, will occur in not less than 5% of patients who are carefully selected as likely to respond and in a much larger number if the selection is less strict. Secondary failure which follows after 6–12 months of satisfactory response may be merely due to growing carelessness over diet or failure to take the tablets regularly. A genuine failure of the pharmacological action of the drug is perhaps better termed secondary resistance. Estimates of the extent to which secondary resistance occurs have varied widely, no doubt because those who do not diet and those who should properly be termed primary failures are not separated.

As one would expect, patients who are slow to respond or do so incompletely are more likely to become resistant than those who are at once perfectly controlled. Once secondary resistance has occurred and other treatment has once more brought the blood glucose down to normal it is hardly ever worth trying sulphonylurea drugs alone for a second time. An apparent response will not be maintained. The only exceptions are patients who temporarily need insulin at the time of an infection or surgical operations and may be able to resume oral treatment successfully once the stress is past.

The mechanism of secondary resistance is not understood but may indicate a natural progression of the diabetic state with a failing capacity of the islets to produce extra insulin. On the other hand, patients who develop secondary resistance are not at that time insulin-dependent, that is to say they can often live for months with uncontrolled diabetes but no major symptoms and no ketosis.

SIDE EFFECTS AND TOXICITY

The enormous scale of treatment with sulphonylureas has confirmed their conspicuous freedom from serious side effects, especially since it has been appreciated that dosage in the early days of treatment was often unnecessarily high. The British diabetologist Arnold Bloom used to say of tolbutamide that it was the safest drug to be introduced to England since coffee arrived from the Levant in the 17th century.

Hypoglycaemia

Hypoglycaemia, although relatively uncommon, is still a significant complication of use. I maintain that it is inappropriate to label it a side effect since glucose-lowering is the main objective of the treatment. Thus it can be termed an exaggerated effect but surely not a side effect.

As a rule it is less severe and less abrupt in onset than that which results from insulin, but severe attacks with coma are seen in elderly patients in a poor state of nutrition. In addition, those who take alcohol in place of a normal meal are unduly susceptible to the hypoglycaemic effect. Severe hypoglycaemic attacks may be prolonged and refractory to treatment so that fatalities have been reported (Asplund, Wiholm and Lithner, 1983; Asplund, Wiholm and Lundman, 1991). Very high serum levels of sulphonylurea have been found in such cases and a failure of detoxication or excretion could well be an important factor. The risk of hypoglycaemia with sulphonylurea is at least great enough to justify a routine warning to patients that they should take food at regular intervals.

Hypoglycaemia due to sulphonylureas is justifiably considered a medical emergency. Of note is that the presentation may be as a stroke and the importance lies in its reversibility with appropriate treatment of the hypoglycaemia. Of course, elderly patients may have a cerebrovascular accident which leaves them lying on the floor of their home undetected. They may lie there long enough for hypoglycaemia to occur. In this situation treatment of the hypoglycaemia will not reverse the hemiparesis. Nevertheless hypoglycaemia presenting as a hemiparesis is sufficiently common to warrant blood glucose measurement in any diabetic patient arriving in Casualty with an apparent cerebrovascular accident. Treatment should not be delayed.

It is still not always appreciated that treatment of sulphonylurea-induced hypoglycaemic coma should be in hospital. Our Casualty Officers get so used to the quick response to intravenous glucose in patients with hypoglycaemic coma from insulin such that the patient may be allowed home shortly afterward. Distressingly, they still fail to make the distinction of sulphonylurea-induced from insulin-induced hypoglycaemia. The patient on a sulphonylurea has gone hypoglycaemic from endogenous insulin. Not only can high levels of sulphonylurea be measured, excessively high levels of insulin are present. Not only that, but by the mechanism of action of sulphonylureas the B cells are sensitized to the secretory effects of glucose. The continued stimulus to insulin production by the circulating sulphonylurea will persist until the latter is metabolized or excreted. Thus relapse into hypoglycaemia is common and predictable after the initial treatment. Indeed, the initial treatment with intravenous glucose bolus then infusion may add to circulating insulin levels. Glucose infusion must be maintained until the sulphonylurea is cleared.

In this situation glucose infusion is being used to replace hepatic glucose output. Prolonged hypoglycaemia is a consequence of suppressed hepatic glucose output and this is more likely to be persistent with a long-acting sulphonylurea. There are cases where the vicious circle of sulphonylurea – hyperinsulinism–exogenous glucose – accentuated hyperinsulinism can only be broken by inhibiting insulin release by an agent such as diazoxide or octreotide (Boyle *et al.*, 1993).

An understanding of the pathophysiology of sulphonylurea-induced hypoglycaemia suggests that glucagon would be inappropriate treatment of the hypoglycaemia. While raising blood glucose it is also a potent secretagogue and will therefore increase insulin levels. Since intravenous glucose will be necessary it makes sense to get on and start giving it at the outset.

Skin rashes

Toxic erythema was reported in about 4.5% of patients treated with chlorpropamide and 3% of those taking tolbutamide. Recent experience would suggest that current figures are considerably lower than these. This may be due to cleaner preparations, reluctance to use high doses or greater care in the choice of suitable patients. There is no doubt that it occurs with all the sulphonylureas and it is sufficiently common to lessen enthusiasm for reporting. The rash has the usual features of a drug eruption and clears rapidly when the sulphonylurea is withdrawn. Porphyria cutanea tarda is also reported with chlorpropamide.

Alcohol intolerance

An interesting and common side effect of chlorpropamide is alcohol intolerance. This consists of intense flushing of the face with variable malaise immediately after taking even very small amounts of alcohol. The flushing is quite obvious to onlookers and may add to the gaiety of a party but is always distressing to the patient, who may have to decide whether to give up alcohol or oral treatment. The frequency of this phenomenon has usually been regarded as low but we found it in 22% of patients having chlorpropamide and in 30% of those who took alcohol (Fitzgerald *et al.*, 1962). No doubt the frankness with which drinking habits are discussed varies somewhat. The similarity of the reaction to that produced by tetraethylthiuram disulphide (Antabuse) has suggested that a similar pharmacological mechanism is responsible and that chlorpropamide inhibits the activity of acetaldehyde dehydrogenase and causes an accumulation of acetaldehyde. This explanation is certainly not adequate in the case of chlorpropamide, as there is no undue accumulation of acetaldehyde in the blood of these patients (Fitzgerald *et al.*, 1962).

You can imagine our distress, having originally described the phenomenon in the 1960s, when Pyke and his colleagues in the 1970s proposed that it was not only a troublesome side effect but identified a subgroup of non-insulin-dependent diabetics. This subgroup was demarcated from the remainder by a tendency to biochemically mild diabetes which did not lead to the development of severe complications. This was clearly an important finding if it could be substantiated. A considerable amount of work was done on the topic; the test was refined; skin temperature was measured; blood acetaldehyde was measured; different groups of patients were studied. Eventually negative findings began to outweigh positive ones and its days as a probable genetic marker were numbered. It remains difficult to explain away the original finding. Explanations have included: a preponderance of diabetics with maturity-onset diabetes of youth (MODY) in the study group; too many patients studied who were on chronic chlorpropamide treatment; and difficulties in defining a flush. In the rush to contradict the King's College Hospital group it may well be that a fragment of interesting and important information has been suffocated along with the rest. After all, no-one has satisfactorily explained why some patients very clearly develop flushing with chlorpropamide and alcohol while others equally clearly do not.

Gastrointestinal upset

This is the commonest side effect and occurs in about 6% of patients treated with first generation sulphonylureas although it is rarely complained of in patients taking second generation sulphonylureas. Excessive dosage certainly increases the incidence. Discomfort after food is the usual complaint and nausea,

constipation or diarrhoea are much less frequent. Taking the tablets after food seems to lessen the chance of this complication.

Liver function

Jaundice which can be ascribed with certainty to the treatment is rare. Liver biopsy in some instances has shown it to be of cholestatic type and these may be accepted as proven cases. It has been reported following tolbutamide, acetohexamide and more frequently with chlorpropamide. The overall incidence with chlorpropamide is about 0.4%, and the jaundice usually begins within the first month of treatment. The majority of reported cases were receiving a dose in excess of 500 mg daily. Abnormalities of liver function tests, jaundice, hepatitis or cholestatic jaundice have been reported with all the sulphonylureas in common use. It is not always clear that a causal relationship may be involved.

Ataxia and muscle weakness

A complaint of transient giddiness or dizziness – in fact, a sensation of unsteadiness – with weakness or lethargy is not rare during sulphonylurea treatment, especially when large doses are used. Although hypoglycaemia may be suggested at first there is no relationship between the symptoms and lack of food and they are often experienced after a meal. Relief by taking sugar should not be accepted as evidence that the symptoms were due to a direct action of the drug on the central nervous system. The complaint may disappear when the dose is reduced.

Leucopenia

A fall in the white cell count to 1000–2000/ mm^3 without agranulocytosis was commonly seen with carbutamide. There are few drugs which have not at some time been associated with marrow damage, and pancytopenia was reported following tolbutamide and fatal marrow aplasia during chlorpropamide treatment. Some effect upon bone marrow or peripheral blood has been reported with all sulphonylureas. Again, causality is in doubt but reports include anaemia (unspecified); haemolytic anaemia; leucopenia; granulocytopenia; thrombocytopenia; pancytopenia; aplastic anaemia.

Weight gain

In practice this is the commonest side effect of sulphonylureas. The extent may be exaggerated, since in a carefully controlled study with intensive dietary input weight gain was about 5% of ideal body weight, which was similar to patients on dietary treatment only (UKPDS, 1983). It is possible that patients have a more relaxed approach to diet when they perceive that tablets are the main agent of treatment, but doubtful that this is the complete explanation. The mechanism is unclear but the weight gain clearly exceeds that which might result from bringing the diabetes under control.

Water handling

The potentiation of antidiuretic hormone effect upon renal tubules by chlorpropamide has been turned to therapeutic advantage in some patients with diabetes insipidus. In others hyponatraemia has resulted in problems and this is particularly so in patients simultaneously taking a thiazide diuretic. Two of the eight patients reported by Zalin *et al.* (1984) experienced epileptiform seizures thought to be a consequence of hyponatraemia. Less well recognized is that certain sulphonylureas, particularly glibenclamide, have a mild diuretic action which may be sufficient to precipitate urinary retention in a predisposed patient.

DRUG INTERACTIONS (TABLE 8.1)

Sulphonylureas are carried in the plasma bound to albumin and any drug which shares

Table 8.1   Drug interactions with sulphonylureas (groups of drugs are asterisked)

- Alcohol
- Azapropazone
- Chloramphenicol
- Cimetidine
- Co-trimoxazole
- Coumarins*
- Cyclophosphamide
- Miconazole
- Monoamine oxidase inhibitors*
- Rifampicin
- Salicylate
- Sulphinpyrazone
- Sulphonamides*
- Tetracyclines*
- Trimethoprim

this transport mechanism may potentiate sulphonylurea effects by displacement. Aspirin, sulphonamides and trimethoprim have all been implicated in severe sulphonylurea-induced hypoglycaemia.

BIGUANIDES

The discovery that guanidine had hypoglycaemic properties was noted by Underhill and Blatherwick (1914). In a study of the effects of parathyroidectomy in dogs a fall in blood glucose concentration accompanied hypocalcaemic convulsions. These observations included elevated concentrations of a substance detected by a colorimetric assay thought to measure guanidine. Following up this finding Watanabe (1918) reported that guanidine injected into rabbits resulted in death from hypoglycaemia. After these early studies guanidine derivatives were sought that combined a hypoglycaemic effect with minimal toxicity. The first of these derivatives were both diguanides, Synthalin A and Synthalin B, and they were introduced into clinical practice in 1926. Doses needed to restore normal blood glucose resulted in intolerable side effects and there appeared a number of case reports of jaundice during

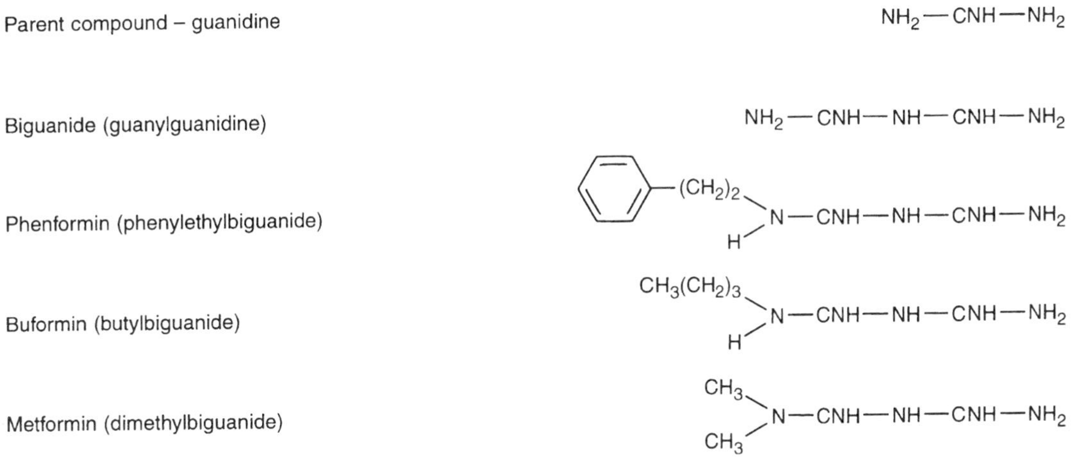

Parent compound – guanidine

$$NH_2 - CNH - NH_2$$

Biguanide (guanylguanidine)

$$NH_2 - CNH - NH - CNH - NH_2$$

Phenformin (phenylethylbiguanide)

Buformin (butylbiguanide)

Metformin (dimethylbiguanide)

Fig. 8.3 Structure of the biguanides.

Synthalin A administration, casting doubts upon the safety of the drug. In retrospect the evidence of hepatic toxicity was less than convincing and it is probable that the lack of interest in the drugs was due more to the recent isolation and clinical use of insulin. The guanidine group occurs in creatinine and arginine, and has been administered extensively without serious toxicity in antimalarial preparations.

The revival of these compounds by Ungar, Freedman and Shapiro (1957) followed pharmacological modifications that led to biguanides which seemed to combine a hypoglycaemic effect with minimal toxicity. Reports of the clinical usage of these compounds began appearing in 1957.

PHARMACOLOGY

Three biguanides have been widely used – phenformin (phenylyethylbiguanide), metformin (dimethylbiguanide) and buformin (butyl-biguanide). Chemically they are quite distinct from the sulphonylureas (Figure 8.3). Metabolism and excretion of the biguanides is different. Phenformin is concentrated in the gastrointestinal tract and liver, where it undergoes hydroxylation, while metformin is concentrated in kidney, pancreas and adrenals, and excreted unchanged.

MODE OF ACTION

The precise mode of action of biguanides has proved difficult to elicit since their introduction into clinical practice. It seems likely that at least three processes are affected.

Firstly, Czyzyk and his colleagues observed decreased glucose absorption in animals and man following biguanide administration (Czyzyk *et al.*, 1968). These findings were confirmed and extended by Creutzfeldt and co-workers (Caspary and Creutzfeldt, 1973), who showed decreased absorption of amino acids and other sugars in addition to glucose.

Secondly, Butterfield, Fry and Whichelow (1961), measuring arteriovenous differences across the human forearm, showed increased peripheral uptake of glucose.

Thirdly, there is a considerable weight of evidence in animal studies that biguanides inhibit hepatic gluconeogenesis. This evidence is difficult to obtain in man, although in normal man decreased lactate uptake and glucose output by the liver is reported (Dietze *et al.*, 1978) and during euglycaemic clamping metformin enhances insulin inhibition of hepatic glucose output (Perriello *et al.*, 1994).

More recent studies have shown an effect of metformin upon insulin receptors and enhancement of postreceptor metabolism of glucose (Lord *et al.*, 1983).

At the cellular level early studies showed an increase in lactate output by liver and muscle with phenformin and inhibition of oxygen uptake. These effects parallel those induced by inhibitors of cellular respiration. The multiplicity of cellular and subcellular effects of biguanides were given a common mode of action by Schafer (1976), who showed that radiolabelled biguanides bound firmly to phospholipid-containing membranes. An important finding in view of later developments was that binding affinity was related to the side-chain attached to the biguanide moiety.

An observation of great interest is the failure of biguanides to lower blood glucose in normal man. In animals there is considerable species differences but the hypoglycaemic dose in a healthy animal is not much lower than the lethal dose. In accord with its lack of effect in normal man is the evidence that the hypoglycaemic effect does not depend upon the presence of islet tissue and is not due to stimulation of insulin secretion. This immediately leads to the possibility that not only are biguanides suitable when insulin stimulation is unwanted, as in obesity, but also to the use of two hypoglycaemic agents, a sulphonylurea and a biguanide, in combination and working in entirely different ways.

THERAPEUTIC USE

It is evident that there is a wide area of application for biguanides in the treatment of non-insulin-dependent diabetic patients, provided a reasonable hypoglycaemic effect can be achieved without major side effects. Some authors (Bailey, 1992) have objected to the use of the term 'hypoglycaemic effect' in describing the effects of biguanides. Justifiably, they point to the lack of effect in non-diabetic subjects and the failure of biguanides to produce hypoglycaemia in diabetic patients. In the light of these considerations the term 'antihyperglycaemic' is preferred to describe their actions.

As the sole treatment of diabetes

The failure of patients to gain weight during treatment with biguanides may be turned to good account in the management of obese patients with uncontrolled diabetes. Biguanides can be regarded as anorexic agents and weight reduction and diabetic control are clearly interrelated. Clarke and Duncan (1968) treated two groups of non-insulin-dependent diabetics who were poorly controlled on diet with either metformin or sulphonylureas. After one year the metformin-treated patients had lost on average 2.7 lb (1.23 kg) while the sulphonylurea treated patients had gained a mean of 11.7 lb (5.32 kg). Similar findings have been reported by the UK prospective study (UKPDS, 1983).

Combination therapy

When secondary resistance to sulphonylurea develops it is sometimes possible to establish control once more by the use of a biguanide, either alone or in combination with the sulphonylurea. The addition of a biguanide to sulphonylurea treatment improves the effect of either drug alone. The adjuvant effect has not been explained but is not apparently due to the side effect of anorexia from the biguanide with improved dieting.

Combination with insulin

The use of biguanides to supplement insulin is more controversial. Many workers have reported a lowering of the insulin dosage and improved stability with this combination. It is true that biguanides can replace a proportion of the insulin requirement but to my mind it is doubtful whether a significant change in the stability of the blood glucose is achieved and it would not be easy to plan a trial that would prove the point. My objection to the treatment is perhaps old-fashioned. I find the management of insulin, diet and all the other variables quite difficult enough in such cases and the addition of another factor increases the problems of doctor and patient. Neither with sulphonylureas nor with metformin can I bring myself to tell a patient that they need insulin because the tablets no longer work and then reintroduce tablets once the patient is on insulin!

METHOD OF USE

Phenformin has been withdrawn in many countries because of the high incidence of lactic acidosis associated with its use (Luft, Schmulling and Eggstein, 1978; Nattrass and Alberti, 1978). Buformin, which was never available in the UK or USA, seems to be akin to phenformin in causing lactic acidosis and it is difficult to justify its use. Metformin remains as the only biguanide currently available in the UK and its introduction into the USA has recently been accepted by the Food and Drugs Administration.

It is supplied as tablets of 500 mg or 850 mg of the hydrochloride. A maximum daily dose of 3 g is recommended, although we would never use such a high dose.

Side effects following its introduction are common and there is an impression that gentle introduction serves to reduce the incid-

ence. Certainly diarrhoea is less common if 850 mg tablets are avoided and the drug is introduced as 500 mg daily for 1 week, then twice daily for the second week, to the normal daily dose three times daily from the third week onwards. As a personal opinion I regard 850 mg tablets as unnecessary and 1500 mg daily the maximum daily dose.

FAILURE TO RESPOND

If insulin-dependent patients are excluded the rate of primary failure to respond to a biguanide is not more than 15%. Secondary failure, apart from the need to abandon treatment because of side effects, certainly does occur but at a much lower rate than with sulphonylureas. This should not imply that biguanides are more potent than sulphonyl-ureas. Rather, it reflects the type of patients selected for biguanide therapy, who tend to be obese and not insulin-deficient.

SIDE EFFECTS

In all reports the incidence of side effects has been high and has necessitated stopping the drug in about 10%. The symptoms at the beginning of treatment are nausea and vomiting, and occasionally diarrhoea. Stopping the drug relieves them within 48 hours at the most. After a month or two of treatment a different set of symptoms may appear including weakness, vague malaise, slight weight loss and a metallic taste in the mouth. The affected patients may not have shown any nausea when they first took the drug. Many of them will deny that their appetite is less or that they have dieted more strictly, so that the loss of weight in the presence of good control is not totally accounted for. Many of these patients fail to thrive, although the blood glucose is normal and there is no keto-nuria. A change to insulin can produce a dramatic improvement and a flood of grati-tude for the restoration of well-being. It is therefore necessary to enquire thoroughly into the patient's story and not to base a decision solely on blood glucose testing or other measures of control.

TOXICITY

Serious toxic effects have been very few with conservative dosage. From the early days of treatment physicians noted a tendency to ketonuria without hyperglycaemia and a rise in the blood lactic acid. Ketonuria is usually attributed to starvation ketosis as a result of anorexia and a low carbohydrate intake. Increased carbohydrate is said to remove it. There is no doubt that hyperketonaemia is one of the many metabolic abnormalities that occur during biguanide treatment (Nattrass *et al.*, 1977, 1979).

Two of the major side effects warrant greater attention, the first because it led to the withdrawal of phenformin and retains some influence over attitudes to metformin prescribing, and the second because it remains unresolved. Soon after the introduction of phenformin into clinical use the occurrence of a severe non-ketotic metabolic acidosis in diabetics was reported. Following this initial report the development of lactic acidosis during biguanide therapy has formed the basis for a number of publications collated by Luft, Schmulling and Eggstein (1978). They analysed 330 cases with an overall mortality of 50% and attempted to identify associated conditions.

A number of conditions can produce lactic acidosis and diabetic patients are at least as prone to these as non-diabetics. The commonest presentation is with hypoxia associated with respiratory failure, cardiovascular collapse or endotoxic shock. It is also found in the absence of hypoxia in association with hepatic disease, alcohol and therapy with salicylates and intravenous feeding solutions. Certain inborn errors of metabolism also produce lactic acidosis.

It is widely reported that diabetes mellitus *per se* can produce lactic acidosis. While there

are good theoretical grounds for expecting this and cases have been reported it is very uncommon unless confused with ketoacidosis, which can have high lactate concentrations at diagnosis. In at least one-third of the cases collected by Luft, Schmulling and Eggstein, there did not appear to be any predisposing condition other than diabetes and biguanide therapy. This may well have been an underestimate, since the distinction between hypoxia producing lactic acidosis and the acidosis itself can be difficult to make. Severe metabolic acidosis may produce hypotension or the prodromal phase of lactic acidosis may lead to severe dehydration, with consequent elevation of plasma creatinine suggesting renal failure.

There are no comparable numbers of reports of diabetics not treated by biguanides who developed lactic acidosis and biguanides are firmly implicated in the pathogenesis. There has been some support for the view that this represents an idiosyncratic response. Luft, Schmulling and Eggstein (1978) identified 15% of cases which occurred within 2 weeks of starting treatment while Cohen and Woods (1976) reported approximately three-quarters of cases occurred within the first 2 months of treatment. I find these arguments unconvincing and prefer the explanation that biguanide therapy was initiated during poor diabetic control induced by the development of an associated illness. In addition, we and many others have consistently shown hyperlactataemia of varying degrees as an accompaniment of biguanide therapy (Nattrass *et al.*, 1977, 1979). Of the 330 cases of Luft, Schmulling and Eggstein (1978), 281 occurred during phenformin therapy, 30 during buformin therapy and only 12 during metformin therapy. This was not a reflection of prescribing volume but represented a real difference between metformin and the other biguanides.

In recent years few cases of lactic acidosis during metformin therapy have been reported and nearly all reflect inappropriate prescribing (Bailey and Nattrass, 1988). The

Table 8.2 Contraindications to metformin therapy

- Ischaemic heart disease
- Peripheral vascular disease
- Chronic obstructive airways disease
- Chronic renal failure
- Chronic liver disease

reduction in incidence may also be due in part to more strict adherence to contraindications to therapy but is not due to a fall in prescribing volume.

It is sensible to avoid metformin prescription when patients have an associated illness which affects either peripheral lactate production or hepatic lactate clearance. These disorders are listed in Table 8.2. Two points warrant emphasis. In view of the renal clearance of metformin and the decline in renal function with age, elderly patients pose special problems. The hypoglycaemic potency of metformin is enhanced by poor clearance and hence withdrawal in elderly patients may be tantamount to a decision to opt for insulin treatment. Secondly, although contraindications may be sought before instigating treatment, they can also develop during treatment. Some will be readily apparent and necessitate changing therapy. Others, such as declining renal function, can be more insidious and some form of monitoring is necessary. Measurement of creatinine clearance annually is impractical but an abnormally elevated serum creatinine, which can reflect a considerable reduction in renal function, should be a clear indication for withdrawing metformin.

Perhaps no study in recent times has aroused so much controversy as the University Group Diabetes Program (1975). Diabetics diagnosed by oral glucose tolerance test were randomly assigned to one of five treatment groups. Initially, six centres were involved although a further six were added 18 months after the start of the study, which coincided with the creation of a phenformin-treated group. The findings in this group were sufficiently alarming to warrant publication of a preliminary report (Knatterud *et al.* 1971) and withdrawal of the drug from the study subjects. An increase in cardiovascular mortality was recorded when compared with two insulin-treated groups and a group given placebo. A major interpretive problem resulted, not from the mortality in the treated groups but from mortality in the placebo group. The overall sex ratio of cardiovascular deaths in the placebo group was 5.3 males to 1 female, which was in stark contrast to findings from the other centres and indeed in the other treated groups. Further argument that the data were unrepresentative was provided by the fact that 70% of the study subjects being female and it was acknowledged that there had been a clear failure of randomisation by sex in assigning subjects to treatment groups. Other flaws in the study have been detailed by Kilo, Miller and Williamson (1980).

Whether the findings have been refuted or remain non-proven is a personal view. They have not been borne out by less rigorous European studies and, since the initial finding was with phenformin, metformin could only be stigmatized by association.

TRADITIONAL TREATMENTS FOR DIABETES

Over 700 traditional treatments for diabetes derived from plants have been described, although many lack critical evaluation in human diabetic patients (Day, 1990). Their use is firmly grounded in history and continues in a number of populations. It is not possible to list all with currently available evidence for a hypoglycaemic effect but fortunately a near-exhaustive review is readily available (Bailey and Day, 1989).

A stroll round a typical garden in Birmingham will reveal numerous plants claimed to have a hypoglycaemic effect. In the vegetable garden cabbage, lettuce, onion, potato and turnip; in the herb garden tarragon, rue, garlic, sage and coriander; in the flower garden periwinkle, purple loostrife, monkshood, lady's mantle, lily of the valley and knotweed. On the edges of the garden, or even in the lawn, can be found dandelion, nettle, burdock and wild carrot while, in the adjacent field is the common edible mushroom, the shaggy cap mushroom (*Coprinas comatus*) and the deadly poisonous death cap mushroom (*Amanita phalloides*).

Major problems with such plant remedies include knowing which part of the plant to eat, the method of preparation, the amount needed for a hypoglycaemic effect and an ability to consume this amount. For example, with garlic, one of the better documented hypoglycaemic effects, a garlic concentrate of 10 g garlic per kilogram body weight is necessary to lower blood glucose.

Some traditional treatments are better known and more widely used than those listed above. The Indian cluster bean has given rise to guar, which delays absorption of glucose, and goat's rue is the origin of hypoglycaemic guanidine derivatives.

The only traditional remedy that significant numbers of patients (5–10%) use in our clinic is the Asian fruit or vegetable karela (*Momordica charantia*). Used as a vegetable, but more strictly a fruit, karela will lower blood glucose concentration in non-insulin-dependent patients (Leatherdale *et al.*, 1981). The aqueous extract or raw fruit may well retain most hypoglycaemic activity but having eaten the cooked form the extreme bitterness which persists would persuade me to avoid the extract or raw fruit at all costs.

It is possible to devise and eat a meal containing a substantial number of alleged hypoglycaemic plants without ill effect (Day and Bailey, personal communication) although, to many Western palates, it might be a once-only experience from the standpoint of taste.

REFERENCES

Asplund, K., Wiholm, B. E. and Lithner, F. (1983) Glibenclamide-associated hypoglycaemia: A report on 57 cases. *Diabetologia*, **24**, 412–417.

Asplund, K., Wiholm, B. E. and Lundman, B. (1991) Severe hypoglycaemia during treatment with glipizide. *Diabetic Med.*, **8**, 726–731.

Bailey, C. J. (1992) Hypoglycaemic, antihyperglycaemic and antidiabetic drugs. *Diabetic Med.*, **9**, 482–483.

Bailey, C. J. and Day, C. (1989) Traditional plant medicines as treatments for diabetes. *Diabetes Care*, **12**, 553–564.

Bailey, C. J. and Nattrass, M. (1988) Treatment – metformin. *Clin. Endocrinol. Metab.*, **2**, 455–476.

Boyle, P. J., Justice, K., Krentz, A. J. *et al.* (1993) Octreotide reverses hyperinsulinemia and prevents hypoglycemia induced by sulfonylurea overdoses. *J. Clin. Endocrinol. Metab.*, **76**, 752–756.

Butterfield, W. J. H., Fry, I. K. and Whichelow, M. (1961) The hypoglycaemic action of phenformin. *Lancet*, **ii**, 563–567.

Caspary, W. F. and Creutzfeldt, W. (1973) Inhibition of intestinal amino acid transport by blood sugar lowering biguanides. *Diabetologia*, **9**, 6–12.

Chow, C. C., Tsang, L. W. W., Sorensen, J. P. and Cockram, C. S. (1995) Comparison of insulin with or without continuation of oral hypoglycemic agents in the treatment of secondary failure in NIDDM patients. *Diabetes Care*, **18**, 307–314.

Clarke, B. F. and Duncan, L. J. P. (1968) Comparison of chlorpropamide and metformin treatment on weight and blood-glucose response of uncontrolled obese diabetics. *Lancet*, **i**, 123–126.

Cohen, R. D. and Woods, H. F. (1976) *Clinical and Biochemical Aspects of Lactic Acidosis*, Blackwell Scientific Publications, Oxford.

Czyzyk, A., Tawecki, J., Sadowski, J. *et al.* (1968) Effect of biguanides on intestinal absorption of glucose. *Diabetes*, **17**, 492–498.

Day, C. (1990) Hypoglycaemic compounds from plants, in *New Antidiabetic Drugs*, (eds C. J. Bailey and P. R. Flatt), Smith-Gordon, London, p. 267–278.

Dietze, G., Wicklmayr, M., Mehnert, H. *et al.* (1978) Effect of phenformin on hepatic balances of gluconeogenic substrates in man. *Diabetologia*, **14**, 243–248.

Feldman, J. M. and Lebovitz, H. E. (1971) Endocrine and metabolic effects of glybenclamide. *Diabetes*, **20**, 745–755.

FitzGerald, M. G., Gaddie, R., Malins, J. M. and

O'Sullivan, D. J. (1962) Alcohol sensitivity in diabetics receiving chlorpropamide. *Diabetes*, **11**, 40–43.

Frank, E., Nothmann, M. and Wagner, A. (1928) Über die Experimentelle und Klinische Wirkung des Dodekamethylendiguanids (Synthalin B). *Klin. Wochenschr.*, **7**, 1996–2000.

Franke, H. and Fuchs, J. (1955) Ein neues antidiabetisches Prinzip: Ergebnisse klinische Untersuchungen. *Deutsche Med Wochenschr.*, **80**, 1449–1452.

Greenfield, M. S., Doberne, L., Rosenthal, M. *et al.* (1982) Effect of sulfonylurea treatment on in vivo insulin secretion and action in patients with non-insulin-dependent diabetes mellitus. *Diabetes*, **31**, 307–312.

Hassall, C. H., Reyle, K. and Feng, P. (1954) Hypoglycin A, B: Biologically active polypeptides from *Blighia sapida*. *Nature*, **173**, 356–357.

Janbon, M., Chaptal, J., Vedel, A. and Schaap, J. (1942) Accidents hypoglycémiques graves par un sulfamidothiazol (le VK 57 ou 2254 RP). *Monpellier Med.*, **21–22**, 441–444.

Jeng, C. Y., Hollenbeck, C. D., Wu, M. S. *et al.* (1991) Changes in carbohydrate metabolism in association with glipizide treatment of type 2 diabetes. *Diabetic Med.*, **8**, 32–39.

Kilo, C., Miller, J. P. and Williamson, J. R. (1980) The crux of the UGDP: spurious results and biologically inappropriate data analysis. *Diabetologia*, **18**, 179–185.

Kilvert, A., FitzGerald, M. G., Wright, A. D. and Nattrass, M. (1984) Newly diagnosed insulin-dependent diabetes mellitus in elderly patients. *Diabetic Med.*, **1**, 115–118.

Knatterud, G. L., Meinert, C. L., Klimt, C. R. *et al.* (1971) Effects of hypoglycemic agents on vascular complications in patients with adult-onset diabetes. *J. A. M. A.*, **217**, 777–784.

Leatherdale, B. A., Panesar, R. K. Singh, G. *et al.* (1981) Improvement in glucose tolerance due to *Momordica charantia* (karela). *Br. Med. J.*, **282**, 1823–1824.

Lord, J. M., White, S. I., Bailey, C. J. *et al.* (1983) Effect of metformin on insulin receptor binding and glycaemic control in Type II diabetes. *Br. Med. J.*, **286**, 830–831.

Loubatières, A. (1944) Analyse du mechanisme de l'action hypoglycémiante du p-aminobenzene-sulfamido-isopropylthiodiazol (2254 RP). *CR Soc. Biol. (Paris)*, **138**, 766–767.

Loubatières, A. (1957) The mechanism of action of the hypoglycemic sulphonamides. A concept based on investigation in animals and in man. *Diabetes*, **6**, 408–417.

Loubatières, A. (1960) Oral hypoglycaemic agents in the treatment of diabetes mellitus. *Proc. Roy. Soc. Med.*, **53**, 595–599.

Luft, D., Schmulling, R. M. and Eggstein, M. (1978) Lactic acidosis in biguanide-treated diabetics. A review of 330 cases. *Diabetologia*, **14**, 75–87.

Nattrass, M. and Alberti, K. G. M. M. (1978) Biguanides. *Diabetologia*, **14**, 71–74.

Nattrass, M., Hinks, L., Smythe, P. *et al.* (1979) Metabolic effects of combined sulphonylurea and metformin therapy in maturity-onset diabetics. *Horm. Metab. Res.*, **11**, 332–337.

Nattrass, M., Todd, P. G., Hinks, L. *et al.* (1977) Comparative effects of phenformin, metformin and glibenclamide on metabolic rhythms in maturity-onset diabetics. *Diabetologia*, **13**, 145–152.

Perriello, G., Misericordia, P., Volpi, E. *et al.* (1994) Acute antihyperglycemic mechanisms of metformin in NIDDM. *Diabetes*, **43**, 920–928.

Pomeranze, J., Fujiy, H. and Mouratoff, G. T. (1957) Clinical report of a new hypoglycemic agent. *Proc. Soc. Exp. Biol. NY*, **95**, 193–194.

Ruiz, C. L., Silva, L. L. and Libenson, L. (1930) Contribucion al estudio sobre la composicion quimica de la insulina. Estudio de algunos cuerpos sinteticos sulfurados con accion hipoglucemiate. *Rev. Soc. Argent. Biol.*, **6**, 134–141.

Schafer, G. (1976) On the mechanism of action of hypoglycemia-producing biguanides. A re-evaluation and a molecular theory. *Biochem. Pharmacol.*, **25**, 2005–2014.

Simonson, D. C., Ferrannini, E., Bevilacqua, S. *et al.* (1984) Mechanism of improvement in glucose metabolism after chronic glyburide therapy. *Diabetes*, **33**, 838–845.

Stowers, J. M. and Sutherland, H. W. (1975) The use of sulphonylurea, biguanides and insulin in pregnancy, in *Carbohydrate Metabolism in Pregnancy and the Newborn*, (eds H. W. Sutherland and J. M. Stowers), Churchill Livingstone, Edinburgh, pp. 205–220.

Sturgess, N. C., Ashford, M. I. J., Cook, D. L. and Hales, C. N. (1985) The sulphonylurea receptor may be an ATP-sensitive potassium channel. *Lancet*, **ii**, 474–475.

UKPDS (1983) UK Prospective Study of therapies of maturity-onset diabetes. 1. Effect of diet, sulphonylurea, insulin or biguanide therapy on fasting plasma glucose and body weight over one year. *Diabetologia*, **24**, 404–411.

Underhill, F. P. and Blatherwick, N. R. (1914) Studies in carbohydrate metabolism VI. The influence of thyreoparathyroidectomy upon the sugar content of the blood and the glycogen content of the liver. *J. Biol. Chem.*, **18**, 87–90.

Ungar, G., Freedman, L. and Shapiro, S. L. (1957) Pharmacological studies of a new oral hypoglycemic drug. *Proc. Soc. Exp. Biol. Med.*, **95**, 190–192.

University Group Diabetes Program (1975) A study of the effects of hypoglycemic agents on vascular complications in patients with adult-onset diabetes. V. Evaluation of phenformin therapy. *Diabetes*, **24**(suppl 1), 65–184.

Watanabe, C. K. (1918) Studies in the metabolic changes induced by administration of guanidine bases. Influence of injected guanidine hydrochloride upon blood sugar content. *J. Biol. Chem.*, **33**, 253–265.

Yki-Jarvinen, H., Kauppila, M. Kujansuu, E. *et al.* (1992) Comparison of insulin regimens in patients with Non-Insulin-Dependent Diabetes Mellitus. *N. Engl. J. Med.*, **327**, 1426–1433.

Zalin, A. M., Hutchinson, C. E., Jong, and Matthews, K. (1984) Hyponatraemia during treatment with chlorpropamide and moduretic (amiloride plus hydrochlorthiazide) *Br. Med. J.*, **289**, 659.

THE HISTORY OF INSULIN

EARLY PANCREATIC EXTRACTS

The initial observation which stimulated the search for insulin is generally credited to Von Mering and Minkowski (1889). They removed the pancreas from a dog and observed the development of diabetes. The animal developed glycosuria, ketonuria, wasting and hyperphagia. They were able to show that neither pancreatic duct ligation nor subtotal pancreatectomy resulted in diabetes. Laguesse (1893) suggested the possibility that the islets secreted a substance into the milieu interieur and the abnormal appearance of the islets in some cases of diabetes described by Opie (1901) made it more likely still. So much so, in fact, that de Meyer (1909) and Schafer (1916) were prepared to christen the unknown substance 'insuline', a name adopted by Banting when in 1922 he finally succeeded in isolating the active secretion of the islets.

In fact the realization of a pancreatic origin for diabetes lies further back in history. The Swiss anatomist Brunner (1683) had also removed the pancreas from dogs and observed polyuria and polydipsia. He was to be remembered however for the glands of the small intestine rather than his contribution to diabetes.

Attempts at making pancreatic extracts for treating diabetes had succeeded up to a point, particularly those of Gley (1905) and Zuelzer (1908) who used the pressed juice of pancreas extracted with alcohol and evaporated to dryness, the residue being dissolved in salt solution. Following intravenous injection in five patients on a constant diet the excretion of acetone, diacetic acid and sugar in the urine decreased or disappeared and the general condition improved. Unfortunately, the injections were followed by severe chills, fever and sometimes vomiting.

Forschbach (1909) used Zuelzer's extract on two patients. In one there was no effect and in the other the result was high fever and anuria for 12 hours. These reactions suggest the effect of protein products rather than hypoglycaemia, as has sometimes been suggested. They were sufficient to discourage further experiments in Germany.

The American diabetologist Allen (1913) also produced a pancreatic extract which, far from correcting diabetes in animals, actually increased glycosuria. He concluded that 'all authorities are agreed upon the failure of pancreatic therapy in diabetes'. In this view he was not alone – both Starling (1920) and Macleod *et al.* (1920), in new editions of their textbooks, regarded the case for a pancreatic hormone as non-proven.

Before citing the work of the Toronto group a few words of consolation should be written for the Romanian physiologist Paulesco. It fell to Paulesco to receive no credit for the discovery of insulin yet in early 1921 he repeatedly presented his work on the antidiabetic action of his pancreatic extract and in June 1921 he described his experiments in detail naming the active principle 'Pancreine' (Paulesco, 1921).

THE DISCOVERY OF INSULIN

Frederick Banting was an orthopaedic surgeon with an interest in physiology! Finding his practice slow to develop after the 1914–18 war he had time to enlist the support of Professor J. J. R. Macleod at the University of Toronto. Macleod recommended Charles Best as a useful chemistry undergraduate who would help Banting in his pancreatic experiments. Beginning in May 1921 and working throughout that summer they performed many experiments involving pancreatic duct ligation in dogs. This led to exocrine gland atrophy and from the remaining tissue they made an aqueous extract. In July 1921 they recorded that the extract lowered blood glucose in diabetic dogs. Later that year came the realization that duct ligation was unnecessary. The method of preparation was refined by J. B. Collip, a protein chemist who joined Banting and Best in late 1921. By January of 1922 they had sufficient confidence in their extract to inject it into a human patient not far from death from his diabetes. The first extract failed to have an effect upon blood glucose but a second extract prepared by Collip lowered blood glucose and cleared glycosuria and ketonuria (Banting, 1922; Banting *et al.*, 1922).

The fascinating story of the discovery of insulin still provokes controversy (Bliss, 1982); jealousies surfaced with the speedy award of a Nobel prize to Banting and Macleod which excluded the more formal recognition of Best and Collip. Although each of the Nobel laureates shared their prize with one of the others a certain unease or dissatisfaction remained.

PROLONGING THE DURATION OF ACTION OF INSULIN

For many years the only insulin preparation available for use was amorphous insulin. Insulin was crystallized by Abel in 1926 and Scott (1934) found that crystallization as the zinc salt was simple and a practical proposition in commercial manufacture. Both amorphous and crystalline insulin were only active for a short time, necessitating frequent injections, and there were soon attempts to prolong the effect by delaying absorption from the injection site.

Initial attempts to prolong action were made by preparing a suspension in oil but the action was irregular. Others added adrenalin to the insulin in an attempt to alter local blood flow and hence absorption. A more appropriate approach was to alter the physical or chemical properties of the insulin molecule. Hagedorn *et al.* (1936) succeeded by the addition of protamine from *Salmo iridius*, which altered the solubility of insulin at pH 7.4 and produced a preparation with a duration of action of about 10 hours. Scott and Fisher (1935) had already shown that the physiological action of insulin was much delayed by the addition of 0.01% of zinc and they prepared protamine zinc insulin, a primarily amorphous precipitate of insulin with protamine and zinc buffered with phosphate. The final development in this preparation was protamine zinc insulin in crystalline suspension, for which a greater stability was claimed.

In 1946 Krayenbuhl and Rosenberg introduced isophane or neutral protamine Hagedorn (NPH) insulin in which a smaller and precise amount of protamine was mixed with zinc-insulin crystals, giving a shorter duration of action than protamine zinc insulin (PZI). This successful preparation overshadowed globin insulin in which globin from beef red cells was substituted for protamine as a retarding agent.

Another major advance was the discovery by Hallas-Moller *et al.* (1952) that the use of acetate rather than phosphate as a buffer made it possible with the addition of zinc to keep insulin in a relatively insoluble crystalline or amorphous form without the use of any added protein. The duration of action of these insulin zinc suspensions varied according to the proportions of amorphous and crystalline preparations. Semilente (amorphous) had an action slightly longer than soluble insulin while ultralente (crystalline) lasted longer than 24 hours. The most successful commercial preparation was lente insulin – three parts semilente to seven parts ultralente with a duration of action of 24 hours.

HIGHLY PURIFIED INSULIN PREPARATIONS

In later years the chemists focussed upon the purification of insulin. Repeated crystallization of insulin was used to reduce the antigenic stimulus but even this preparation contained many foreign compounds. Conventional commercial insulin preparations could be shown to contain many impurities including other pancreatic hormones in small amounts as well as insulin molecules inadvertently modified in the preparation. These included arginine-insulins, desamido-insulin, ethylester insulins and proinsulin. These impurities resulting from the manufacturing process were held responsible for the production of antibodies in patients using conventional preparations (Bloom *et al.*, 1979). The development of a purification process, based on ion-exchange chromatography (Schlichtkrull *et al.*, 1972) which could be applied commercially led to the production of monocomponent insulins. These were followed by single peak or similarly named insulins; all the names indicating that when subjected to disc gel electrophoresis or similar separation technique the preparations revealed only one component or a single peak of pure chemical insulin.

HUMAN INSULIN

Having demonstrated an ability to produce the pure chemical commercially it seemed logical that the next step would be to move from beef or pork insulin to the commercial production of human insulin. From the outset it was clear that two of the possible methods would be unlikely to lead to commercial viability. Extraction of insulin from human pancreata and total synthesis of insulin were both performed in the 1960s. The former method has been used to produce standards for radioimmunoassay and as the

Table 9.1 Differences in amino acid sequence between insulins from different species

| | Location | | |
Species	A8	A10	B30
Bovine	Alanine	Valine	Alanine
Porcine	Threonine	Isoleucine	Alanine
Human	Threonine	Isoleucine	Threonine

international standard. Small amounts produced by total chemical synthesis were sufficient only for limited experiments in animals and a few volunteers (Markie and Albrecht, 1977).

More recently bacterial synthesis of insulin and conversion of porcine to human insulin have been successful commercially. In 1979 Goeddel *et al.* synthesized human A and B chains in *E. coli*. Chemically synthesized codons were inserted into plasmid DNA and, under appropriate conditions, large quantities of A and B chains were produced. After purification of the insulin chains they were combined to produce human insulin.

Minor amino acid differences exist between beef, pork, and human insulin (Table 9.1). The porcine/human difference, only in the C-terminal amino acid of the B chain proved irresistible as a target for the protein chemists. They were able to replace the B-30 amino acid alanine of porcine insulin with threonine, thus semi-synthesizing human insulin (Markussen, 1984). This latter approach failed to solve the problem of supply of porcine insulin and proved a temporary solution now replaced by biosynthesis using genetic engineering in yeast.

The structure of insulin

Insulin is a protein with a molecular weight of around 6000. For human insulin the molecular weight is 5807 Da. The structural formula was revealed by a remarkable piece of arduous and largely individual research by Sanger and his colleagues (Sanger, Thompson and Kitai, 1955; Ryle *et al.*, 1955) and is

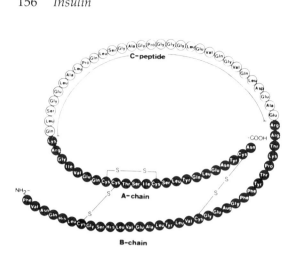

Fig. 9.1 The structure of human proinsulin.

shown in Figure 9.1 The two polypeptide chains of 21 and 30 amino acids are joined by two disulphide links, A7 to B7 and A20 to B19 and there is one intra-chain A6 to A11 connecting the cysteine components. These links contain all the sulphur in the molecule and are essential for the physiological action of insulin.

Proteins such as insulin, however, are three-dimensional structures and this has been identified by X-ray analysis (Adams *et al.*, 1969). In this three-dimensional structure certain amino acids are buried while others on the surface have specific functions. Of particular importance are the dimer and hexamer forming residues and the receptor binding surface. Removal of the terminal of the B-chain, e.g. B22-B31, virtually abolishes insulin action, reducing its potency to about 1% and evidence from patients with mutant insulin supports the view of the importance of the area around the two phenylalanines at B24 and B25.

Potential routes of administration

Hydrolysis of insulin destroys its activity and for this reason it is without effect when given by mouth. Sublingual and nasal absorption, though slight, have been demonstrated, but pulmonary, rectal, vaginal and scrotal administration have been tried in vain. Attempts to overcome the enzyme digestion by the use of a gelatin capsule covered with cellulose plastic material have given irregular results. Experimental work suggests great difficulty in getting insulin across the intestinal mucosa, although the possibility exists in theory. Experimentally insulin injected into the submucous layer of the intestine or into the mesenteric veins retains full activity.

Recently there has been a resurgence of interest in intranasal administration of insulin as an alternative to invasive subcutaneous injections. The major point of interest is in the speed of absorption of insulin given in this way. Absorption is fast from the nasal mucosa and the peak of insulin in the circulation is found 10–23 minutes after a sniff (Bruce *et al.*, 1991; Drejer *et al.*, 1992). An enhancer of absorption is needed to enhance transport of the peptide across the mucosal membrane. Bile salts, non-ionic polyethylene, fusidic acid derivative and phospholipid have been used. The major drawback appears to be bioavailability, which is low: around 5–10%.

It seems difficult to increase bioavailability without increasing the second problem, which is nasal irritation. Nevertheless interest in the preparation is likely to continue, since insulin dynamics more closely mimic the physiological response to a meal than can be obtained with subcutaneous insulin (Jacobs *et al.*, 1993).

GENETICALLY ENGINEERED INSULIN ANALOGUES

While some have pursued different ways of administering insulin in an attempt to mimic normal physiology more closely others have concentrated upon the insulin molecule. It might have been thought that, with the production of highly purified human insulin, the protein chemists would have little further to contribute in the management of diabetes. Not so! The techniques of genetic engineering allow an almost infinite number of modified insulin molecules to be produced.

An initial aim has been to modify the molecule such that dimerization and hexamer formation is reduced or abolished. It is clear that this can be achieved with only minor changes to the amino acid structure of the molecule. Genetically engineered insulin analogues which have altered dimerization surfaces can be absorbed two to three times faster than soluble insulin (Brange *et al.*, 1988; Vora *et al.*, 1988). LYSPRO (Lys(B28), Pro(B29))-human insulin is an insulin analogue in which the natural sequence of amino acids at B28, B29 is inverted, leading to a reduced capacity for self-association. Therefore it manifests monomeric behaviour in solution, binds zinc less avidly and has a faster pharmacodynamic action consistent with rapid absorption (Howey *et al.*, 1994; Trautmann, 1994). Similar faster onset of action is found with human insulin B28 Asp (Heinemann *et al.*, 1993).

In theory it is possible to set the desired profile for an insulin analogue and produce a number of compounds which might meet the requirements. Very-short-acting insulins or longer-acting insulins which could provide constant basal levels without peaks of absorption are readily imagined and already being developed. In the longer term it could theoretically be possible to produce a genetically engineered analogue which could be given by mouth and retain activity. This would involve identifying digestion sites and modifying the amino acids at these sites; perhaps changing some amino acids to change the chemical composition of the fragments that are produced in digestion; and hopefully leaving a peptide fragment which retains some insulin-like activity yet can cross the intestinal mucosa.

COMMERCIAL PREPARATIONS OF INSULIN

The international standard unit of insulin is the amount of a crystalline preparation needed to lower the blood glucose of a normal 24-hour fasting rabbit weighing 2 kg from 6.7 mmol/l (120 mg/dl) to 2.5 mmol/l (45 mg/dl) within 5 hours. The international standard of comparison is a preparation of zinc insulin crystals containing 22 units per milligram. The biological potency of bovine and porcine insulins is practically the same. Indeed the fourth international standard of insulin was a mixture of the two species insulins. Human insulin has the same potency in rabbits as animal insulins but there are minor differences in timing between the species. This has led to a new generation of highly purified insulin standards, the International Standards for Bovine, Porcine and Human Insulin. At the same time, *in vivo* bioassay has been complemented by HPLC methods to check purity as well as strength.

Insulin is supplied in vials, cartridges or pre-loaded pens at a concentration of 100 units/ml. In some parts of the world strengths of 40 units/ml and 80 units/ml are the standard commercial preparations.

There are various species differences, porcine, bovine and human being readily obtainable, although the future of bovine looks uncertain. There is little point in supplying a list of available insulins; such a list would be outdated in a very short time as manufacturers strive for novelty and market share or simply rationalization of the product range.

The traditional method for grouping insulins is not by species or method of manufacture but rather by duration of action. The major classes have been short-acting, intermediate-acting, long-acting and preset mixtures.

Short-acting insulins, often called soluble or neutral insulin, contain insulin in a solution with a preservative such as phenol or para-aminobenzoate. Early preparations used an acid medium to achieve stability but improvements in preparation technique have allowed a shift to neutral solutions, which are less painful on injection. Short-acting insulins are absorbed from tissue depots at a lower rate than would be anticipated. This is due to dimer and hexamer formation at injection sites. Hexamer formation utilizes zinc drawn from surrounding tissues and dissociation of the hexamer is necessary for absorption.

The distinction between intermediate-acting and long-acting insulins has become less clear since the introduction of highly purified human insulins. The longest-acting insulins, ultralente and protamine zinc insulin, have been shortened in action by different means. Ultralente human insulin clearly has a shorter duration of action than conventional ultralente due both to species change and enhanced purification. Attempts to clean up protamine zinc insulin have had only limited success and the purity, along with the chemical properties of excess protamine, have left it lagging behind the porcine zinc or isophane insulins in the extent of its clinical use.

Insulins with a longer duration of action are required to dissociate from their retardant before absorption. Protamine is cleared from insulin before absorption and zinc insulins disassociate at the injection site. The rates of these processes determine the production of the short-acting insulin, which is then absorbed.

Premixed insulins have proved popular with the prescriber and the consumer for convenience. The 30/70 mixtures of quick- to intermediate-acting insulin are relatively safe in the hands of a patient unable to mix their own insulins while introduction of a wider range of premixed insulins, 10/90, 20/80, etc. have virtually obviated the need for patients to do any mixing of insulins in the syringe.

FACTORS INFLUENCING ABSORPTION OF INSULIN

In addition to the type of insulin injected a number of other factors contribute to the absorption characteristics of the insulin.

As far as species of insulin is concerned human insulin absorption seems to proceed at a slightly higher rate than bovine or porcine insulin injection. This is true for soluble and protamine insulins and particularly for zinc insulins.

A large dose of insulin shows a tendency to slower absorption but some of this effect is offset by increasing the concentration of the injected fluid.

The site of injection clearly influences the rate of absorption. Subcutaneous injection into the abdominal wall is absorbed faster than subcutaneous injection into the arm, which in turn is absorbed quicker than thigh or buttock subcutaneous injection.

Injecting into the intramuscular space increases the rate of absorption compared with subcutaneous injection while, as would be anticipated, intravenous injection obviates a need for absorption.

Changes at the site of injection can have marked effects upon absorption. Injections into the thigh, when followed by a hot bath or vigorous leg exercise increase the rate of absorption through alteration in blood flow. Conversely, adrenalin, by reducing blood flow, slows absorption. Interestingly, this is true during adrenalin infusions designed to achieve circulating levels of adrenalin as found in moderately stressful situations (Fernqvist, Gunnarsson and Linde, 1988).

Many insulin-treated diabetic patients are not sufficiently well controlled for the above factors to have an impact but in those well-controlled an awareness of these factors is important. Similarly, systematic enquiry may reveal an influence by one of the factors in an unexplained hypoglycaemic episode.

INDICATIONS FOR INSULIN

The decision to use insulin is not difficult when the patient presents in diabetic keto-acidosis. Nor should there be great soul-searching in a young patient with intense symptoms and acute weight loss leaving the patient underweight. Occasionally, a middle-aged patient will present with acute symptoms of diabetes and weight loss but may still be obese at presentation. In this situation sulphonylureas are likely to fail and insulin should be used. A mental note may be made to review the selection of therapy after 2 or 3 months, when treatment by diet or oral agents may be successfully substituted.

Faced with one of the above patients the physician is attempting to second-guess the type of diabetes which the patient has without any of the aetiological evidence. In the absence of information on HLA status, viral antibodies or islet cell antibodies, tests which are rarely performed in the clinic as opposed to in research studies, we are trying to identify type 1 diabetes. The only information available is a collection of indirect clues, the symptoms and signs, which reflect an underlying pathogenesis.

Thirst and polyuria simply indicate diabetes mellitus and not the type of diabetes, although the acuteness of the symptoms may suggest type 1 diabetes. By far the most useful sign is weight loss and greatest consideration is given to this. Appreciable weight loss implies loss of fat and fat breakdown can be confirmed by finding ketone bodies in the urine. Since fat breakdown is inhibited by low levels of insulin it is clear that if fat breakdown is occurring even these low levels are not being reached, despite the hyperglycaemic stimulus to insulin secretion, and therefore the patient is significantly insulin-deficient. It should be noted also that the spurious argument that ketonuria may be due to fasting is demolished by the presence of hyperglycaemia, which would stimulate insulin secretion if the pancreas was capable

of responding. Fat breakdown always indicates an inability to secrete even small amounts of insulin and hence severe insulin deficiency. In the best tradition of dogmatic medical sayings such as the previous sentence it is necessary to acknowledge one important exception to this rule.

Increased circulating ketone bodies and ketonuria can be found in the presence of amounts of insulin sufficient to control blood glucose. This occurs when a catabolic response accompanies a severe illness. Thus patients on the coronary care unit or intensive care unit suffering from a myocardial infarction or overwhelming infection may, under normal day-to-day living, have sufficient circulating insulin to achieve good control of blood glucose on diet or tablets. With the catabolic response to their illness, however, hyperglycaemia and ketonuria develop and if neglected diabetic ketoacidosis may ensue. The mechanism is an inability to increase insulin secretion both from adrenergic inhibition of insulin secretion and from poor secretory reserve in the face of increased insulin resistance due to high circulating concentrations of catabolic hormones. Although the mechanism for producing ketonuria is different there should be no room for doubt that this patient requires insulin treatment.

Insulin is required also when other forms of treatment fail to control diabetic symptoms. When thirst, asthenia or weight loss continue in spite of diet or oral treatment, insulin is undoubtedly needed. When the problem is that of hyperglycaemia and constant glycosuria without symptoms and there is evidence that the diet is being adequately followed it is wise to press the patient to accept insulin. There is danger of sudden deterioration under the stress of infection or injury (an argument which patients usually understand) and insulin is a safeguard against the risk, apart from the possible effect of improved control on the development of complications.

In old age diabetes is often unresponsive to dieting so that the idea of insulin should not be put aside. In fact the problem is an individual one and the decision to use insulin rests on the clinical findings – the symptoms and the appearance of the patient, which should be supplemented rather than replaced by the laboratory data.

Diabetes at every age is infinitely variable; there are children with mild diabetes which can be controlled by dietary restriction; a stout, middle-aged patient may occasionally develop severe ketosis; aged patients quite often have urgent thirst and lassitude. It is possible to generalize, however, to the extent of saying that all children and nearly all adults diagnosed under the age of 40 need insulin if not grossly overweight.

CONTRAINDICATIONS

These rarely have to be considered. It is obviously undesirable for those who could be controlled by dieting and these patients usually maintain an excessive weight with insulin allied to gluttony. It is at times unwise to provide a potent weapon of manipulation, which as, insulin is, to those who may relish the advantage this gives them in manipulating their situation. Occasionally the introduction of insulin treatment may threaten livelihood such as the loss of a vocational driving licence with subsequent unemployment. In the insulin-dependent patient there is, of course, no alternative but when the problem is of poor control on tablets it may be tempting to prolong the period of inadequate control and continue the oral therapy.

The possibility that insulin plays a part in the development of diabetic vascular complications has been put forward (Stout, 1987) but is not generally accepted, although in the development of atheroma it remains a field of intense debate.

THE PRACTICAL USE OF INSULIN

Diet arrangements are necessarily individual and the insulin dose should be adapted to the patient's normal habits rather than forcing a new mode of life on him/her in the interests of a chosen insulin scheme.

QUICK-ACTING INSULIN

As insulin in the normal subject is secreted in response to a rise in blood glucose level, an ideal preparation would release insulin into the circulation with each meal. The early users of insulin gave injections before each meal of the day and occasionally an extra dose at midnight to cover the long fasting period of sleep. This severe regimen of four or even five daily injections was effective and was particularly well suited to the temporary management of severe hyperglycaemia during a period of complication such as an infection.

In many respects, and as in other aspects of diabetes, the wheel has come full circle, with a resurgence of interest in multiple injections.

Quick-acting insulin injected before breakfast and again before the evening meal, as the only two injections of insulin per day, is not much in favour today. In the past it was described as the best treatment for diabetes of moderate severity but this was always a far from universal view. If by moderate severity is meant that the patient retains appreciable endogenous insulin secretion then twice-daily quick-acting insulin may be appropriate. The rationale is that it covers the hyperglycaemia from at least two of the three meals while residual insulin secretion is sufficient to account for maintenance of blood glucose overnight. The regimen should then be contrasted with an alternative approach of twice-daily intermediate-acting insulin to provide a basal level of insulin during the day and overnight while endogenous secretion responds to mealtime stimuli. As with much of the advice in the use of insulin the ability of the patient to mount an endogenous insulin response remains most important. If, therefore, we try to apply the above logic to non-insulin-dependent patients who are poorly controlled on maximum doses of sulphonylurea – i.e. their insulin secretory ability must be severely compromised – we find that neither regimen produces normoglycaemia although preprandial short-acting insulin may give better results than a single daily injection of long-acting insulin (Paterson *et al.*, 1991).

Undoubtedly, one of the underlying reasons for the success of twice-daily quick-acting insulin in the past was the antigenic nature of the injected insulin. Most patients had demonstrable antibodies to insulin, which bound injected insulin. The net effect was to convert quick-acting insulin into a bound depot and the release of this from the antibody had the characteristics of a longer-acting insulin. These attributes have become apparent since the introduction of highly purified insulins and it is unusual to see long-standing insulin-dependent diabetics maintaining the same degree of control on twice-daily quick-acting insulin, which is highly purified, as they had with twice-daily quick-acting conventional bovine insulin.

Current activity is directed towards modifying the insulin molecule to give more speedy absorption from subcutaneous injection sites as with LYSPRO Human Insulin (see above).

LONG-ACTING AND INTERMEDIATE-ACTING INSULINS

Single daily injections of a long-acting insulin are no longer appropriate in patients where the level of diabetic control is important. To produce good control a single daily injection needed to be combined with a regimented life such that meals were similar in content and at identical times from day to day. That this did not have to be so in so many patients was because their level of control fell below an acceptable standard. In other words, a patient did not develop hypoglycaemia when

lunch or dinner was late because they were still hyperglycaemic at that time.

Protamine zinc insulin, either as a single dose or combined in a once-daily injection with quick-acting insulin is rarely used today. When it is used it is necessary to be aware of the problems created by the excess of protamine. Mixing in the syringe results in a change in the soluble insulin, converting about half in a 1:1 mixture from soluble to long-acting. Attempts to draw both insulins into one syringe can also affect the composition of soluble in the ampoule. Injection of even small amounts of PZI into the soluble ampoule can prolong the action of soluble. It is perhaps true to say that in the few remaining patients using this regimen it is difficult to know the exactness of the insulin prescription. All that can be ensured is that the patient repeats exactly the same procedure for drawing up and injecting each day.

The other long-acting insulin has strong advocates – not as the sole injection each day, nor even with one dose of quick-acting insulin, but with two- or three-times-daily quick-acting. The theoretical goal is fasting normoglycaemia brought about by ultralente given the previous night or even morning. Turner's group have stressed the reproducibility of fasting blood glucose measurement in non-insulin-dependent diabetics (Turner *et al.*, 1977). In this group of patents, it is argued, it may only be necessary to reduce fasting blood glucose to produce a diurnal profile not far removed from normal. When glucose excursions after meals are excessive, injections of quick-acting insulin can be introduced to the regimen.

Isophane insulins remain popular. They are particularly suited to the twice-daily regimen of mixtures of short- and intermediate-acting insulins. The use of a once-daily insulin mixture is less prevalent and probably owed much of its efficiency to the antibody-generating effect described above. Whether modern-day isophanes are even suited to maintaining normoglycaemia overnight when given in the morning is debatable, but to my mind doubtful. It is even asking rather a lot for an injection at 6.00 pm to hold down blood glucose at 8.00 am next morning without some peak of absorption occurring around midnight with a risk of hypoglycaemia. Better results have been obtained with isophane given before bedtime rather in the morning in non-insulin-dependent patients (Seigler, Olsson and Skyler, 1992). Isophanes are popular in the Western world and are probably marginally preferred to zinc insulins.

The lente family of insulins enjoyed a long run of popularity in the UK. Semilente and ultralente in 30/70 proportion as lente or in individualized proportions have had considerable success, which continues through Monotard. This insulin is more patently a twice-daily insulin than was conventional lente insulin.

Of all the premixed insulins available I am particularly attracted to the 50/50 mixture. In studies using the artificial endocrine pancreas (Biostator®) to assess insulin requirement over 24 hours it is clear that about half the insulin is needed to cover meals and half to maintain basal blood glucose. This suggests that a 50/50 mixture would be the most physiological and appropriate. That the 50/50 mixture has not been used more widely is, I am sure, due to a reluctance to increase the proportion of the dose given as quick-acting for fear of hypoglycaemia.

The biphasic insulin Rapitard must surely be shortly for extinction. Indeed, one of the quarrels with the insulin manufacturers is that insulins are rarely withdrawn; the range is added to! This accusation is quite unfair, since any attempt by a manufacturer to withdraw an insulin has always met resistance from patients who feel it is well-suited to them, or from their doctors who feel that they should not disturb good control in the patient.

STARTING INSULIN

Much has been written on the respective merits of starting insulin in the patient's home or in hospital. Protagonists of home stabilization point to the more realistic lifestyle of the patient at home and the putative psychological advantages, particularly for a child, of remaining in the bosom of the family. Opponents suggest a benefit of being able to concentrate upon learning to the exclusion of other aspects of life.

The paramount consideration is safety and this should never be conceded to dogma. Cases with significant ketonuria are only safe to treat at home if the doctor and others are able to give a good deal of time every day to the problem. Without adequate community backup a great disservice can be done to the patient by shouting loudly for home stabilization. Similarly, if the best offer for in-patient stabilization is a bed on a general medical ward surrounded by severely ill patients this course of action will do the patient no favours. In practice few patients are admitted to an inpatient bed to start insulin in the modern era. The growth in facilities and staff to educate patients on a day-attendance basis has rendered admission unnecessary. Only with heavy ketonuria does one's nerve tend to fail and the patient is admitted.

The aims of starting insulin are twofold: firstly to improve diabetic control and secondly to attempt to imbue a degree of independence in the patient. At the end of the process it would be appropriate to have good diabetic control but as important is that the patient can inject, knows the diet, appreciates the relation of diet, exercise and insulin, and can cope with hypo- and hyperglycaemia.

It must be emphasized that there is no way of telling how much insulin per day will be needed by an individual patient. No calculation from age, body weight, diet, blood glucose or glycosuria can help. The prescription is an empirical one based on experience but always likely to be proved wrong. While the dose is empirical the regimen need be less so. Here again the patient is the guide. Once-a-day insulin may be sufficient to relieve symptoms in a 70-year-old but would be inappropriate in a youngster facing a lifetime of diabetes. Clearly, a tailored regimen is needed yet some general guidelines have to be set down based on the aims of treatment.

THE AIMS OF INSULIN TREATMENT

The aims of treatment must be defined. In essence these revolve around the degree of blood glucose control that is thought appropriate in the particular patient. Constantly there lurks in the shadows the knowledge that overenthusiastic use of insulin increases the risk of hypoglycaemia. Goals may be set as follows.

1. The aim is normoglycaemia at best or good blood glucose control at worst, to delay onset of complications.
2. The aim is to keep the patient symptom-free without necessarily achieving normoglycaemia, a goal suitable for the elderly, the infirm or those with considerable residual insulin secretion.

There is some merit in always starting insulin as quick-acting insulin frequently, 4–6-hourly. This allows the patient plenty of practice at injecting, obviates the need or temptation to give a big dose of insulin initially and reduces blood glucose gradually. It is wise not to exceed 24 units of insulin in the first 24 hours, split among the injections.

An alternative is to commence treatment with twice-daily intermediate-acting insulin or a preset mixture. An initial daily dose of 12 units in the morning and 8 units in the evening is appropriate and this can be increased by 4 units next day depending upon the response. Adjusting treatment requires that diet be sorted out quickly. The hospital system does not allow careful mimicry of daily

life but a good diabetes educator or ward sister will always moderate the regimentation. Similarly, physical activity should be encouraged.

Many physicians aim to produce a mild hypoglycaemic attack during the initial period of treatment so that the patient will be quite clear about the nature of symptoms and their rapid relief by sugar.

In the past there have been advocates of an initial dose in adults of 30–40 units of insulin, especially in the presence of ketonuria. There are, as already stated, not a few insulin-sensitive subjects who would become hypoglycaemic within two to three doses at this level, perhaps even with their first dose – not the best introduction to the benefits of insulin treatment. Our experience has been that 20 units is occasionally excessive. Sometimes there is evidence of a rapid response in fasting blood glucose so that a reduction of dose has to be considered. More often, the blood glucose is slightly reduced and the symptoms are partially relieved, in which case an increase of 4 units can be made. Commonly, there is no obvious effect from 16 units daily; it is then possible to raise the dose more rapidly – by 8 units at least. The position is reviewed daily at the outset and then every few days until blood glucose control is achieved.

In newly diagnosed insulin-dependent patients during the initial phase of treatment the diabetes often comes under control with surprising ease, and a remarkably stable situation is soon achieved with a dose of up to 40 units of insulin daily. The urine is constantly sugar-free and the blood glucose normal but there are no hypoglycaemic episodes. Where the insulin dose is small the variety seems to matter very little. Unfortunately this happy state seldom lasts for more than 1 or 2 years. Gradually, control becomes less easy or there may be a sudden deterioration following an acute infection – thereafter there is no return to this honeymoon state of easy diabetes.

Table 9.2 Definitions of metabolic control

	Good	Acceptable	Poor
Fasting blood glucose (mmol/l)	4.4–6.7	< 7.8	> 7.8
Post-prandial blood glucose (mmol/l)	4.4–8.9	< 10.0	> 10.0
Glycated proteins	< mean + 2 s.d.	< mean + 4 s.d.	> mean + 4 s.d.

CONTROL OF BLOOD GLUCOSE

I am conscious, both in writing and talking of diabetes, of the lack of precision in the use of the word 'control' and other related terms. To write that non-insulin-dependent diabetic patients on oral agents 'poorly controlled, or with persistent hyperglycaemia', should be changed to insulin treatment is a meaningless statement without some point of reference for the terms. Normoglycaemia is one such point but if hyperglycaemia – blood glucose above the normal range – is to be equated with poor control then we may have to admit that 99% of diabetic patients are poorly controlled.

While strictly accurate this may be less than helpful in practice and realistic goals must be set. Unless insulin delivery in the patient is intimately linked to prevailing blood glucose concentration, obtaining and maintaining euglycaemia may be an unattainable goal in the majority of patients using insulin. Synchronizing insulin delivery from a subcutaneous depot with glucose delivery from the gut following a meal is well-nigh impossible. The rapid absorption of quick-acting insulin from subcutaneous sites cannot match the speed of insulin secretion in response to a secretory stimulus of the non-diabetic. Nor should we forget the handicap imposed by peripheral administration of insulin in the diabetic patient as opposed to portal delivery in the normal subject. These factors mitigate against the ability to achieve euglycaemia and must influence our views on control of blood glucose.

Alberti and Gries (1988), on behalf of the European NIDDM Policy Group, have set targets for metabolic control in non-insulin-dependent diabetic patients. These are summarized in Table 9.2 for blood glucose and glycated proteins. The original publication includes targets for cholesterol, triglycerides and HDL-cholesterol. Because of wide differences in measurement and reference ranges for glycated proteins between laboratories these definitions are given with reference to the local reference range. While these standards can be applied to non-insulin-dependent diabetic patients treated with insulin, applying them to insulin-dependent patients would be using them out of context in a manner for which they were not intended. Nevertheless, they give some idea of the thinking behind the description of control as acceptable or poor.

LOCAL REACTIONS TO INSULIN

INSULIN ALLERGY

Modern insulin preparations normally cause no local reactions. Occasionally, local skin sensitization is seen which is seldom seriously troublesome. The reaction consists of a stinging or itching sensation with redness and minor degrees of swelling and tenderness at the injection site. It is difficult to know whether the response is to insulin species, protein used to prolong action or the diluent in the vial. Most insulin manufacturers will supply testing kits, which rarely give a clear-cut answer.

General symptoms such as nausea, vomiting and circulatory collapse are not recorded with purified human insulins, although anaphylactic shock has occasionally been reported with conventional insulins.

Generalized allergic skin reactions are occasionally seen with human insulin. The antibody responsible for the skin reaction is usually IgE and is distinct from insulin antibodies of IgG class. Insulin resistance and skin reaction are not necessarily associated. Most local reactions cease spontaneously after 2–4 weeks of continued injections and are not sufficiently severe to interrupt treatment. When they persist for a longer period they are apt to disappear for no obvious reason, a fact that is significant in assessing the value of treatment. Antihistamine drugs are useless, although inevitably used often enough, and systemic steroids are hardly justified, although the inclusion of hydrocortisone in the insulin might be considered in a severe case. Changing the brand of insulin is occasionally effective. Desensitization by repeated intradermal doses of insulin gives results which are at best uncertain, although the method has been repeatedly recommended by writers who, one suspects, have never themselves used it.

LIPODYSTROPHY

The term 'lipodystrophy' includes the loss of subcutaneous fat – lipoatrophy – and localized excess of fat tissue – lipohypertrophy. The incidence of the former has declined dramatically with the use of highly purified insulins although it is still seen occasionally even in patients using human insulin. Lipohypertrophy is less likely to be commented upon by the patient.

Lipoatrophy

This is local disappearance of subcutaneous fat, usually at the site of insulin injection. The lesion may appear occasionally in areas in which an injection has never been given and has been reported in patients giving other protein injections. The extent ranges from slight hollowing of the tissues to deeply troughed areas, although the latter are rarely

seen nowadays. Estimates of its incidence with conventional insulin ranged from 1% to 55%, no doubt reflecting methods of enquiry and assessment. When highly purified porcine insulins were introduced the incidence of lipoatrophy fell sharply and with human insulin the incidence is at the 'worthy of a case report' stage. Slight lipoatrophy may regress if the site is not injected for a time and highly purified human insulin should be prescribed if any other was being used.

Lipohypertrophy

This lesion ultimately forms a large subcutaneous mass, not attached to skin as is a lipoma. The lesion might reasonably be regarded as a local effect of insulin and almost always occurs in response to repeated injection into the same site. Disappearance at least of minor degrees of hypertrophy, can occur if the site is avoided for a while. It is not always easy to persuade patients to accept this since the fatty area is often totally pain-free at injection. It is acknowledged that injection into the lipohypertrophy renders insulin absorption somewhat unpredictable.

OTHER LOCAL REACTIONS

The majority of other problems of sites of injection are due to faulty technique. Localized purpura may occur, especially in those prone to inject areas that cannot be seen by the patient, such as buttocks. Occasionally, abscess formation and ulceration is seen with repeated injections into one area.

INSULIN ANTAGONISTS

Substances that reduce the action of insulin are by definition antagonists. They can be divided into intrinsically useful compounds and antibodies. In the former group would be those compounds whose effect upon metabolism is such as to reduce the effectiveness of insulin, such as the catabolic hormones glucagon, adrenalin, cortisol and growth hormone and the metabolites non-esterified fatty acids and ketone bodies.

Circulating insulin antibodies to injected insulin still occur with the use of highly purified and human insulins but as a clinical problem its importance has declined. In newly diagnosed diabetics treated from the onset with highly purified insulins about 60% develop antibodies but of such low titre as to be of little importance. Previously reported high titres of insulin antibodies in patients treated with conventional insulins are not equalled with modern-day treatment. Many studies have shown that titres in such patients decline rapidly when a change to highly purified insulins is made. Despite these changes it is apparent that diabetic patients continue to require more units per day than would be predicted from secretory rates of the pancreas. This is probably more correctly ascribed to insulin resistance developing as part of the disease rather than the injected insulin.

CHRONIC INSULIN RESISTANCE

The original definition of clinical insulin resistance as a daily requirement of more than 200 units per day is outmoded. It was based upon a calculation that a completely depancreatectomized man would require 200–300 units each day. Estimates of the daily secretion of the pancreas have come down and down and are currently held to be 26–30 units per day. Thus insulin resistance is present in all patients who require more than this as a daily dose. This definition is not helpful since the majority of insulin-deficient patients require in excess of this. Why this should be so is unclear and indeed it is not certain that such a finding is worldwide. The average daily dose in our clinic is about 50 units per day.

Several factors may influence such a figure. Obese patients require higher daily doses of insulin, as would be expected from the calculated daily secretion rates in obese patients (Polonsky, Given and Van Cauter, 1988). It also appears that many injections in the course of the day use less insulin in total than a single daily injection. Physicians will be familiar with the improvement in control that follows splitting a once-daily dose to a twice-daily dose without an increase in units given. In part this must be due to changes in insulin metabolism that occur.

The major cause of insulin resistance, however, must lie in the natural history of treated insulin-dependent diabetes. We have shown an impaired hypoglycaemic effect and anti-lipolytic effect of insulin in patients treated for more than 5 years compared with those recently diagnosed (Singh, Palma and Nattrass, 1987). Others have reported similar findings for the hypoglycaemic effect. The mechanism for this is uncertain but may well lie in peripheral injection of insulin.

Occasional patients have been reported with a massive requirement for insulin who are otherwise apparently normal insulin-dependent diabetic patients. Such patients are rare and tend to gravitate to centres with a particular interest in the problem. Perhaps that is why I have not encountered a patient with this problem. Doses of up to 3000 units per day have been recorded in an attempt to obtain control of blood glucose. Provided it can be ensured that insulin is being injected the implication is of a failure of absorption from the injection site, possibly as a result of insulin breakdown at the site.

ACUTE INSULIN RESISTANCE

Chronic insulin resistance, i.e. resistance maintained over months and years, excludes the insulin resistance of infection, and ketoacidosis. Both states are accompanied by elevated circulating concentrations of anti-insulin hormones, which reduce effectiveness of insulin. Additionally, in ketoacidosis the acidosis *per se* contributes to a lessening of the effect of insulin. Provided sufficient insulin is given the effect is readily overcome and massive insulin resistance is rarely seen. Usually it can be predicted, where a patient in ketoacidosis is also given large doses of corticosteroids.

EXCESSIVE USE OF INSULIN

The studies of Somogyi, starting in 1938 and summarized in his paper of 1959 made an important contribution to our understanding of excessive insulin action. He observed that in some patients who had defied all attempts to control their blood glucose with insulin there was a distinct pattern in the record of urinary sugar output, suggesting that excessive glycosuria was an aftermath of hypoglycaemia. It seemed possible that depression of blood glucose by insulin provoked a powerful correcting mechanism which could bring about a prolonged and substantial hyperglycaemic phase. Especially important was the demonstration that the initial fall in blood glucose did not have to reach such a level as to produce symptoms of hypoglycaemia. This was in accord with clinical and experimental evidence that increased secretion of adrenalin and of corticosteroids could be provoked by a degree of hypoglycaemia short of that which produced clinical symptoms. The critical level at which an increase in adrenalin secretion could be shown was about 4.4 mmol/l (80 mg/dl), with blood sugar measured by a method not specific for glucose. Using a specific method for measuring glucose this level has been set at 3.8 mmol/l (68 mg/dl) (Mitrakou *et al.* 1991). Thus the situation could be envisaged in which insulin caused a fall in blood glucose insufficient to elicit symptoms of hypoglycaemia but sufficient to bring into play counter-regulatory mechanisms which would initiate a phase of hyperglycaemia. If treatment was directed to the elimination of hyperglycaemia an increase in dose of insulin would aggravate the situation.

Belief in the existence of the Somogyi phenomenon has fluctuated, with a pattern akin to the swings in blood glucose it describes. A popular diagnosis in the 1970s (Bruck and MacGillivray, 1974; Travis, 1975; Tattersall, 1977), more latterly it has disappeared from the literature. Many instances exist where poor blood glucose control at home on 60 units of insulin per day becomes good control in hospital on 30 units per day. Not often is it necessary to invoke the Somogyi phenomenon as an explanation – more often it is clearly a feature of dietary regulation.

BRITTLE DIABETES

Inclusion of this topic at this particular place in the volume betrays my views on a contentious subject. The term is reported to have been coined by Woodyat (1937) to describe the situation of patients whose control is always insecure, with rapid swings between hypoglycaemia and ketoacidosis. It is a difficult phase in the life of an insulin-dependent patient, fortunately occurring in only a small number of patients. The area is contentious, not as to whether the condition occurs, but as to whether it signals a particular type of diabetes.

Haunz (1950) found six brittle diabetics in a series of 310, half of whom needed insulin, over a period of 2 years. He thought these patients were often mentally depressed, with reactions of futility and frustration, for obvious and rather justifiable reasons. They tended to drift from physician to physician in a vain search for the one who knew the whole answer.

As with any loosely defined condition, prevalence figures are hard to come by. Gill, Walford and Alberti (1985), writing from a centre with interest in brittle diabetes, estimate a considerably lower prevalence of 1–5 per 1000.

Patients are recognizable by the total disruption that their diabetes brings not only to their own lives but also to the lives of their families. Tattersall (1977), in an oft-quoted definition, described 'insulin-dependent diabetics whose lives are constantly disrupted by episodes of hypo- or hyperglycaemia, whatever the cause'. Put like that no-one could deny the existence of the labile diabetes that is described. It is the final phrase which serves to confuse. The over-riding concern is whether, when patients with a recognizable cause for their labile diabetes are excluded, any remain with a specific type of diabetes that could be described as being brittle. From the wealth of publications on the topic it is clear that a small number of patients remain, although it is unclear whether there is no cause other than the type of diabetes or whether a cause exists but is unidentified.

Mention must be made at this stage of the natural tendency of doctors to believe what they are told by the patient. It is difficult to accept that a patient may be deliberately deceiving by word and behaviour for protracted periods of time. The last brittle diabetic I saw was sent to us after more than 12 months in hospital elsewhere in the country. Her stay with us was brief and stormy. Rapid swings in blood glucose despite intravenous insulin occurred, punctuated by episodes of sepsis. It was our nursing sister who suggested we should measure the concentration of insulin in the syringe just before it was empty. Rather better than this, since insulin was diluted in saline we could simply measure sodium concentration at the beginning of the infusion and the end. It rapidly became clear that saline, and hence insulin, was disappearing from some of the syringes during the infusion. I mention this young woman not to show how clever we are in Birmingham but to illustrate two important points. When we sent her back to the referring centre our explanation of her brittleness was greeted with incredulity. It could not be accepted that they had been deceived for 12 months and clearly we had made errors! Only in later publications from that centre did I notice an acceptance of our

findings. The second point made by the story is that insulin was not missing from every syringe. The assumption should not be made that manipulation is going on constantly. It is clearly intermittent and, indeed, becomes unnecessary for long periods, for example when an introduced infection leads to a septicaemia.

I agree with the view that there are people with brittle personalities who have insulin-dependent diabetes. I find little support for a biochemically specific type of diabetes that is characterized by being brittle. Conversation some years later with reformed characters is instructive revealing the extent of their deviation from the prescribed treatment at a time when diabetes could be used as a tool to attract attention and interest. The role of centres with a special interest in the condition is difficult if they are not to perpetuate the state by answering the needs of the patient for interest and attention.

FUTURE TREATMENTS

In writing of future treatments it is acknowledged that some patients will already have received treatment by some of the methods outlined but I have labelled them as part of the future treatment of diabetes because they are not readily available to all diabetics. In addition, not all of them may be widely applicable.

ALTERNATIVE METHODS OF DELIVERING EXOGENOUS INSULIN

Intraperitoneal insulin delivery

Experience of intraperitoneal insulin delivery is limited to a few centres. It has usually been linked to continuous infusion by external or implantable pump and used, although not exclusively, in difficult-to-control brittle diabetics. Others in whom it has been used include those patients held to have massive resistance to subcutaneous and intramuscular insulin.

The rationale for this method of treatment is that there may be partial insulin absorption into the portal system, leading to more physiological insulin pharmacokinetics. Selam *et al.* (1985) reported on its use in 40 insulin-dependent diabetic patients treated for from 1 month to more than 2 years. Good control of diabetes was obtained but side effects were frequent. There was one episode of peritonitis, 12 hypoglycaemic comas and seven hyperglycaemic episodes. Pump and catheter survival rates were only 46% and 70% at 1 year. They concluded that their results were obtained mainly through careful selection of patients, intensive education and, only possibly, through more physiological insulin delivery.

Glucose-controlled insulin infusion system

Many would think the next major step in the treatment of diabetes with insulin has to be some means of linking insulin delivery to the prevailing blood glucose concentration. If this could be done successfully then hypoglycaemia would cease to be a major problem linked to tight control of blood glucose.

In fact a prototype system has been around for some years but results have been only moderately successful. The glucose-controlled-insulin-infusion-system (Biostator®) developed by Life Science Instruments, a division of the Miles Company of Elkhart, IN, was devised as a system incorporating a blood-sampling system leading to a glucose sensor; a computer; and an infusion system. Blood was sampled through a double-lumen cannula with heparinized saline pumped down the outer lumen and blood diluted with the heparinized saline pumped back to the glucose sensor. The glucose sensor was based on a glucose oxidase immobilized enzyme system which gave rapid results for blood glucose concentration. These results were used by the computer on the basis of preprogrammed algorithms to calculate rates of infusion. The algorithms could take into account not only the absolute glucose concentration but also the rate of change. The computer controlled a pump with options to infuse saline, insulin or glucose. These were administered intravenously.

It was clear that with two intravenous cannula sites any treatment could only be short-term but it was also clear that good control of blood glucose equating with normoglycaemia could be obtained in these short studies. The overwhelming problem, apart from the size of the equipment, was the difficulty of sampling for any length of time and this is a running sore in glucose sensor research. About a week was the maximum a sensor would work before platelet and fibrin deposition rendered it of no further use.

Continuous subcutaneous insulin infusion

The feedback device described above constitutes a 'closed loop' system. In other words, the loop is closed from withdrawal of blood to infusion. An alternative approach is to use an 'open loop' system. In this type of system intermittent blood samples are taken and analysed, and on the basis of the results the infusion rate of a pump is altered manually.

Continuous subcutaneous insulin infusion (CSII) was a technique popularized in the 1970/80s by a number of groups in Europe and the USA. The underlying idea was that a continuous infusion of insulin at a constant or basal rate should be infused subcutaneously and that this should be supplemented by boluses of insulin with meals, thus mimicking normal physiology. Use of this infusion system should also lead to more freedom in size and timing of meals.

The initial pumps were rather simple machines which soon led to the development of more sophisticated programmable pumps. Users tended to be highly motivated. Some groups have reported extensive experience of this approach to treatment (Chanteleau *et al.*, 1989).

A number of problems were noted with their use, which has resulted in a decline in popularity. These range from relatively minor problems such as skin infections at the site of access, through hypoglycaemia from attempts at tight control, to diabetic keto-acidosis as a consequence of pump failure. Because of the possibility of pump failure in particular and problems in general the system was demanding of time from the patient and time and resources from the clinic supervising the treatment. Most clinics with a number of patients on this therapy had a doctor and/or a nurse on call all the time.

REPLACING ENDOGENOUS INSULIN

Pancreatic transplantation

Pancreatic transplantation in insulin-dependent diabetic patients began in the late 1960s at the University of Minnesota with the use of vascularized segmental grafts in uraemic patients who were also receiving a kidney. A high morbidity and mortality resulted from technical problems and difficulties in the diagnosis and treatment of rejection and it was not until the late 1970s, when the newer immunosuppressive agents such as cyclo-sporin A arrived, that interest in the technique was reawakened. From an annual rate of transplant of between one and eight before 1978 the rise since that time has been exponential. About two-thirds of patients have received a combined kidney and pancreas graft; one-sixth, a pancreas after a kidney; and in the remaining one-sixth a pancreas only.

Initial techniques used ductal ligation or injection in an attempt to destroy exocrine tissue, since in early transplants there was a high incidence of complications, particularly infection, associated with exocrine secretion. Recently, exocrine drainage has been used to overcome this problem, with the main site of drainage the bladder. This does not interfere with the gastrointestinal tract and has the added advantage of allowing early identification of rejection by monitoring urinary amylase.

Successful transplantation of a pancreas results in correction of hyperglycaemia. Subtle defects of the regulation of carbohydrate metabolism persist but the life of the patient is revolutionized. In the mid-1980s successful graft function at 1 year was of the order of 40–60%. More recently some centres have reported 70% 1-year graft survival rates, with patient survivals of 90%, with a total number of patients from 1987 onward of over 2000. Technical failure accounts for 15% from thrombosis, infection, pancreatitis and leakage.

Islet cell transplantation

Islet cell transplantation is an inherently more attractive prospect than organ transplantation. Unfortunately it shows no signs of becoming as successful! The current problems lie mainly in the harvesting of the islets. In isolating islets from a donor pancreas high yields can be obtained but the price paid is low purity. High purity preparations tend to result in low yields such that sufficient islets for one recipient necessitates two to four donors. Of the limited number of transplants that have been done the islet survival figures are not known but they do not begin to approach those of pancreatic transplant. In theory one of the attractive options with islets would be to encapsulate them in such a way that they were not exposed to immune attack. This goal has also proved elusive.

REFERENCES

Abel, J. J. (1926) Crystallisation of insulin. *Proc. Nat. Acad. Sci.* **12**, 132–136.
Adams, M. J., Baker, E. N., Blundell, T. L. *et al.* (1969) Structure of rhombohedral 2 Zinc insulin crystals. *Nature*, **224**, 491–495.
Alberti, K. G. M. M. and Gries, F. A. (1988)

Management of non-insulin-dependent diabetes mellitus in Europe: a consensus view. *Diabetic Med.* **5**, 275–281.

Allen, F. M. (1913) *Glycosuria and Diabetes*, Harvard University Press, Cambridge, MA.

Banting, F. G. (1922) The internal secretion of the pancreas. *J. Lab. Clin. Med.*, **7**, 251–256.

Banting, F. G., Best, C. H., Collip, J. B. *et al.* (1922) Pancreatic extracts in the treatment of diabetes mellitus. *Can. Med. Ass. J.*, **12**, 141–146.

Bliss, M. (1982) *The Discovery of Insulin*, McClelland & Stewart, Toronto.

Bloom, S. R., Adrian, T. E., Barnes, A. J. and Polak, J. M. (1979) Autoimmunity in diabetics induced by hormonal contaminants of insulin. *Lancet*, **i**, 14–17.

Brange, J., Ribel, U., Hansen, J. E. *et al.* (1988) Monomeric insulins obtained by protein engineering and their medical implications. *Nature*, **333**, 679–682.

Bruce, D. G., Chisholm, D. J., Storlien, L. H. *et al.* (1991) Meal-time intranasal insulin delivery in type 2 diabetes. *Diabetic Med.* **8**, 366–370.

Bruck, E. and MacGillivray, M. H. (1974) Post-hypoglycemic hyperglycemia in diabetic children. *J. Pediatr.*, **84**, 672–680.

Brunner, J. C. (1683) In: *Experimenta Nova Circa Pancreas*, Amstelaedami.

Chantelau, E., Spraul, M., Muhlhauser, I. *et al.* (1989) Long term safety, efficacy, and side effects of continuous subcutaneous insulin infusion treatment for type 1 (insulin-dependent) diabetes mellitus: a one centre experience. *Diabetologia*, **32**, 421–426.

Drejer, K., Vaag, A., Bech, K. *et al.* (1992) Intranasal administration of insulin with phospholipid as absorption enhancer: pharmacokinetics in normal subjects. *Diabetic Med.*, **9**, 335–340.

de Meyer, J. (1909) Action de la secretion interne du pancreas sur different organs et en particulier sur la secretion renale. *Arch. Fisiol.*, **7**, 96–99.

Fernqvist, E., Gunnarsson, R. and Linde, B. (1988) Influence of circulating epinephrine on absorption of subcutaneously injected insulin. *Diabetes*, **37**, 694–701.

Forschbach, J. (1909) Zur Pathogenese des Pankreas-Diabetes. *Arch. Exp. Path. Pharmak. Leipzig*, **60**, 131–153.

Gill, G. V., Walford, S. and Alberti, K. G. M. M. (1985) Brittle diabetes – present concepts. *Diabetologia*, **28**, 579–589.

Gley, E. (1905) Quoted by Hoet, J. P. (1953)

Gustave Edouard Laguesse; his demonstration of the significance of the islands of Langerhans. *Diabetes*, **2**, 322–328.

Goeddel, D. V., Kleid, D. G., Bolivar, F. *et al.* (1979) Expression in *Escherichia coli* of chemically synthesised genes for human insulin. *Proc. Nat. Acad. Sci. USA*, **76**, 106–110.

Hagedorn, H. C. Jensen, B. N., Krarup, N. B. and Wodstrup, I. (1936) Protamine insulinate. *J. A. M. A.*, **106**, 177–180.

Hallas-Moller, K., Jersild, M., Petersen, K. and Schlichtkrull, J. (1952) Zinc insulin preparations for single daily injection. Clinical studies of new preparations with prolonged action. *J. A. M. A.*, **150**, 1667–1671.

Haunz, E. A. (1950) An approach to the problem of the 'brittle' diabetic patient. *J. A. M. A.*, **142**, 168–173.

Heinemann, L., Heise, T., Jorgensen, L. N. and Starke, A. A. R. (1993) Action profile of the rapid acting insulin analogue: human insulin B28Asp. *Diabetic Med.* **10**, 535–539.

Howey, D. C., Bowsher, R. R., Brunelle, R. L. and Woodworth, J. R. (1994) [Lys(B28), Pro(B29)]-human insulin. *Diabetes*, **43**, 396–402.

Jacobs, M. A. J. M., Schreuder, R. H., Jap-A-Joe, K. *et al.* (1993) The pharmacodynamics and activity of intranasally administered insulin in healthy male volunteers. *Diabetes*, **42**, 1649–1655.

Krayenbuhl, C. H. and Rosenberg, T. H. (1946) Crystalline protamine insulin. *Rep. Steno Memorial Hospital and Nordisk Insulin Laboratorium*, **1**, 60–73.

Laguesse, E. (1893) Sur la formation des ilots de Langerhans dans le pancreas. *C. R. Soc. Biol. Paris*, **9** (serie 5), 819.

Macleod, J. J. R., Pearce, R. G., Redfield, A. C. and Taylor, N. B. (1920) *Physiology and Biochemistry in Modern Medicine*, 3rd edn, C. V. Mosby, St Louis, MO.

Markie, F. and Albrecht, W. (1977) Biological activity of synthetic human insulin. *Diabetologia*, **13**, 293–295.

Markussen, J. (1984) Production of human insulin, in *Recent Advances in Diabetes 1*, (eds M. Nattrass and J. V. Santiago), Churchill Livingstone, Edinburgh, p. 45–53.

Mitrakou, A., Ryan, C., Venemen, T. *et al.* (1991) Hierarchy of glycemic thresholds for counter-regulatory hormone secretion, symptoms and cerebral dysfunction. *Am. J. Physiol.*, **260**, E67–E74.

Opie, E. L. (1901) On the relation of chronic interstitial pancreatitis to the islands of Langerhans and to diabetes mellitus. *J. Exp. Med. (Balt.)*, **5**, 397–428.

Paterson, W., Wilson, M., Kesson, K. M. *et al.* (1991) Comparison of basal and prandial insulin therapy in patients with secondary failure of sulphonylurea therapy. *Diabetic Med.* **8**, 40–43.

Paulesco, N. C. (1921) Recherches sur le rôle du pancreas dans l'assimilation nutritive. *Arch. Intern. Physiol.* **17**, 85–109.

Polonsky, K. S., Given, B. D. and Van Cauter, E. (1988) Twenty-four-hour profiles and pulsatile patterns of insulin secretion in normal and obese subjects. *J. Clin. Invest.*, **81**, 442–448.

Ryle, A. P., Sanger, F., Smith, L. F. and Kitai, R. (1955) The disulphide bonds of insulin. *Biochem. J.*, **60**, 541–556.

Sanger, F., Thompson, E. O. P. and Kitai, R. (1955) The amide groups of insulin. *Biochem. J.*, **59**, 509–518.

Schafer, E. A. (1916) *The Endocrine Organs; An Introduction to the Study of Internal Secretion*, Longmans, Green, London, p. 128.

Schlichtkrull, J., Brange, J., Christiansen, A. H. *et al.* (1972) Clinical aspects of insulin-antigenicity. *Diabetes*, **21**(suppl 2), 649–656.

Scott, D. A. (1934) Crystalline insulin. *Biochem. J.*, **28**, 1592–1602.

Scott, D. A. and Fisher, A. M. (1935) The effect of zinc salts on the action of insulin. *J. Pharmacol.*, **55**, 206–221.

Seigler, D. E., Olsson, G. M. and Skyler, J. S. (1992) Morning versus bedtime isophane insulin in type 2 (non-insulin dependent) diabetes mellitus. *Diabetic Med.* **9**, 826–833.

Selam, J. L., Slingeneyer, A. and Saeidi, S. *et al.* (1985) Experience with long-term peritoneal insulin infusion from external pumps. *Diabetic Med.* **2**, 41–44.

Singh, B. M., Palma, M. and Nattrass, M. (1987) Multiple aspects of insulin resistance: comparison of glucose and intermediary metabolite response to incremental insulin infusion in IDDM subjects of short and long duration. *Diabetes*, **36**, 740–748.

Somogyi, M. (1959) Exacerbation of diabetes by excess insulin action. *Am. J. Med.*, **26**, 169–191.

Starling, E. H. (1920) *Principles of Human Physiology*, Lea, Philadelphia, PA.

Stout, R. W. (1987) Insulin and atheroma – an update. *Lancet*, **i**, 1077–1079.

Tattersall, R. B. (1977) Brittle diabetes. *Clin. Endocrinol. Metab.*, **6**, 403–419.

Travis, L. B. (1975) 'Over control' of juvenile diabetes mellitus. *Southern Med. J.*, **68**, 767–771.

Trautmann, M. E. (1994) Effect of the insulin analogue [LYS(B28),PRO(B29)] on blood glucose control. *Horm. Metab. Res.*, **26**, 588–590.

Turner, R. C., Mann, J. I., Simpson, R. D. *et al.* (1977) Fasting hyperglycaemia and relatively unimpaired meal responses in mild diabetes. *Clin. Endocrinol.*, **6**, 253–264.

Von Mering, J. and Minkowski, O. (1889) Diabetes mellitus nach Pankreas-exstirpation. *Arch. Exp. Path. Pharmakol.*, **26**, 371–387.

Vora, J. P., Owens, D. R., Dolben, J. *et al.* (1988) Recombinant DNA derived monomeric insulin analogue: comparison with soluble human insulin in normal subjects. *Br. Med. J.*, **297**, 1236–1239.

Woodyat, R. T. (1937) Diabetes mellitus, in *A Textbook of Medicine* (ed. R. L. Cecil), W. B. Saunders, Philadelphia, PA, p. 620–650.

Zuelzer, G. L. (1908) Ueber Versuche einer specifischen Ferment-therapie des Diabetes. *Z. Exp. Path. Ther.*, **5**, 307–318.

Diabetic ketosis, acidosis, ketoacidosis, diabetic precoma and diabetic coma are all terms used to describe the grave metabolic illness which is the end result of severe untreated diabetes. Ketoacidosis can be defined clinically by the presence of overbreathing and chemically by the presence of gross ketonaemia in association with a reduction in bicarbonate level to 15 mmol/l or less. Earlier reports attempting to distinguish ketosis, as a bicarbonate level between 15 and 20 mmol/l, from ketoacidosis, where bicarbonate is less than 15 mmol/l, are of very limited value. These figures define the degree of acidosis but do not indicate the gravity of the patient's plight, which may be determined by loss of fluid and electrolytes.

The more precise definition of ketoacidosis as severe uncontrolled diabetes requiring emergency treatment with intravenous fluids and insulin with a blood ketone body concentration > 5 mmol/l (Alberti, 1974) is only useful clinically and biochemically in retrospect since in most centres ketone bodies are rarely measured as part of the routine clinical biochemistry service.

PATHOGENESIS

A degree of insulinopenia is an absolute requirement for any form of ketonaemia. Where confusion often arises is in the finding that the insulin deficiency is often more relative than absolute (Schade et al., 1981). Thus, even in severe diabetic ketoacidosis, the patient's serum usually contains some measurable amount of insulin. This amount is insufficient for the needs of metabolism in the patient and is relatively deficient in the

light of an increased drive from anti-insulin or catabolic hormones. The increased catabolic effect upon metabolism is the second factor in the development of ketonaemia and, if unchecked, ketoacidosis.

The net result of insulin deficiency and catabolic hormone excess is unrestrained hepatic glucose output combined with decreased glucose uptake by peripheral tissues leading to hyperglycaemia (Miles et al., 1980). Concomitant with the changes in glucose there is mobilization of non-esterified fatty acids from adipose tissue, enhanced hepatic ketogenesis and decreased peripheral utilization of ketone bodies (Owen et al., 1977).

THE ROLE OF CATABOLIC HORMONES IN THE DEVELOPMENT OF KETOACIDOSIS

It is clear that in diabetic ketoacidosis there are markedly increased circulating levels of glucagon, catecholamines, cortisol, and growth hormone (Schade et al., 1981; MacGillivray, Bruck and Voorhess, 1981). Indeed, rises in these hormones suggest a common mechanism by which precipitating illnesses result in ketoacidosis. Insulin withdrawal experiments in hypophysectomized and pancreatectomized patients have demonstrated the importance of these hormones in prompting a rise in ketone bodies (Barnes et al., 1977, 1978).

The effects upon metabolism of the catabolic hormones have been the subject of intense investigation over the last few years.

Effects upon glucose metabolism (Table 10.1)

The predominant acute effects upon glucose metabolism result from catecholamines and

Table 10.1 Effects of catabolic hormones upon metabolism in diabetic ketoacidosis (+ = stimulatory; 0 = no effect; − = inhibitory)

	Catecholamines	*Glucagon*	*Cortisol*	*Growth hormone*
Liver				
Glycogenolysis	+++	++	0	0
Gluconeogenesis	+	+++	+++	+
Ketogenesis	+	++	+	+
Muscle				
Glucose uptake	−	0	− −	−
Ketone body	−	?	?	?
Adipocyte				
Glucose uptake	−	0	− −	−
Lipolysis	+++	0	++	+

glucagon. In diabetic ketoacidosis catecholamines may be increased up to sevenfold while glucagon is raised four- to fivefold. In normal man a major role for glucagon and catecholamines is the stimulation of hepatic glucose output. Traditionally catecholamines do this by stimulating hepatic glycogen breakdown while glucagon acts mainly through stimulation of gluconeogenesis, but both hormones may affect each process. The time course of action of catecholamines is acute and prolonged. With glucagon, however, although the onset of action is rapid the effect upon glucose production is not prolonged and there is a return to basal values of hepatic glucose output despite raised glucagon levels – the 'evanescent' effect of glucagon (Felig, Wahren and Hendler, 1976).

The effects of these hormones on peripheral tissues is less clear. In particular, it has proved difficult to demonstrate a peripheral effect of glucagon, which may mean that even if one occurs it is of little biological meaning. In contrast, there is evidence that catecholamines decrease glucose uptake in the periphery (Rizza *et al.*, 1980).

The diabetogenic effect of corticosteroids is well recognized yet the effects upon glucose metabolism are delayed compared with glucagon and catecholamines. This is probably due to a prerequisite for cellular entry and subsequent regulation of DNA and RNA synthesis. Thus the action of cortisol to stimulate gluconeogenesis and hence hepatic glucose output is through increased activity of gluconeogenic enzymes, particularly phosphoenolpyruvate carboxykinase (Wicks, 1971). In addition there is an increased supply to the liver of gluconeogenic precursors lactate and pyruvate prompting gluconeogenesis (Johnston *et al.*, 1980).

In the periphery cortisol decreases glucose uptake. This occurs as a direct effect but when insulin is present, insulin-stimulated glucose uptake is decreased, which may in part result from the potent inhibitory effect of cortisol on insulin binding to its receptor (Olefsky *et al.*, 1975).

The role of the anterior pituitary, and in particular growth hormone, in promoting hyperglycaemia has long been recognized (Houssay and Biasotti, 1930). In normal man or even in non-diabetic man many of the effects are not apparent because of simultaneous effects upon insulin secretion. Where this is absent, however, there can be little doubt that growth hormone is hyperglycaemic. In the insulin withdrawal studies referred to above, hypophysectomized patients showed a slower rise in blood glucose than diabetics in whom the pituitary was intact. Similarly, abolition of insulin secretion in normal man with somatostatin allows the hyperglycaemic effect of administered growth hormone. Hyperglycaemia results from both decreased peripheral uptake of glucose (Zierler and Rabinowitz, 1963) and increased hepatic production.

Effect upon fat metabolism (Table 10.1)

Catecholamines have a potent effect upon lipolysis, stimulating release of glycerol and non-esterified fatty acids. Numerous studies demonstrate this effect both *in vitro* and *in vivo* and, importantly, catecholamines present in raised amounts can overcome the inhibitory effect of insulin upon lipolysis. In contrast glucagon has little peripheral effect on the fat cell in physiological amounts. In pharmacological concentrations lipolysis is stimulated but these concentrations exceed those seen pathophysiologically even in diabetic ketoacidosis. Cortisol does not promote lipolysis *in vivo* in normal man and in Cushing's syndrome NEFA levels are normal (Johnston *et al.*, 1980). In diabetic insulin deficient man, however, there is a marked rise in non-esterified fatty acids, suggesting that cortisol does overcome the inhibitory effect of insulin upon lipolysis (Schade, Eaton and Standefer, 1978). Growth hormone stimulates lipolysis but the effect is delayed (Gerich *et al.*, 1976).

In the liver glucagon has important major effects upon ketogenesis. Using numerous techniques – e.g. hepatic vein catheterization and/or exogenous hormone infusion – it is clear that there is a direct ketogenic effect of glucagon. Indeed the effect has been used in the elucidation of the mechanism of ketogenesis. Likewise, catecholamines promote hepatic ketogenesis independent of the lipolytic effect. Thus, provided there is adequate supply of non-esterified fatty acids, glucagon and catecholamines are strongly ketogenic (Schade and Eaton, 1979). Cortisol increases circulating ketone bodies to a greater effect than would be predicted from the rise in NEFA, confirming a ketogenic effect. Similarly growth hormone raises ketone body concen-

trations and this is apparent before the rise in NEFA.

In addition to direct metabolic effects a number of other factors should be taken into account. Firstly, it has to be borne in mind that the panoply of effects due to catabolic hormone excess are intrinsically mixed with the effects of insulin deficiency and contribute to the insulin deficiency as well as the insulin antagonism. Adrenalin is a potent inhibitor of insulin secretion through an alpha-adrenergic effect (Porte and Williams, 1966).

Secondly, there is the permissive action of cortisol. It is clear that in adrenalectomized animals the catabolic effects of catecholamines, glucagon and growth hormone are reduced and the full effect can be restored by cortisol replacement. This permissive effect of cortisol may well be as important as any direct effect upon metabolism.

Thirdly, there is a tendency to concentrate upon the effects of the hormones upon intermediary metabolism. It is likely, however, that the stress response to illness or trauma has evolved in such a way to be beneficial to the organism. In addition to their effects upon substrate supply the physiological effects should not be forgotten. Thus the cardiovascular effects of catecholamines are beneficial in the markedly dehydrated patient, contributing an inotropic effect.

THE ROLE OF INSULIN DEFICIENCY IN THE DEVELOPMENT OF KETOACIDOSIS

The catabolic drive alone is insufficient to produce diabetic ketoacidosis. Abnormalities of glucose tolerance may result, as evidenced by hyperglycaemia following myocardial infarction, but even in these patients it is unclear whether transient diabetes occurs in normal patients or only in those with a tendency to diabetes: an unmasking of diabetes. A relative insulin deficiency is necessary for the development of diabetic ketoacidosis. Catecholamine-induced inhibition of insulin secretion contributes to this but a basic inability to secrete insulin despite major increases in blood glucose is necessary.

An important point to grasp is the differential sensitivity of different metabolic processes to the effect of insulin. Lipolysis is inhibited by relatively small amounts of insulin, as is hepatic glucose production, yet stimulation of peripheral glucose uptake by insulin requires relatively large amounts of insulin. Thus raised levels of non-esterified fatty acids and ketone bodies are metabolic markers of low circulating insulin concentrations. In patients with diabetic ketoacidosis plasma insulin is measurable, with a mean in published studies of around 10 mU/l, which is equivalent to or greater than normal subjects after an overnight fast. Clearly in diabetic patients with a blood glucose of 20–30 mmol/l (360–540 mg/dl) this figure is inappropriately low and indicates a major diminution in insulin secretion.

Effects upon glucose metabolism

Insulin is the major regulator of blood glucose concentration influencing both glucose production by liver and kidney and glucose utilization by a number of tissues, including the major metabolic tissue of muscle.

Net release of glucose by the liver is reduced by insulin through an inhibition of glycogen breakdown and gluconeogenesis, while there is a promotion of glycogen storage. The precise sites of action of insulin in these processes have defied elucidation, with a concomitant disappointment that the mechanism is obviously more complex than the glucagon- or catecholamine-induced changes in a second messenger like cyclic AMP. Recent progress in delineating the events that follow the binding of insulin to its receptor have shed light on this area (see Chapter 2).

There is a dose dependency for the inhibition of hepatic glucose output, where an effect is apparent at a circulating insulin of 10 mU/l and complete suppression occurs at

100 mU/l. It should be noted that in normal life complete suppression of hepatic output does not occur and data has been obtained only during glycaemic clamping with simultaneous glucose infusion in order to maintain normoglycaemia. In the periphery insulin stimulates glucose uptake into muscle, which is about 85% of total uptake, and adipocyte, which accounts for a further 10%. A number of tissues do not require insulin for glucose uptake (see below). The specific site of action is a further area of intensive investigation.

Effects upon fat metabolism

The influence of insulin upon fat metabolism is apparent at two specific sites. Insulin is a potent inhibitor of release of fatty acids from adipose tissue and directs the fate of these within the liver.

Triglyceride breakdown to non-esterified fatty acids and glycerol occurs in the basal state and is enhanced by catabolic hormones. While lipolysis is not totally suppressed by insulin basally, small rises in insulin will decrease hormone-stimulated lipolysis.

The fate of non-esterified fatty acids within the liver is influenced by insulin and glucagon. The intrahepatic inhibition of ketogenesis by insulin has proved elusive to document and it may be that the relative proportions of fatty acids going into triglyceride or ketone bodies are determined by insulin/glucagon ratios in portal blood.

A third site of insulin action is a possibility and this lies in stimulation of peripheral ketone metabolism by insulin. The relative ketonaemia of fasting versus diabetic ketoacidosis indicates a defect of peripheral ketone clearance in the latter. Our own studies suggest that ketonaemia is cleared more quickly in ketoacidosis if large amounts of insulin are given in the post-initial treatment phase but since additional glucose must also be given it is difficult to ascribe this effect to insulin or glucose or a combination of the two (Krentz *et al.*, 1989).

THE OVERALL METABOLIC CHANGES IN KETOACIDOSIS

The maintenance of a normal blood glucose concentration relies upon a fine balance between glucose production by the liver (and a lesser extent the kidney) and uptake of glucose by peripheral tissues. The major regulators of these processes are circulating glucose concentration, circulating insulin concentration and levels of catabolic hormones.

Hepatic glucose production both from glycogen degradation and through gluconeogenesis is exquisitely sensitive to inhibition by insulin (Felig and Wahren, 1971). Importantly, it is also influenced by circulating glucose concentration (Soskin and Levine, 1946). Using either hepatic vein catheterization techniques or isotopically determined rates of glucose production it has been shown that diabetic patients have normal or raised hepatic glucose production rates. In ketoacidosis normal values are found, although the variation between subject is considerable. The teleological function of hepatic glucose production is the maintenance of a normal fasting blood glucose concentration and thus, in the presence of a markedly raised circulating glucose, a normal production rate is inappropriately high. Both glycogen breakdown and accelerated gluconeogenesis contribute to the enhanced glucose output (Figure 10.1).

The rise in blood glucose is accentuated by the decrease in peripheral extraction (Figure 10.1). Certain tissues such as liver, brain, red blood cells, renal medulla and retina do not require insulin for glucose uptake and even in muscle and adipocyte there is a glucose-stimulated glucose uptake independent of an insulin-stimulated effect. It is apparent that total body uptake is markedly decreased in the absence of insulin, with the implication

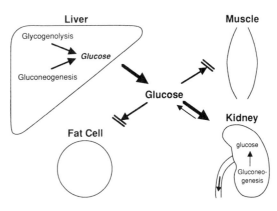

Fig. 10.1 Changes in glucose metabolism in the development of diabetic ketoacidosis.

that glucose effects alone are unable to maintain normoglycaemia. The rise in blood glucose may be attenuated by urinary glucose loss but this is counterbalanced by an increased glycolysis in non-insulin-dependent tissue, leading to higher lactate and pyruvate levels. These prompt hepatic gluconeogenesis and there is thus increased Cori cycle activity.

In the adipocyte there is a constant cycle of triglyceride breakdown and reesterification of fatty acid. For reesterification, synthesis of alpha-glycerophosphate from glucose is necessary since adipocytes lack glycerol kinase. The only fate of glycerol is therefore release, transport to the liver and utilization in gluconeogenesis or glycolysis. Reesterification will be decreased, therefore, when adipocyte uptake of glucose is impaired, in addition to the stimulation of triglyceride breakdown by catabolic hormones. Non-esterified fatty acid levels are raised in diabetic ketoacidosis although the rise is ameliorated by hepatic uptake. Uptake of fatty acids by the liver is along a concentration gradient with no modifying factors. Three fates await fatty acids within the liver. They can be reesterified to triglyceride and released as VLDL, oxidized to acetyl CoA and enter the Krebs cycle, or partially oxidized to the ketone bodies (Figure 10.2).

Beta-oxidation of fatty acids is intramito-

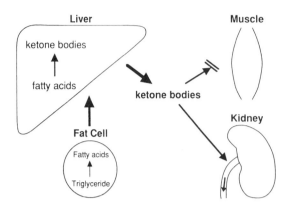

Fig. 10.2   Changes in fat metabolism in the development of diabetic ketoacidosis.

chondrial and the mitochondrial membrane contains two obligatory enzymes. Carnitine acyl transferase I is located on the inner aspect of the outer membrane and converts the fatty acid CoA derivative to a carnitine-linked compound. Carnitine acyltransferase II splits carnitine from the molecule as it transverses the inner membrane, allowing fatty acyl CoA to pass into the mitochondrion (McGarry and Foster, 1980). Subsequent oxidation releases acetyl CoA, which condenses to acetoacetyl CoA and then acetoacetate. Acetoacetate is in equilibrium with 3-hydroxybutyrate and release into the circulation occurs. Liver is deficient in enzymes capable of metabolizing ketone bodies and oxidation is therefore peripheral. Spontaneous decarboxylation of acetoacetate forms acetone.

Precise regulation of this process is unclear, although malonyl CoA is a contender for a major site. This is the first committed intermediate of the triglyceride synthesis pathway and helps explain the long-apparent relationship of ketogenesis with the fed or fasted state. There is evidence that glucagon acts at the malonyl CoA site, promoting ketogenesis.

Ketone bodies can be advantageous fuels under certain circumstances but in ketoacidosis there is a maximum rate of utilization. Exceeding concentrations at which this

rate operates accelerates the rise, although urinary loss is enhanced. In addition to ketonuria the breath is also an excretory pathway, as can be detected in the classic smell of acetone.

SUMMARY

The consequences of insulin deficiency and catabolic hormone excess upon metabolism follow logically from the preceding discussion. There is increased glucose production and decreased glucose utilization. Hyperglycaemia leads to increased urinary loss, of glucose, of water and of electrolyte. Oral intake cannot be maintained at the level of urinary loss and dehydration ensues.

Enhanced lipolysis, ketogenesis and decreased ketone clearance lead to a metabolic acidosis with vomiting, abdominal pain, Kussmaul respiration and the characteristic odour of exhaled acetone. The pH decreases until acidosis, renal failure or respiratory failure lead to coma and/or death.

THE CAUSES OF KETOACIDOSIS

Infection is the most frequently identified cause of ketoacidosis in the diabetic (Table 10.2). The second cause – omission or reduction of the insulin dose – is often associated with infection in the following sequence. An acute infection leads to anorexia or vomiting; because the dietary intake is inadequate insulin is reduced or not given – all too often on the advice of a doctor – at the very time when the need for insulin is greater than usual as a result of the infection.

Ketoacidosis as the presentation of type 1 diabetes is, unfortunately, relatively common. Pinkney *et al.* (1994) found that 16% of children were in severe ketoacidosis at diagnosis, with a further 10% with mild to moderate ketoacidosis.

Omission of insulin as a result of emotional disturbance or neglect was the commonest cause of ketoacidosis in known diabetics in

Table 10.2 Precipitating causes of diabetic ketoacidosis at General Hospital, Birmingham 1971–1990 (% in brackets)

Years	Number of episodes	Infection	Insulin error with no other obvious cause	New diagnosis of diabetes	Miscellaneous identified causes	No cause identified
1971–1975	262	82 (31.3)	21 (8.0)	26 (9.9)	18 (6.9)	115 (43.9)
1976–1980	226	62 (27.4)	23 (10.2)	28 (12.4)	21 (9.3)	92 (40.7)
1981–1985	259	74 (28.6)	36 (13.9)	22 (8.5)	30 (11.6)	97 (37.5)
1986–1900	163	57 (35.0)	23 (14.1)	15 (9.2)	23 (14.1)	45 (27.6)

the series of Cohen *et al.* (1960) but has not been nearly as common as infection in our experience (Nattrass and Hale, 1984). It is true that certain patients, often identified by their repeated admission to hospital in diabetic coma, are emotionally unstable and show a wilful inability to adjust their treatment to prevent ketoacidosis, but they form a small group, which includes the rare case of suicide. There are others whose diabetes is genuinely too difficult for some patients of average ability to handle successfully and this may be the case with girls at the menarche and women during pregnancy, presumably as a result of hormonal disturbances.

It is doubtful if overeating by itself is a factor in precipitating ketoacidosis. Overeating, particularly of food or drink rich in carbohydrate, will enhance hyperglycaemia but, provided insulin is continued or sufficient insulin can be secreted, then lipolysis and ketogenesis will not increase. Such a clinical situation occurs in hyperosmolar non-ketotic diabetic coma. Overeating to the extent deserving of the label 'bingeing', and when accompanied by vomiting, may result in the rise in catabolic hormones necessary for the development of ketoacidosis. Short-term fasting has been implicated in the pathogenesis of euglycaemic ketoacidosis (Burge, Hardy and Schade, 1993).

Vomiting or fasting causes unnecessary confusion in interpreting the presence of ketone bodies in diabetic patients. The ketosis of fasting is a result of the fall in insulin levels. In the diabetic, therefore, when hyper-

glycaemia is present to stimulate insulin secretion, coexisting hyperglycaemia and hyperketonaemia always indicate insulinopenia.

The substitution of oral hypoglycaemic agents for insulin is an infrequent but avoidable cause of ketoacidosis, usually resulting from the error of believing that a small daily insulin dose means that the diabetes does not really require insulin.

Trauma is often given as a precipitating cause of diabetic ketoacidosis but for some peculiar reason it is virtually absent in our own series. I would like to think that it is because of excellent cooperation between the diabetic team and the trauma or general surgeon, but suspect this is a half-truth.

Likewise, patients with coexistent myocardial infarction and diabetic ketoacidosis are few in our own series although important for the high mortality that results.

It is always worth exploring the possibility of simple technical errors if the cause of ketoacidosis is not readily apparent. Enquiry may reveal a leaking syringe, that dosage instructions have been misinterpreted, or that insulin is being omitted either by the patient or by the nurse.

THE CLINICAL PRESENTATION

The best measure of the severity of diabetes is the time it takes for ketoacidosis to develop when insulin treatment is omitted. In the most severe cases this period is only a few hours and comparatively minor disturbances of control may lead rapidly to diabetic coma.

In the less severe it requires prolonged deficiency of insulin treatment or a major catabolic drive to produce the same effect.

SYMPTOMS (TABLE 10.3)

The symptoms of ketoacidosis can develop insidiously over many days, but the average history extends over 36 hours and in rare cases the time from the onset of symptoms is as short as 6 hours. On the whole those with a long history respond best to treatment and those with a very short acute onset should be watched more carefully.

At first there are all the symptoms of acute diabetes – thirst, polyuria and lassitude – followed by anorexia, nausea and vomiting. Diarrhoea is commonly mentioned but is not confirmed on arrival in hospital or explained by investigation, so that the common diagnosis of gastroenteritis at the onset is usually meaningless. Severe abdominal pain is common and may have to be distinguished from the pain of an acute abdominal emergency. In this differentiation the history of vomiting preceding the pain is often helpful and the improvement when ketoacidosis is treated is rapid. Some patients are aware of breathless-ness at quite an early stage of the illness before air hunger is apparent, while a few are unaware of their abnormal breathing even when it is quite obvious on inspection. The development of stupor and coma follows but the patient is usually quite lucid even when hardly rousable.

SIGNS (TABLE 10.3)

The milder cases may not appear to be seriously ill except to one who is familiar with the normal appearance of the patient. Those with severe ketoacidosis look ill and present the features so well described by Kussmaul in 1874. He noted pallor, coolness of the face and body, abdominal tenderness, rapid and feeble pulse and especially deep breathing (*grosse Atmung*). This air hunger, in which it is the depth rather than the rate of breathing that strikes the observer, is quite different from the rapid shallow breathing of pneumonia and is a most important physical sign. We have used it to define the clinical diagnosis of ketoacidosis and it is certain that patients who have air hunger are in need of insulin, while the disappearance of this sign is good evidence of response to insulin treatment. Occasionally, in a deeply unconscious patient, air hunger may be replaced by shallow breathing, an unfavourable and usually terminal phenomenon.

The breath smells of acetone, which has been likened to new-mown hay, stale beer or a room in which apples have been kept. The latter seems to me the best simile but my nose fails me every time, while my predecessor admitted to being slower to detect the odour of acetone than many junior students and nurses. Some are apparently able to pick up very low concentrations in the breath, while others, like us, can hardly even recognize this useful sign.

The general appearance is often characteristic, for the eyes are sunken and the skin is flushed and pink yet dry, inelastic and cool. The body temperature is usually 37°C or

Table 10.3   Clinical features of diabetic ketoacidosis

Symptoms	Thirst, polyuria, nocturia
	Lassitude
	Blurred vision
	Leg cramps
	Anorexia, nausea, vomiting
	Abdominal pain
	Breathlessness
Signs	Pallor
	Dehydration
	Tachycardia
	Acidotic respiration
	Drowsiness, confusion, coma
	Abdominal tenderness
	Gastric distension with splash
	Acetone on the breath
	Hypovolaemic shock

below even in the presence of infection. The tongue is dry and has a dirty brownish coating, the pharynx is beefy and stringy saliva may be seen in the mouth, while the teeth are covered by a dry deposit. The abdomen may be tender in any quadrant, gastric distension with a splash is common and the stomach contents may contain altered blood (Hirsch, 1960). The pulse is always rapid but in the more severe cases it becomes feeble, with a fall in blood pressure, collapse of the superficial veins and capillary stasis. Under these circumstances gangrene of the skin over pressure areas may develop quickly.

Drowsiness is the rule and when coma occurs it is of serious significance. In general, however, stupor or coma are not reliable guides to the severity of the ketoacidosis because a patient with severe ketoacidosis can be alert and clear-headed. Less than 25% of patients are in coma, 25% are fully conscious and orientated and the remaining 50% have some disturbance of consciousness (Alberti and Nattrass, 1978). Sometimes the patient may be very restless or even maniacal. The tendon reflexes are depressed or absent but the plantar responses usually remain flexor until a very late stage.

URINE FINDINGS (TABLE 10.4)

In striking contrast to the obvious dehydration is the common finding that the bladder contains a large volume of very pale urine, which contains from 2–10 g/dl of glucose and gives an immediate strongly positive nitroprusside reaction for acetoacetate. Owing to the presence of glucose the specific gravity is high – at least 1030 – but the osmolarity is much above that of the hyperosmolar serum – about 500 mosmol/l – indicating defective renal conservation of water. In part this is due to the osmotic effect of glucose, but low renal blood flow and potassium depletion also impair the renal tubular concentrating mechanisms. In late cases the renal circula-

Table 10.4 Investigations in diabetic ketoacidosis

Investigation	Abnormality
Urine glucose	High
Urine ketones	High
Blood ketones	High
Blood glucose	Raised to markedly high Occasionally euglycaemia
Plasma sodium	Low, normal or raised
Plasma potassium	Low, normal or raised
Plasma bicarbonate	Low
Blood hydrogen ion	High
Blood pH	Low
P_aCO_2	Low

tion fails and oliguria or anuria supervene, in which case ketones may be absent from the residual bladder urine. Proteinuria, usually slight, is invariably found in severe ketoacidosis and is of the type found in renal tubular damage. Microscopic examination shows numerous granular and hyaline casts.

SERUM CHEMISTRY

Examination of the blood before treatment shows some striking abnormalities. Table 10.5 shows the figures in 30 patients.

The degree of hyperglycaemia does not always correlate well with the severity of the ketoacidosis. Even at a level of blood glucose as low as 20 mmol/l (360 mg/dl) acidosis can be well marked, while a patient with a blood glucose above 50 mmol/l (900 mg/dl) may walk into hospital. Hyperglycaemia does not account entirely for the extreme hyperosmolarity of the plasma, which is also due to the accumulation of ketones, urea and sometimes sodium.

The bicarbonate level does not always correspond with the clinical severity of the ketoacidosis but the blood pH is a more valuable guide. If the pH is not below 7.3 it is certain that it is mild; if it is below 7.0 it is certainly very severe. Very low figures may be inaccurate if the capillary sample is taken

Table 10.5 Biochemical abnormalities at presentation of diabetic ketoacidosis

	Mean	*Range*	*Normal*
Blood glucose (mmol/l)	37	16–76	4.0–7.2
Blood pH	7.06	6.85–7.20	7.38–7.46
Blood bicarbonate (mmol/l)	7	2–15	22–26
Blood total ketone bodies (mmol/l)	12.4	9.2–18.6	0.02–0.38
Blood lactate (mmol/l)	3.2	1.0–12.3	0.3–1.3
Plasma sodium (mmol/l)	130	124–156	134–144
Plasma potassium (mmol/l)	5.2	3.4–6.1	3.4–5.3

from an area of stasis in a patient with circulatory failure.

There are no quick, readily available quantitative methods for the determination of plasma ketones, which can be present to the extent of 10–30 mmol/l in severe ketoacidosis. A simple semiquantitative technique, however, exists in the application of the sodium nitroprusside test to plasma. A Ketostix strip only has to be dipped quickly into plasma and the purple colour is read after 15 seconds by comparison with a colour chart. A three-plus reaction, and usually a two-plus reaction, indicates severe hyperketonaemia as the cause of the acid–base changes and is reliable as a semiquantitative guide. A negative plasma Ketostix reaction prompts a search for some other cause for the illness, such as salicylate poisoning, lactic acidosis, vascular accidents or overwhelming infections.

The nitroprusside reaction is specific for acetoacetate and does not react with 3-hydroxybutyrate. The ratio of these two ketone bodies reflects the mitochondrial hepatic redox state and is therefore influenced by other acidotic states or the mitochondrial metabolism of agents such as alcohol. It has been suggested that occasional cases of 3-hydroxybutyrate ketoacidosis are seen where the urine or plasma gives a negative Ketostix reaction. Since the ratio of 3-hydroxybutyrate/acetoacetate rises in any acidotic condition I doubt that 3-hydroxybutyrate ketoacidosis is a real entity.

FLUID AND ELECTROLYTE LOSSES

The extent of the fluid and electrolyte losses in ketoacidosis were studied in detail as early as 1933 by Atchley *et al.* Insulin was withdrawn from two volunteers and renal losses of water and various electrolytes were measured. Butler *et al.* (1947) made similar measurements and Nabarro, Spencer and Stowers (1952) carried out balance studies during treatment and recovery. Their findings are summarized in Table 10.6.

In considering these figures as a guide to replacement therapy it must be remembered that continuing renal losses in the early phases of treatment have to be added. From these results and some of their own Martin, Smith and Wilson (1958) calculated the immediate replacement needs as water 70–120 ml/kg, sodium 7–10 mmol/kg, chloride 5 mmol/kg and potassium 3 mmol/kg. Sodium and potassium were lost both as the result of the osmotic diuresis and some vomiting. Water losses were equally divided between extracellular

Table 10.6 Estimates of the fluid and electrolyte deficiency in patients with diabetic ketoacidosis

	Atchley et al., 1933	*Butler et al., 1947*	*Nabarro, Spencer and Stowers, 1952*
Water (litres)	5.0	7.0	4.6
Nitrogen (g)	34.8	40.0	38.8
Sodium (mmol)	300	217	500
Potassium (mmol)	385	273	347
Chloride (mmol)	110	142	390

and intracellular fluid. Restoration was divisible into three overlapping phases – water was rapidly absorbed by the cells as the blood glucose and therefore extracellular osmotic pressure fell; extracellular fluid loss was made good at the same time with massive sodium retention which may have become intracellular. In the second stage, lasting several days, potassium, magnesium and phosphorus were restored and finally after some weeks nitrogen losses were made good (Nabarro, Spencer and Stowers, 1952).

WHITE BLOOD CELLS

There is always a polymorphonuclear leucocytosis, which may be as high as 50 000/mm^3 even in the absence of infection and is attributed to a non-specific response to dehydration.

DIFFERENTIAL DIAGNOSIS

The diagnosis on clinical grounds is usually easy if a history is available. Previously unrecognized diabetes, usually in elderly patients, presents a more difficult problem and may only be suspected by the acetone in the breath or a routine test of the urine. The coma due to a cerebral vascular accident in a diabetic patient may be associated with hyperglycaemia but the ketonaemia is slight and the pH level is unaffected.

Hypoglycaemia seldom deceives an experienced observer. The history is quite different from that of ketoacidosis, air hunger is absent and dehydration is not a feature. After severe hypoglycaemic attacks ketonuria is the rule but ketonaemia is slight.

Other causes of hyperglycaemic acidosis may have to be considered if only small amounts of ketone bodies are present in blood and urine. Lactic acidosis and the acidosis of chronic renal failure are the commonest. Alcoholic ketoacidosis may also occur while severe salicylate overdosage may present a picture that closely resembles that of diabetic ketoacidosis with air hunger and prostration.

Both lactic acidosis (Marliss *et al.*, 1970) and alcoholic ketoacidosis (Thompson *et al.*, 1986) may present difficulties in diagnosis because of effects on the ratio of 3-hydroxybutyrate to acetoacetate.

TREATMENT (TABLE 10.7)

Diabetic ketoacidosis threatens life and there is no place for hesitation or half-measures in treatment once the diagnosis is certain. Speed in initiating treatment is essential; constant medical, nursing and laboratory attention are necessary and the guidance of a physician experienced in the management of this emergency is invaluable. Where such experience and facilities are available low mortality rates can be achieved, which means that lives are saved. There is no place for a routine treatment and attempts to lay down such merely represent an attempt to pass on experience. Detailed flow charts should never be followed slavishly at the expense of careful clinical review. Certain guides in treatment can be laid down, which are summarized in a later section. The important decisions are how much fluid, of what composition and at what rate; how much potassium, how much insulin and by which route?

FLUID

There is no satisfactory formula from which to calculate the extent of fluid and electrolyte depletion. A patient of average size with clinical evidence of severe dehydration may be assumed to have a deficit of about 3 litres of extracellular fluid and a similar volume of cell water (Nabarro, Spencer and Stowers, 1952). Replacement must be intravenous in every case. The setting up of the intravenous infusion can be technically difficult because of collapsed veins and it must always be remembered that the veins may be needed again at a future date. Between 2 and 3 litres of fluid should be given in the first 4 hours followed by a further litre every 2–4 hours

Table 10.7 Treatment of diabetic ketoacidosis

---

1. **Fluid**
   a) Type
   Saline (150 mmol/l) ('isotonic'; 'normal'; 0.9%) unless indications for an alternative type are
      present
   Saline (75 mmol/l) ('hypotonic'; 'half-normal'; 0.45%) if plasma sodium greater than 150 mmol/l
   5% glucose ('5% dextrose') when blood glucose less than 14 mmol/l
   Bicarbonate (highly irritant in concentrated form – use weakest solution available, e.g. 1.4%) give
      100–150 mmol over 30 minutes if pH < 7.0 (see text).
   b) Rate
      Initial replacement rate: 1 l/hour for 4 hours
                                   1 l/2 hours for 4 hours
                                   1 l/4 hours for 12 hours
2. **Potassium**
   Dosage based on measurement of plasma potassium
   If < **3.5 add 40 mmol KCl** to each litre of infusion fluid
   3.5–5.5 add 20 mmol KCL to each litre of infusion fluid
   If > 5.5 withhold potassium infusion
3. **Insulin**
   Use only quick-acting insulin
   a) Intravenous infusion
   5–10 u/h initially until blood glucose less than 14 mmol/l then **2–5 u/h**
   b) Intramuscular
   20 units immediately then **5–10 u/h** until blood glucose < 14 mmol/l then **2–5 u/h**

---

depending upon the response of the patient and the extent of the urinary output. The ideal composition of the replacement fluid has been debated for many years, a debate which continues. Should it be isotonic or hypotonic? and should bicarbonate be used? or even lactate-containing solutions?

The fluid and electrolyte lost by the patient is not isotonic and consequently at presentation osmolarity is raised. The argument about hypotonic or isotonic replacement fluid is not strictly appropriate, since both are hypotonic to the patient. Sodium 150 mmol/l / chloride 150 mmol/l is probably the most used and most appropriate fluid for initial rehydration. The immediate use of 5% glucose is undesirable because the prolongation of hyperglycaemia aggravates renal water losses. Occasionally it might be necessary to use 5% glucose from the outset if the patient has euglycaemic ketoacidosis or if the blood glucose at presentation is between 10 and 15 mmol/l (180–270 mg/dl). Alternatives to isotonic saline may also be sought if the presenting plasma sodium is greater than 150 mmol/l. In this situation it might be considered appropriate to start rehydration with hypotonic saline, always bearing in mind the reservations on the use of this solution outlined below.

It should be stressed that these exceptions to the normal guidelines occur infrequently and the first response should be to reach for the isotonic saline. There is little to commend the use of lactate-containing solutions. When metabolized, lactate generates alkali and the use of these solutions was only appropriate in the pre-bicarbonate era.

It is important to monitor the clinical state of the patient with care. Pulmonary oedema may be precipitated, not only in those cases where its occurrence might be predicted but occasionally it is seen in young people during rehydration where there is no reason to suspect ischaemic heart disease. In the elderly a strong case can be made for insertion of a central venous catheter but in our experience, while trained and training doctors in cardiology or anaesthetics will pass such tubes with impunity, there appears a natural reluctance within the ranks of diabetologists in training.

Great care must be taken to record urinary losses. The NPU of the nursing record (not passed urine) is unacceptable and it is far more important to measure urine loss accurately than to withhold urinary catheterization because of a vague worry of introducing infection. Oliguria is a bad prognostic sign, with almost certain doom if fluid is continued. It is thus important to know whether fluid rests in the bladder or whether there is true oliguria. At the other end of the spectrum it is necessary to know whether the volume excreted exceeds the volume infused. Such a situation is likely to occur in elderly patients when infusion is proceeding with care. Further dehydration under the eyes of the attending physicians is deserving of reproof.

Markedly hypotonic saline solution may be infused from time to time. It is rarely necessary in diabetic ketoacidosis but is commonly required in hyperosmolar coma. Solutions containing sodium 30 mmol/l are probably best avoided and it is wise to fix an upper limit on the amount of 75 mmol/l sodium solution infused. There is no doubt that haemolysis, which may particularly affect the limb or have further effects upon the kidney, does occur with overenthusiastic use of hypotonic solutions, which currently restricts us to less than 2 litres. The indication for infusing hypotonic saline is invariably a rise in sodium to > 150 mmol/l during treatment. It is important to be aware of the sharp rise in sodium concentration which can occur when treatment starts. At presentation some methods of measuring plasma sodium concentration give falsely low values due to circulating lipid. Sodium, contained in plasma water but not plasma lipid, is measured in plasma water but expressed per litre (water + lipid).

Insulin treatment clears lipid, allowing an apparent marked rise in sodium. Newer techniques for measuring sodium, such as ion-specific electrodes, circumvent this problem.

POTASSIUM

Plasma potassium must be measured immediately the diagnosis is suspected. Marked hyperkalaemia may be present and may lead to the demise of the patient as treatment is being started. For this reason, and despite the fact that plasma potassium may be normal or low at presentation, it is usually unwise to give potassium supplements before measurement of plasma potassium.

Potassium falls rapidly with treatment of ketoacidosis. Rehydration without potassium, and movement of potassium into cells, are the major factors, while bicarbonate, if used, exacerbates the fall. Potassium should be given with the aim of maintaining normokalaemia. Standard medical texts consistently underestimate the amounts needed per litre or per day. Monitoring is important since it leads to alterations in potassium infusion rates, which may vary from 10 to 20 or 40 mmol/l. Potassium may be discontinued once the patient resumes eating and drinking. It is rarely necessary to prolong supplementation with oral potassium.

BICARBONATE

Controversy over the use of bicarbonate continues. On the one hand it is argued that severe acidosis (generally argued as pH less than 7.0 but more appropriately here pH < 6.8) can result in terminal respiratory depression or circulatory collapse. On the other hand, while 100 mmol infused in the early stages of treatment may partially correct hyperpnoea, there is little to suggest a useful metabolic effect. Indeed, on the contrary we have suggested that bicarbonate may delay metabolic correction (Hale, Crase and Nattrass, 1984). In addition, there is a risk of overcorrection of the acidosis, leading to alkalaemia, the promotion of potassium excretion by bicarbonate, creation of a paradoxical acidosis of the cerebrospinal fluid (Posner and Plum, 1967) and an adverse effect upon the oxyhaemoglobin dissociation curve (Ditzel and Standl, 1975).

The effect upon potassium excretion may be turned to advantage faced with life-threatening hyperkalaemia and is probably the only indication for bicarbonate administration. Having stated that so dogmatically the reader should be aware of the all-persuasive nature of one's own research as the context for the previous sentence.

INSULIN

The case for large doses of insulin (200–300 units) to treat diabetic ketoacidosis, so eloquently argued by Malins in the first edition of this book, has passed into folklore. Constant infusion of small amounts of insulin or intermittent intramuscular injection of small doses is routinely practised. The introduction of low-dose insulin regimens met stern resistance in its early days and many were prepared to argue for the continuation of larger doses. That this case continued to be made was not due to fears of inadequate treatment in the majority of patients. It was readily apparent that small doses would inhibit fat breakdown and hepatic glucose production. Rather, there was a worry that the patient with insulin resistance would respond inadequately, and the partial response would be detected only slowly, risking morbidity and mortality. The counter was to double infusion rate or hourly dose and eventually the debate has resolved.

In 1968 Malins wrote 'temporary insulin resistance in ketosis, requiring hundreds or even thousands of units, is not common but has been described many times'. The mechanism of insulin resistance was not understood. All patients in ketoacidosis are insulin-resistant, requiring doses of insulin that would make normal people comatose. Yet the mas-

sive insulin resistance described is now so rare as to cast doubt upon its occurrence. Was it more an apparent than real phenomenon with much of the insulin lost in the urine? Certainly the occasional case reported by junior staff now as displaying insulin resistance is rarely convincing and has to be apparent rather than real.

It must always be remembered that the initial fall in glucose is due to insulin and rehydration and a reluctant fall is often due to inadequate rehydration rather than insulin resistance. It is likely that the purity of insulin, with concomitant reduction in antibody production, results in an absence of the type of patient presenting with high antibody titres when infused or injected insulin was rapidly bound to the antibody without obvious action. Nevertheless insulin resistance (massive) if it exists at all is rare and can often be expected, for example, in a patient taking large doses of corticosteroids.

Rapid-acting insulin is always used in the treatment of ketoacidosis. Table 10.7 shows the commonly used regimens. Small variations from these are of little consequence other than to the pride of the deviser. It would seem logical that a regimen should be tailored either to a relatively instant circulating concentration of insulin at the low–mid physiological range, or that if a high concentration is to be achieved this should be early when blood glucose is high rather than later when blood glucose has fallen. It is important to check from time to time that the patient is receiving insulin as prescribed. Hourly intramuscular insulin means 60, not 90, minutes between injections. Infusion systems may become blocked or disengaged. Patients do not do well when insulin is infused into the bedding.

CHANGES DURING TREATMENT

Since a major aim in treatment of diabetic ketoacidosis is to lower ketone bodies and hence decrease the acidosis it is important to continue insulin even when blood glucose has fallen. Insulin is a potent inhibitor of lipolysis and hence ketogenesis, but clearly further administration when glucose has fallen requires covering with glucose infusion. Thus when blood glucose falls below 14–15 mmol/l (252–270 mg/dl) the infusion fluid is changed to 5% glucose. At this time the insulin regimen may be changed to 2-hourly intramuscular or even 4-hourly subcutaneous, the latter on the assumption that rehydration is almost complete. The combination of insulin and 5% glucose infusion almost certainly completely inhibits hepatic ketogenesis. Some advocate the change to 10% glucose with more insulin following the suggestion that this enhances clearance of ketone bodies. Our own studies (Krentz *et al.*, 1989) indicate that ketone bodies fall more rapidly with this regimen although there is no difference in effect upon pH and bicarbonate. Whether relapse into ketoacidosis is less likely is unknown but it is clear that premature cessation of frequent small amounts of insulin may have just this result. The choice of 14–15 mmol/l (252–270 mg/dl) at which to make these changes is somewhat arbitrary allowing the fall in glucose to level out and being a convenient point of measurement on the glucose reagent strip with which response to treatment is monitored. Certainly hypoglycemia should be avoided.

MONITORING

It cannot be overstressed that monitoring involves regular assessment of the clinical state of the patient. Although important to know the latest blood glucose and electrolytes it cannot be sufficient to detail changes in treatment by telephone. Fortunately, the majority of patients with diabetic ketoacidosis recover but the attending physician should not be lulled into a false sense of security by successful treatment of 10 consecutive 15–30-year-olds, especially when the next patient is 79 years old. The potential for

things to go wrong during treatment is great and of major concern is that disaster may intervene with enormous haste. Approximately 50% of deaths attributable to diabetic ketoacidosis occur in the active stage of treatment and there is therefore scope for improvement in mortality figures. Unfortunately in this group it is often impossible to identify a precise cause of death and most series, including our own, contain deaths under an unhelpful heading such as 'metabolic'.

Of the dangers during treatment, hypokalaemia is paramount. Any reduction in mortality from diabetic ketoacidosis in recent years must be due in part to greater awareness of hypokalaemia and a concentration upon replacement therapy. Monitoring of the plasma potassium should be done 2–4-hourly, a demand which causes few problems with current clinical biochemistry methodology. During treatment, change in the size of the T waves on lead II of the ECG is a good indicator of potassium status and may help sequentially to see the effect of treatment modifications. Whether it truly is a better guide to intracellular potassium status, as claimed by some, may be debated. Nevertheless hypokalaemia should and must be avoided otherwise dysrhythmias and asystole become a real possibility.

There can be little doubt that hypoglycaemia is less common with the use of frequent low-dose insulin administration. It should be possible to avoid it completely, especially since the result may be so devastating. Patients who tolerate acute hypoglycaemic episodes with apparent impunity may be less successful in outcome when hypoglycaemia follows marked hyperglycaemia. The explanation may be linked with that used to account for cerebral oedema. There is little excuse for not measuring the blood glucose at least hourly with reagent strips and 4-hourly by a true blood glucose method.

The degree of acidosis is assessed by measuring pH, $P_a\text{CO}_2$, and HCO_3 at presentation. There is little need to monitor changes further unless there is reason to suppose a non-response. Our results suggest that even when ketones are high initially pH is normal after 12 hours, although bicarbonate may take longer.

PRECIPITATING CAUSE

The search for a precipitating cause should be undertaken at presentation. Myocardial infarction is particularly important to detect since it influences fluid infusion and mortality.

Infection, the commonest identifiable cause, presents no difficulty when a carbuncle is apparent or where a classic history of a urinary tract infection is obtained. When it is less clear-cut, however, there are many sources of confusion. Pyrexia is rarely present upon arrival at the hospital while a leukocytosis is of little specificity for infection in this situation. In turn, how infection is defined will influence the number of patients in whom the attributable cause is infection. Authorities will vary – most would agree that the urine should be microscoped and cultured; a few would go as far as me in advocating a couple of blood cultures (and more where specifically indicated); some swab the throat, where a search for *Candida* may be rewarding; while a few zealots would have every orifice swabbed.

OTHER MEASURES

For want of a better term, 'other measures' includes a variety of considerations during treatment which have no common theme.

It is self-evident that hypoxic patients should have oxygen and occasionally assisted ventilation may be necessary, either when acute or chronic respiratory disease is associated with the ketoacidosis or when pulmonary oedema occurs during treatment.

Reference has been made to the gastric

splash that can be heard. Occasionally a patient will vomit the huge residue that may be present in the stomach, aspirate and die. This is probably the best example of a preventable cause of mortality yet it occurs in only 1 in 100–300 patients. Insertion of a nasogastric tube might prevent this yet a note of caution is warranted. Although only 25% of patients are in coma 50% have some disturbance of consciousness. The risks of passing nasogastric tubes in these patients cannot be underestimated and care should be taken that we do not increase morbidity and mortality in this way. In the comatose patient it is possible to get away without passing a nasogastric tube but it is clearly tightrope walking and justifiable only if successful. In these patients a tube should be passed after endotracheal intubation.

Anticoagulation is advocated by some, based on their experience of digital gangrene occurring in ketoacidosis. It is certainly true that disseminated intravascular coagulation occurs in ketoacidosis (Timperley, Preston and Ward, 1974) but in our experience gangrene is rare. Currently we would not anticoagulate patients routinely but would not ignore other medical considerations.

Plasma expanders are also advocated for hypotension (< 80 mmHg systolic blood pressure). As with other aspects of their use the reasoning is incorrect. Ketoacidosis is characterized by both intracellular and extracellular dehydration, and fluid that repletes both compartments should be used.

The identification of infection in all series as a major precipitating cause has led to the suggestion that antibiotics should be given routinely to all patients. Others would argue that this is unnecessary.

As in most other areas of medicine good treatment records are of major importance. They should include time, fluids given, blood and urine monitoring, laboratory results and clinical state. Our own sheet is far from ideal (Figure 10.3) but helps considerably.

NAME WARD REGISTRATION No. CONSULTANT DATE

TIME	INSULIN	INTRAVENOUS FLUIDS	TOTAL INFUSED	ADDED POTASSIUM	TOTAL	ORAL FLUIDS	URINE			VOLUME TOTAL	VOMIT	TEMP	PULSE	B/P	BLOOD GLUCOSE	LABORATORY RESULTS			STATE OF PATIENT
							TOTAL	SUGAR	ACETONE							BLOOD GASES	UREA & ELECTROLYTES	OTHER	

Fig. 10.3 A record sheet for the treatment of diabetic ketoacidosis.

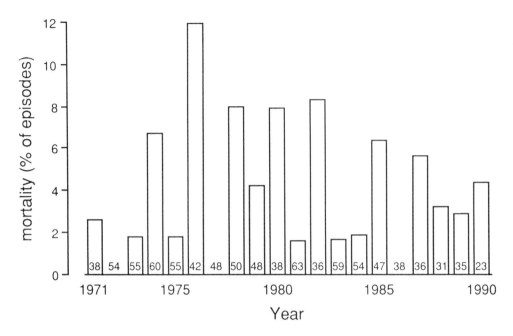

Fig. 10.4 Mortality of patients with diabetic ketoacidosis expressed as percentage of episodes for 1971–1990.

MORTALITY

Comparative mortality rates are difficult to find in the literature. There is a natural reluctance to publish rates that fall below those obtained in centres with a special interest in the condition. It is necessary to have a substantial number of episodes in any series recording mortality since it is relatively easy to have 60 episodes successfully treated before two deaths bring realism to experience. Mortality rates can also be 'adjusted' by exclusion of certain patients. Should a patient dying in ketoacidosis in the emergency room before treatment has commenced be included in the series? Should a patient dying before discharge from an admission in ketoacidosis be included when the metabolic upset may have been corrected weeks before the death? Our own figures (Figure 10.4) include anyone arriving at the hospital whether treatment had been commenced or not and includes deaths before discharge from an admission with the diagnosis of ketoacidosis even if death occurred weeks later.

The annual mortality rate clearly varies widely but over the 20 years 1971–1990 our overall mortality was 3.9 per 100 episodes. The major identifiable causes of death are cardiac events, infections and thromboembolic events such as pulmonary embolus or saddle embolus. Every series contains a number of deaths where no cause is readily identifiable even at post-mortem. These constitute about one-third of our deaths but are concentrated in the early years of the series of 930 episodes depicted in Figure 10.4.

COMPLICATIONS OF TREATMENT

Some of the things that can go wrong during treatment have been referred to above. Others, of less clear pathogenesis, are dealt with here.

FOOT DROP

Occasionally, unilateral or bilateral foot drop may follow diabetic ketoacidosis. It is often difficult to date the onset of the foot drop as coincident with development or treatment. It is probably less than adequate to ascribe it to poor nursing where the test of good/poor nursing is probably how quickly it is detected. It may be part of the vessel sludging of keto-acidosis leading to lateral peroneal paresis as a mononeuritis. I am less than convinced that this can be safely promised to the patient as completely reversible with time, although some improvement may be expected.

CEREBRAL OEDEMA

Cerebral oedema is an uncommon complication occurring during the treatment of keto-acidosis but can be devastating in its effect. Few diabetologists have much experience of recognizing and treating it, although those dealing with children and young adults feel it is commoner in their patient age-group. In a typical case an apparently successful early response to treatment is followed by a sudden deterioration particularly in the state of consciousness. Diagnosis is difficult because at this time other biochemical variables may be changing rapidly, blood glucose is falling, the acidaemia is being corrected and potassium is changing.

Coma at presentation of diabetic ketoacidosis carries a poor prognosis. In one of our series (Soler *et al.*, 1973) the mortality was 19% in these patients. There is a correlation between the degree of depression of the sensorium and extracellular hyperosmolarity (Guisada and Arieff, 1975). During initial treatment cerebrospinal fluid pressure is high as blood osmolarity falls (Clements *et al.*, 1968). These extra osmoles in the brain have been labelled 'idiogenic' to disguise their unidentified nature. In animal experiments (Arieff and Kleeman, 1973, 1974) the osmotic pressures in the two compartments will equilibrate provided blood glucose is not lowered beyond about 14 mmol/l (252 mg/dl) leading to the suggestion that water will not move into the brain provided blood glucose is not lowered rapidly beyond 14 mmol/l (Arieff, 1980). Unfortunately these observations in animals are not confirmed in humans (Rosenbloom *et al.*, 1980). Nor could Rosenbloom *et al.* (1980) confirm other postulated mechanisms from their series, such as hyponatraemia, infusion of hypotonic solutions or raised cerebrospinal fluid pressure. The cause, therefore, remains obscure and if avoidance of the uncommon complication is not possible the only safeguard remains a high index of suspicion when the clinical appearances ensue. Whether early use of mannitol and dexamethasone after an empirical diagnosis will improve outcome is unclear.

PULMONARY OEDEMA

Also labelled 'adult respiratory distress syndrome' this is another uncommon complication during treatment of ketoacidosis. As with cerebral oedema the cause is unknown, and diagnosis may be difficult since respiratory symptoms may be assumed to originate from the acidaemia. The key feature is that after an initial good response symptoms of dyspnoea worsen and there is tachypnoea and cyanosis. Hypoxia can be confirmed and chest X-ray shows pulmonary infiltrates. Provided it is diagnosed, modification of fluid therapy and assisted ventilation can improve the outlook.

HYPEROSMOLAR NON-KETOTIC DIABETIC COMA

After diabetic ketoacidosis, hyperosmolar non-ketotic coma is the next commonest of the hyperglycaemic comas. It has some marked differences in presentation and pathogenesis, not all of which can be fully explained. Profound dehydration and hyperglycaemia, often with blood glucose concentration in excess of 50 mmol/l (900 mg/dl), are present but acidosis and ketonaemia are absent. It has been suggested that the hyperosmolarity suppresses peripheral lipolysis (Gerich *et al.*, 1973) or that the catabolic hormone levels are lower than in ketoacidosis (Lindsay, Faloona and Unger, 1974), thus explaining the absence of ketosis.

The majority of patients we see with hyperosmolar coma are elderly or Afro-Caribbean. There is often a history of the quenching of thirst with drinks rich in glucose. Other precipitating factors include diuretics, beta-blockers, corticosteroids, phenytoin and cimetidine. Not all black patients present with this type of hyperglycaemic coma. A significant number present in diabetic ketoacidosis despite appearing to have non-insulin-dependent diabetes (Banerji *et al.*, 1994).

Clouding of consciousness or coma are common and the occasional patient presents with focal neurological signs or fits. Many patients are moribund on admission to hospital and others show profound dehydration and hypotension. Nearly a third of our patients are newly diagnosed diabetics at presentation.

The diagnosis is confirmed by the markedly raised blood glucose, absence of acidosis and a plasma osmolarity of greater than 340 mosmol/l. The latter may be measured directly in the laboratory or calculated from the formula $2 \times$ (plasma Na + K concentration) + plasma glucose concentration + plasma urea concentration, always providing these concentrations are millimoles per litre.

Treatment is identical to that of ketoacidosis although problems may arise with a plasma sodium at presentation or in the early phase of treatment of greater than 150 mmol/l. It is probably wise, even in this case, to restrict the infusion of hypotonic saline in accordance with the guidelines in the previous section, i.e. a maximum of 2 litres.

Hyperosmolar non-ketotic coma is approximately one-tenth as common as ketoacidosis but the mortality is considerably higher. In our recent series the mortality approached one-third (Krentz and Nattrass, 1991). Thromboembolic complications during treatment contribute to this but the benefits of routine anticoagulation remain doubtful.

Insulin treatment may be advised for a few months but patients usually recover sufficient endogenous insulin secretion to make a trial of diet or diet plus oral agents worthwhile. I have little doubt that this should not be rushed. Because it is known that these patients may not need insulin there is a temptation to try oral agents within a day or two of recovery. This serves only to create confusion, since a patient failing a trial of tablets at this stage may be committed to long-term insulin yet the reason for the failure may have more to do with the partial recovery from a metabolic insult than a true inability of the B cells to produce insulin. Better to commit the patient to a 2–3-month period of insulin treatment with a promise of review at the end of that time. On review it is usually abundantly clear whether insulin is truly needed or if the record of persistently normal blood or urine tests and normal glycated protein measurements indicate a real likelihood of a response to diet and/or tablets.

LACTIC ACIDOSIS

Lactic acidosis is the least common form of hyperglycaemic coma. Of course, diabetic patients are at no less risk of Type A lactic acidosis associated with tissue hypoxia from hypovolaemia or endotoxic shock but this need not be associated with hyperglycaemia. The more specific, Type B lactic acidosis (Cohen and Woods, 1976), which may be associated with diabetes *per se* or with biguanide therapy, is seen infrequently.

Occasional patients with diabetes do present with a hyperglycaemic coma without significant ketonuria and not in renal failure. These patients are usually insulin-dependent. They do not necessarily have a major degree of macrovascular or microvascular disease, although it might be anticipated that both these complications could lead to significant tissue hypoxia. Dehydration is a presenting feature, as is hypotension, although the role of hypotension is difficult to assess; clearly it can lead to lactic acidosis but the acidaemia can also result in hypotension.

Making the diagnosis depends on an appreciation that the degree of acidosis – often profound – is out of proportion to the degree of ketonaemia or ketonuria – usually mild. This raises the question as to the ion that is being generated in equimolar amounts to the hydrogen ion. Measurement of blood lactate by the laboratory rapidly confirms the diagnosis. It is wise to take a diagnostic cut-off of 5 mmol/l and to keep in mind that an elevated blood lactate concentration is a frequent accompaniment of ketoacidosis. In the latter situation treatment of the ketoacidosis will lead to resolution of the hyperlactataemia.

Biguanide-induced lactic acidosis has declined dramatically since the withdrawal of phenformin (Bailey and Nattrass, 1988). Sporadic cases occur with metformin although nearly all reports are of patients in whom there were contraindications to the use of metformin. The commonest of these has been renal impairment when accumulation of metformin and an increased risk of lactic acidosis would be entirely predictable. It is unclear how many episodes of lactic acidosis go unrecognized when patients on metformin experience acute onset of a condition predisposing to lactic acidosis such as myocardial infarction.

The prognosis for a patient with lactic acidosis is poor. The mortality rate is about 50%, mainly reflecting the serious underlying condition but also the absence of effective treatment. Reducing agents such as ascorbic acid have been tried without convincing benefit.

Apart from correcting any underlying condition the mainstay of treatment continues to be sodium bicarbonate infusion. Unlike ketoacidosis when 150 mmol of bicarbonate is a therapeutic dose, amounts exceeding 2000 mmol may be given in lactic acidosis. Since a similar amount of sodium must be given it may be necessary to resort to dialysis to remove some of the sodium. The rationale for this treatment is that in severe acidosis the liver is a lactate-producing organ while at normal pH the liver utilizes lactate. Thus, correcting the acidosis should improve lactate clearance. Controlled trials of this treatment are unavailable and are probably not possible from the infrequent nature of the condition. I am pessimistic of its value and indeed would hesitate to advise its use except under the strictest supervision and guidelines. It is not a treatment to be indulged in by a passing junior doctor without sound advice from someone more senior.

REFERENCES

Alberti, K. G. M. M. (1974) Diabetic ketoacidosis – aspects of management, in *Tenth Advanced Medicine Symposium*, (ed. J. G. Ledingham), Pitman Medical, Tunbridge Wells, p. 68–82.

Alberti, K. G. M. M. and Nattrass, M. (1978) Severe diabetic ketoacidosis. *Med. Clin. N. Am.*, **62**, 799–814.

Arieff, A. I. (1980) Treatment of metabolic derangements in diabetic coma. Idiogenic osmoles, in *Diabetes 1979*, (ed. W. K. Waldhausl), Excerpta Medica, Amsterdam, p. 689–692.

Arieff, A. I. and Kleeman, C. R. (1973) Studies on mechanisms of cerebral edema in diabetic comas. *J. Clin. Invest.* **52**, 571–583.

Arieff, A. I. and Kleeman, C. R. (1974) Cerebral edema in diabetic comas. *J. Clin. Endocrinol. Metab.*, **38**, 1057–1067.

Atchley, D. W., Loeb, R. F., Richards, D. W. *et al.* (1933) On diabetic acidosis. A detailed study of electrolyte balances following the withdrawal and reestablishment of insulin therapy. *J. Clin. Invest.*, **12**, 297–326.

Bailey, C. J. and Nattrass, M. (1988) Treatment – metformin. *Clin. Endocrinol. Metab.*, **2**, 455–476.

Banerji, M. A., Chaiken, R. L., Huey, H. *et al.* (1994) GAD antibody negative NIDDM in adult black subjects with diabetic ketoacidosis and increased frequency of human leukocyte antigen DR3 and DR4. *Diabetes*, **43**, 741–745.

Barnes, A. J., Bloom, S. R., Alberti, K. G. M. M. *et al.* (1977) Ketoacidosis in pancreatectomized man. *N. Engl. J. Med.*, **296**, 1250–1253.

Barnes, A. J., Kohner, E., Bloom, S. R. *et al.* (1978) Importance of pituitary hormones in aetiology of diabetic ketoacidosis. *Lancet*, **i**, 1171–1174.

Burge, M. R., Hardy, K. J. and Schade, D. S. (1993) Short term fasting is a mechanism for the development of euglycemic ketoacidosis during periods of insulin deficiency. *J. Clin. Endocrinol. Metab.*, **76**, 1192–1198.

Butler, A. M., Talbot, N. B., Burnett, C. H. *et al.* (1947) Metabolic studies in diabetic coma. *Trans. Ass. Am. Physicians*, **60**, 102–109.

Clements, R. S., Prockop, L. D. and Winegrad, A. I. (1968) Acute cerebral oedema during treatment of hyperglycaemia. An experimental model. *Lancet*, **ii**. 384–386.

Cohen, A. S., Vance, V. K., Runyan, J. W. and Hurwitz, D. (1960) Diabetic acidosis: an evaluation of the cause, course and therapy of 73 cases. *Ann. Intern. Med.*, **52**, 55–86.

Cohen, R. D. and Woods, H. F. (1976) *Clinical and Biochemical Aspects of Lactic Acidosis*, Blackwell, Oxford.

Ditzel, J. and Standl, E. (1975) The oxygen transport system of red blood cells during diabetic ketoacidosis and recovery. *Diabetologia*, **11**, 255–260.

Felig, P. and Wahren, J. (1971) Influence of endogenous insulin secretion on splanchnic glucose and amino acid metabolism in man. *J. Clin. Invest.*, **50**, 1702–1711.

Felig, P., Wahren, J. and Hendler, R. (1976) Influence of physiologic hyperglucagonemia on basal and insulin-inhibited splanchnic glucose output in normal man. *J. Clin. Invest.*, **58**, 761–765.

Gerich, J., Penhos, J. C., Gutman, R. A. and Recant, L. (1973) Effect of dehydration and hyperosmolarity on glucose, free fatty acid and ketone body metabolism in the rat. *Diabetes*, **22**, 264–271.

Gerich, J. E., Lorenzi, M., Bier, D. M. *et al.* (1976) Effects of physiologic levels of glucagon and growth hormone on human carbohydrate and lipid metabolism. *J. Clin. Invest.*, **57**, 875–884.

Guisada, R. and Arieff, A. I. (1975) Neurologic manifestations of diabetic comas: correlation with biochemical alterations in the brain. *Metabolism*, **24**, 665–679.

Hale, P. J., Crase, J. and Nattrass, M. (1984) Metabolic effects of bicarbonate in the treatment of diabetic ketoacidosis. *Br. Med. J.*, **289**, 1035–1038.

Hirsch, M. L. (1960) Gastric hemorrhage in diabetic coma. *Diabetes*, **9**, 94–96.

Houssay, B. A. and Biasotti, A. (1930) La diabetes pancreatica de los pirros hipofisoprivos. *Rev. Soc. Argent. Biol.*, **6**, 251–296.

Johnston, D. G., Alberti, K. G. M. M., Nattrass, M. *et al.* (1980) Hormonal and metabolic rhythms in Cushing's syndrome. *Metabolism*, **29**, 1046–1052.

Krentz, A. J. and Nattrass, M. (1991) Diabetic ketoacidosis, non-ketotic hyperosmolar coma and lactic acidosis, in *Textbook of Diabetes*, (eds J. C. Pickup and G. Williams), Blackwell Scientific Publications, Oxford, p. 479–494.

Krentz, A. J., Hale, P. J., Singh, B. M. and Nattrass, M. (1989) The effect of glucose and insulin infusion on the fall of ketone bodies during treatment of diabetic ketoacidosis. *Diabetic Med.* **6**, 31–36.

Kussmaul, A. (1874) *Deutsch. Arch. Clin. Med.*, **14**, 1–46, cited in Major, R. H. (1932) *Classic Descriptions of Diseases*, Charles C. Thomas, Springfield, IL, p. 200.

Lindsay, C. A., Faloona, C. R. and Unger, R. H. (1974) Plasma glucagon in nonketotic hyperosmolar coma. *J. A. M. A.*, **229**, 1771–1773.

McGarry, J. D. and Foster, D. W. (1980) Regulation of hepatic fatty acid oxidation and ketone body production. *Ann. Rev. Biochem.*, **49**, 395–420.

MacGillivray, M. H., Bruck, E. and Voorhess, M. L. (1981) Acute diabetic ketoacidosis in children: role of the stress hormones. *Pediatr. Res.*, **15**, 99–106.

Marliss, E. B., Ohman, J. L., Aoki, T. T. and Kozack, G. P. (1970) Altered redox state obscuring ketoacidosis in diabetic patients with lactic acidosis. *N. Engl. J. Med.* **283**, 978–980.

Martin, H. E. Smith, K. and Wilson, M. L. (1958) The fluid and electrolyte therapy of severe diabetic acidosis and ketosis. *Am. J. Med.*, **24**, 376–389.

Miles, J. M., Rizza, R. A., Haymond, M. W., and Gerich, J. E. (1980) Effects of acute insulin deficiency on glucose and ketone body turnover in man. *Diabetes*, **29**, 926–930.

Nabarro, J. D. N., Spencer, A. G. and Stowers, J. M. (1952) Metabolic studies in severe diabetic ketosis. *Q. J. Med.*, **21**, 225–248.

Nattrass, M. and Hale, P. J. (1984) Clinical aspects of diabetic ketoacidosis, in *Recent Advances in*

Diabetes 1, (eds M. Nattrass and J. V. Santiago), Churchill Livingstone, Edinburgh, p. 231–238.

Olefsky, J. M., Johnson, J., Liu, F. *et al.* (1975) The effects of acute and chronic dexamethasone administration on insulin binding to isolated rat hepatocytes and adipocytes. *Metabolism*, **24**, 517–527.

Owen, O. E., Block, S. B., Patel, M. *et al.* (1977) Human splanchnic metabolism during diabetic ketoacidosis. *Metabolism*, **26**, 381–398.

Pinkney, J. H., Bingley, P. J., Sawtell, P. A. *et al.* (1994) Presentation and progress of childhood diabetes: a prospective population-based study. *Diabetologia*, **37**, 70–74.

Porte, D. and Williams, R. H. (1966) Inhibition of insulin release by norepinephrine in man. *Science*, **152**, 1248–1250.

Posner, J. B. and Plum, F. (1967) Spinal-fluid pH and neurologic symptoms in systemic acidosis. *N. Engl. J. Med.*, **277**, 605–613.

Rizza, R. A., Cryer, P. E., Haymond, M. W. and Gerich, J. E. (1980) Adrenergic mechanisms for the effects of epinephrine on glucose production and clearance in man. *J. Clin. Invest.* **65**, 682–689.

Rosenbloom, A. L., Riley, W. J., Weber, F. T. *et al.* (1980) Cerebral edema complicating diabetic ketoacidosis in childhood. *J. Pediatr.*, **96**, 357–361.

Schade, D. S. and Eaton, R. P. (1979) Pathogenesis of diabetic ketoacidosis – a reappraisal. *Diabetes Care*, **2**, 296–306.

Schade, D. S., Eaton, R. P., Alberti, K. G. M. M. and Johnston, D. G. (1981) *Diabetic Coma*, University of New Mexico Press, Albuquerque, NM.

Schade, D. S., Eaton, R. P. and Standefer, J. (1978) Modulation of basal ketone body concentration by cortisol in diabetic man. *J. Clin. Endocrinol. Metab.*, **47**, 519–528.

Soskin, S. and Levine, R. (1946) *Carbohydrate Metabolism: Correlation of Physiological, Biochemical, and Clinical Aspects*, University of Chicago Press, Chicago, IL, p. 250.

Soler, N. G., Bennett, M. A., FitzGerald, M. G. and Malins, J. M. (1973) Intensive care in the management of diabetic ketoacidosis. *Lancet*, **i**, 951–954.

Thompson, C. J., Johnston, D. G., Baylis, P. H. and Anderson, J. (1986) Alcoholic ketoacidosis: an underdiagnosed condition. *Br. Med. J.*, **292**, 463–465.

Timperley, W. R., Preston, F. E. and Ward, J. D. (1974) Cerebral intravascular coagulation in diabetic ketoacidosis. *Lancet*, **i**, 952–956.

Wicks, W. D. (1971) Differential effects of glucocorticoids and adenosine 3',5'-monophosphate on hepatic enzyme synthesis. *J. Biol. Chem.*, **246**, 217–223.

Zierler, K. L. and Rabinowitz, D. (1963) Roles of insulin and growth hormone, based on studies of forearm metabolism in man. *Medicine*, **42**, 385–402.

It has been known since the time of Claude Bernard that the blood sugar could be reduced in experimental animals as a result of exhaustion of hepatic glycogen. Similarly, after hepatectomy in dogs Mann and Magath (1921) found a gradual fall of blood sugar to very low levels. This hypoglycaemia was accompanied by a fairly clear-cut set of manifestations which could be readily reversed by giving intravenous glucose.

Recognition of hypoglycaemia in man, however, had to wait until reliable methods for the estimation of blood glucose on small samples were published. Porges (1910) is credited with the first clinical report of a patient with Addison's disease in whom the blood sugar fell as low as 1.8 mmol/l (33 mg/dl). Joslin (1921) published three cases of diabetes in whom exhaustion of hepatic glycogen on the low carbohydrate diets of the Allen era was associated with a fall in blood sugar to as low as 2.2 mmol/l (40 mg/dl).

Banting and Best found that large doses of their extract of pancreas invariably produced hunger, hyperexcitability, fear and finally convulsions and, from Mann and Magath's work, were immediately able to recognize these effects as being due to hypoglycaemia. As soon as insulin was available for treatment similar symptoms were observed in man (Banting, Campbell and Fletcher, 1923), and the correlation of symptoms with blood glucose levels was noted.

The correct methods of management and treatment of the insulin reaction as well as the occurrence of unexpected fatalities were all described in Campbell and Macleod's (1924) massive review on insulin.

The widespread vogue of insulin therapy for schizophrenia, first in small doses as a method of improving nutrition and later for the therapeutic effects of the coma, led to a considerable experience of hypoglycaemia in non-diabetic patients. It soon became apparent that there was a wide variation in the individual response of blood glucose to injected insulin, some patients going into coma on as little as 40 units and others who had received insulin for some time requiring several hundred units to achieve the same effect. The therapy also emphasized the potentially dangerous character of deep hypoglycaemic coma, which had an appreciable mortality even under controlled conditions in hospital.

Simultaneously with the observations on hypoglycaemia in diabetic patients reports appeared on the occurrence of spontaneous hypoglycaemia in patients who did not have diabetes. Harris (1924) described some non-diabetic patients with hypoglycaemia and considered that they might have endogenous hyperinsulinism and Wilder *et al.* (1927) described the first laparotomy undertaken for spontaneous hypoglycaemia at which a carcinoma of the islets of Langerhans was found. Since then a large variety of causes of spontaneous hypoglycaemia in both adults and children have been recognized, of which hyperinsulinism from islet cell adenoma or carcinoma is only one. Hypoglycaemia can be associated with large tumours, is a feature of some endocrine diseases and occurs with alcohol and severe liver disease. Spontaneous hypoglycaemia is sometimes found in children linked with leucine sensitivity and is part of the syndromes of familial fructose and galactose intolerance as well as some glycogen storage diseases.

DEFINITION

Using a method which determines true glucose, the lowest values found on capillary samples taken fasting and 2 hours after 50 g of glucose were about 2.8 mmol/l (50 mg/dl) in 345 normal people of all ages (Report of a Working Party of the College of General Practitioners, 1963).

In 12-hour studies with half-hourly sampling we found the fifth centile for blood glucose measured by a specific glucose assay to be 3.3 mmol/l (60 mg/dl). These results were obtained under more physiological conditions when subjects ate their normal meals during the study but the majority of the subjects were young people. In another study of 169 elderly normal patients (65 years or over) the lowest random blood glucose found was 2.5 mmol/l (45 mg/dl) (Kilvert, 1987). Although these patients were normal in the sense of being non-diabetic, the presence of other illnesses did not exclude them from the study. We have suggested, therefore, that values below 2.5 mmol/l (45 mg/dl) can always be regarded as abnormal and those between 2.5 and 2.8 mmol/l (45 and 50 mg/dl) should be viewed with suspicion in non-diabetic patients and are of questionable normality in diabetic patients.

Older methods for measuring blood 'glucose' such as the Folin and Wu, and Hagedorn and Jensen techniques measure a variable amount of reducing substance other than glucose and a value below 3.1 mmol/l (55 mg/dl) is acceptable evidence of hypoglycaemia.

A strict definition of hypoglycaemia is clearly of importance in identifying those non-diabetic patients in whom further investigation is indicated. It loses some of its meaning, however, when applied to the diabetic patient. In this situation the concern is whether treatment should be offered to raise blood glucose. In a patient who is taking insulin it may well be appropriate to advise oral intake of carbohydrate when the blood glucose is well above the level of the definition and

certainly this will be so if it is some time to the next meal or if exercise is contemplated. In addition, there is some variation in the level of blood glucose at which symptoms of hypoglycaemia appear in insulin-dependent diabetic patients, suggesting that there is no one blood glucose level above which is normoglycaemia and below which the patient can be rigidly termed hypoglycaemic.

It must be understood also that by no means all patients develop recognizable hypoglycaemic symptoms at or below these levels. This is especially true of children, who may behave quite normally when the blood sugar by the older methods is no more than 1.7 mmol/l (30 mg/dl). If, on the other hand, the blood glucose is unexpectedly high during an alleged hypoglycaemic attack the explanation may be that clinical recovery has lagged behind the rise in blood glucose from its lowest point (Figure 11.1, 11.2).

RELATIVE HYPOGLYCAEMIA

While some normal subjects and even diabetic patients may be apparently normal with biochemical hypoglycaemia, other diabetic patients will describe hypoglycaemic symptoms at normal blood glucose levels. The term 'relative hypoglycaemia' has been applied to this situation, although it is far from satisfactory. Hypoglycaemic symptoms at such times are supposedly due to a rapid fall in blood glucose as a result of insulin action. It is suggested that a drop from a level of 25 mmol/l (450 mg/dl) to one of 7 mmol/l (125 mg/dl) in a period of half an hour or less may provoke symptoms by the speed of the fall. The topic is important because of the frequency with which one has to decide whether bizarre symptoms in a patient taking insulin are due to the effects of hypoglycaemia or not. I have never seen a convincing demonstration of this phenomenon and am fortified in my scepticism by the agreement of Joslin *et al.* (1946). The evidence for the occurrence of relative hypoglycaemia has

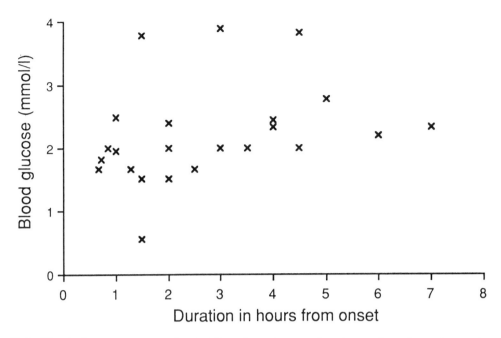

Fig. 11.1   Blood glucose concentration in 23 patients in a confused state from hypoglycaemia.

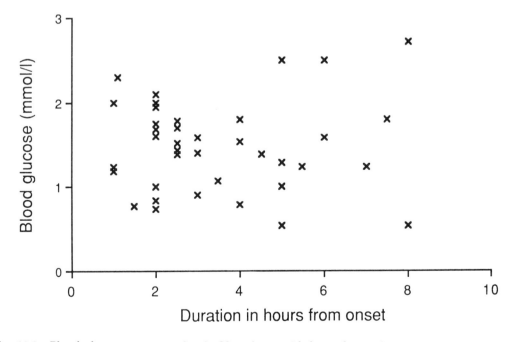

Fig. 11.2   Blood glucose concentration in 38 patients with hypoglycaemic coma.

never been fully presented and since there are many other explanations for pseudo-hypoglycaemic symptoms the concept seems better discarded.

PATHOPHYSIOLOGY OF HYPOGLYCAEMIA

Hypoglycaemia produces symptoms which are partly due to cerebral starvation of glucose – neuroglycopenic symptoms – and partly due to physiological responses – autonomic or neurogenic symptoms. Adequate defence against hypoglycaemia is crucial to the survival of normal man. Teleologically it is easy to see the importance of an adequate response to hypoglycaemia. Thousands of years ago when feasting–fasting rather than regular supply of meals was the nutritional norm, hypoglycaemia developing at an inappropriate time might well turn man from hunter into prey.

CEREBRAL EFFECTS OF HYPOGLYCAEMIA

The brain is the most important recognition site of hypoglycaemia. In dogs a model has been described whereby the brain and the body of the dog can be perfused separately. If blood glucose supply is maintained to the brain while the rest of the body is starved of glucose the counter-regulatory response is almost absent (Biggers *et al.*, 1989).

In man and many other animals it is held that glucose is the only readily available substrate for supplying the energy requirements of the brain. Glycogen stores in mammalian brain are almost negligible and therefore glucose must be supplied from the blood. Extraction of glucose from the blood by brain is by facilitated glucose transport via the glucose transporter, GLUT 1. Transport is not normally rate-limiting but when the external supply drops it becomes so because of an inability to increase glucose uptake urgently. This fall in cerebral metabolism

is held to be important in stimulating the counter-regulatory response.

There may also be an adaptive mechanism which operates chronically. In studies of normal subjects kept moderately hypoglycaemic for 2 days by insulin infusion the response to acute hypoglycaemia at the end of this time was impaired, occurring at a blood glucose concentration of 2.5 mmol/l (36 mg/dl) rather than 3.6 mmol/l (65 mg/dl). During the studies rates of cerebral glucose utilization were measured. In the first study a fall in cerebral glucose metabolism preceded the hormonal responses; in the second rates were preserved to the lowest blood glucose (Boyle *et al.*, 1994).

It is true that during prolonged fasting the brain adapts to the use of ketone bodies but these substrates have little part to play during normal daily life and it is clear that adapting to ketone body utilization takes some time (Owen *et al.*, 1967).

The main effect of hypoglycaemia upon the brain, therefore, is to initiate a counter-regulatory response in order to prevent the next sequence of effects on the brain of cognitive dysfunction.

COUNTER-REGULATION

Increased circulating 'sympathins' during insulin-induced hypoglycaemia were noted soon after the introduction of insulin, and an increase in plasma adrenalin levels following hypoglycaemia in both dogs and man has since been confirmed many times. Concurrently there is also a depletion of the adrenal medullary stores. It is caused by hypoglycaemia rather than insulin since it is abolished when hypoglycaemia is prevented by the simultaneous administration of glucose.

Adrenalin release is a protective mechanism since it acts to phosphorylate liver and muscle glycogen and raise the blood glucose level. The response does not depend on an intact pituitary and is unaffected by transection of the midbrain, indicating that neural pathways from the hypothalamus are not essential. It is blocked by adrenal denervation and also by removal of the thoracic and upper lumbar spinal cord in dogs.

Release of adrenalin is not the only factor in counter-regulation. Release of glucagon, which also acts upon phosphorylase of liver converting glycogen to glucose, also plays an important role. It may well be the more important stimulus to restoring normal blood glucose levels. If both glucagon and adrenalin responses are impaired recovery of blood glucose concentration is severely impaired.

Hypoglycaemia is also a potent stimulus to the rapid release of growth hormone and adrenal corticosteroids. In the presence of a defective glucagon and adrenalin response these hormones cannot totally compensate and it is likely that their role is of importance in prolonged hypoglycaemia.

While initially the glucagon and adrenalin responses act to raise blood glucose through mobilization of glycogen this is rapidly followed by an increase in gluconeogenesis. Catecholamines also increase rates of lipolysis and increased non-esterified fatty acids are found. These may serve to impair glucose uptake into muscle, making more available for brain uptake. The hormonal response may also contribute to an impaired peripheral uptake of glucose, although this effect is likely to be relatively minor.

A tremendous body of work has accumulated on defining the thresholds at which the various responses to hypoglycaemia occur (Schwartz *et al.*, 1987; Mitrakou *et al.*, 1991). The sequence of events can be summarized thus. Glucagon and adrenalin secretion occur in response to a fall in arterialized venous plasma glucose to 3.8 mmol/l (68 mg/dl); growth hormone secretion also occurs at around this level but cortisol secretion requires a fall to 3.2 mmol/l (58 mg/dl); symptoms are felt at 3 mmol/l (54 mg/dl); and cognitive dysfunction is found at 2.7 mmol/l (49 mg/dl).

ELECTROLYTE CHANGES

Insulin had been available for only a short time before it became evident that its administration produced a decrease in serum inorganic phosphate. A similar fall follows fructose administration, which does not require insulin for entrance into the cell. The fall in blood phosphate, therefore, is likely to be a consequence of the rapid entrance of hexoses into cells. During hypoglycaemia there is also a fall in serum potassium. The reasons for this change seem complex but adrenalin release is important, because hypokalaemia does not occur in hypoglycaemic demedullated rats. The electrocardiographic changes found in hypoglycaemia, consisting of diminished T waves, depressed ST segments and prolongation of the Q–T interval, are thought to be due to a fall in serum potassium.

GASTRIC SECRETION AND PERIPHERAL BLOOD FLOW

Insulin-induced hypoglycaemia has a marked effect on gastric secretion. The action is a complex one and consists of an initial phase of inhibition followed by a sharp rise dependent upon vagal stimulation. The latter reaction has been found useful as a test of the effectiveness of vagotomy, but is otherwise without practical effects in diabetic patients. Muscle and skin blood flow is increased in the forearm in hypoglycaemia – a response which cannot be entirely accounted for by adrenalin release.

KETONE FORMATION

Collip (1923) first pointed out the effect of hypoglycaemia as a stimulus to ketone formation in rabbits. McPherson *et al.* (1958) showed a fivefold increase in splanchnic ketone production 3–4 hours after experimental hypoglycaemia was induced by insulin in normal subjects. In clinical practice transient ketonuria is found some hours after insulin reactions, but serum ketones do not accumulate to the extent of producing an acidosis. This effect is due to the release of catecholamines, leading to enhanced lipolysis and increased non-esterified fatty acids, the precursors of ketones. Adrenalin is known to be a potent lipolytic agent and the non-esterified fatty acid increase stimulated by hypoglycaemia can be prevented by adrenergic blocking agents.

CLINICAL ASPECTS

Patients who have to take insulin nearly all agree that their greatest problem is hypoglycaemia. Those of us who treat diabetes would certainly agree that our own dislike of insulin, if we had to use it on ourselves, would be related to the fear of such attacks. It is, indeed, quite probable that the reason why patients are so reluctant to be put on insulin is less a distaste for the needle than the reputation of insulin as a cause of comas and fainting turns, a part of the folklore of every suburb.

The frequency of hypoglycaemia is usually underestimated because the victims have a curious tendency to forget or deliberately minimize the frequency of their attacks; a talk with the family may discover an alarming situation which the patient has not even mentioned at his routine visit. We questioned 100 patients with diabetes of varying duration who were a random sample of those taking insulin; 24 of them had lost consciousness on at least one occasion and 65 had experienced minor attacks short of losing consciousness. Only 11 had never had hypoglycaemic attacks at all.

Asymptomatic hypoglycaemia is even commoner. Gale and Tattersall (1979) observed blood glucose concentrations of < 2.0 mmol/l (36 mg/dl) in 56% of 39 insulin-dependent diabetic patients in whom blood sampling was performed during the night.

Pramming *et al.* (1991) found that their insulin-dependent diabetic patients had an average of 1.8 episodes of symptomatic hypoglycaemia per week while estimates of severe hypoglycaemia vary wildly according to the population studied and the definition of severe hypoglycaemia.

Under the more controlled conditions of the Diabetes Control and Complications Trial (DCCT Research Group, 1991) further daunting figures emerged. It must be remembered that patients with a history of recurrent severe hypoglycaemic episodes were excluded from the outset. With a definition of severe hypoglycaemia as episodes that required assistance, even if only oral carbohydrate was taken, the rates were 19 per 100 patient years in the conventionally treated group and 62 per 100 patient years in the intensive treatment group.

CAUSES OF HYPOGLYCAEMIA

Blood glucose level is the net result of the amount of glucose entering the blood minus the amount leaving the blood. It follows therefore that reducing the amount going into the blood or increasing the amount leaving the blood, without a compensatory change in the other variable, must lead to a fall in blood glucose concentration.

The more common situations in which hypoglycaemia occurs are listed in Table 11.1. The most common cause is delay or omission of a meal, particularly during the active part of the day, so that the importance of a strict timetable cannot be overemphasized, especially for those who drive cars. The man who

Table 11.1 Causes of hypoglycaemia

Delay or omission of a meal
Unplanned exercise
Irregular absorption of carbohydrate from the gut
Alcohol
Menstruation
Malice
Change in injection site

is hurrying to get home for a late meal and has no carbohydrate to hand is in some danger.

Unusual exertion is next in frequency. Typically, the effort of mowing the lawn on Sunday morning is too great a contrast with the weekday of the sedentary worker. This problem affects farmers, whose physical work varies greatly from day to day. In them it may be necessary to vary the insulin dose considerably as well as increasing the car- bohydrate on active days. In general it is unplanned physical exercise that causes problems. Many insulin-dependent diabetic patients have played strenuous sports such as soccer or rugby, even at the highest level, without major problems from hypogly- caemia. The weekend golfer soon learns to adjust insulin and/or carbohydrate in order to complete a round.

The relationship of exercise and hypogly- caemia should be clearly explained as part of the patient's education. Plans can be made for avoiding hypoglycaemia and it should never deter patients from regular exercise. Physical effort cannot always be predicted: for instance, a car wheel may have to be changed. It is then essential to have an emergency supply of carbohydrate available.

Gastric stasis resulting from autonomic neuropathy can lead to irregular absorption of carbohydrate and unpredictable variations in the blood glucose level.

Alcohol intake may cause hypoglycaemia and certainly arouses fears of hypoglycaemia. This has to be due partly to our inability to predict the effects of alcohol. Since beer and most mixers contain carbohydrate as sugar as well as alcohol a hyperglycaemic stimulus would be expected. Alcohol, however, inhibits hepatic formation of glucose and is therefore a hypoglycaemic agent. The extent to which a hyper- or hypoglycaemic response may be predicted varies not only from patient to patient but within a patient from day to day. This makes logical advice exceedingly difficult. Beyond not drinking to excess, and ensuring a

carbohydrate intake before bed after consum- ing alcohol, we have little to offer. Experi- enced patients are well able to detect our own uncertainties in such areas. At least it is no longer recommended that patients consume low carbohydrate/high alcohol beers, but whether the low carbohydrate/low alcohol beers will alter the risk is not yet known.

Menstruation is associated with changes in diabetic control, presumed to reflect alterations in insulin sensitivity. Certainly there are effects upon insulin receptors and postreceptor events during the menstrual cycle. For many women this means hyperglycaemia preceding the onset of menses unless insulin dose is adjusted. There is a group of female insulin- dependent patients in whom the start of a period is preceded by a tendency to hypogly- caemia. Fortunately the majority display a degree of predictability which allows evasive action.

Deliberate overdosage with insulin has to be thought of when hypoglycaemia occurs repeatedly in a patient with a psychopathic personality. Even those of healthy mind are not always above enjoying an attack and a good feed of confectionery, but malingerers have more complex motives which may be difficult to elicit.

When all causes are considered there re- mains the occurrence of a hypoglycaemic attack out of the blue. This can be distressing for the patient, previously stable for many months, who ends up in the Casualty Department. The patient is rightly keen for an explanation so that it can be avoided next time and the degree to which this is pursued often serves only to expose the doctor's inadequacies. There are some minor reasons which should be sought but in my experience they are rarely fruitful and do not convey much certainty of a causal role.

Had there been a change in injection sites? It is generally appreciated that absorption of insulin is affected by a number of factors, including site of injection. A switch of site from leg or abdomen to arm will lead to an increase in absorption, as will a change from a lipohypertrophic area to a normal area.

In my experience, not many patients have a hypoglycaemic episode while bathing, although a warm perfusate will speed absorption.

Inadequate shaking of a bottle of long-acting insulin will alter the characteristics of the injected insulin. In turn this will produce a contrast between the end of one bottle and the beginning of the next.

Most readers will be able to expand this list, knowing of one patient who ascribes an otherwise unexplained hypoglycaemic attack to a semi-plausible chain of events.

RECURRENT HYPOGLYCAEMIA

At times a patient with previously well controlled diabetes will begin to experience recurrent hypoglycaemic attacks. These may be due to repeated errors of the paragraph above but it may be necessary to look further afield (Table 11.2).

The majority of newly diagnosed insulin-dependent diabetic patients retain the ability to secrete small amounts of insulin in the short term. This remission phase, while being difficult to define biochemically, is quite often blatantly obvious from the patient's progress. Once controlled there is often a progressive reduction in the need for insulin, even to zero, and great vigilance must be exercised in adjusting the dose at frequent intervals.

The same is true of patients who are recovering from an infection that has increased

Table 11.2 Causes of recurrent hypoglycaemia

- Recovery of endogenous insulin secretion
- Reduction in titre of antibodies to insulin
- Declining renal function
- Development of other endocrine disease, e.g. hypopituitarism, Addison's disease, myxoedema
- Anorexia
- Anorexia nervosa and/or bulimia
- Manipulation

the insulin requirement, while anyone who returns to active life from immobilization in hospital is likely to need less insulin. For this reason stabilization under conventional hospital conditions is often pointless unless adequate physical activity can be provided.

Change in the type or species of insulin can lead to a gradual fall in insulin antibody titre. With less of the injected dose bound on absorption, hypoglycaemia is a risk. The greatest fall in antibodies is likely when conventional beef insulin is changed for highly purified human insulin but any change should be sought in a patient with recurrent episodes of hypoglycaemia.

Some confusion can and has arisen through insulin manufacturers retaining the same name for insulin from different species and it is not unknown for pharmacies to dispense porcine instead of human insulin or *vice versa*. It is self-evident, therefore, that an inspection of the vial may be necessary.

Recurrent hypoglycaemia may occur with declining renal function. It is clear that the insulin resistance of uraemia is insufficient in the diabetic to counter the loss of glucose production from renal gluconeogenesis and the alteration in insulin half-life in renal failure.

Diabetics are no less likely to develop other systemic illness than their non-diabetic counterparts. A major systemic illness may lead to a persistent decrease in calorie intake from anorexia. The development of an endocrine disease which leads to loss of one or more of the counter-regulatory hormones may also lead to recurrent hypoglycaemia. Indeed, the latter may raise the first suspicion of the onset of endocrine disease. Occasional patients develop anorexia nervosa or other eating disorder. Fortunately the numbers are few, since they may present major problems in the management of both diet and insulin.

SYMPTOMS

The symptoms of hypoglycaemia vary greatly but the pattern of the attack tends to be the same every time for an individual so that the earliest manifestation is easily recognized by the patient. This rule is not, of course, inviolable and patients are sometimes thrown by symptoms of a hypoglycaemic attack that does not follow their regular pattern.

Symptoms are attributable to neuroglycopenia and autonomic stimulation. Within the latter category the symptoms attributable to adrenalin release are the most obvious but some symptoms result from a cholinergic stimulus. They consist of shaking, sweating, anxiety, hot and cold feelings, hunger, weakness and palpitation. Shaking or trembling is the most common of all. A characteristic warning for some patients is the onset of paraesthesiae around the lips and tongue; a sensation which is unusual from any other cause and is therefore of some diagnostic value. Headache, blurred vision and double vision are also common, while nausea and vomiting may occur in isolation and can be confused with symptoms of early ketosis.

Rarer symptoms include visual, auditory and olfactory hallucinations, altered colour vision and hemianopia. Changes in mood and behaviour are often the earliest indication of an attack, although not recognized by the patient. Irritability and talkativeness in one who is normally taciturn, depression and reticence in a cheerful extrovert, may be well known to the family of a diabetic and their offer of sugar at this stage is often resented and violently rejected. This curious state of mind has been described to me more than once as like having a dual personality, one that is aware of the need for sugar and the other that wants only to be left in peace. Sometimes behaviour may seem normal but the patient later has no recollection of his attack. In the absence of corrective treatment drowsiness and coma follow the period of confusion. The progression may be rapid so that the patient falls and may be injured.

SIGNS

Sweating and pallor are early signs of hypoglycaemia while tremor of the hands may be obvious. The speech is often slurred and repeated yawning, grimacing and smacking of the lips are less common. The picture at times may closely resemble that of acute alcoholic intoxication, including pupil changes and rotatory nystagmus. All grades of disturbance of consciousness are possible from mild confusion to manic violence and deep coma. The most common picture is one of quiet unconsciousness. The patient appears to be asleep but is unrousable. The skin is warm and usually bathed in sweat, the pulse full and rather fast with occasional ventricular ectopic beats as a result of hyperadrenalism. The systolic blood pressure is slightly raised and the pulse pressure increased. The state of the pupils varies with the degree of coma, the tendon reflexes are depressed, but the plantar responses always extensor even in the lightest coma.

A confusing variant is the attack with focal signs in the nervous system which may mimic any type of intracranial catastrophe. Hemiplegia is quite common and it may be quite impossible to distinguish the coma with stertorous breathing and obvious paralysis of one side of the body from that of cerebral thrombosis or haemorrhage. Recovery, when glucose is given intravenously, is usually rapid and complete but the localized weakness may recur in subsequent attacks. This manifestation of hypoglycaemia probably indicates the presence of a local vascular deficiency which is compensated but cannot withstand the added effect of glucose deprivation.

Convulsions are not uncommon, especially in children, but have no special significance. Epileptics who also have diabetes and take insulin may have fits provoked by hypoglycaemia but this is by no means invariably the case as some of them fail to have a fit even in a severe hypoglycaemic attack.

DIAGNOSIS

In most cases the diagnosis can be suspected from a knowledge of the fact that the patient is on insulin or oral hypoglycaemic drugs coupled with the circumstance that symptoms of mental confusion have appeared rapidly in someone apparently in good health before a meal or after undue exertion. However, the diagnosis depends upon finding a low blood glucose and it is extremely important to take a blood sample whenever the diagnosis is in doubt before giving any treatment. If glucose promptly restores the patient to normal and there is no question of any other disease being present the blood sample can always be thrown away, but if there is any doubt it may turn out to be invaluable and may save fruitless investigation. If the blood glucose is above 2.8 mmol/l (50 mg/dl), hypoglycaemia as a cause of unconsciousness is unlikely, unless treatment has already been given or the patient has been unconscious for some hours.

The most common difficulties in differential diagnosis lie in distinguishing hypoglycaemia from neurotic disorders, strokes, epilepsy and alcoholic intoxication, especially if no history of treatment for diabetes can be obtained. If there is doubt then giving glucose after taking a blood sample is a good diagnostic test. If this promptly restores the patient to normal, hypoglycaemia is the likely diagnosis.

Hypoglycaemia should rarely be confused with diabetic ketoacidosis and I am consistently irritated by undergraduate textbooks that list the differential diagnosis of the two conditions side by side. Typical cases of either condition bear no resemblance to one another. Coma is present in only 20% of patients in ketoacidosis, Kussmaul respiration should not be confused with that seen in hypoglycaemia, and dehydration is not a feature of hypoglycaemia.

Despite this, the error is not uncommon, most often arising from failure to get a proper history, which may be inevitable with a patient in coma; or failure to examine the patient, which is neither inevitable nor excusable. In addition, bedside tests for blood glucose, done in the heat of the moment, are not beyond giving a false result. An old-fashioned urine test, if a specimen can be obtained, will show the heavy glycosuria and ketonuria of ketoacidosis. In hypoglycaemia there is usually no glycosuria but there may be as much as 1%. At the end of an attack ketonuria may be considerable as fat catabolism is stimulated by counter-regulatory hormones.

The importance of correct diagnosis is emphasized by the occasional case of hypoglycaemic coma treated by insulin. This dangerous mistake is often due to ordering treatment by telephone in ignorance of the full facts, but I have known a patient treated in this way in spite of his own protests while still conscious, and on a second occasion while in coma. Each time he was revived with considerable difficulty.

TREATMENT

Attacks can be prevented by strict attention to the timing of meals, the quantity of carbohydrate and the insulin administration technique, while knowledge of the effects of exercise is invaluable. Spontaneous recovery from hypoglycaemia may occur within a few minutes with the aid of rest but this should never be necessary if sugar or carbohydrate in some form is always carried. At the first symptom 10 g (2 teaspoonfuls) of sugar should be taken, preferably in water to speed absorption. If there is no improvement in five minutes the dose should be repeated. If only biscuits or bread are available the effect is much more gradual. Sometimes very large amounts of carbohydrate are necessary but more often they are given impatiently because full recovery does not take place at once. Even at rest a period of 10–15 minutes is often needed. Heavy glycosuria follows such enthusiastic treatment and it may be necessary to reduce the carbohydrate in the diet at subsequent meals on that day, whereas after taking only 10–20 g of sugar the meals should not be altered.

Unconscious patients require intravenous glucose and 50 ml of 50% glucose will immediately raise the blood glucose by at least 5.5 mmol/l (100 mg/dl). Glucose in a solution of this concentration is viscous and difficult to inject through a narrow-bore needle. Care should be taken to prevent the escape of glucose solution around the vein because it is a tissue irritant and attempts to inject an irrational or violent patient should never be made unless there are assistants to keep the arm steady.

If no intravenous glucose is available glucagon is an alternative. It can be given subcutaneously or intramuscularly in a dose of 1 mg. The intravenous route is not recommended since it can induce vomiting. Patients' relatives can be taught to give glucagon subcutaneously; many already have experience of giving the occasional insulin injection to the patient. Glucagon mobilizes glycogen from the liver but will only raise blood glucose by approximately 2 mmol/l (36 mg/dl) which may be sufficient to raise consciousness level to allow oral intake. It should always be followed by oral carbohydrate when this is achieved. It is not invariably successful, however, and intravenous glucose is still the treatment of choice. In addition, the knee-jerk response of 'if hypoglycaemia then give glucagon' is to be avoided. Glucagon is inappropriate in sulphonylurea-induced hypoglycaemia and non-diabetic hypoglycaemia because of its insulin-stimulating properties. While intravenous glucose will also stimulate insulin release at least it provides a simultaneous and substantial supply of substrate. The place of glucagon seems to be for patients in whom it is difficult or not possible to give intravenous glucose, for use by relatives of those patients who have frequent sudden hypoglycaemic attacks, particularly if they live far from medical help, and to provide considerable reassurance to patients undertaking unusual ventures.

RECOVERY

In mild hypoglycaemia oral glucose should promote complete recovery in 10–15 minutes. Some patients recover spontaneously from coma – a not uncommon story from those who live alone. Many improve without treatment while on their way to hospital (Table 11.3).

There are few more dramatic results of treatment in medicine than the instant revival of a deeply unconscious patient when intravenous glucose is given, and resident staff are apt to be disappointed if this miracle is not achieved in every case. However, although some immediate response to treatment is the rule, complete recovery is often delayed for as long as an hour. In a few cases the clearing of consciousness is much slower and hospital admission becomes necessary. It is then particularly important to have substantiated the diagnosis by measuring the blood glucose prior to treatment and further tests may be necessary lest there is a tendency for hypoglycaemia to recur.

It is often difficult to explain why the patient fails to improve although the blood glucose has been restored. Prolonged coma, the occurrence of convulsions and the degenerative changes of old age are definite factors.

Table 11.3 Recovery time in 78 consecutive patients with hypoglycaemia brought to hospital as emergencies (77 patients were on insulin, one was on chlorpropamide)

	No.	%
Spontaneous recovery	16	20
Complete recovery within 10 min of intravenous glucose administration	26	33
Recovery within 10 min and 1 h	29	37
Recovery within 1 and 12 h	5	6
Over 12 h	2	3

IRREVERSIBLE BRAIN DAMAGE

Considering the large number of patients who have major insulin reactions it is uncommon to see evidence of permanent brain damage. Focal neurological signs and even decerebrate posturing may resolve speedily with treatment.

Delayed recovery from coma may take several days and yet seem to be complete in that the capacity to carry out exacting intellectual work is unimpaired. Persistence of focal signs such as hemiplegia is especially rare, but dementia of minor degree is probably more common than we think, because the defect may only be apparent on a searching test. In a few cases it is quite obvious and permanent. There are some who after many attacks suffer a subtle deterioration in personality similar to that which follows prefrontal leucotomy.

FATAL CASES

Death from hypoglycaemia is uncommon but not rare. In the follow-up study of young diabetic patients diagnosed before the age of 31 from the Steno Hospital Deckert, Poulsen and Larsen (1978) found that 3% of the deaths could be attributable to hypoglycaemia. In the British Diabetic Association survey of factors contributing to deaths of diabetics under 50 years of age (Tunbridge, 1981), 4% of 448 deaths were due to hypoglycaemia. All but one of the patients were taking insulin. In half the patients blood glucose was measured and confirmed hypoglycaemia, which was the presumptive diagnosis in the other patients. Most of the patients had either personality problems or psychiatric disorders.

Malins (1968) kept full records of 14 patients attending our clinic in whom the diagnosis was established by all clinical criteria and the absence of any alternative cause of death at autopsy. In six the histology of the brain was consistent with the established findings of pathological studies (Lawrence, Meyer and Nevin, 1942). Eight of the patients were over 60 years of age and in them the circumstances of the fatal attack were similar – a substantial dose of a long-acting insulin, poor nutrition, a nocturnal attack and the absence of an alert member of the family so that the coma was not seen or treated for at least 5 hours. The six younger patients were more disturbing. Two were pregnant women and in both of them the maximum period of coma was known to be 3 hours before adequate and continued treatment was begun.

It is clear, therefore, that it is not easy to state a minimum period of coma that will threaten life, for coma lasting 3 hours can kill while an attack of apparently similar severity lasting 6–10 hours may leave no permanent mark. Of course, the state of the blood glucose throughout the period of coma is practically never documented and there may in fact be wide differences between the levels in attacks of clinically identical character. One lesson emerges – that hypoglycaemic coma is to be regarded as an extreme emergency.

The pathological changes found in the brain in fatal cases are not particularly specific and resemble those due to anoxic damage from any cause. There is widespread degeneration and necrosis of neurones, with corresponding macroglial and microglial proliferation. The cortex, caudate nucleus and putamen are areas most severely affected while changes in the cerebellum and brain stem are less marked (Lawrence, Meyer and Nevin, 1942). The frequently prolonged nature of the terminal coma in these patients, plus the often associated severe hypoxia which may be experienced, makes it difficult to interpret the specificity of the pathological changes.

CHANGE IN CHARACTER OF HYPOGLYCAEMIC SYMPTOMS WITH INCREASING DIABETES DURATION

R. D. Lawrence (1941) seems to have been the first to point out how commonly changes in

the symptomatology of insulin-induced hypoglycaemia occur as the years of treatment
proceed. At first it is the rule that patients feel
and easily recognize minor premonitory
symptoms, such as sweating, tremulousness
and paraesthesiae around the mouth and use
these symptoms as a warning to take food
or sugar. Many conscientious patients even
welcome such mild attacks, regarding them
as a sign that their diabetes is well controlled.
As the years of insulin life go on, sometimes
after only 5–10 years, the type of reaction
changes, the premonitory autonomic symptoms are missed and the attack proceeds
directly to the more serious manifestations
affecting the central nervous system. In
Lawrence's words:

A patient instead of becoming shaky,
sweaty or hungry if his meal is unduly late
becomes suddenly confused or obstreperous,
creates a scene and refuses sugar. Another,
accustomed to drive a car and usually
warned of hypoglycaemia by slight diplopia,
becomes suddenly wild and unbalanced in
his driving. Yet another, instead of being
awakened at night by palpitations – his
warning to take sugar – goes straight into
convulsions and cannot reach his sugar.

HYPOGLYCAEMIC AWARENESS

One most plausible explanation for this
phenomenon favoured for many years was
that diabetic neuropathy led to failure of
the neurogenic stimulus responsible for the
secretion of adrenalin so that not only was
the patient deprived of some warning symptoms but also of a stimulus to hepatic glucose
output. It is clear however that adrenalin and
noradrenalin responses to hypoglycaemia are
not reduced in the presence of autonomic
blockade, indeed they may even be exaggerated (Towler *et al.*, 1993). Rather it is the
symptoms of sweating, tremor and tachycardia that subjects fail to appreciate under these
conditions.

In recent years autonomic neuropathy as a
cause for hypoglycaemic unawareness has
fallen from favour. Ryder *et al.* (1990) could
find no direct relationship between the two in
23 insulin-dependent diabetic patients while
Hepburn *et al.* (1990) performed cardiovascular autonomic function tests on 226 insulin
treated diabetics. Cardiovascular tests were
abnormal in similar proportions of patients
who had either hypoglycaemic awareness or
hypoglycaemic unawareness.

The loss of hypoglycaemic awareness can
be a source of considerable distress in experienced diabetic patients. Just as the doctor is
tempted to invoke loss of autonomic responses
as a possible explanation so the patient will
already have reviewed their recent life for
change that may offer explanation. In recent
years the many changes in insulin preparations have provided possible explanations for
the patient. The change from conventional
insulin to highly purified insulins, from beef
to pork insulin, and from animal to human
insulins have all been invoked at one time or
another. While it is apparent that the change
from beef insulin to porcine or human insulin, particularly in those patients with a high
daily dose requirement, can prompt hypoglycaemia there are no logical grounds for
blaming a loss of symptoms on this change.

The loss of hypoglycaemic warning symptoms reported by some patients using human
insulin has recently been drawn somewhat
forcibly to the physician's attention by threats
of legal action. It is exceedingly difficult to
know whether human insulin is directly
implicated. As mentioned above the changes
in insulin preparation through the years have
often provoked the claim of lost warning
symptoms since changing insulin. Not only
did some patients report lost warning with
change from beef to porcine or from conventional to highly purified but also from U40 or
U80 to U100 insulin – a change in concentration only of injected insulin.

The average diabetologist has only clinical
experience to go on. Since there was no *a priori*

case for linking the introduction of human insulin to loss of hypoglycaemic warning no long-term studies have been performed to confirm or refute the hypothesis. Clinical experience is notoriously open to bias. In our clinic I have heard the claim often enough for me to be convinced of some likelihood of the link being established. My senior colleague, however, who sits in the same clinic and sees the same assortment of patients and problems, remains much more sceptical of a causal link.

Evidence for a change in symptoms with use of human insulin is far from strong. Retrospective questionnaire surveys, with all their problems, first raised the issue (Berger and Althaus, 1987; Teuscher and Berger, 1987). In double-blind crossover studies hunger and sweating are less common initial symptoms of hypoglycaemia, and restlessness and lack of concentration are more frequently reported (Berger *et al.*, 1989; Egger *et al.*, 1991). It has been argued that hunger and sweating alert the patient to a need for sugar whereas restlessness and loss of concentration impair the ability to realize the need. It should be appreciated that this is not an absolute difference between treatments – for example, in the study of Egger *et al.* (1991) reporting of hunger as initial symptom was 33% when taking human insulin and 42% when taking porcine insulin – 22 patients were studied. I have not found the published literature particularly helpful or convincing, in contrast to the excellent summary of the published studies provided by Nelleman Jorgensen, Djgaard and Pramming (1994). They collated 39 clinical studies and 12 epidemiological studies on human insulin and hypoglycaemia and concluded that from a large number of studies in a large number of patients there was 'overwhelming evidence' that human and porcine insulins do not provoke different hormonal responses to hypoglycaemia; that they do not cause different symptoms of hypoglycaemia; and that the incidence of hypoglycaemia does not differ with human,

as opposed to porcine, insulin. I suspect we are in for a lengthy debate at least in the UK – hopefully it will not be in the courtroom!

One theory propounded by way of explanation involves the development of symptoms as a result of the rate of fall of blood glucose rather than as a function of an absolute level. Highly purified insulins, it is argued, can accentuate the rate of fall because 'free' insulin concentrations can be achieved quicker. Our own suggestion some years ago that the presence of insulin-binding antibodies provides a depot that works against rapid swings in insulin levels has been invoked to support this view. The argument cannot be extended to a change from highly purified animal insulins to human insulin, when many studies have shown similar rates of fall of blood glucose.

The list of probable causes of loss of hypoglycaemic warning signs has been added to recently by the finding that tight blood glucose control using intensified insulin regimens may increase the risk. Asymptomatic hypoglycaemia in patients using such regimens is three times more common (Lager *et al.*, 1986), as is severe hypoglycaemia (DCCT Research Group, 1987). Amiel *et al.* (1988) showed that intensified insulin treatment is associated with a lowering of blood glucose level at which physiological responses to hypoglycaemia are triggered; from 3.7 mmol/l (67 mg/dl) before intensive treatment to 2.6 mmol/l (47 mg/dl) after 6 months' intensive treatment. The counter-regulatory hormonal response was also reduced during the second test but the blood glucose level at which cerebral function was impaired was not altered in these patients, remaining around 2.8–3.0 mmol/l (50–54 mg/dl). The important consequence of this arrangement is that the order of appreciation is reversed. From the situation where autonomic responses clearly occur before cognitive dysfunction providing protection against the latter the situation develops where cognitive function is the first manifestation of hypoglycaemia

(Amiel *et al.*, 1991). There is evidence that loss of awareness resulting from tight glucose control and impaired endocrine responses is reversible with a relaxation of the goals of control (Cranston *et al.*, 1994; Fanelli *et al.*, 1994).

Modification of counter-regulatory response and symptoms in normal subjects has been shown by a preceding episode of hypoglycaemia. Heller and Cryer (1991) observed responses on successive days of subjects undergoing 2 hours of hypoglycaemia and found both symptomatic and hormonal responses reduced on the second day. Continuing this line of work Veneman *et al.* (1993) induced asymptomatic nocturnal hypoglycaemia in normal volunteers and found an increased threshold (that is a greater degree of hypoglycaemia, reduced autonomic and neuroglycopenic symptoms, counter-regulatory hormone response and cognitive dysfunction) during subsequent acute hypoglycaemia.

OTHER ASPECTS OF HYPOGLYCAEMIA IN DIABETES

SPONTANEOUS HYPOGLYCAEMIA AS AN EARLY MANIFESTATION OF DIABETES

Difficult to prove but impressive to the clinician is the number of patients who give a history of one or more episodes suggestive of hypoglycaemia in the few months prior to diagnosis of diabetes. The subject was first brought forward by Allen (1953) who, in the course of an investigation into the causes of obesity preceding the onset of diabetes, was struck by the fact that many of his patients had episodes of hunger, weakness, sweating, trembling and irritability which were relieved by eating. Seltzer, Fajans and Conn (1956) reported 110 patients with diabetic glucose tolerance tests whose blood glucose dropped to hypoglycaemic levels between the third and fifth hour following the glucose. Many of

these patients had complained of hypoglycaemic symptoms. Lloyd (1964) recorded the case of the child of a diabetic mother who was admitted to hospital following a convulsion and found to have a blood glucose of 2.6 mmol/l (46 mg/dl). Clinical diabetes developed soon afterwards.

It is certainly true that symptoms very suggestive of hypoglycaemia are not rare a few months before the finding of glycosuria leads to the diagnosis of diabetes, but the proof is lacking because the blood glucose is not estimated. The early stages of non-insulin-dependent diabetes are marked by a sluggish initial release of insulin by the islets, which ultimately respond with excessive insulin production. It is the final phase that could theoretically induce hypoglycaemia. The hyperinsulinism is prompted by a decreased ability to dispose of a glucose load, which casts doubts upon this theory, and it is notable how difficult it can be to reproduce either symptoms or measured hypoglycaemia under controlled conditions.

Prediabetic hypoglycaemia is also reported in patients subsequently insulin-dependent. The observation that some patients have antibodies to insulin at diagnosis may explain some of these cases. Antibodies can bind and release insulin and the time of release may be inappropriate for the blood glucose level. Other cases of antibodies responsible for spontaneous hypoglycaemia are reported but the numbers are few (Hirata, 1977).

OVER-TREATMENT WITH INSULIN

The powerful stimulus provided by hypoglycaemia to rebound hyperglycemia and ketonaemia can mislead the physician into further increases of insulin dosage. The features of this syndrome were emphasized by Somogyi (1959). The situation can cause considerable confusion and is poorly defined. It is discussed further in Chapter 9.

CARDIOVASCULAR DISEASE

There were a number of case reports in the literature of the early 1930s to suggest that hypoglycaemia in diabetic patients with coronary artery disease may precipitate attacks of angina or even coronary thrombosis. Clinical experience has not supported these early claims and although hypoglycaemia in those with coronary artery disease is best avoided it does not often precipitate serious cardiac ischaemia. There is a suggestion that hypoglycaemia in suitably compromised patients may precipitate cardiac arrhythmias.

NEUROPATHY AS THE RESULT OF HYPOGLYCAEMIA

As well as permanent cerebral damage it has been found that prolonged hypoglycaemia is sometimes a cause of peripheral neuropathy, which was described by Williams (1955). The cases were all patients with insulinomas and the characteristic findings were weakness and wasting of distal muscles, particularly the hands, sometimes with paraesthesiae. Similar events were reported following insulin coma therapy. Acute exacerbation of peripheral neuropathy may follow instigation of good control in insulin-dependent diabetic patients without overt hypoglycaemia.

ATTEMPTED SUICIDE WITH INSULIN

Given the power to manipulate insulin and the numerous reports of manipulation to produce recurrent ketoacidosis or instability of control, attempted suicide with insulin is uncommon and successful suicide even rarer. In a successful event, however, the diagnosis may be difficult to substantiate, compounded by post-mortem glucose metabolism. It is possible that suicide by injection is unpopular or that the apparent certainty of death as viewed by the patient discourages attempts. We have reported attempted suicide in six patients from our own clinic (Hale *et al.*, 1985),

setting a lower limit of 100 units administered as the marker of a serious attempt. All patients made a complete recovery without permanent cerebral damage, even when the dose taken exceeded 500 units.

The biochemical management poses special problems but they do not warrant the panic which is the occasional reaction. Of course, the dose is never known with certainty even if an amount is offered by a conscious patient, but above a certain level the amount taken is largely irrelevant. Hepatic glucose production is maximally inhibited by circulating insulin concentrations of 100 mU/l, which are reached after a subcutaneous injection of 100 units of quick-acting insulin. Further reduction of blood glucose then depends upon stimulation of peripheral disposal. The maximal effect of insulin is produced when only 15% of receptors are occupied by insulin. Thus a dose–response relationship only comes into play up to a maximally effective dose. Studies during glucose clamping illustrate this phenomenon. With circulating insulin concentrations of 400 mU/l or 1200 mU/l there were no differences between glucose infusion rates to maintain normoglycaemia (De Fronzo *et al*, 1983). Despite the massive increase in insulin concentration, 0.06 mmol/kg/min glucose (10.5 mg/kg/min) was sufficient to maintain normoglycaemia. Thus in a 70 kg man, 42 g glucose per hour, i.e. 1 litre of 5% glucose, will maintain normoglycaemia. At a circulating concentration of 100 mU/l, glucose uptake is approximately 50% maximal equivalent to an infusion of 21 g/h (500 ml 5% dextrose).

The half-life of circulating insulin is 5 min and after complete absorption a concentration of 10 000 mU/l will fall to 100 mU/l in 35 mins. Obviously this decay curve is influenced by continuing absorption, especially when long-acting insulin is used, but on such occasions circulating insulin levels will be lower in addition to persistent. In the light of these considerations we recommend that after an initial bolus of glucose a 5% glucose infusion is used. The rate and duration will depend upon the type of insulin used and the feedback from blood glucose monitoring but maximum rates are predictable. Stronger glucose solutions may be reserved for patients in whom the amount of fluid is a consideration. I doubt whether excision of the injection site (Campbell and Ratcliffe, 1982) is ever justified.

LEGAL IMPLICATIONS OF HYPOGLYCAEMIA

Hypoglycaemia and the law make for uneasy bedfellows in a number of areas. At one extreme is the episode of severe prolonged hypoglycaemia described above. Such patients invariably end up on intensive therapy units with life or perhaps more accurately vital functions maintained by machinery. The difficulties of predicting recovery have been alluded to and gradual recovery to normal consciousness may occur over a time period of 1 week. Clearly, therefore, vital functions may have to be maintained in the early phase of recovery. Difficulties arise, however, when no recovery is apparent at this time yet respiration can be maintained almost indefinitely. Every series of patients in a persistent vegetative state contains some in which hypoglycaemia was the underlying cause (Jennett and Dyer, 1991). In the United States the courts have been involved in similar cases in deciding who can take a decision and what that decision should be. In the United Kingdom, the confused position is well set out by Jennett and Dyer (1991) and summarized by their phrase 'leaving doctors and families in a legal vacuum'.

Of greater concern to the majority of patients and doctors is the position regarding insulin-dependent diabetics driving. Does the risk of hypoglycaemia lead to a greater number of road traffic accidents? In a 5-year retrospective study comparing drivers who were insulin-dependent with non-diabetic drivers Stevens *et al.* (1989) recorded

accident rates of 23% and 25% respectively. Songer *et al.* (1988) performed a case-control study of 127 insulin-dependent diabetic patients and 127 non-diabetic siblings in Pittsburgh. They found no overall increase in accidents in diabetic drivers although the association of being female and diabetic did lead to a significantly greater number of accidents than being a female non-diabetic. This study was conducted by questionnaire, with no account of accident type or severity. Other studies have found different problems in design, with both increased and decreased frequency of traffic incidents reported in the diabetic population.

It is clear, however, that occasional road traffic accidents occur when the driver was hypoglycaemic. The specific charge brought by the police can vary according to circumstances although I am unimpressed by some recent attempts I have encountered to make the charge 'driving while under the influence of drugs' (i.e. insulin).

Hypoglycaemia may be an attempted defence by a patient against criminal or civil charges. This is a most difficult area where there often seem to be discrepancies between the letter of the law and a successful defence. Physicians have considerable difficulties in assessing a defence and one can predict with some certainty that any expert evidence will be challenged by the argument that since you were not present you cannot speak with certainty of the diagnosis. Since it is likely that all the professionals in court were elsewhere at the time it is relatively easy to subdue the irritation of the challenge. The major error that can be made is to adopt the approach that the behaviour at the time of the incident was so bizarre that the patient must have been hypoglycaemic. This attitude has to be rejected. After all the majority of thefts, wife- or husband-beatings and road-traffic accidents occur with people who are normoglycaemic. The alleged behaviour must always be viewed in the context of the patient's more normal self and it is a sensible precaution when invited to attend as an expert witness to seek interviews with others who know the patient well in addition to the accused.

Central to the use of hypoglycaemia as a defence is the concept of automatism, referred to by one of our law lords as a 'quagmire of the law seldom entered save by those in desperate need of some kind of defence'. While this is perhaps unfair to diabetic patients it sets the scene rather nicely. An automatism is an act carried out in an altered state of consciousness during which consciousness, volition and memory are impaired, although muscle tone, posture and automatic movements remain intact (Fenton, 1972). This medical definition may be interpreted as covering hypoglycaemia, and complex manoeuvres can be carried out while hypoglycaemic. I have heard of a man who drove his car for more than 5 miles while hypoglycaemic with ultimately tragic consequences. Even without blood glucose measurement there can be little doubt that he was hypoglycaemic for some time preceding the final accident, from the reports of eye witnesses.

The definition of automatism in legal terms is somewhat different to the medical definition. The law recognizes sane and insane automatisms and in both the act occurs unconsciously while the mind is absent. The law recognizes that cerebral tumours or atherosclerosis are internal causes creating insane automatisms. Hypoglycaemia from injected insulin lies within the extrinsic causes as sane automatisms. An anomalous situation exists, therefore, whereby hypoglycaemia resulting from an insulinoma is an insane automatism while if the cause is injected insulin it is a sane automatism.

The doctrine of *mens rea* (the guilty mind) is central to English law: not only to have committed the act but to have done so willingly. Thus if the act occurred during an automatism then the defence must prevail. The expert witness, therefore, has considerable power in this situation and an even greater responsibility to exercise that power.

There are times when such power is unwelcome, being unmatched by the certainty or otherwise of the opinion. There have been calls for revision of the law and in particular the division into sane and insane automatism (Fenwick, 1986). The major anomaly is the view that insane automatism is likely to recur while sane automatism is not. Clearly, the latter is not the case in insulin-dependent diabetic patients. Currently diabetic patients enjoy this distinction and indeed would find it difficult otherwise to lead normal lives.

REFERENCES

Allen, O. P. (1953) Symptoms suggesting prodromal stage of diabetes mellitus. *Ohio State Med. J.*, **49**, 213–215.

Amiel, S. A., Sherwin, R. S., Simonson, D. C. and Tamborlane, W. V. (1988) Effect of intensive insulin therapy on glycemic thresholds for counterregulatory hormone release. *Diabetes*, **37**, 901–907.

Amiel, S. A., Pottinger, R. C., Archibald, H. R. *et al.* (1991) Effect of antecedent glucose control on cerebral function during hypoglycemia. *Diabetes Care*, **14**, 109–118.

Banting, F. G., Campbell, W. R. and Fletcher, A. A. (1923) Further clinical experience with insulin (pancreatic extracts) in the treatment of diabetes mellitus. *Br. Med. J.*, **1**, 8–12.

Berger, W. G. and Althaus, B. U. (1987) Reduced awareness of hypoglycemia after changing from porcine to human insulin in IDDM. *Diabetes Care*, **10**, 260–261.

Berger, W., Keller, U., Honegger, B. and Jaeggi, E. (1989) Warning symptoms of hypoglycaemia during treatment with human and porcine insulin in diabetes mellitus. *Lancet*, **i**, 1041–1044.

Biggers, D. W., Myers, S. R., Neal, D. *et al.* (1989) Role of brain in counterregulation of insulin-induced hypoglycemia in dogs. *Diabetes*, **38**, 7–16.

Boyle, P. J., Nagy, R. J., O'Connor, A. M. *et al* (1994) Adaptation in brain glucose uptake following recurrent hypoglycemia. *Proc. Nat. Acad. Sci. USA*, **91**, 9352–9356.

Campbell, W. R. and Macleod, J. J. R. (1924) Insulin. *Medicine*, **3**, 195–308.

Campbell, I. W. and Ratcliffe, J. G. (1982) Suicidal insulin overdose managed by excision of insulin injection site. *Br. Med. J.*, **285**, 408–409.

Collip, J. B. (1923) The occurrence of ketone bodies in the urine of normal rabbits in a condition of hypoglycemia following the administration of insulin – a condition of acute acidosis experimentally produced. *J. Biol. Chem.*, **55** (suppl), 38–39.

Cranston, I., Lomas, J., Maran, A. *et al.* (1994) Restoration of hypoglycaemia unawareness in patients with long-duration insulin-dependent diabetes. Lancet, **344**, 283–287.

DCCT Research Group (1987) Diabetes Control and Complications Trial (DCCT): results of feasibility study. *Diabetes Care*, **10**, 1–9.

DCCT Research Group (1991) Epidemiology of severe hypoglycemia in the Diabetes Control and Complications Trial. *Am. J. Med.*, **90**, 450–459.

Deckert, T., Poulsen, J. E. and Larsen, M. (1978) Prognosis of diabetics with diabetes onset before the age of thirty-one. *Diabetologia*, **14**, 363–370.

De Fronzo, R. A., Ferrannini, E., Hendler, R. *et al.* (1983) Regulation of splanchnic and peripheral glucose uptake by insulin and hyperglycemia in man. *Diabetes*, **32**, 35–45.

Egger, M., Davey Smith, G., Teuscher, A. U. and Teuscher, A. (1991) Influence of human insulin on symptoms and awareness of hypoglycaemia: a randomised double blind crossover trial. *Br. Med. J.*, **303**, 622–626.

Fanelli, C., Pampanelli, S., Epifano, L. *et al.* (1994) Long-term recovery from unawareness, deficient counterregulation and lack of cognitive dysfunction during hypoglycaemia, following institution of rational, intensive insulin therapy in IDDM. *Diabetologia*, **37**, 1265–1276.

Fenton, G. W. (1972) Epilepsy and automatism. *Br. J. Hosp. Med.*, **7**, 57–64.

Fenwick, P. B. C. (1986) Automatism and the law. *Br. J. Hosp. Med.*, **36**, 397.

Gale, E. A. M. and Tattersall, R. B. (1979) Unrecognized nocturnal hypoglycaemia in insulin-treated diabetes. *Lancet*, **i**, 1049–1052.

Hale, P. J., FitzGerald, M. G., Wright, A. D. and Nattrass, M. (1985) Attempted suicide by insulin administration. *Pract. Diabetes*, **2(1)**, 42–44.

Harris, S. (1924) Hyperinsulinism and dysinsulinism. *J. A. M. A.*, **83**, 729–733.

Heller, S. R. and Cryer, P. E. (1991) Reduced neuroendocrine and symptomatic responses to subsequent hypoglycemia after 1 episode of hypoglycemia in nondiabetic humans. *Diabetes*, **40**, 223–226.

Hepburn, D. A., Patrick, A. W., Eadington, D. W. *et al.* (1990) Unawareness of hypoglycaemia in insulin-treated diabetic patients: prevalence and relationship to autonomic neuropathy. *Diabetic Med.*, **7**, 711–717.

Hirata, Y. (1977) Spontaneous insulin antibodies and hypoglycaemia, in *Diabetes. Proceedings of the IX Congress of the International Diabetes Federation*, (ed. J. S. Bajaj), Excerpta Medica, Amsterdam, pp. 278–284.

Jennett, B. and Dyer, C. (1991) Persistent vegetative state and the right to die: the United States and Britain. *Br. Med. J.*, **302**, 1256–1258.

Joslin, E. P. (1921) Practical lessons for physicians and patients in diabetes. *Med. Clin. N. Am.*, **4**, 1723–1732.

Joslin, E. P., Root, H. F., White, P. *et al.* (1946) *The Treatment of Diabetes Mellitus*, 8th edn, Lea & Febiger, Philadelphia, PA, p. 388.

Kilvert, J. A. (1987) MD thesis, University of London.

Lager, I., Attvall, S., Blohme, G. and Smith, U. (1986) Altered recognition of hypoglycaemic symptoms in Type I diabetes during intensified control with continuous subcutaneous insulin infusion. *Diabetic Med.*, **3**, 322–325.

Lawrence, R. D. (1941) Insulin hypoglycaemia. Changes in nervous manifestations. *Lancet*, **ii**, 602.

Lawrence, R. D., Meyer, A. and Nevin, S. (1942) The pathological changes in the brain in fatal hypoglycaemia. *Q. J. Med.*, **35**, 181–201.

Lloyd, J. K. (1964) Diabetes mellitus presenting as spontaneous hypoglycaemia in childhood. *Proc. Roy. Soc. Med.*, **57**, 1061–1063.

McPherson, H. T., Werk, E. E., Myers, J. D. and Engel, F. L. (1958) Studies on ketone metabolism in man. II. The effect of glucose, insulin, cortisone and hypoglycemia on splanchnic ketone production. *J. Clin. Invest.*, **37**, 1379–1393.

Malins, J. M. (1968) *Clinical Diabetes Mellitus*, Eyre & Spottiswoode, London, p. 439.

Mann, F. C. and Magath, T. B. (1921) The liver as a regulator of the glucose concentration of the blood. *Am. J. Physiol.*, **55**, 285–286.

Mitrakou, A., Ryan, C., Venemen, T. *et al.* (1991) Hierarchy of glycemic thresholds for counterregulatory hormone secretion, symptoms and cerebral dysfunction. *Am. J. Physiol.*, **260**, E67–E74.

Nellemann Jorgensen, L., Dejgaard, A. and Pramming, S. K. (1994) Human insulin and hypoglycaemia: a literature survey. *Diabetic Med.*, **11**, 925–934.

Owen, O. E., Morgan, A. P., Kemp, H. G. *et al.* (1967) Brain metabolism during fasting. *J. Clin. Invest.*, **46**, 1589–1595.

Porges, O. (1910) Ueber Hypoglykämie bie Morbus Addison, sowie bei nebennieren-lösen Hunden. *Z. Klin. Med.*, **69**, 341–349.

Pramming, S., Thorsteinsson, B., Bendtson, I. and Binder, C. (1991) Symptomatic hypoglycaemia in 411 type 1 diabetic patients. *Diabetic Med.*, **8**, 217–222.

Report of a Working Party appointed by the College of General Practitioners (1963) Glucose tolerance and glycosuria in the general population. *Br. Med. J.*, **2**, 655–659.

Ryder, R. E. J., Owens, D. R., Hayes, T. M. *et al.* (1990) Unawareness of hypoglycaemia and inadequate hypoglycaemic counterregulation: no causal relation with diabetic autonomic neuropathy. *Br. Med. J.*, **301**, 783–787.

Schwartz, N. S., Clutter, W. E., Shah, S. D. and Cryer, P. E. (1987) Glycemic thresholds for activation of glucose counterregulatory systems are higher than the threshold for symptoms. *J. Clin. Invest.*, **79**, 777–781.

Seltzer, H. S., Fajans, S. S. and Conn, J. W. (1956) Spontaneous hypoglycemia as an early manifestation of diabetes mellitus. *Diabetes*, **5**, 437–442.

Somogyi, M. (1959) Exacerbation of diabetes by excess insulin action. *Am. J. Med.*, **26**, 169–191.

Songer, T. U., LaPorte, R. E. & Dorman, J. S. *et al.* (1988) Motor vehicle accidents and IDDM. *Diabetes Care*, **11**, 701–707.

Stevens, A. B., Roberts, M., McKane, R. *et al.* (1989) Motor vehicle driving among diabetics taking insulin and non-diabetics. *Br. Med. J.*, **299**, 591–595.

Teuscher, A. and Berger, W. G. (1987) Hypoglycaemia unawareness in diabetics transferred from beef/porcine insulin to human insulin. *Lancet*, **ii**, 382–385.

Towler, D. A., Havlin, C. E. Craft, S. and Cryer, P. (1993) Mechanism of awareness of hypoglycemia. *Diabetes*, **42**, 1791–1798.

Tunbridge, W. M. G. (1981) Factors contributing to deaths of diabetics under fifty years of age. *Lancet*, **ii**, 569–572.

Veneman, T., Mitrakou, A., Mokan, M. *et al.* (1993) Induction of hypoglycemia unawareness by asymptomatic nocturnal hypoglycemia. *Diabetes*, **42**, 1233–1237.

Wilder, R. M., Allan, F. N., Power, M. H. and Robertson, H. E. (1927) Carcinoma of the islands of the pancreas. *J.A.M.A.*, **89**, 348–355.

Williams, C. J. (1955) Amyotrophy due to hypoglycaemia. *Br. Med. J.*, **1**, 707–708.

DIABETES AND PREGNANCY

It is often said that pregnancy in the diabetic woman was rare before the introduction of insulin. No doubt women with severe diabetes rarely became pregnant but the incipient mild diabetes, especially affecting obese women during pregnancy and making up nearly one-quarter of all cases referred to our antenatal clinic, must have been common enough in those days. A woman with diabetic symptoms and a sweet-tasting urine which recurred in three successive pregnancies was described by Bennewitz in 1828; one of the infants was large and died at birth.

The prevalent view in the 19th century was summarized by Blott (Peel, 1972): that true diabetes was inconsistent with conception. This view was challenged by Duncan (1882), who reported 22 pregnancies in 15 women with the loss of nine babies and concluded that diabetes may develop during pregnancy and cease with the termination of pregnancy, recurring some time afterwards; that hydramnios is common; that pregnancy is very liable to be interrupted by the death of the fetus; and that the dead child is often enormous.

Williams (1909) collected 66 cases from prior to 1909, reporting one-eighth of the pregnancies ending in abortion and one-third in stillbirth. Maternal mortality was high, with 27% of mothers dying at labour or post-partum and a further 22% dying within 2 years. Similarly daunting figures were reported by DeLee (1920), who wrote that sterility was common but that, when it did occur, the pregnancy ended in abortion or premature labour in one-third and when it went to term the infant often died at or soon after birth. The overall perinatal mortality he calculated

at two-thirds. Maternal mortality was also high with about one-third of mothers dying in diabetic ketoacidosis.

The introduction of insulin therapy brought about a dramatic reduction in maternal mortality but had less immediate impact upon perinatal mortality, which has declined more gradually.

METABOLIC CHANGES IN NORMAL PREGNANCY

Fasting blood glucose concentrations decrease with normal pregnancy. The lowest levels are reached by about 12 weeks of gestation and stay at this value throughout the remainder of pregnancy. In contrast there is a small increase in fasting insulin levels, which is mainly restricted to the third trimester. After oral glucose or mixed meals blood glucose concentration is higher in pregnancy than in the non-pregnant state and there is an increased insulin response.

Basal levels of serum circulating amino acids are reduced in pregnancy and there is also a reduced response to a mixed meal. Freinkel and Metzger (1972) showed that when pregnant and non-pregnant women were fasted blood levels of amino acids fell more rapidly in the pregnant women. Alanine fell by 63% in 24 hours while in non-pregnant women the fall was only 41% by 48 hours. This heightened state of nitrogen conservation they termed 'accelerated starvation' and concluded that the fasting fall in blood glucose in pregnancy could result from a diminution of gluconeogenic substrate supply.

The changes in female metabolism during pregnancy are mediated through changes in the hormonal milieu. In addition to alterations in circulating insulin, glucagon suppressibility by glucose is enhanced in the third trimester. Serum progesterone increases gradually from luteal phase levels throughout pregnancy, as does oestradiol and prolactin. Human placental lactogen (HPL) increases throughout pregnancy while human chorionic gonadotrophin achieves a peak at 10 weeks gestation and shows only small variations thereafter. Progesterone raises fasting levels of insulin and enhances the insulin response to meals without lowering blood glucose levels while oestrogens increase insulin responses and lower glucose. HPL impairs glucose tolerance.

METABOLIC CHANGES IN DIABETIC PREGNANCY

Many authors have looked for differences in circulating hormones between diabetic and non-diabetic pregnant women. For the hormones of pregnancy it is surprising that so many differences have been sought and claimed. Most agree that prolactin is not different but higher values in diabetic pregnancy for oestrogens, progesterone, chorionic gonadotrophin and HPL are claimed. Progesterone is higher in late pregnancy, oestradiol in the second and third trimesters, chorionic gonadotrophin higher and HPL higher throughout or in late pregnancy.

The differences between levels in diabetic and non-diabetic pregnant women, while statistically significant, are likely to be only marginally biologically significant, as shown by the fact that the mean value for groups of diabetic patients lie well within the normal range. The difficulty the diabetic woman has in altering insulin secretion (or administration) during these major hormonal changes is likely to be the primary cause of the differences in metabolism between pregnant and non-pregnant. In other words, the severity of the patient's diabetes will, in a major way, or at least in part, determine the metabolic

change that occurs. It is probably true to say that this has not been considered sufficiently in many published studies. The result, of course, is contradictory and often confusing findings in the literature.

GLYCOSURIA IN PREGNANCY

Glycosuria increases during pregnancy. This has been confirmed with newer test methods specific for glucose and it is not an erroneous finding based upon non-specific tests for reducing substances. In nearly all women glucose excretion doubles and is much more in nearly half the population of normal women. Even in high excretors (>3 g/day) there is only a poor correlation with meals and the appearance of glucose may be episodic. The excretion of glucose reflects the change that occurs in the glomerular filtration rate, which increases by one-third to one-half in normal pregnancy. The maximal rate of re-absorption of glucose by the renal tubules however, does not increase from about 1.7 mmol/min (300 mg/min), resulting in urinary loss.

While the finding of glycosuria in pregnancy is common it should not be ignored. Fine (1967) examined the urine of 700 normal subjects with a glucose–oxidase test. Two populations were suggested. The largest, 91% of patients, showed a gaussian distribution, with a range of 0.06–0.83 mmol/l (1–15 mg/dl). The remaining 9% excreted quantities ranging from 0.83–170 mmol/l (15 mg–3 gm/dl). He went on to test 1000 urines from pregnant women. A greater proportion of pregnant women (4.9%) had less than 0.06 mmol/l (1 mg/dl) glucose, 46% had 0.11–0.5 mmol/l (2–9 mg/dl) and 26% had greater than 0.83 mmol/l (15 mg/dl).

Glycosuria of pregnancy is often noted to disappear with delivery. This reflects reports from the era of low-sensitivity, non-specific urine testing. As Fine (1967) has shown, a significant proportion of the normal population has glycosuria detectable by sensitive specific methods. Thus the concept of glycosuria of pregnancy is one based upon the sensitivity of the particular test which is used, and has little meaning. Sensitive specific methods only serve to reduce the threshold at which glycosuria becomes apparent.

THE SIGNIFICANCE OF GLYCOSURIA

Abnormal glucose tolerance tests have been recorded in as many as 80% of pregnant women. Such high figures are dependent upon criteria of normality at the time of the investigation and the commonest abnormality in the past has been a 2-hour blood glucose exceeding 6.7 mmol/l (120 mg/dl). This may well reflect an alteration in absorption of glucose, since the intravenous glucose tolerance test is normal in these cases and the coefficient of glucose assimilation is usually enhanced in pregnant women.

A more realistic estimate of the prevalence of abnormal glucose tolerance in pregnancy is that of O'Sullivan (1961), who applied stringent diagnostic criteria to the standard glucose tolerance test and studied a large population. He calculated that abnormal glucose tolerance tests would be found in 1 in 116 (0.86%) of pregnant women. In the Birmingham survey (Report of a Working Party appointed by College of General Practitioners, 1962), using similar criteria, the prevalence of abnormal glucose tolerance in 2647 women aged 20–39 was calculated to be 1 in 529 (0.19%). Allowing for possible differences between the populations studied it seems that there is a significant increase in abnormal glucose tolerance in pregnancy.

Fine (1967) performed glucose tolerance tests in 374 pregnant women with glycosuria. Most of the women had normal glucose tolerance with glycosuria (94%); 5% had a high peak value (> 10 mmol/l; 180 mg/dl) but a normal 2-hour value and 1% had diabetes.

Thus, since glycosuria is common during pregnancy but diabetes uncommon, it is probably best interpreted as a physiological finding. The high proportion of women detected show a tiny incidence of diabetes and this has led to the suggestion that glycosuria alone is a poor indication for further investigation and even if systematically investigated has a relatively low yield.

Current practice still favours investigation of glycosuria although if there are no symptoms and no history of unexplained fetal loss, a large baby, or diabetes in the family, a single blood glucose 1–2 hours after a meal is sufficient. Where these points in the history are positive a glucose tolerance test is performed.

SCREENING FOR DIABETES IN PREGNANCY

The illogicality of screening by testing the urine in pregnancy allied to the development of rapid bedside tests for blood glucose surely points to all pregnant women having blood glucose measured as is done for haemoglobin.

A number of solutions have been put forward to detect diabetes in pregnancy. The glucose tolerance test will remain the confirmatory test, unless frank diabetes is present, but what is needed is a screening test that indicates a high probability of diabetes. As in any screening test, it should have a good pick-up rate, or conversely it should miss only a tiny proportion of women with diabetes, and it should also generate a good proportion of positive confirmed cases.

First to be considered are clinical risk factors. The major ones are listed in Table 12.1. An

Table 12.1 Clinical risk factors for diabetes in pregnancy

1. Family history of diabetes in first-degree relative
2. Prepregnancy obesity (> 20% above ideal body weight)
3. Previous baby weighing > 4.5 kg at birth

Table 12.2 Additional risk factors for diabetes in pregnancy

1. Previous baby weighing < 2.5 kg at birth with no known cause
2. Previous obstetric history of pre-eclampsia, hydramnios, unexplained stillbirth, repeated spontaneous abortion

appreciable problem with clinical risk factors is the frequency with which they occur in the non-diabetic population. Approximately one-third of women from an indigenous population which was unselected had one risk factor. In other words there is a high occurrence rate which, when put to the oral glucose tolerance test, does not give an overly large confirmation rate.

Additional risk factors (Table 12.2) have been suggested by some authors but it is likely that they indicate diabetes only when one of the primary factors (Table 12.1) is present.

Fasting or postprandial blood glucose concentration has been suggested as an initial screening test. This sort of investigation is highly dependent upon the definition of diabetes, which has been modified in recent years. Previous rates of pick-up should be considered in the light of the temporal criteria.

For reasons outlined above the fasting blood glucose measurement is unlikely to be a useful screening test in pregnancy. Compared with the non-pregnant state there is a fall in fasting glucose. It should be pointed out that criteria for abnormality, either fasting or 2 hours post-glucose, as laid down by the WHO, make no allowance for change in pregnancy and they may therefore be of doubtful application. O'Sullivan (1984) found that 2% of patients had a fasting blood glucose > 5.0 mmol/l (90 mg/dl), which does not suggest that, with the inconvenience of measuring fasting blood, such a test would be a useful screen for diabetes.

Postprandial blood glucose measurement is highly dependent upon time from the last meal unless used in a structured way. In a group of 1500 pregnant women without signs or symptoms of diabetes, nearly 7000 blood glucose measurements gave a mean of 4.6 mmol/l (83 mg/dl) and a 95% confidence limit of 6.3 mmol/l (113 mg/dl). An abnormal value was found in 11.6% of patients. Of these 5.7% had an abnormal glucose tolerance test (Stangenberg, Persson and Nordlanden, 1985). As with many similar studies, glucose tolerance tests were not performed on the initial negatively screened patients and the proportion of missed patients is not known. Lind and Anderson (1984) found 1.4% of pregnant women with an abnormal postprandial blood glucose. Of the original population of 2400 patients, two had diabetes and four impaired glucose tolerance. This low detection rate of abnormal glucose tolerance is partly a result of the criteria used but may also reflect the fact that glucose tolerance tests were performed in only a very few of the screened population (less than 2%). Thus there seems a distinct possibility that either fasting blood glucose or 2-hour postprandial blood glucose leaves a significant proportion of patients with diabetes undetected.

Few studies can rival those of O'Sullivan. High levels of sequential recruitment, systematic and painstaking investigation and adequate follow-up have all combined to produce the best-founded and most applicable data. Using the rather non-specific Somogyi–Nelson method for measurement of blood glucose the screening level has been set at 7.2 mmol/l (130 mg/dl). This would translate to a lower value using the more specific glucose–oxidase or hexokinase methods for glucose measurement.

A considerable literature has built upon the use of glycated proteins in the diagnosis of diabetes. In general terms (Chapter 5) these tests function poorly in detecting anything other than frank diabetes and their use in pregnancy is almost certainly inappropriate.

Table 12.3 Diagnostic criteria for diabetes in pregnancy

			Blood glucose mmol/l			
Author	*Glucose load*	*Sample*	*Fasting*	*1 h*	*2 h*	*3 h*
Malins, 1968	50 g	Plasma	6.1	10.0	6.7	–
O'Sullivan and Mahan, 1964	100 g	Blood	5.0	9.2	8.1	6.9
Abell and Beischer, 1975	100 g	Capillary plasma	5.2	9.2	7.1	5.9
Hatem *et al.*, 1988	(a) 75 g	Plasma	4.9	8.8	7.5	
	(b) 75 g	Plasma	4.9	11.0	9.6	
WHO, 1985	75 g	Blood	⩾ 6.7	–	⩾ 10.0	
	75 g	Plasma	⩾ 7.8	–	⩾ 11.1	

(a) Second trimester; (b) third trimester.

CRITERIA FOR AN ABNORMAL GLUCOSE TOLERANCE TEST

It is interesting to compare the criteria for abnormality of the glucose tolerance test in pregnancy 20 years ago with today's recommendations (Table 12.3). Current recommendations, using venous whole blood, are fasting glucose equal to or greater than 6.7 mmol/l (120 mg/dl) and 2-hour equal to, or greater than 10 mmol/l (180 mg/dl) (WHO, 1985).

These criteria should have reduced the incidence of gestational diabetes. If so, this may be correct and some patients may have been unnecessarily labelled gestational diabetic. Not totally in keeping with this view is that when O'Sullivan *et al.* (1973), applying their stricter interpretation, identified 187 pregnancies with an abnormal glucose tolerance test, they found a fourfold increase in perinatal mortality. Furthermore, women identified in this way were followed up 16 years later when 60% had abnormal glucose tolerance (O'Sullivan, 1975).

Timing of testing is important since the glucose tolerance test may be abnormal in the second and third trimester when it was normal in the first and unless diagnosed during the pregnancy there is little chance of post-partum diagnosis. O'Sullivan (1961) found that 93% of 146 women with abnormal tests during pregnancy reverted to normal glucose tolerance within 6 months of delivery.

THE DIABETIC MOTHER

The specific risks of pregnancy in diabetic mothers arise from difficulty in controlling the diabetes and from the effects of pregnancy upon diabetic complications. The principles of diabetic management are the same as for any other time in her career, with the added advantage for the physician that careful explanation of the need for good control almost inevitably ensures cooperation to a limitless degree. It is valuable to be as sure as we are of the impact of control upon outcome, and this has exceeded our certainty of more long-term effects of control until recently.

The change in insulin requirement as pregnancy advances increases the chances of poor control and even diabetic ketoacidosis. The latter is relatively rare in current practice, with a sharp reduction in incidence from 20 years ago. This is likely to be a consequence of closer supervision of the mother, with the drive for greater control. Hyperemesis increases instability and electrolyte and water loss increase the risk of diabetic ketoacidosis.

The need for tight control of blood glucose with much manipulation of insulin dose increases the risk of hypoglycaemia. Occasionally, profound and irreversible hypoglycaemic coma occurs for reasons that do not seem entirely adequate in terms of insulin taken and deficiency of food intake. There is no definite evidence that hypoglycaemia is harmful to the fetus in the early weeks of pregnancy. A teratogenic effect has been suspected but a history of hypoglycaemia is no more common in pregnancies that result in congenital defects than in those that do not. This is in contrast to ketoacidosis occurring during pregnancy, when the fetal loss rate is said to be 50%.

It has already been noted that diabetes may appear during pregnancy and disappear entirely after delivery, so that it is not surprising that pregnancy usually aggravates diabetes that is already manifest. Nevertheless, the insulin dosage is unchanged or even lowered in about one-quarter of the patients throughout the pregnancy. These changes have no clear relation to the chance of survival of the fetus except in so far as they influence the degree of control of the diabetes. During the first trimester the need for insulin is often slightly reduced and there is a tendency to hypoglycaemia due to the nausea and vomiting which interfere with the dietary intake. When the need for insulin increases it does so usually at two periods in the pregnancy – about the 15th and about the 29th week – although there is often a continuous rise between these points. From the 30th week until delivery the dose tends to be constant, but after delivery the insulin requirement falls immediately to the prepregnancy level; in fact so rapidly that the insulin prescription on the day of delivery has to be calculated with this in mind. The use of oestrogens to suppress lactation increases the need for insulin quite significantly but only while the treatment is being given. There is certainly a higher fetal loss in pregnancy if it is associated with a big increase in insulin dosage than if there is no such rise, but it is impossible to say whether this is merely due to the difficulty of achieving good control of the diabetes when the insulin prescription is being changed at frequent intervals. In 235 consecutive patients treated with insulin throughout pregnancy we found there were 67 who needed no significant change in

insulin dose and the fetal loss in this group was three (4.5%). A total of 168 patients had to make a substantial increase and they suffered a fetal loss of 28 (16.7%).

MICROVASCULAR COMPLICATIONS

Retinopathy

This is common enough in pregnancy but scrutiny of the eye is likely to be more searching than at other times and the incidence cannot be compared with that in women who are not pregnant without suitable qualification. There is no doubt that the lesions may appear first during pregnancy, that regression or progression of established retinopathy may occur, and that alarming progression may happen, although this is rare. Early reports indicated progression of simple retinopathy in about 20% of patients and of retinitis proliferans in about one-third.

The practice of attempting tight control of blood glucose has influenced changes during pregnancy. Phelps *et al.* (1986) demonstrated progression of retinopathy in those patients with the highest blood glucoses during pregnancy, and in those in whom glucose showed the greatest fall from the prepregnant level. Larinkari *et al.* (1982) observed that women with retinopathy that progressed in pregnancy had higher blood glucose levels in the first, but not the second or third, trimester than women with no progression of their retinopathy. Similarly, this may be interpreted as women with the greatest fall in blood glucose showed progression.

Following delivery changes tend to regress, although intraretinal abnormalities and abnormalities detected by fluorescein angiography remain. Soft exudates developing during pregnancy tend to regress.

Neovascularization at the start of pregnancy is an ominous sign. Almost all progress without treatment and there is a real risk of a major bleed unless photocoagulation is performed. Visual loss from rupture of new vessels does not, of course, clear after pregnancy.

Some guidance can be given from the prepregnant state. If retinopathy is absent at the beginning of pregnancy it may develop during pregnancy in about 10% of women. This is likely to be microaneurysm only. Obviously the risk in any single patient will also relate to the duration of diabetes. If background retinopathy is present at onset of pregnancy the prognosis is only slightly worse for the development of further microaneurysms and haemorrhages. Some progress to proliferative retinopathy (about 5%). When proliferation is present before pregnancy the outlook without treatment is bleak. When retinopathy is quiescent for long periods before pregnancy there is rarely any change.

Photocoagulation should be performed if necessary during pregnancy. Before this treatment was available about one-quarter of women with proliferative retinopathy in pregnancy had significant vitreous haemorrhage. The success of photocoagulation in pregnancy is similar to the non-pregnant results.

Nephropathy

Information upon the course of diabetic nephropathy is largely based on indirect methods of assessment. Proteinuria is the earliest clinical sign and this is scanty or intermittent except in advanced nephropathy. Infections should be absent if proteinuria is to be ascribed to nephropathy. The assumption that most patients with duration of diabetes in excess of 10 years have glomerular capillary damage appears to be borne out by the studies of pregnant women (Kitzmiller *et al.*, 1981; Jovanovich and Jovanovich, 1984). Broadly speaking, women with presumed nephropathy will have had diabetes for 10–14 years (one-quarter), 15–19 years (one-half), 20+ years (one-quarter).

Hypertension in this situation is indicative of advanced disease and the customary relationship of nephropathy and retinopathy

holds. Hypertension and proteinuria may point to more rapid progression of retinopathy in these women. The possibility of anaemia in advanced cases should not be overlooked.

Among diabetic women, those with microalbuminuria before pregnancy have an exaggerated rise in albumin excretion during pregnancy. Both groups return to prepregnant levels within 12 weeks of delivery (Biesenbach *et al.*, 1994). With nephropathy established before conception the progress during pregnancy may be marked. Certainly proteinuria may increase. Proteinuria of 3–6 g/day in the first trimester was found in 12% patients. By the third trimester 35% patients were excreting this amount. In the third trimester 17% excreted > 6 g/day (Kitzmiller *et al.*, 1981; Jovanovich and Jovanovich, 1984). Such losses may lower serum albumin, causing oedema.

Despite these figures it is difficult to argue a deleterious effect of pregnancy on nephropathy. Control populations have been studied less extensively and the rate of deterioration in those who excrete >3 g/day and are not pregnant may be considerable. Current views would support enthusiastic treatment of hypertension and pre-eclampsia for the mother's health.

Neuropathy

By contrast with retinopathy and nephropathy the literature on neuropathy and pregnancy is scanty. Nerve entrapment syndromes may occur, as they can in the non-diabetic population. Cases are recorded of pregnancy in patients with autonomic neuropathy with a successful outcome. Parenteral nutrition may be necessary if upper gastrointestinal symptoms dominate.

Atherosclerosis

The existence of overt coronary artery disease in a young woman planning pregnancy is

Table 12.4   White classification of diabetes in pregnancy (White, 1949)

Class	Age at onset of diabetes	Duration of diabetes	Complications present
A	Age at which pregnant	During pregnancy	None
B	> 20 years	0–9 years	None
C	10–19 years	10–19 years	None
D	< 10 years	> 20 years	Background retinopathy
F	Any	Any	Nephropathy
R	Any	Any	Proliferative retinopathy
H	Any	Any	Macrovascular disease

rare. Anecdotal evidence supports the undesirability of pregnancy.

CLASSIFICATION OF DIABETES IN PREGNANCY

The condition of the diabetic mother on entering pregnancy has a profound influence on the outcome. Thus some logical classification of diabetes in pregnancy is necessary if sound advice is to be given on likely success of a pregnancy and if results between centres are to be compared. Any classification can be quarrelled with but the one which has best stood the test of time is that promulgated by Dr Priscilla White (White, 1949). This is based on the age of onset of diabetes, duration and the presence of complications (Table 12.4).

In general, classes B–R refer to patients with insulin-dependent diabetes and, as would be anticipated, perinatal mortality increases from class B through R. Class A as a specific group of patients works less well. As originally suggested it was to include women in whom the diagnosis of diabetes was made from a glucose tolerance test 'which deviates but slightly from normal'. Such a definition allows an effect from redefinition of diagnostic levels for a glucose tolerance test. More importantly it leads into the difficult area of gestational diabetes. Strictly speaking gestational diabetes is a pregnancy-related diabetes, which remits after delivery. It is thus a retrospective diagnosis. Furthermore the diagnosis of diabetes during pregnancy may not be synonymous with onset of diabetes during pregnancy. We are acutely aware of this in our Asian population, where non-insulin-dependent diabetes may be present before pregnancy but be first diagnosed during pregnancy. This type of diabetes, of course, does not remit after delivery.

Complications and outcome

Undoubtedly the major concern for fetal outcome is the presence of diabetic nephropathy. Results have improved somewhat in recent years. Oppe, Hsia and Gellis (1957) reviewed 83 pregnancies in 41 women with nephropathy, reporting miscarriage in 28, therapeutic abortion in eight, stillbirth in six and neonatal death in 13. More recent evidence on perinatal survival suggests that it is as high as 90%. Pregnancy is reported in women on continuous ambulatory peritoneal dialysis and following transplantation. In the main these have been successful although other complications, particularly vascular disease, should be taken into account.

OBSTETRIC COMPLICATIONS

The pathogenesis of specific obstetric complications in the diabetic mother is difficult to elucidate. Are they a feature of the disease itself or a reflection of inadequate diabetic control? The decreased incidence of many of the complications with closer supervision of the confinement testifies to the major contribution to morbidity of the latter.

Pyelonephritis

It is generally stated that pyelonephritis is commoner in the diabetic than the non-diabetic population although definitive studies are lacking. While there are reasons for doubting this it is certain that when infection occurs it is more severe in the diabetic patient. The overall incidence in diabetic pregnancy has been put at 4–5% and it is associated with an increased perinatal mortality. Suggestions that the presence of complications is likely to be associated with pyelonephritis are not confirmed and nor is the claim of a decreased incidence in recent years. As pyelonephritis is a common finding in normal pregnancy it presents a serious problem in diabetic patients and must contribute to the incidence of premature labour and neonatal death.

Hydramnios

Hydramnios is a common feature of diabetic pregnancy. Minor degrees of this condition are difficult to assess so that it is not surprising to find a reported incidence varying from 3% to 30%. Our recent experience would confirm a figure midway between the two although ascertainment depends upon criteria, the diligence with which these criteria are applied, and the increasing use of ultrasound. The particular make-up of the diabetic population also influences numbers, with an incidence of about 5% in gestational diabetes and nearly 20% in the remainder.

There is no doubt that it is commoner in diabetic women than in non-diabetic women (Lufkin *et al.*, 1984). There is no obvious correlation between incidence and age, duration, severity and control. Minor degrees seem to be quite unimportant but tense hydramnios which may develop acutely is a serious threat to the fetus. It is most often seen from the 29th to the 34th week and is an absolute indication for strict rest and supervision for the remainder of the pregnancy. The cause of hydramnios in diabetes is unknown. There

is no relationship between amniotic fluid volume and glucose concentration. Furthermore of diabetic mothers with hydramnios there is no other aetiological factor except diabetes in about 85% (Lufkin *et al.*, 1984).

The perinatal mortality rate is increased partly as a result of the association of hydramnios and congenital defect and partly from preterm labour. There is just a suggestion that rates of hydramnios are decreasing, although the deficiencies of a historical control period must be acknowledged.

Hypertension

Control studies of the incidence of hypertension in diabetic pregnancy are difficult to perform. The uselessness of measuring blood pressure immediately after a long discussion between doctor and patient on risks, importance of control and likely outcome is readily apparent. Nor can the chronic effects of such a discussion be discounted on repeated visits to the antenatal clinic. Where comparisons have been undertaken hypertension, including chronic and pregnancy-induced, has been found to be two to three times as common in diabetic as in non-diabetic mothers. Within the diabetic population the rates rise from 15% in gestational diabetes to 30% in those with major complications.

MATERNAL MORTALITY

The death in ketosis of seven out of 57 mothers in the Joslin Clinic series from 1898–1922 indicates the risk to the mother at that time. Since insulin became available maternal death-rates are reported to be little above those for non-diabetics. No doubt the greater care bestowed on the diabetic woman throughout pregnancy compensates for the increased risk from diabetic ketosis, hypoglycaemia, renal disease and even coronary atheroma. There is a tendency, however, for published figures to present the situation in the best light since, in the main, only centres with a special interest in the problem collect and publish their data.

Interesting and relatively recent data from the USA indicate that maternal mortality continues to be higher in the diabetic woman than in the non-diabetic. Some of this is preventable but in Class H women it remains high. Gabbe, Mestman and Hibbard (1976) reported deaths from haemorrhage, keto-acidosis, sepsis and hypoglycaemia giving an overall mortality of 115/100 000 – more than 10 times the overall maternal mortality in the US in the mid-70s.

SUBSEQUENT DIABETES

It is of some interest to know the number of gestational diabetic women who subsequently progress to frank diabetes. A number of studies have been directed at this area and there is uniform agreement that the percentage progressing to diabetes is high. O'Sullivan (1984) in 24 years of follow-up found that 75% of gestational diabetics progressed to either frank diabetes or impaired glucose tolerance and persistent obesity was a determining factor in this progression. The actual figure is dependent upon criteria of diagnosis and in view of the strict criteria for blood glucose set by O'Sullivan it may be an underestimate.

In the same study O'Sullivan (1984) produced worrying results for cardiovascular risk factors and morbidity in previous gestational diabetics. He reported a three- to fivefold increase in myocardial infarction and angina compared with control subjects.

THE PLACENTA

Claude Bernard was aware of the important metabolic function of the placenta and suggested it might act as the fetal liver. The early placenta has a marked ability to synthesize glycogen *in vitro* but this activity gradually decreases and is absent at term. Concurrently the ability of the placenta to produce glucose

decreases and the ability of the liver increases.

It is clear that glucose crosses the placenta and that the transfer is via a transport mechanism. It is also clear that there is a system for the proteolytic inactivation of insulin in human placental tissue, which may be similar to the insulinase system in the liver. Studies with ^{131}I-labelled insulin indicate that the placenta contributes a substantial barrier to the free flux of insulin from mother to fetus. It is also apparent that this system works in reverse manner, since injection of large doses of insulin into the blood of fetal rabbits close to term produces no significant fall in the maternal blood glucose.

These observations were employed by Pedersen (Pedersen and Osler, 1961) to explain the increased birth weight of the fetus from a diabetic mother. Raised maternal blood glucose, whether from undiagnosed or inadequately treated diabetes, leads to a raised fetal blood glucose. The rise in fetal blood glucose is checked by increased fetal secretion of insulin. Thus the fetus is hyperglycaemic and hyperinsulinaemic.

The placenta is heavier than normal in diabetic pregnancy as a result of hyperplasia. Pathological changes are non-specific – small infarcts can be found but their frequency seems to be that of the non-diabetic woman. The immunology of the diabetic placenta has been extensively studied with the rather unexciting findings of increased complement and immunoglobulin deposition.

EFFECTS UPON THE FETUS

The weight of the fetus seems to be the same as of normal infants until the 28th week of pregnancy but then often increases more rapidly so that the mean weight at term is 0.22–0.45 kg (8 oz–1 lb) more than that of the fetus of a non-diabetic mother. There is a tendency, as in normal infants, for size to increase slightly with parity of the mother. Long duration and probably greater severity of diabetes are associated with a decrease in birth weight.

The weight gain of the fetus in the first half of gestation owes much to genetic factors and it is only in the second half of pregnancy that the nutritional and hormonal factors come into play.

The belief that a rise in maternal blood glucose provokes excess activity of the fetal islets of Langerhans was derived from the very thorough studies of Osler and Pedersen (1960) and Farquhar (Baird and Farquhar, 1962). The islets of the large babies who die are commonly hyperplastic and the degree of hyperplasia is related to the birth weight. Baird and Farquhar (1962) found a greater tolerance than normal to a glucose load in the newborn infants of diabetic women, suggesting that they were truly oversecreting. Pedersen and Osler (1961) found the blood glucose higher in women who had big babies than in those who had babies of normal weight. This concept has been extended following observations of increased maternal circulating concentrations of other nutrients, non-esterified fatty acids and amino acids. The latter in particular are capable of crossing the placenta and stimulating insulin secretion. In general, animal experiments support the hyperinsulinaemia hypothesis although many of them have been conducted with insulin concentrations of little clinical relevance.

THE COMPOSITION OF THE NEWBORN INFANT

Osler and Pedersen (1960) studied the body composition of 122 newborn infants of diabetic mothers and compared them with 122 controls. The maturity of diabetic infants as judged by ossification and the excretion of water, electrolytes and nitrogen corresponded to their chronological age or less. They were grossly overweight on account of a surplus of fat and to a lesser degree of carbohydrate stores in tissues and organs.

Ultrasound study of the developing infant suggests that growth is accelerated in insulin-sensitive tissues rather than in tissues not sensitive to insulin. The organs principally showing organomegaly are liver, heart and adrenal. It is of some interest that brain does not figure in this list, and indeed tends to be of lesser weight in diabetic infants than in non-diabetic infants. If the hyperglycaemia is the stimulus to hyperinsulinaemia then there is reason to expect that non-insulin-sensitive tissues would share in the organomegaly.

Islet cell hypertrophy and hyperplasia has been a feature in most reports. It is most striking in the largest infants and appears to involve the B cells. Increased insulin content of the fetal pancreas has also been reported.

An alternative explanation for the macrosomia might lie with the insulin-like growth factors. Both IGF-1 and IGF-2 can exert effects qualitatively similar to insulin upon glucose transport, oxidation, glycogen synthesis, amino acid transport and fat oxidation, in addition to effects upon DNA, RNA, and protein synthesis. The effect of insulin upon cell growth, division and differentiation appears to be mediated via different receptors to those for intermediary metabolism. These receptors show a high affinity for insulin-like growth factors and indeed IGF-1 and IGF-2 have a degree of structural homology with insulin. In general insulin interacts weakly with IGF receptors and IGFs react weakly with insulin receptors. The latter has been explored in human pregnancy, with no correlation between maternal or fetal IGF levels and birth weight. A more likely but theoretical consideration would lie with hyperinsulinaemia promoting a growth effect through interaction with IGF receptors.

MANAGEMENT OF DIABETES IN PREGNANCY

GESTATIONAL DIABETES

A precise definition of gestational diabetes remains difficult. Strictly speaking it has to be considered unsatisfactory to define it as the onset or first recognition of diabetes in pregnancy, thus lumping together new diabetes and undiagnosed diabetes. Similarly, gestational diabetes should remit after pregnancy otherwise the patient has fully expressed diabetes.

Not enough attention has been paid to characterization of the different types of diabetes that may be recognized in pregnancy. The classification of White has been extensively used in studies of gestational diabetes. Class A of the White classification was originally chemical diabetes during pregnancy requiring only dietary treatment. Neither of these criteria are particularly useful, chemical diabetes having been relegated to limbo with the redefinition of diabetes and diet-alone therapy being swallowed up in the quest for yet tighter control of blood glucose by introducing insulin.

Some workers have attempted to refine the original Class A to A1 and A2, separating the categories on the basis of fasting blood glucose of 5.8 mmol/l (105 mg/dl) while others have relegated insulin-treated patients to Class B. Such attempts have not received universal acceptance.

With diagnosis achieved some consideration can be given to management. This is based upon the concept that above a certain degree of hyperglycaemia perinatal mortality and morbidity is increased. Quite what this critical hyperglycaemic level is remains in doubt but most centres strive to keep preprandial blood glucose levels of < 5.5 mmol/l (100 mg/dl) and a mean blood glucose level of < 6.7 mmol/l (120 mg/dl). In most large series of gestational diabetics perinatal morbidity is increased even with these aims of control.

Diet is the main agent of therapy and only when this fails is insulin considered. Most of the evidence concerning diet testifies to the importance of calorie intake in determining the degree of hyperglycaemia rather than the amount of carbohydrate, although the type of carbohydrate clearly plays a role in swings

of blood glucose. In pregnancy there is less scope for restriction of calorie intake since weight gain in pregnancy is desirable. This allows scope only for relatively minor alterations in type of intake. Advice follows the outlines agreed for dietary treatment of diabetes.

Some feedback on the success or otherwise of the regimen is necessary. It is no longer sensible to make a case for persisting with urine testing for glucose. Variable alterations in renal threshold within and between pregnancies leave little scope for the precise information that is necessary. If not urine testing, then blood glucose monitoring – leaving the questions how often per day, at what times and how many days per week. As a minimum there should be one day of testing per week with measurements before and 2 hours after two main meals. The 0200 h measurement advocated for patents on insulin is to detect hypoglycaemia and is therefore not necessary in the gestational diabetic treated only by diet.

Interpretation by the physician should consider the likelihood of this being the best day of the week for the patient and thus failure to meet the criteria of control should always cause concern. Failure on consecutive weeks will demand some intensification and this will usually mean insulin therapy. There is a tendency for control to deteriorate around the 15th or 29th week of pregnancy.

Early suggestions of the teratogenicity of sulphonylurea drugs have not been borne out and successful use of sulphonylureas in pregnancy has been reported. The major worry has been fetal islet cell hyperplasia, resulting in neonatal hypoglycaemia, and even proponents of sulphonylureas restrict the dosage used to a low therapeutic level. Metformin has also been used. With the exception of diehard sulphonylurea users, of whom there are few, most people opt for insulin if dietary regimen fails.

Various regimens have been used and there probably is not a right or wrong regimen. Lowering the fasting blood glucose with a nocturnal injection of intermediate-acting insulin may be sufficient to achieve 24-hour control. Twice-daily intermediate-acting insulins with or without a quick-acting insulin would be the choice of many people, although pen-injection devices have largely superseded that regimen. Some people have suggested an initial dose of insulin of 30 units or more, arguing that pregnancy is a time of major insulin resistance. Such haste seems unnecessary and a lower starting dose is preferable. Patients find it difficult to forgive, and a major blow is dealt to their confidence, if hypoglycaemia results from their first insulin injection.

Obstetric monitoring

Gabbe *et al.* (1977) reported 261 gestational diabetic pregnancies with normal fasting blood glucose throughout pregnancy. About one-quarter of these had other risk factors such as previous stillbirth or pre-eclampsia. Only the latter group were monitored antepartum, with daily oestriol measurement and weekly contraction stress tests. In the remainder the perinatal mortality was 19/1000, which is similar to the general population. Based on this it was suggested that this particular group of diabetics did not need special antepartum monitoring unless another risk factor was present or they reached 40 weeks.

With current definitions of diabetes the patient with fasting euglycaemia may have impaired glucose tolerance in pregnancy rather than diabetes and, without other risk factors, need little in the way of specialized treatment or monitoring. Certainly there seems little indication to deliver the infant before term unless other risk factors are present. I suspect that opinion is split on whether a gestational diabetic should be allowed to go over term.

INSULIN-DEPENDENT DIABETES

Most established diabetic women who get pregnant will already be on insulin. For the remaining few they will almost definitely need insulin for the duration of the pregnancy and perhaps thereafter. Only those with impaired glucose tolerance before pregnancy and the few with maturity-onset diabetes of young people stand much chance of negotiating pregnancy on diet only.

There is no doubt that resistance to the action of insulin is a feature of pregnancy and it is to be expected that insulin requirement will rise as pregnancy progresses. Presumably most of the insulin resistance is hormonally mediated and insulin requirement might be expected to be linked with increased hormonal secretory patterns. The most important guide, however, will always be the degree of blood glucose control achieved by a particular dose of insulin. In this respect home monitoring of blood glucose has a crucial role to play. The concept of good metabolic control in pregnancy requires that specific targets of blood glucose levels are set and hopefully achieved. What are these targets to be? The study of Karlsson and Kjellmer (1972) established a relationship between the degree of control and perinatal mortality. An average third trimester blood glucose level of > 8.3 mmol/l (150 mg/dl) was associated with a perinatal mortality of 24% whereas 5.5–8.3 mmol/l (100–150 mg/dl) was associated with a mortality of 15% and < 5.5 mmol/l (100 mg/dl) with 3.8% mortality. Other studies have supported this claim but varied methods of obtaining an average blood glucose level have been used. Karlsson and Kjellmer (1972) used three daily determinations at unspecified times while others have used different combinations of fasting and postprandial measurements.

Some attempt has been made to approach the problem in a more systematic way using 12- or 24-hour profiles with samples at fixed times. Gillmer *et al.* (1975) took hourly samples over 24 hours in insulin-dependent diabetics and in controls. Under optimum conditions they found a mean diurnal blood glucose level of 5.9 mmol/l (106 mg/dl) in the diabetic women compared with 4.7 mmol/l (85 mg/dl) in non-diabetics. During the day-time period the respective values were 6.5 mmol/l (117 mg/dl) and 4.7 mmol/l (85 mg/dl). The average daily value hides important information upon the variation around the mean figure and this was found to be greater in the insulin-dependent diabetics.

Other groups have pursued this approach using intensive home blood glucose monitoring (Jovanovich *et al.*, 1980), continuous subcutaneous insulin therapy (Potter, Reckless and Cullen, 1980; Kitzmiller *et al.*, 1985) and intensified conventional therapy (Coustan *et al.*, 1986). These studies confirm the clinical finding that tight metabolic control is feasible in pregnant diabetics. This is often described as resulting from increased motivation of the mother toward the outcome of her pregnancy, yet even the best-motivated non-pregnant diabetics can rarely achieve such standards of control. Thus with the evidence from perinatal mortality and the general move towards good diabetic control, allied to the demonstrable feasibility of good diabetic control, euglycaemia seems synonymous with the drive towards tight control. This means preprandial blood glucose concentrations of less than 5.5 mmol/l (100 mg/dl) and 2-hour postprandial concentrations of < 6.7 mmol/l (120 mg/dl).

Diet

The recommendations for the diet of pregnant women have progressed from the era of calorie restriction. An optimum weight gain of 0.9–1.8 kg (2–4 lb) in the first trimester followed by 0.25–0.5 kg (0.5–1 lb) per week to term is recommended. Thus the optimum weight gain in pregnancy is 10–13.7 kg (22–30 lb). The average non-diabetic pregnant women will achieve this with a daily calorie intake of around 1800–2300 cal (30–35 cal/kg ideal body weight). Within this framework 50% of the calories are provided by carbohydrate, 15–20% by protein and the remain-

der from fat, with the accepted concentration upon saturated fats (10%) and polyunsaturated fats (10%) and dietary fibre intake.

Insulin treatment

Methods of insulin treatment show a continued advance and all are feasible in pregnancy. Intensified conventional regimens, multiple injections with pen devices and continuous subcutaneous insulin infusion (CSII) have all been used to good effect. The popularity of CSII in the early 1980s has been largely replaced by enthusiasm for multiple injection regimens, to the relief of many who found the technique time-consuming and not widely applicable. Although tried in pregnancy it has never been popular, which may be due to the good results obtained in other, less rigorous and time-consuming, ways.

The aim of insulin treatment in any diabetic patient is to mimic normal insulin secretion. In normals insulin is secreted into the portal circulation at all times. A basal secretion acts mainly upon the liver, inhibiting hepatic glucose production yet allowing sufficient glucose output by the liver to supply peripheral non-insulin-sensitive tissues. Rapid rises in insulin secretion, which occur with meals, further inhibit glucose output while peripheral insulin levels reach concentrations that stimulate insulin dependent glucose uptake into tissues such as muscle and fat. Regulation in this way is precise and serves to keep blood glucose concentrations within relatively narrow limits.

At present little can be done to replace portal secretion of insulin and peripheral administration must suffice. This results in the loss of the normal 2:1 ratio of portal: peripheral concentrations. Imitating normal secretory patterns has this disadvantage and possibly a further disadvantage in that no quick-acting insulin can yet produce the rapid peaks of endogenously secreted insulin.

A single injection of intermediate- or long-acting insulin is rarely adequate, meeting the

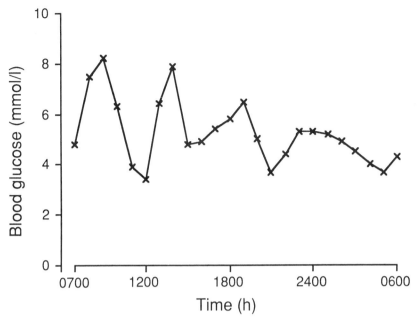

Fig. 12.1 Blood glucose concentrations over 24 hours in a 21-year-old insulin-dependent diabetic woman who was 28 weeks pregnant. Treatment was by twice-daily injections of a mixture of quick- and intermediate-acting insulin before breakfast and before the evening meal.

needs of the pregnant woman only if she still has considerable endogenous production of insulin. The minimum regimen is twice-daily insulin, which is most likely to be a mixture of a quick-acting and an intermediate-acting insulin. This type of regimen can give very good control of blood glucose (Figure 12.1) (Coustan, Berkowitz and Hobbins, 1980). A useful reference point is that two-thirds of the daily dose should be given in the morning and the remaining third before the evening meal and that one-third of each injection should be quick-acting. These proportions have been widely accepted in the non-pregnant diabetic although all clinicians will know the wide variety of regimens that come to be used in patients. Information on the relative proportions of insulin requirement obtained in studies using the glucose-controlled insulin infusion systems put the relative proportions of quick-acting to intermediate-acting as 1:1. The pattern of the physiological

alteration of the glucose tolerance test in pregnancy would suggest that these proportions would be more appropriate in pregnancy but direct evidence is lacking.

Whenever 24-hour studies of blood glucose are undertaken it becomes apparent that pre-breakfast is the most difficult time to control on this type of regimen. Whether this is because of an inadequate duration of action of intermediate-acting insulin, rises in hormones antagonistic to insulin during the night, rises in other metabolites during the night or combinations of these factors is not really apparent. The temptation is always to increase the pre-dinner intermediate-acting insulin to achieve better morning control. The consequence of this is to provide peak concentrations from absorption of intermediate-acting insulin in the early hours of the morning, with hypoglycaemia around 0200 h. A better solution in the non-pregnant is to move the evening intermediate-acting insulin to just before bedtime, leaving a three-injection regimen. Jovanovich *et al.* (1980) obtained good results with this regimen in 10 insulin-dependent diabetic women in pregnancy. The logical extension of this type of regimen is to give three quick-acting insulin injections before main meals, with bedtime intermediate-acting insulin. This regimen is gaining in popularity in the non-pregnant due to the increased feasibility and simplicity of pen injection devices.

Continuous subcutaneous insulin infusion remains a possibility in the pregnant diabetic. All pumps deliver a basal rate of insulin, with the facility for boluses with meals, which can be preprogrammed with the more technological and expensive pumps. Potter, Reckless and Cullen (1980) and Rudolf *et al.* (1981) obtained good results in this way. Potter, Reckless and Cullen (1980) studied eight diabetic women after optimum conventional insulin and after 5–55 days of CSII. The average blood glucose over 24 hours (hourly samples during the day and 2-hourly at night) was 6.2 mmol/l (112 mg/dl) on conventional treatment and 5.9 mmol/l (106 mg/dl) on CSII. Both maximum excursion and M value, a measure of variation in swings, were comparable on the two regimens. Rudolf *et al.* (1981) undertook CSII in seven insulin-dependent diabetic women from 10–29 weeks of pregnancy through to delivery. Glycated haemoglobin levels were normalized and swings in blood glucose reduced compared with conventional therapy. After stabilization, insulin requirement rose by 2.5 units per week on average. Coustan *et al.* (1986) compared multiple injections and CSII on a randomized trial basis. Provided with the same back-up support no difference could be found for glycated haemoglobin, mean blood glucose or fetal outcome. Hypoglycaemic episodes on the two regimens were also similar. Currently, therefore, there is little reason to advocate CSII, while the reporting of diabetic ketoacidosis in non-pregnant patients through undetected pump failure

must cast doubts upon widespread use in pregnancy when the accelerated starvation of the pregnant may increase the risk.

BLOOD GLUCOSE MONITORING

No amount of fiddling with an insulin regimen can replace adequate feedback information from home blood glucose monitoring. Reliable information is required upon which to base adjustments in dose. To this end 7-point blood glucose profiles are the preferred programme of testing – before and 2 hours after the three main meals and either before bed or at 2–3 am. This latter time point is necessary because of the recognition of asymptomatic hypoglycaemia occurring in the early morning.

Langer and Mazze (1986) evaluated the reliability of patient records during diabetic pregnancy. Using memory meters, unbeknown to patients they compared the memory with the patient's record. There were significant discrepancies in two-thirds of patients, with the record showing less variability and a tendency to lower values. Overall the difference was only of the order of 0.5 mmol/l (9 mg/dl), which does not testify to collective deviousness among our patients. Glycated haemoglobin or fructosamine is used in conjunction with blood glucose monitoring. It appears possible to obtain normal values of these variables in pregnancy contrasting with the non-pregnant state. Much of the adjustment in insulin dose is now carried out as outpatients. Clearly patients new to insulin or requiring intensive education may benefit from a few days in the ward. Every effort should be made to involve the patient in self-management. It is anomalous to leave dietary responsibility with the patient yet not allow responsibility for minor adjustments of insulin dose. Part of the continuing educational process is the 2-weekly visit to the clinic, which allows objective assessment and evaluation of obstetric progress.

Only failure to achieve treatment goals is

considered a diabetic reason for admission although obstetric considerations may supervene. Persson *et al.* (1984) compared outpatient management from 32 to 36 weeks followed by admission, to admission at 32 weeks. No substantial differences emerged between the two programmes for fetal outcome or for maternal blood glucose levels. Joint diabetic/obstetric clinics are widely advocated and most people give some acknowledgement of their role in reducing fetal mortality. We have adopted that practice for many years now although there are practical difficulties in small centres where there may only be one or two diabetic pregnancies at any one time.

MANAGEMENT OF LABOUR AND DELIVERY

GESTATIONAL DIABETES

In gestational diabetic women with no obstetric complications and a record of good control throughout pregnancy there is little indication for preterm delivery. Whether such patients should be allowed to go over term is debatable. Any suspicion of macrosomia alters this recommendation and increases the likelihood of caesarean section. Shoulder dystocia is the major worry with the large baby although, except in unusual circumstances, a trial of labour may be allowed. The situation in UK is less defensive than that of the USA, where caesarian section is recommended for estimated fetal weights in excess of 4.5 kg (10 lb).

INSULIN-DEPENDENT DIABETES

The move to deliver insulin-dependent diabetic women at 36 weeks gestation balanced the probability of fetal loss after that stage with an increased risk of respiratory distress syndrome. Improvements in management have decreased the potential fetal loss after 36 weeks such that the risk of respiratory distress is unwarranted in the absence of indications other than diabetes. It should be stressed that allowing the diabetic mother to proceed to term should not be by omission but only contemplated 1) when other contra-indications are absent and 2) with full support and assessment, using the means available which have led to the reduction in mortality. Drury *et al.* (1983), in 129 pregnancies excluding gestational diabetics, allowed women to go to term where possible; 85% delivered between 38 and 40 weeks with a perinatal mortality rate of 3.1%. The aim throughout pregnancy was euglycaemia. One conclusion of this study might be that close expert scrutiny of the pregnancy can go some way to replacing modern technology, upon which the rest of us need to rely.

Antepartum monitoring using a battery of tests, oestriol measurement, fetal movement records, stress tests and accurate dating with ultrasound serve to identify risks of fetal jeopardy and also serve to restrain the eager deliverer when the risk of fetal harm is low. Where preterm delivery is considered, measurement of fetal lung surfactants will indicate the risk of respiratory distress. In general, therefore, uncomplicated diabetic pregnancy with good control of blood glucose throughout may proceed to term and vaginal delivery. Where other obstetric complications coexist – hypertension, growth retardation – or when diabetes has been poorly controlled and macrosomia is a risk, preterm delivery should be contemplated. The optimum time for this will be the balance of compromised continuance, reflected in monitoring tests, versus risks of prematurity. An inclination of the woman to go over term when uncomplicated should not be favoured and attempted induction should be started.

The mode of delivery creates argument among those interested in the subject. Published reports indicate rates for caesarian section of 19%–83% (!) in recent years. Interestingly, the rate of 19% was obtained by Drury *et al.* (1983), in the study referred to above. With careful monitoring and greater attention to diabetic control most pregnancies can proceed to spontaneous labour with vaginal delivery or induced labour with vaginal delivery or caesarean section.

Coexisting medical problems may leave little alternative to caesarean section. Shoulder dystocia is a real risk in a macrosomic fetus. In babies weighing more than 4.5 kg (10 lb) approximately 10% may experience shoulder dystocia. Macrosomia is not easily estimated by current ultrasound techniques but should be seen less often with the concentration upon diabetic control.

MANAGEMENT OF DIABETES DURING LABOUR AND DELIVERY

Euglycaemia is a reasonable and attainable aim in diabetic labour. Hyperglycaemia is associated with increased fetal lactate levels, acidosis and death in animals, while in women infused with large quantities of glucose before caesarean section fetal acidosis is documented. Also, the risk of neonatal hypoglycaemia is increased by maternal hyperglycaemia stimulating fetal hyperinsulinism before delivery.

Various regimens for glucose and insulin administration during labour have been used in the past. I would contend that all regimens based upon subcutaneous insulin are outmoded. West and Lowy (1977) used infusion of glucose and insulin to manage labour. Other groups have subsequently published similar regimens. There is some argument about the optimal infusion rate, with West and Lowy (1977) using 8.3 g/h glucose with 1–2 units per hour of insulin. Lower rates of glucose infusion have been used: 5–6 g/h, sometimes with no insulin. Where these pointless arguments exist a rule would be to fall back on simplicity – 100 ml/h of 5% or 10% glucose with 1–2 units per hour of insulin.

A glucose-controlled insulin infusion system has been used during labour (Figure 12.2) (Nattrass *et al.*, 1978). Wide variation in insulin requirement was noted despite glucose infusion rates of 10 g/h or less. These findings confirm the importance of monitoring blood glucose during labour.

Whatever the situation – spontaneous labour, induced labour, emergency or planned caesarean section – insulin and glucose infusions are a convenient and useful means of controlling diabetes during labour and delivery.

POST-DELIVERY AND LACTATION

Following delivery the insulin requirement of the mother falls abruptly. We found, using a glucose-controlled insulin infusion system, that this fall occurred immediately after delivery (Nattrass *et al.*, 1978). This remains so even when breast-feeding is established. There is no contraindication to breast-feeding by the diabetic mother, although practical considerations may make for difficulties. The separation of mother and baby, with the infant being cared for on a special unit, may discourage some mothers. An increased calorie intake should be allowed if breast-feeding is successful but the effect of this upon insulin requirement is offset by glucose conversion into lipid by lactating mammary gland. Insulin requirement will rise, however, if the mother should acquire a breast infection.

PERINATAL MORTALITY AND MORBIDITY (TABLE 12.5)

BIRTH INJURY

A consequence of fetal macrosomia is the increased tendency to birth trauma and asphyxia. Haust (1981) examined 95 infants at post-mortem from diabetic mothers: 32 had clinically significant cerebral petechiae, or intracranial bleeding. Hypoxia at birth and birth trauma contributed equally.

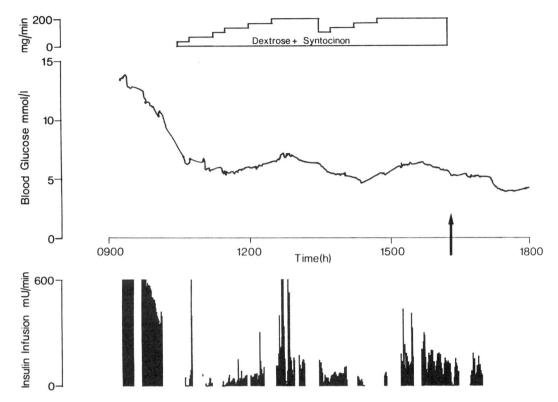

Fig. 12.2 Blood glucose concentration and the rate of insulin infusion by a glucose-controlled insulin infusion system during labour and delivery (marked by arrow) induced with syntocinon infusion in dextrose. (Source: Nattrass *et al.*, 1978, with permission.)

Table 12.5 Perinatal problems in the infant of the diabetic mother

- Birth injury
- Asphyxia neonatorum
- Congenital malformations
- Hypoglycaemia
- Hyperbilirubinaemia
- Hypocalcaemia
- Polycythaemia
- Respiratory distress syndrome

ASPHYXIA

Gamsu (1978) found asphyxia in 35% of infants born to diabetics and half of these required intubation. Asphyxia is attributed to the technical difficulties of delivering a large infant and these problems also give rise to

direct injury. Fractures of the clavicle and humerus and facial palsies are the most frequently encountered.

CONGENITAL MALFORMATIONS

It is relatively well established that congenital malformations are commoner in the infants of diabetic mothers. Pedersen, Tygstrup and Pedersen (1964), in a large study, carefully controlled, found malformations in 6.4% of a diabetic group and 2.1% of the control group. In those who died there were malformations in 19.5% of the diabetic group and 6.6% of the control group.

The seeds for congenital malformations are sown at a time early in pregnancy and in many cases before pregnancy is recognized.

It is to be expected that the early environment for the fetus will exert an influence on its development. The view that exogenous insulin or sulphonylureas might be teratogenic has not held up and it is currently felt that hyperglycaemia or other metabolic abnormality of inadequately treated diabetes is the primary agent. Furthermore, in mapping fetal development the critical time would appear to be prior to the seventh week of pregnancy (Kucera, 1971).

Some confirmation of the association of hyperglycaemia and congenital malformations has come from studies of glycated haemoglobin in early pregnancy. Leslie *et al.* (1978) reported a significantly higher incidence of major congenital anomalies in the offspring of diabetic women who had elevated glycated haemoglobin levels, and others have confirmed this. If, apart from an association, there is any causal role for the metabolic abnormalities, strict control around conception and in the early weeks would be expected to lower the incidence. A number of groups have reported that this is so. Fuhrmann *et al.* (1983) attempted good control prior to conception and noted a fall in birth defects from 7.5% to 0.8%. Similar results were obtained by a number of groups.

Other factors are likely to play a part in the incidence of malformations in offspring of diabetic mothers, particularly when vascular disease or nephropathy is present. Perhaps the best epidemiological data is from North America where Chung and Myrianthopoulos (1975) analysed outcome of 372 pregnancies in gestational diabetics, 577 in established diabetics and 47 000 non-diabetic pregnancies. In the non-diabetic women 8.4% of offspring had malformations while in established diabetics this was 17.6%. This latter figure may be excessively high, as a result of awareness of the problem in diabetics or increased reporting of minor malformations. The figure is certainly higher than our own malformation rate and that of others in Europe. Somewhat surprisingly, the rate of malformation reported in non-diabetic women is also considerably less than the American series.

In gestational diabetics the situation is confused, with some authors reporting increased malformation rates although others report no increase. Scrupulous prepregnancy assessment is needed to avoid biasing results of gestational diabetics by inclusion of undiagnosed diabetics.

Types of malformation

There is a wide spread of congenital malformations in the diabetic child (Table 12.6) and it is doubtful if there is any specific defect associated with diabetes.

Abnormalities of the central nervous system include anencephaly, meningocele and myelomeningocele, and microcephaly. Kucera (1971) and Chung and Myrianthopoulos (1975) reported six- to eightfold increases in anencephaly versus meningocele. Some groups have reported an excessive increase in holoprosencephaly, a rare defect, in insulin-dependent diabetics within a general increase in neural tube defects.

Table 12.6   Major congenital anomalies

1. **Cardiovascular**
   Transposition; ventricular septal defect; coarctation; hypoplastic left ventricle; single ventricle; patent ductus arteriosus; pulmonary atresia; pulmonary stenosis
2. **Skeletal**
   Sacral agenesis or hypoplasia; pes equinovarus; limb hypoplasia; laryngotracheomalacia
3. **Neural tube defects**
   Anencephaly; microcephaly; holoprosencephaly; meningocele; meningomyelocele
4. **Gastrointestinal**
   Tracheo-oesophageal fistula; duodenal atresia; Meckel's diverticulum; Hirschsprung's disease; anorectal atresia
5. **Renal**
   Renal agenesis; polycystic kidney; duplex ureter; hydronephrosis

Of the major cardiac anomalies ventricular septal defect, coarctation, single ventricle and transposition are all seen with pulmonary atresia, stenosis and patent ductus arteriosus. A fivefold increase in congenital heart disease has been reported, and a relationship with duration and vascular complications (Pedersen, Tygstrup and Pedersen, 1964).

Renal agenesis and polycystic kidneys are well recognized, as are duplex ureters and hydronephrosis. These may be associated with duodenal atresia, Meckel's diverticulum or Potter facies.

In addition to Meckel's diverticulum and duodenal atresia, anorectal atresia, Hirschsprung's disease and tracheoesophageal fistula occur.

Among skeletal abnormalities are found sacral agenesis, hypoplasia or hypoplastic limbs, also pes equinovarus. All occur at an increased rate in diabetics but do occur in non-diabetics and thus it is incorrect to consider the caudal regression syndrome as pathognomonic.

HYPOGLYCAEMIA

The hyperinsulinism that results in macrosomia is responsible not only for morbidity associated with the large baby, such as birth injury, but also has important direct consequences. Coming up to delivery the fetal blood glucose level is similar to the maternal blood glucose level and the latter therefore determines the stimulus to the fetal islet. If this is excessive, removal of the glucose source at delivery leaves the fetus grossly overinsulinized. Hypoglycaemia is an inevitable consequence of this picture. Even in normal infants blood glucose falls rapidly after birth, particularly in the premature infant. This fall, which is exaggerated in the infant of the diabetic mother, reaches a nadir about 1–1.5 hours after birth. Newborn babies have difficulty explaining they are hypoglycaemic and may tolerate the episode without symptoms. Others will let it be known that all is not well though excessive crying, jitteriness, twitching, hypotonia and, rarely, convulsions. Quite what constitutes a hypoglycaemic level of blood glucose is difficult to say since 14% of normal babies will drop their blood glucose to < 1.7 mmol/l (30 mg/dl). Nevertheless, hourly blood glucose estimation in the first 3 hours should be undertaken, with laboratory confirmation if bedside testing suggests a level of less than 2.2 mmol/l (40 mg/dl). Treatment may be instigated if blood glucose is less than 1.7 mmol/l (30 mg/dl). Bolus injections of hypertonic glucose should not be given since they perpetuate hyperinsulinism. Similar reservations should be expressed about the use of glucagon, where the insulin-stimulating properties are often forgotten or ignored. Certainly the recommended paediatric dose of 300 µg/kg is far too high and it is not surprising that it results in a large increase in blood glucose. Adrenalin, which inhibits insulin secretion in addition to prompting glycogen background, is not advisable because of cardiovascular effects. Early initiation of oral feeding is probably the best approach, if it can be got away with but where this is not possible a slow intravenous glucose infusion of 5–6 mg/kg/min is appropriate. With adequate monitoring hypoglycaemia is rarely a cause of serious trouble in the neonate although there are occasional babies with recurrent hypoglycaemia for the first couple of days of life.

HYPERBILIRUBINAEMIA

Jaundice is another frequent accompaniment of diabetic birth. This is not solely as a result of prematurity but occurs more commonly even when gestational age is matched. The underlying reason is obscure, although the tendency to polycythaemia and haemolysis may play a part. More likely is the lack of glucose supply to form glucuronic acid available for conjugation. As with all jaundiced neonates kernicterus must be avoided.

HYPOCALCAEMIA

Hypocalcaemia occurs more frequently in this group of neonates. Quite why this should occur is not known. Hyperparathyroidism in the mother has been implicated as has hyperglucagonaemia in the neonate but neither explanation is convincing. Coexisting acidosis will disguise the tendency to hypocalcaemia, which may be precipitated by correction of the acidosis.

POLYCYTHAEMIA

Similarly, the pathogenesis of polycythaemia remains obscure. Relative asphyxia will exacerbate this. Exchange transfusion may be used with a plasma expander.

RESPIRATORY DISTRESS SYNDROME

Respiratory distress syndrome has declined in recent years coincident with allowing a longer gestation in the diabetic pregnancy. Where delivery at or before 36 weeks is unavoidable the lecithin/sphingomyelin ratio is of value in assessing fetal lung maturity. A L/S ratio of > 2 in amniotic fluid virtually precludes major problems with respiratory distress. Some groups have suggested that a ratio greater than 3 is more appropriate, since ratios of 2 do not guarantee a normal level of phosphatydylglycerol. There is also a suggestion that the incidence is decreasing, independent of gestational age, and it is difficult to remember the major problem that it presented. Gellis and Hsia (1959) found hyaline membrane disease at post-mortem as the only abnormality in 73 of 104 cases. These babies appear well at birth, although the respiratory rate may be somewhat raised. Within 6–8 hours respiratory distress is evident, with rapid grunting respiration and rib

retraction. The child is listless or irritable with twitching and occasionally convulsions. This condition may progress to respiratory failure and death within 48 hours, or it may gradually improve. Associated with this distress, or occurring as an isolated symptom, are cyanotic attacks of sudden and often unexpected onset. Breathing slows and even ceases for a minute while the pulse slows markedly. The attacks are usually brief and when isolated are never fatal. Generally speaking the respiratory distress syndrome does not begin more than 24 hours after birth and ceases to cause anxiety when the infant is 48 hours old.

LATER STUDIES

The prognosis of the neonatal period after the first few days is good.

Many neurological conditions have been linked with children of diabetic women. Certainly there is ample reason to expect an increased incidence from macrosomia and birth trauma, neonatal hypoglycaemia and hyperbilirubinaemia. Whether an increased incidence will be observed with tighter standards of metabolic control for the mother remain to be seen.

In a much quoted, but little read, study Churchill, Berendes and Nemore (1969) purported to show a relationship of intellectual impairment with ketonuria during pregnancy and support for this view was given by Stehbens, Baker and Kitchell (1977). Persson and Gentz (1984) failed to confirm this finding when they followed up infants of insulin-dependent diabetic mothers born between 1969 and 1972. More recently, Rizzo *et al.* (1990) observed inverse correlations between fasting blood glucose and glycated haemoglobin with newborn behaviour assessments.

There is no relationship between maternal hypoglycaemia, neonatal hypoglycaemia and reduction in IQ but Rizzo *et al.* (1991) reported an inverse correlation with fasting 3-hydroxybutyrate concentration in the second and third trimesters.

THE DEVELOPMENT OF DIABETES IN THE CHILD

All diabetics know that diabetes runs in families and potential parents often ask the risks of diabetes in the child.

Diabetes would be expected to occur with abnormal frequency in the offspring of diabetic mothers and must surely do so, although earlier reports failed to distinguish between insulin-dependent and non-insulin-dependent diabetes in the mother and in the offspring, assuming a single aetiology. In general the parents are concerned about the risk of insulin-dependent diabetes and recent figures can be quoted with some confidence.

The risk of insulin-dependent diabetes in the child of a diabetic mother is of the order of 1–2%. In situations where there is conjugal diabetes this risk is increased to 2–3%.

PREPREGNANCY AND CONTRACEPTION

Contraception for insulin-dependent women has been made unnecessarily complex by well intentioned researchers. The combined oestrogen/progesterone pill is questioned on two accounts. Firstly, the increased thrombotic episodes resulting from pill use, which are well established, cast doubt upon whether the oestrogen-containing pill should be used in a disease associated with atheroma. Steel and Duncan (1978) reported five serious episodes in 136 diabetic patients who had taken the pill compared with one in a control group of 180 who had never taken the pill. The risk of thromboembolism in women taking a combined contraception pill is reduced by decreasing the oestrogen content. The second worry has concerned the effects of a pill upon metabolism in the insulin-dependent diabetic. Clinical experience shows that about one-fifth of women will require adjustment of insulin dose, the majority by a small increase and a few by a large increase (> 20 U). Most experimental studies show a degree of insulin resistance in pill users, due mainly to an

effect upon glucose utilization. There is also an increase in fatty acids and ketones of relevance to early reports of ketoacidosis in women using the pill. Neither of these considerations outweighs the advantages of the contraceptive pill in young women with insulin-dependent diabetes, although prolonged use into the mid-thirties or use in the presence of long duration and overt vascular disease must be carefully considered.

Use of the intrauterine contraceptive device has been controversial in diabetic women since reports appeared of high failure rates. Steel and Duncan (1978) reported a failure rate of more than one-third in a small number of women with all IUCDS *in situ*. Others have not agreed with these findings. Skouby and Molsted-Pedersen (1982) reported only one pregnancy and one infection in 105 women.

Steel and Duncan (1981) have reported good results with the progesterone-only pill.

Sterilization is the ultimate in contraception and may be requested by couples when they have completed a family. The only extra concern is the husband with insulin-dependent diabetes, when there is likely to be an effect of diabetes upon life expectancy. Frank discussion of this may be difficult but is important in reaching a decision on tubal ligation or vasectomy.

PREPREGNANCY CLINICS

The acknowledgement of the importance of diabetic control around conception and in the early weeks of pregnancy has instigated a rush to establish prepregnancy clinics. The object of such a clinic is to address better diabetic control before the pregnancy begins and it is a testament to our failure in the diabetic clinic that we need specialized clinics in which to do this. Disposition of physician time in this way with cooperation of the patient can improve control before pregnancy, as indeed it can in any group of patients incorporated into such a programme or study. Early results suggest a reduction in congenital anomalies in such a group (Fuhrmann *et al.*, 1983), although it should not be forgotten that patients who will attend and conform to such a clinic are a self-selecting group.

REFERENCES

Abell, D. A. and Beischer, N. A. (1975) Evaluation of three-hour oral glucose tolerance test in detection of significant hyperglycemia and hypoglycemia in pregnancy. *Diabetes*, **24**, 874–880.

Baird, J. D. and Farquhar, J. W. (1962) Insulin-secreting capacity in newborn infants of normal and diabetic women. *Lancet*, **i**, 71–74.

Biesenbach, G., Zazgornik, J., Stoger, H. *et al.* (1994) Abnormal increases in urinary albumin excretion during pregnancy in IDDM women with pre-existing microalbuminuria. *Diabetologia*, **37**, 905–910.

Chung, C. S. and Myrianthopoulos, N. C. (1975) Factors affecting risks of congenital malformations, II. Effect of maternal diabetes on congenital malformations. *Birth Defects*, **11**, 23–38.

Churchill, J. A., Berendes, H. W. and Nemore, J. (1969) Neuropsychological deficits in children of diabetic mothers. *Am. J. Obstet. Gynecol.*, **105**, 257–268.

Coustan, D. R., Berkowitz, R. L. and Hobbins, J. C. (1980) Tight metabolic control of overt diabetes in pregnancy. *Am. J. Med.*, **68**, 845–852.

Coustan, D. R., Reece, E. A., Sherwin, R. S. *et al.* (1986) A randomized clinical trial of the insulin pump vs intensive conventional therapy in diabetic pregnancies. *J.A.M.A.*, **255**, 631–636.

DeLee, J. B. (1920) *The Principles and Practice of Obstetrics*, 3rd edition, W. B. Saunders, Philadelphia, PA.

Drury, M. I., Stronge, J. M., Foley, M. E. and MacDonald, D. W. (1983) Pregnancy in the diabetic patient: timing and mode of delivery. *Obstet. Gynaecol.*, **62**, 279–282.

Duncan, J. M. (1882) On puerperal diabetes. *Trans. Obst. Lond.*, **24**, 256–285.

Fine, J. (1967) Glycosuria of pregnancy. *Br. Med. J.*, **i**, 205–210.

Freinkel, N. and Metzger, B. E. (1972) 'Accelerated starvation' and mechanisms of conservation of maternal nitrogen in pregnancy. *Isr. J. Med. Sci.*, **8**, 426–439.

Fuhrmann, K., Reiher, H., Semmler, K. *et al.* (1983) Prevention of congenital malformations in infants of insulin-dependent diabetic mothers. *Diabetes Care*, **6**, 219–223.

Gabbe, S. G., Mestman, J. H., Freeman, R. K. *et al.* (1977) Management and outcome of class A diabetes mellitus. *Am. J. Obstet. Gynecol.*, **127**, 465–469.

Gabbe, S. G., Mestman, J. H. and Hibbard, L. T. (1976) Maternal mortality in diabetes mellitus. An 18-year survey. *Obstet. Gynaecol.*, **48**, 549–551.

Gamsu, H. R. (1978) Neonatal morbidity in infants of diabetic mothers. *J. Roy. Soc. Med.*, **71**, 211–222.

Gellis, S. S. and Hsia, D. Y. (1959) The infant of the diabetic mother. *Am. J. Dis. Child.*, **97**, 1–41.

Gillmer, M. D. G., Beard, R. W., Brooke, F. M. and Oakley, N. W. (1975) Carbohydrate metabolism in pregnancy. Part 1: Diurnal plasma glucose profile in normal and diabetic women. *Br. J. Med.*, **3**, 399–404.

Hatem, M., Anthony, F., Hogston, P. *et al.* (1988) Reference values for 75 g oral glucose tolerance test in pregnancy. *Br. Med. J.*, **296**, 676–678.

Haust, M. D. (1981) Maternal diabetes mellitus – effects on the fetus and placenta, in *Perinatal Diabetes* (eds R. H. Naeye and J. Kissane) Williams & Wilkins, Baltimore, MD, p. 201.

Jovanovich, R. and Jovanovich, L. (1984) Obstetric management when normoglycemia is maintained in diabetic pregnant women with vascular compromise. *Am. J. Obstet. Gynecol.*, **149**, 617–623.

Jovanovich, L., Peterson, C. M., Saxena, B. B. *et al.* (1980) Feasibility of maintaining normal glucose profiles in insulin-dependent pregnant diabetic women. *Am. J. Med.*, **68**, 105–112.

Karlsson, K. and Kjellmer, I. (1972) The outcome of diabetic pregnancies in relation to the mother's blood sugar level. *Am. J. Obstet. Gynecol.*, **112**, 213–220.

Kitzmiller, J. L., Brown, E. R., Phillippe, M. *et al.* (1981) Diabetic nephropathy and perinatal outcome. *Am. J. Obstet. Gynecol.*, **141**, 741–751.

Kitzmiller, J. L., Younger, M. D., Hare, J. W. *et al.* (1985) Continuous subcutaneous insulin therapy during early pregnancy. *Obstet. Gynaecol.* **66**, 606–611.

Kucera, J. (1971) Rate and type of congenital anomalies among offspring of diabetic women. *J. Reprod. Med.*, **7**, 73–82.

Langer, O. and Mazze, R. S. (1986) Diabetes in pregnancy: evaluating self-monitoring performance and glycemic control with memory-based reflectance meters. *Am. J. Obstet. Gynecol.*, **155**, 635–637.

Larinkari, J., Laatikainen, L., Ranta, T. *et al.* (1982) Metabolic control and serum hormone levels in relation to retinopathy in diabetic pregnancy. *Diabetologia*, **22**, 327–332.

Leslie, R. D. G., John, P. N., Pyke, D. A. and White, J. M. (1978) Haemoglobin A1 in diabetic pregnancy. *Lancet*, **ii**, 958–959.

Lind, T. and Anderson, J. (1984) Does random blood glucose sampling outdate testing for glycosuria in the detection of diabetes during pregnancy. *Br. Med. J.*, **289**, 1569–1571.

Lufkin, E. G., Nelson, R. L., Hill, L. M. *et al.* (1984) An analysis of diabetic pregnancies at Mayo Clinic, 1950–79. *Diabetes Care*, **7**, 539–547.

Malins, J. M. (1968) *Clinical Diabetes Mellitus*, 1st edn, Eyre & Spottiswoode, London.

Nattrass, M., Alberti, K. G. M. M., Dennis, K. J. *et al.* (1978) A glucose-controlled insulin infusion system for diabetic women during labour. *Br. Med. J.*, **2**, 599–601.

Oppe, T. E., Hsia, D. Y. and Gellis, S. S. (1957) Pregnancy in the diabetic mother with nephritis. *Lancet*, **i**, 353–354.

Osler, M. and Pedersen, J. (1960) The body composition of newborn infants of diabetic mothers. *Pediatrics*, **26**, 985–992.

O'Sullivan, J. B. (1961) Gestational diabetes. Unsuspected asymptomatic diabetes in pregnancy. *N. Eng. J. Med.*, **264**, 1082–1085.

O'Sullivan, J. B. (1975) Long-term follow-up of gestational diabetes, *Early Diabetes in Early Life. Third International Symposium*, (eds R. A. Camerini-Davalos and H. S. Cole), Academic Press, New York.

O'Sullivan, J. B. (1984) Subsequent morbidity among gestational diabetic women, in *Carbohydrate Metabolism in Pregnancy and the Newborn*, (eds H. W. Sutherland and J. M. Stowers), Churchill Livingstone, Edinburgh.

O'Sullivan, J. B. and Mahan, C. M. (1964) Criteria for the oral glucose tolerance test in pregnancy. *Diabetes*, **13**, 278–285.

O'Sullivan, J. B., Mahan, C. M., Charles, D. and Dandrow, R. V. (1973) Screening criteria for high-risk gestational diabetic patients. *Am. J. Obstet. Gynecol.*, **116**, 895–900.

Pedersen, J. and Osler, M. (1961) Hyperglycemia as the cause of characteristic features of the foetus and newborn of diabetic mothers. *Dan. Med. Bull.*, **8**, 78–83.

Pedersen, I. M., Tygstrup, I. and Pedersen, J. (1964) Congenital malformations in newborn infants of diabetic women. *Lancet*, **i**, 1124–1126.

Peel, J. (1972) A historical review of diabetes and pregnancy. *J. Obstet. Gynaecol.*, **79**, 385–395.

Persson, B. and Gentz, J. (1984) Follow-up of children of insulin-dependent and gestational diabetic mothers. *Acta Paediatr. Scand.*, **73**, 349–358.

Persson, B., Bjorko, O., Hansson, U. and Strangenberg, M. (1984) Neonatal management, 1983, in *Carbohydrate Metabolism in Pregnancy and the Newborn*, (eds H. W. Sutherland and J. M. Stowers), Churchill Livingstone, Edinburgh, pp. 133–143.

Phelps, R. L., Sakol, P., Metzger, B. E. *et al.* (1986) Changes in diabetic retinopathy during pregnancy. *Arch. Opthalmol.*, **104**, 1806–1810.

Potter, J. M., Reckless, J. P. D. and Cullen, D. R. (1980) Subcutaneous continuous insulin infusion and control of blood glucose concentration in diabetics in third trimester of pregnancy. *Br. Med. J.*, **280**, 1099–1101.

Report of a Working Party Appointed by the College of General Practitioners (1962) A diabetes survey. *Br. Med. J.*, **1**, 1497–1503.

Rizzo, T. Freinkel, N., Metzger, B. E. *et al.* (1990) Correlations between antepartum maternal metabolism and newborn behavior. *Am. J. Obstet. Gynecol.*, **163**, 1458–1464.

Rizzo, T., Metzger, B. E., Burns, W. J. and Burns, K. (1991) Correlations between antepartum maternal metabolism and intelligence of offspring. *N. Engl. J. Med.*, **325**, 911–916.

Rudolf, M. C. J., Coustan, D. R., Sherwin, R. S. *et al.* (1981) Efficacy of the insulin pump in the home treatment of pregnant diabetics. *Diabetes*, **30**, 891–895.

Skouby, S. O. and Molsted-Pedersen, L. (1982) Intrauterine contraceptive devices for diabetics. *Lancet*, **i**, 968.

Strangenberg, M., Persson, B. and Nordlanden, E. (1985) Random capillary blood glucose and conventional selection criteria for glucose tolerance testing during pregnancy. *Diabetes Res.*, **2**, 29–33.

Steel, J. M. and Duncan, L. J. P. (1978) Serious complications of oral contraception in insulin-dependent diabetics. *Contraception*, **17**, 291–295.

Steel, J. M. and Duncan, L. J. P. (1981) The progestogen only contraceptive pill in insulin dependent diabetes. *Br. J. Fam. Plan.*, **6**, 108–110.

Stehbens, J. A., Baker, G. L. and Kitchell, M. (1977) Outcome at ages 1, 3, and 5 years of children born to diabetic women. *Am. J. Obstet. Gynecol.*, **127**, 408–413.

West, T. E. T. and Lowy, C. (1977) Control of blood glucose during labour in diabetic women with combined glucose and low-dose insulin infusion. *Br. Med. J.*, **1**, 1252–1254.

White, P. (1949) Pregnancy complicating diabetes. *Am. J. Med.*, **7**, 609–616.

WHO (1985) Diabetes mellitus. Report of a WHO study group. *Technical Series Report 727*. World Health Organization, Geneva.

Williams, J. W. (1909) The clinical significance of glycosuria in pregnant women. *Am. J. Med. Sci.*, **137**, 1–26.

The first reference to childhood diabetes in the English literature is probably that by Richard Morton (1637–1698). He called it diabetes infantalis (1689) and the description is quoted by Underwood (1799): 'He speaks of it as the effect of irritation from teething, and as a family disorder, having been fatal to all the male children in one, except the last infant, to whose assistance he was called at the commencement of the thirst and increased secretion of urine; which was sweet as in the diabetes of adults.'

The US physician Jacobi (1830–1919) described a more rapid course in infants and children than in adults, terminating more readily in coma and death (Jacobi, 1896). Both Morton and Jacobi were able to try dietary modification; Morton used milk mixed with Islington chalybeate water; Jacobi, milk and alkalis (the latter a mixture of iodoform, arsenic, bromide, salicylate of sodium in an alkaline beverage).

Joslin, Root and White (1925) reported results in 300 patients (children to young adults) before and immediately after the introduction of insulin. Of 164 patients diagnosed before the availability of insulin only 12 survived and the mean survival time in the other 152 was 2.4 years. Of the 130 patients who received insulin 10 died.

PREVALENCE AND INCIDENCE

Diabetes is uncommon in children when compared with the number of adults with the disease. Among paediatric disorders, however, it is relatively common with an incidence in the USA of 14.8 per 100 000 compared with childhood cancers (12.2/100 000) and cystic fibrosis (3.1/100 000).

The mean age at onset is around 8 years and the commonest age of incidence 11–12 years (Diabetes Epidemiology Research International Group, 1988) although a slight difference in age of onset between the sexes is reported; 10–12 years for girls and 14–15 for boys.

There are marked differences in incidence of insulin-dependent diabetes in children and young people between countries and even within countries. Finland, with an annual incidence of 28.6 per 100 000, and Sardinia, where the incidence also approaches 30, currently lead the league table, whereas Poland, France, Cuba and Japan, all have an incidence of less than 5 per 100 000 (LaPorte et al., 1985). Within the UK the variation is 8–21 per 100 000 of the under-16-years population (Patterson et al., 1988), the overall incidence being 7.7/100 000. There is also an impression, and some evidence to support it in the literature, that insulin-dependent diabetes in children is increasing. This seems particularly true in Finland but is also reported for the UK (Stewart-Brown, Haslum and Butler, 1983).

The overall prevalence in the USA is 1.73/1000, with a countrywide variation from 0.6–2.5/1000.

AETIOLOGY

The majority of patients with diabetes in infancy and childhood have insulin-dependent diabetes, that is, in aetiological terms, type 1 diabetes. Occasional cases are part of a particular inherited syndrome (Chapter 3) or result from pancreatic damage occasioned in cystic fibrosis, thalassaemia or by surgery for nesidioblastosis.

The hereditary nature of insulin-dependent diabetes is well established (Chapter 1) and has been shown to be firmly based, although not exclusively, in the HLA system.

Identification of precipitating factors has proved more elusive. No special features have been demonstrated in the life history of children prior to the onset of their diabetes, although recently the introduction of dairy products at a young age has come under suspicion (Virtanen *et al.*, 1993). The birth weight is average and obesity is not unduly common. The recognition of the relationship of mumps to subsequent insulin-dependent diabetes by Gundersen (1927) has influenced the view of viruses as potential precipitating factors. Circumstantial evidence favouring viruses has come from the British Diabetic Association register of childhood diabetes in the UK. This confirms a seasonal incidence, peaks of incidence with age and increased incidence of antibodies to Coxsackie B4 (Bloom, Hayes and Gamble, 1975). At best the age and seasonal information depends upon a similar pattern emerging for viral infection in the non-diabetic population. Peaks at the age of 4 and 12 have been interpreted as exposure to new pools of viruses with change in schooling.

It is likely that these data have been over-interpreted. A prerequisite for association is the concept of rapid onset of the disease such that time since diagnosis closely approximates time since onset. Yet it is known that the prodromal phase may be up to 2 years (Gorsuch *et al.*, 1981), which may cloud recognition of an associated precipitating factor. Laboratory evidence for the role of viruses is more convincing (Szopa *et al.*, 1993).

Islet cell antibodies have been identified in the serum of children at increased risk of insulin-dependent diabetes predating the development of diabetes (Gorsuch *et al.*, 1981). While these have a strong predictive influence, for example islet cell antibodies present in a first-degree relative of an insulin-dependent diabetic predict that 75% will progress to diabetes in 5 years, it is not inevitable that islet-cell-antibody-positive children will proceed to insulin-dependent diabetes; indeed it has been shown that children identified as antibody-positive may revert to antibody-negative during follow-up without developing diabetes (Tarn *et al.*, 1988). Other antibodies which have been identified are insulin antibodies, which do not seem to be predictive without islet cell antibodies, and GAD (glutamic acid decarboxylase) antibodies. The latter appear to be a family of proteins of different sizes.

PREVENTION AND INTERVENTION

There is an enthusiasm for the prevention of type 1 diabetes which causes me some concern. Nevertheless it must receive serious consideration since it is a popular subject attracting funding, publicity and invitations to lecture worldwide!

It is unfortunate that the term prevention has been used loosely, and it is doubly unfortunate that some of the studies have applied less than rigorous methodology even to the extent of omitting a control group. Prevention must refer to the stage where the disease is not manifest. Once the diagnosis of insulin-dependent diabetes has been made it is too late for prevention but intervention at this stage may alter the natural history of the disease.

PREVENTION OF DIABETES

There is no serious suggestion that the whole population can be treated to prevent diabetes. Thus the first step in prevention is to identify individuals in whom the risk of progression to insulin-dependent diabetes is high. It must be high enough to outweigh any side effects of the means of prevention. In this respect, therefore, it is not an absolute but related to potency and lack of side effects of these agents. There is not even a suggestion that we can screen the general population. If this were to be done on a genetic marker, of which Asp 57 could be most appropriate, it is clear that in Sweden, for example, 2% of children are Asp homozygous and 20% are Asp 57 heterozygotes.

The protagonists of prevention argue that markers are available which identify those with a strong probability of progression to diabetes. These include genetic markers but particular attention has been paid to immunological markers. Among first-degree relatives of insulin-dependent diabetic patients 1 in 50 have high titres of islet cell antibodies (ICA) and approximately one-third of relatives who are positive for ICA have other markers, e.g. high titres of insulin autoantibodies or the metabolic marker of impaired first-phase insulin release.

Against this must be set certain disadvantages in this approach. The majority of type 1 diabetes occurs in the general population and not in the families of type 1 diabetics. Only 10% of children and young adults with recent-onset type 1 diabetes have a first-degree relative with the disease (Dahlquist *et al.*, 1989). In Sweden the cumulative incidence rate for under 15s is 0.4%, i.e. 400 of 100 000 children born each year will develop insulin-dependent diabetes. Intervention in families therefore will affect 40 cases only, leaving 360 unidentified. If we turn to the marker in otherwise healthy children the frequency of ICA exceeds the disease by a factor of 20; for example, in Sweden 3% are ICA-positive but the prevalence is only 0.15% (Landin-Olsson, Karlsson and Dahlquist, 1989).

Clearly it will be necessary to use additional markers for the disease if significant numbers of patients with a high probability of progression to diabetes are to be identified. The current approach (Figure 13.1) is to use markers stepwise with clear identification of the risk of progression.

The baseline risk for insulin-dependent diabetes is 0.08% with a negative family history and 1.5% over 5 years if there is a positive family history. With a positive family history and when ICA are strongly positive (defined by reference to JDF units) the risk is 37% over 5 years; with low titres it is 5%; and in the strongly positive group if aged less than 40 years the risk is 42% but aged greater than 40 it is only 12%. The possibility exists for taking this group with a family history, high titres of ICA, and aged less than 40 and further refining the risk by including presence or absence of insulin autoantibodies; or of antibodies to glutamic acid decarboxylase; presence or absence of Asp 57; and attenuated first-phase insulin response.

This last criterion leaves me uneasy. If first-phase insulin response is deficient can the aim be prevention or is it simply an early intervention approach? Certainly it is clear that if ICA are strongly positive and there is some loss of first-phase insulin response 100% will progress to diabetes in 3.5 years.

EARLY INTERVENTION STUDIES

Intervention at an early stage of insulin-dependent diabetes is based on the premise that the disease is an immune disorder and that therapy aimed at the immune attack upon the islets can alter the development or at least retard the progression of the disease. A number of immune strategies are available and can be considered. These include: non-specific agents such as azothioprine and/or corticosteroids; non-specific immunomodulators such as BCG; semi-specific immunotherapy with cyclosporine A; specific immunotherapy by induction of antigen tolerance; anti-inflammatory agents such as nicotinamide; B-cell modification with insulin prophylaxis; and other approaches such as exclusion of antigens like cows' milk protein. Some of these approaches have undergone clinical trials.

Probably the first attempt at intervention on any rational basis and with half-decent

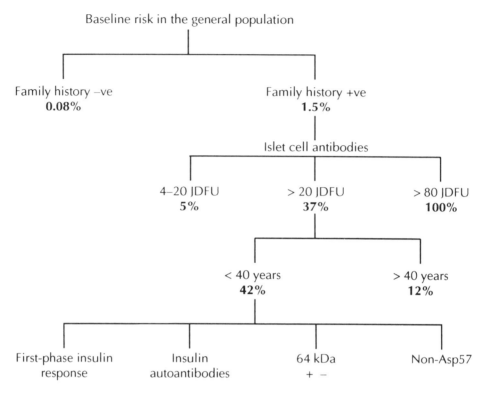

Fig. 13.1 Strategy for identifying individuals at high risk for the development of insulin-dependent diabetes.

methodology was by Ludvigsson *et al.* (1983). They took 10 children diagnosed with insulin-dependent diabetes between 1979 and 1980 who were aged 11–16 and compared them with a second group of 17 patients diagnosed 1976–1980. The intervention group had plasmapheresis on four occasions over the period of 4–11 days after diagnosis. One month later plasma C-peptide was greater in the intervention group, and the difference between the groups was even more marked at 3, 9 and 18 months for fasting C-peptide concentrations and in the maximum response to a standardized meal.

It is well recognized that insulin can prevent insulitis in the NOD mouse and in Wistar rats. On the basis of this information it has been thought appropriate to examine the role of insulin prophylaxis in early interven-tion studies. In five pre-diabetic humans with a normal oral glucose tolerance test but a predicted time to onset of the disease of 2.5 years, twice-daily subcutaneous ultralente insulin was given in a dose of less than 0.2 u/kg and insulin (soluble) was given every 9 months. In the group receiving insulin, none had developed diabetes after 2.5 years while in those who declined to participate (a not altogether satisfactory control group) six out of seven developed overt disease in 27 months (Keller, Eisenbarth and Jackson, 1993).

If nicotinamide is coadministered with streptozotocin it can prevent the development of diabetes in the experimental animal. The mechanism is thought to be through inhibition of poly (ADP-ribose) synthetase and the net effect is to restore islet NAD content. In addition to decreasing B-cell damage it increases insulin synthesis and B-cell regeneration. Following the demonstration that it is effective *in vitro*, in the NOD mouse and in some pilot studies, a number of larger trials have been performed. Elliott and Chase (1991) used it in individuals with a high ICA titre (> 80 JDU) and with a first-phase insulin response of 31 mU/l (mean 1 minute + 3 minutes, which is less than the fifth centile). Nicotinamide, in a dose of 150–300 mg per year of age per day (to a maximum of 3 g/day), was given to 14 patients and their results compared with eight historical controls. All of the controls developed diabetes but only one of the 14 treated patients did so. In contrast, studies in Denmark and Minnesota have shown no beneficial effects.

Harrison *et al.* (1985) published their results from Melbourne on the treatment of 13 patients with symptoms for less than 12 weeks by azothioprine (2 mg/kg) and 11 controls. Two patients withdrew from the treated group, three dropped out at 6 months and two reduced the dose of azothioprine. Remission, defined as withdrawal of insulin for 1 week, a fasting blood glucose of less than 7 mmol/l (126 mg/dl) with or without oral therapy, occurred in seven of 13 in the treated group compared with only one of 11 controls. In the group who were given azothioprine, post-glucagon C-peptide secretion was greater in the seven responders than the six non-responders.

In a follow-up study the Australian group studied 49 'children' aged 2–20 years. They failed to find any difference in insulin dose, control or C-peptide and none of the children were in remission at 1 year (Cook *et al.*, 1989).

In a pilot study 41 patients were given cyclosporin A 10 mg/kg/day for 2–12 months. When the drug was given within 6 weeks of diagnosis 16 of 30 patients gained a remission but if it was used after 6 weeks from diagnosis only two of 11 did so (Stiller *et al.*, 1984). Following on from this the Canadian–European randomized controlled study of cyclosporin A included 188 patients aged 9 to 35 years, who were less than 6 weeks from diagnosis and with symptoms for less than 14 weeks; they were given the same dose of cyclosporin A. Remission was defined as a C-peptide of greater than 0.6 nmol/l or off insulin treatment with preprandial blood glucose of less than 7.8 mmol/l (140 mg/dl). Of the treated group 24 (33%) met these criteria but in the untreated group only 10 (21%) entered remission (Canadian–European Randomized Control Trial Group, 1988).

Currently in Finland, where the incidence of insulin-dependent diabetes has risen dramatically in recent years, a primary prevention trial by nutritional intervention is under way. The object is avoidance of cows' milk protein in the first 9 months of life in siblings and babies of patients with insulin-dependent diabetes.

To summarize the prospects for success, azothioprine looks to be of only moderate efficacy. Even when combined with corticosteroids, as it has been in some centres, the results at 1 year are disappointing in terms of patients off insulin. Is a short period off insulin an aim in itself? Is a greater C-peptide (or C-peptide/glucose ratio – always suspicious if an arbitrary and meaningless ratio is used to show benefit!) sufficient end in itself?

Cyclosporine appears to have an effect on preserving B-cell function but the responses at best appear to be transient. In addition, the side effects of cyclosporine A are not negligible, especially nephrotoxicity which is a concern. Cyclosporine A also leads to peripheral insulin resistance and it seems somewhat illogical to use a drug that causes insulin resistance in the early phase of a disease of diminished insulin secretion.

Results with nicotinamide are mixed and large trials are planned. Whether the evidence to date would support their performance is in the eye of the beholder! At least nicotinamide appears to be without unpleasant side effect.

Which leaves us rather neatly with insulin prophylaxis or early treatment with insulin. It seems rather ironic to think that the most appropriate early treatment may be that which has been in use for 50 years.

CLINICAL FEATURES

The onset is commonly acute, with emphasis on thirst and polyuria. Enuresis may be the presenting complaint. Since the report of thirst at once suggests diabetes the diagnosis is not usually long delayed and was made within 30 days in over half the children of Danowski (1957). In 32% of Danowski's series, however, it was only routine testing of the urine in a child who was unwell that revealed the diabetes. It is not clear whether this figure has been altered in recent years by greater awareness of diabetes among parents and physicians. Certainly, in our series of 611 patients with diabetic ketoacidosis of all ages there remain a substantial number of patients who present in diabetic ketoacidosis at diagnosis (Nattrass and Hale, 1984). While traditionally this is interpreted as an acute onset it must undoubtedly be true that there is a contribution from delay in diagnosis by the doctor, or down/playing of minor symptoms by a patient or even a parent.

Weight loss is always an important presenting feature of insulin-dependent diabetes for reasons set out elsewhere. Loss of protein and fat reserves clearly indicates insulinopenia.

Nor is the child spared the other typical presentations of insulin-dependent diabetes – balanitis and pruritus, blurring of vision or infection, particularly abscesses.

More specific to children is the rather more chronic presentation, which presumably reflects partial preservation of islet cell function. Thus a child will occasionally present with failure to thrive when physical development shows a drift downward in height and weight centiles.

DIAGNOSIS

When typical symptoms are present a random blood or plasma glucose will usually give ample confirmation of the diagnosis. Glycosuria is common in children, however, and it may be necessary to resort to a glucose tolerance test if the clinical findings are indefinite. It is not sufficient to dismiss the diagnosis of diabetes on the ground that typical symptoms are absent. Where a glucose tolerance test is necessary it must be performed under the strict conditions applicable also to those performed in adults (WHO, 1985). Before the glucose tolerance test the child should be free from infection, fully active and taking a normal diet. The only divergence allowed from a test in an adult lies in the dose of glucose used, which may be calculated at 1.75 g per kilogram of body weight to a maximum of 75 g.

Children quite often have ketonuria when unwell in the absence of glycosuria. The pathogenesis in this 'fasting' state is that lowered oral intake allows a slight decline in circulating glucose. In turn, this leads to a decline in the secretion of insulin, thus allowing mobilization of fat depots. Non-esterified fatty acids are transported to the liver where the altered insulin: glucagon ratio favours their conversion into ketone bodies. Thus, the finding of ketonuria shows a normal physiological or pathophysiological response to a reduced oral intake or fasting. It should be stressed that this explanation does not hold if the blood glucose is raised. Raised blood glucose will stimulate insulin secretion, inhibit fat breakdown and abolish ketonuria. Thus at presentation of diabetes with hyperglycaemia, fasting or vomiting is not the explanation of the ketonuria; the underlying reason is always insulin deficiency.

TREATMENT

PRESENTATION IN DIABETIC KETOACIDOSIS

About one-quarter of the children who develop insulin-dependent diabetes have an initial presentation in diabetic ketoacidosis (Pinkney *et al.*, 1994). The child who presents in ketoacidosis will require immediate treatment with intravenous fluids and insulin.

The principles of treatment are as outlined in Chapter 6 with the modifications described below for volumes of fluid, potassium supplements and doses of insulin, which are made in the light of the size of the patient.

ACUTE PRESENTATION NOT IN DIABETIC KETOACIDOSIS

For the child who is showing heavy ketonuria, but is not vomiting nor dehydrated and is well enough to take a full diet, the first injection of insulin can be given before the evening meal or next morning before breakfast.

A single daily injection of a long-acting insulin can be used from the start and may be felt to be particularly suitable for children under the age of 5 or 6. Children above the age of 6 may require, or benefit from, or find more suitable, more than one injection of insulin per day from diagnosis.

While long-acting insulin as a single injection may be effective at first and control is sometimes surprisingly good for the first 12–18 months it should be made clear that two or more injections per day will eventually be required. Indeed, there is nothing which compels the use of a single daily injection of long-acting insulin from diagnosis and it may be appropriate to use two, or multiple, insulin injections. Pen-injection devices have so revolutionized insulin administration, making it easier and less traumatic, that there is little justification for using any other means of administration whether multiple or only one injection is given.

The initial dose is based on body weight rather than the height of the blood glucose, being about 0.5 units/kg/day. This is a safe starting dose designed to avoid immediate hypoglycaemia but may well be an underestimate of requirement, which may approach 1 unit/kg/day, especially in those children who show no evidence of a partial remission.

Brush (1944) advocated the use of maximal doses of insulin in the initial stabilization of diabetic children, ignoring the occurrence of moderately severe hypoglycaemia produced by several daily injections. Within a month the majority of the children were well controlled by a single daily dose of 2–8 units. The achievement of a limited period of partial remission, often possible with less strenuous methods, hardly justifies this form of management. More recently others have attempted to induce a partial remission, claiming success with intensive insulin treatment in the early stages of treatment (Mirouze *et al.*, 1978).

DIET

Following the introduction of insulin there was a cautious change from the high fat, low carbohydrate and low calorie diets of Allen (1917) to a more normal intake. Favourable results were soon reported with a low fat, high carbohydrate diet and there were even some prepared to extend such a regime to allow the children to choose both the quantity and composition of the food they wished to eat, on condition that the food was not different from that of normal healthy children. Sweets, cakes and sugar were included. An essential part of this treatment was the use of three or even four injections of soluble insulin which the patients were said to prefer to single injections of long-acting insulin, because they feared a restriction of diet. A fairly common finding was that children ate about the same amount of the same things daily, and therefore many were tempted to allow a normal diet corresponding to that of non-diabetics of the same age, usually with three injections of insulin a day.

Meanwhile there was no lack of physicians who insisted on a measured diet with strict control of carbohydrate, protein and fat, the carbohydrate being not more than 40% of the total calorie allowance. In accordance with the trends in diets for diabetic adults this approach won the day and became the prevalent attitude for decades. Restriction was the dominant approach; restriction of carbohydrate, which led to restriction of calories, and always children were subjected to restriction of many foods enjoyed by their non-diabetic peers, particularly mono- and disaccharide foods and drinks.

Only in recent years has the wheel come full circle with a liberalization of diet which has followed the general reappraisal of diets for diabetic patients. Most physicians would attempt to persuade children to follow the same diet as older insulin-dependent patients.

It is self-evident that the diet prescription must be made out for each child individually and the details will be dictated to a great extent by the intelligence and good sense of the child and the parents. A diet designed for a diabetic child must have an adequate calorie content to allow growth and physical activity. Total calorie intake is probably the single most important factor in the child's diet and is often overlooked in the obsession with carbohydrate intake. In other respects the diet is bound to be nutritionally correct so that the vitamin supplements so often recommended are unnecessary.

The following general rules may be used. The calorie content should be approximately 25 kilocalories per kilogram of body weight at age 1, 20 kilocalories per kg at age 5, 15 kilocalories per kg at age 10 and 12 kilocalories per kg at age 15. Alternatively, one may allow 1000 kilocalories at 1 year with an additional 100 kilocalories for each succeeding year of age.

It has been calculated that the average normal child takes 50% of the day's calories as carbohydrate, 15% as protein and 35% as fat. Undoubtedly these proportions become more difficult to maintain if mono- and disaccharides are excluded from the diet. Nevertheless they represent ideal proportions for the insulin-dependent child. Just how good compliance is or how realistic is the prescription, is unknown. Undoubtedly there are children of upper- or middle-class

parents who can tolerate the 50% of energy as carbohydrate with predominance upon high-fibre sources. Equally, such a diet may be nonsense to some children in the context of the normal eating habits of their family.

A sensible plan is to explain these principles of a normal diet and its composition to the mother. The three main meals are made approximately equal, with extra feeds as required, especially last thing at night. Approximately the same amount is eaten at the same time each day but the quantities need not be measured.

A yet more liberal and realistic approach would be to allow a proportion of the carbohydrate to be taken as mono- or disaccharides. Evidence that this is harmful to blood glucose control, as opposed to teeth, is extremely difficult to find.

EDUCATION

Immediately after diagnosis there is a lot of information to be taken in by child and family. Either or both will need to be taught the basic principles of insulin and its administration, diet and monitoring. Some simple guidelines are also necessary on the warning signs of hypoglycaemia and how to respond to them, and what to do if the child becomes ill and hyperglycaemic. Further reinforcement of these messages will be needed, along with more detailed discussion of other aspects of diabetes.

INITIAL STABILIZATION

Initial stabilization of the newly diagnosed child is a topic capable of arousing passionate debate. Some argue that hospital is an inappropriate place for this, not only because it is an unrealistic lifestyle, which it certainly is, but also because it is best for the child to be left in the bosom of the family at this time. I do not know the correct response to this argument. Some parents are grateful that they did not have to cope immediately with the child and diabetes but had a short time when they could come to terms with the idea. But such responses and alleged studies of such responses are artificial to the point of absurdity. There is often a fierce loyalty of patients and parents to the doctor and they will not want to decry the methods of the doctor to a passing psychologist. Thus there will always be a tendency to support what they have experienced and since it is not possible for one family to experience both home and hospital stabilization, common sense indicates that we should be wary of any particular claim. Of one thing I am sure – that the safety of the patient should not be compromised. Home stabilization demands the availability of considerable resources to visit and advise. If these are not available then it is folly to jeopardize safety.

SUBSEQUENT COURSE OF DIABETES

REMISSION

Striking improvement of diabetes when it is first treated with insulin is common enough and familiar to all who treat a large number of patients. Not so well known is the fact that this remission was recognized before the days of insulin and can sometimes be achieved by intense dietary restriction.

The memorable examples of remission, however, are seen in patients who urgently need insulin at the time of diagnosis but immediately after control is established are able to reduce the dose progressively. Insulin requirement may fall to less than 0.3 units/kg/day and sometimes it may be possible, within a week or two, to stop it altogether. Indeed this action may be prompted by the occurrence of hypoglycaemia even on the smallest dose. Because relapse is virtually certain most physicians try to maintain daily insulin treatment but the proportion of children who could live without insulin for a time may be around 30%.

The explanation of remission is not ob-

vious. Patients with acute diabetes even when they develop ketosis may have measurable circulating insulin in their plasma (Schade *et al.*, 1981) and there is evidence that the pancreatic insulin supplies are not yet exhausted at this stage. If the islets are examined within a few weeks of the onset in such patients there is often a normal appearance. Traditionally, therefore, remission is ascribed to recovery of B-cell function as the 'stress' of the hyperglycaemic stimulus is relieved. In biochemical terms this may support the view that prolonged hyperglycaemia transiently impairs B-cell function – a so-called glucotoxic phenomenon.

Some patients show no evidence of remission or a poor and short-lived (measured in months) response may be seen. In others it may last for 5 years. After this variable period and often gradually and almost imperceptibly, but occasionally following an infection, the diabetes relapses, control deteriorates and insulin requirement rises.

Once the initial phase of easy treatment is over it may no longer be possible to maintain adequate control with a single injection and combinations of short- and intermediate-acting insulins twice daily; premixed insulins; or short-acting before the three main meals with intermediate-acting before bed are preferred. The total daily dose will show a rise to around 0.8–1.2 units/kg/day. There is no one dosage scheme suitable for all children but an understanding of the time of action of the various insulins is essential and at all times the spread of carbohydrate in the diet must be taken into account.

SELF-INJECTION

By the age of 8 a child should be able to inject insulin without help or supervision. Obviously there are individual variations but it is justifiable to press for self-injection by this age and to override the tortuous and often ingenious arguments which parents bring forward in favour of doing it themselves.

Unfortunately, this age tends to coincide with the age at which a single daily injection of insulin becomes inadvisable or inadequate. Thus the child may have to cope simultaneously with a change to self-injection and a change of regimen.

MANAGEMENT OF CHILDHOOD DIABETES

The care of the diabetic child is exacting and time consuming and should only be undertaken by those who are prepared to provide a constant service at all times. The support of a hospital clinic or specialist advice in case of emergency is almost essential and regular visits to a clinic have a function in putting the problem into perspective. Children and parents learn from each other and are comforted to find that their difficulties are not unique.

The task of the physician, alongside other members of the health-care team, is to educate the family in the handling of insulin, the details of diet, and the planning of the day's timetable, with especial regard to exercise. If there is enough insulin at work exercise often has a profound effect in lowering blood glucose, but if the dose is inadequate physical activity may make control worse. Urine testing or home blood glucose monitoring should be a regular routine carried out every day, once or twice before a meal. Blood glucose monitoring is to be preferred, although a potential lifetime of finger pricking cannot be an attractive prospect. Nevertheless urine testing is often perceived by the child as 'dirty', with blood glucose measurement the chosen method of monitoring. The results should be recorded in a diary in which other events are noted, especially hypoglycaemic attacks with their time of onset and intercurrent illness. In a family who have been appropriately educated minor adjustments of insulin dosage can and should be made without medical advice in the light of monitoring, but the necessity of urgent action in the event of an acute infection has to be stressed. In particu-

lar one should stress repeatedly the importance of maintaining the insulin dose when vomiting occurs and of testing the urine for ketones. Most of the disastrous attacks of ketoacidosis in children result from reducing or omitting insulin because no food is being taken.

Good judgement is needed to achieve a positive response in the child and the parents. The child must trust the physician while at the same time developing self-reliance and initiative. At some periods a firm rein is called for while at others, and especially around puberty, regimentation may provoke emotional crises.

Summer camps for diabetic children have been very successful in the USA and Britain. Under good conditions of physical activity group instruction is given easily. More important, the weak pick up habits of self-reliance from those who are well adjusted. It is notable that almost every child is able to inject insulin without supervision by the end of the camp session.

PROBLEMS WITH CONTROL

Despite all the attempts of dieticians, nurses and doctors a reasonable degree of blood glucose control in children and adolescents is difficult to achieve (Hocking, Rayner and Nattrass, 1986; Hocking *et al.*, 1986; Simell *et al.*, 1993). This is traditionally ascribed to the unpredictable lifestyle of the youngster or dietary indiscretion yet most studies suggest that it is not the daytime glucose excursions that present the major problem. Rather it is the almost insurmountable problem of obtaining normoglycaemia after an overnight fast (Figure 13.2). Quite why this should be so is not obvious and may be multifactorial.

In pathophysiological terms the role of the dawn phenomenon has received most attention. This is the name given to the rise in blood glucose which occurs from about 0600 h onwards as a result of the rise in cortisol and other hormones starting a couple

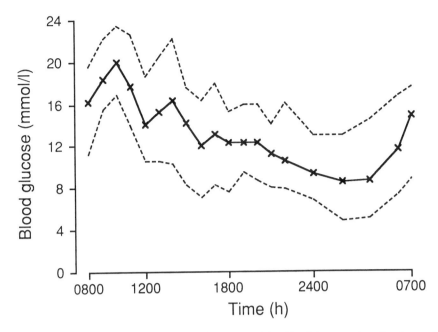

Fig. 13.2 Median blood glucose concentration (✕———✕) in 28 adolescent insulin-dependent diabetic patients (aged 10.8–17.4 years; mean 13.8 years) taking their normal daily dose of insulin. Main meals were eaten at 0800 h, 1200 h and 1800 h with snacks at 1000 h, 1500 h and 2100 h. Dashed lines represent 25th and 75th centiles.

of hours earlier. This occurs in non-diabetic people when the effect is counteracted by increased insulin secretion. When this physiological response is denied hyperglycaemia results.

Secondly, attention has been drawn to asymptomatic hypoglycaemia occurring during the night (Simell *et al.*, 1993) sufficient to elicit a counter-regulatory response. This was analogous to the Somogyi effect and is so called; it is also called rebound hyperglycaemia. The awareness that this might be commoner than supposed has followed home blood glucose monitoring studies and overnight monitoring studies in pregnant women. It is clear that blood glucose may fall to levels of 2 mmol/l (36 mg/dl) during the night in pregnant women without producing hypoglycaemic symptoms. It is by no means clear that in these patients a counter-regulatory response follows but extrapolation has been made to

the non-pregnant situation with an argument that counter-regulatory response can lead to early-morning hyperglycaemia and ketonaemia.

A unifying hypothesis for these explanations can be found in Jones *et al.* (1991). They reported differences in the glycaemic thresholds which triggered counter-regulatory responses. Children without diabetes evoked an adrenalin response at a blood glucose level of 3.9 mmol/l (70 mg/dl), 0.7 mmol/l (12.6 mg/dl) higher than the level at which the response was triggered in non-diabetic adults. Children with diabetes (average age 14 years) who were poorly controlled (very! – average HbA₁ 15% compared with a mean ± 2 S. D. of 4.8 ± 1.0% in non-diabetic children) had even higher glycaemic thresholds for counter-regulation at 4.9 mmol/l (88 mg/dl). Similar findings were reported for the stimulus to growth hormone secretion. If these findings were widely applicable in childhood or adolescence then their contribution to metabolic instability would be significant.

It can be extremely difficult to know with certainty whether early-morning hyperglycaemia and ketonaemia arises from too much or too little insulin. If there is any doubt then the correct advice will be a reduction in insulin. Early-morning hyperglycaemia will also arise from inadequate insulinization overnight. This seems to me to be a far commoner explanation than rebound hyperglycaemia. The studies which we have performed in adolescents almost uniformly show poor blood glucose control overnight yet attempts to improve blood glucose over this period lead to little success. Young patients and their parents are acutely worried about hypoglycaemia occurring during sleep, as evidenced by the responses of children at British Diabetic Association camps. Fear of not waking up is very real and leads to resistance to increasing overnight insulin dose.

The fact remains that the majority of young people with insulin-dependent diabetes are poorly controlled and methods of improving control, particularly aimed at allowing a normoglycaemic start to the day, are urgently needed. Studies of blood glucose monitoring in children or 12- and 24-hour studies have all indicated the extent of the poor control in these age groups. It cannot be surprising therefore that complications develop later in life; rather, it is surprising that some people do well with slow onset of complications.

EMERGENCY TREATMENT

INTERCURRENT ILLNESS

During acute intercurrent illness such as the specific fevers, upper respiratory infections and gastroenteritis, the control of diabetes may be quickly lost and it is best to give quick-acting insulin in frequent small doses with simple carbohydrate feeds of 40 g each after each injection. Sweetened milk drinks are often better tolerated than glucose, which

is apt to cause vomiting. Home blood glucose measurement and urine testing for ketones should be regularly performed during the acute illness and expert help sought earlier rather than later. Insulin should not be discontinued despite the argument that oral calorie intake is reduced. The likely requirement is for a increase in insulin dose. It is important to avoid dehydration, which results from increased fluid loss through the skin when the child has a temperature, vomiting or diarrhoea. Glycosuria will also enhance fluid losses. When careful monitoring and alterations to insulin dose are unsuccessful in preventing vomiting, dehydration or heavy ketonuria then the development of overt diabetic ketoacidosis is a clear risk and the child will almost certainly require hospitalization.

DIABETIC KETOACIDOSIS

The development of diabetic ketoacidosis is a most serious situation. Despite improvements in treatment of the condition it still carries significant morbidity and mortality. The latter is around 6% in centres with a special interest in the management of ketoacidosis and most of this is concentrated in the elderly. Nevertheless, occasional deaths in diabetic ketoacidosis are seen in children and young adults and rightly when these occur they spread an aura of doom and gloom.

The clinical presentation of the child in ketoacidosis does not differ from the presentation of the adult with the exception that the onset may be notably acute. Abdominal pain may confuse more in this age group.

Diagnosis must be confirmed immediately by laboratory blood glucose measurement, the finding of ketonuria, and pH and blood gases estimation to identify a metabolic acidosis. There is no real differential diagnosis although salicylate poisoning in a child under 3 years can result in a metabolic acidosis with hyperglycaemia. Diabetic ketoacidosis should never be confused with hypoglycaemia on the clinical presentation.

Treatment must be instigated without delay. The principles are the same as for the adult: rehydration; correct and maintain electrolyte balance; and correct the metabolic abnormalities with insulin; and units anticipating patients in ketoacidosis needing treatment should have protocols in place. The following is a brief account of treatment and is not intended to supersede a more detailed protocol as set out by Greene (1991).

As in the adult isotonic saline is the preferred fluid for rehydration. Paediatricians are rightly concerned about volume of fluid given since even small amounts under- or overestimated may be a significant deviation in a small child. It is helpful in calculating volume replacement if some estimate of the patient's weight can be obtained. Rather complicated regimens have been devised in an attempt to avoid overhydration (Greene, 1991). An estimate of fluid deficit, the daily fluid requirement and urinary and other losses are taken into account to calculate infusion rates.

Potassium administration is undertaken intravenously, titrated against regular plasma potassium measurement.

Intravenous insulin should be given at a rate of 0.1 units/kg/h.

As with adult physicians there is still some use of bicarbonate by paediatricians treating ketoacidosis. Reservations about this are expressed in Chapter 6 and I know of no convincing report of its beneficial use in children.

In all probability careful supervision, which includes clinical and biochemical monitoring, is the most important consideration in producing a successful outcome. Treatment protocols are most useful but they are not to be slavishly followed without due regard to clinical and biochemical progress. The protocol must be constantly amended in the light of the progress of the individual patient being treated. Blood glucose should be checked hourly and electrolytes 2–4-hourly. Bedside

measurement of blood glucose may be insufficient to monitor progress and laboratory estimations are then necessary.

When blood glucose has fallen to 14 mmol/l (250 mg/dl) rehydration is continued with 5% glucose and the insulin infusion rate is halved.

It has been suggested that cerebral oedema occurs more commonly during the treatment of children with ketoacidosis than during the treatment of adults (Nattrass and Hale, 1984). It is an extremely rare complication in adults and fortunately rare in children. The clinical picture is fairly characteristic with clinical improvement occurring after treatment of ketoacidosis is commenced, which is abruptly terminated by a catastrophic collapse. Because it is rare few people have experience of the condition and it is not diagnosed. Delay in instigating treatment is probably disastrous, although immediate treatment is not a guarantee of a wholly successful outcome. Duck and Wyatt (1988) reported their collection of patients who suffered brain herniation during diabetic ketoacidosis and it makes for depressing reading.

HYPOGLYCAEMIA

Attacks of severe hypoglycaemia with loss of consciousness occur relatively commonly in diabetic children. Pinkney *et al.* (1994) reported severe hypoglycaemia within 4 years of diagnosis in one-quarter of their children and in 15% this necessitated hospital admission. The annual risk of a child experiencing one attack has been put at between 6% and 16% (Bergada *et al.*, 1989; Daneman *et al.*, 1989). It is tempting to blame the search for tighter control of the diabetes for this high figure but it has also been argued that this need not be so provided the move to tight control is accompanied by careful monitoring, greater parental involvement and strong support from the health-care team. In addition, episodes of severe hypoglycaemia occur more commonly in those patients who also have hospital admissions for hyperglycaemia or ketoacidosis (Pinkney *et al.*, 1994).

Although in poorly controlled children the counter-regulatory response is evoked at blood glucose concentrations higher than non-diabetic children it is also true to say that the converse is true. In many children, it is not clear whether these are the well controlled, the level of blood glucose at which symptoms of hypoglycaemia appear is lower than in the adult so that it is not rare for a child to behave normally with a blood glucose of only 1.7–2.2 mmol/l (31–40 mg/dl). As with adults, however, the threshold at which adrenergic or neuroglycopenic symptoms develop is tremendously variable. Special problems arise in young children before the age at which they recognise hypoglycaemia. Excessive irritability, hunger, sweating and abdominal pain may give the clue. Neuroglycopenia may precipitate convulsions.

The question often arises of whether the child should be made to experience hypoglycaemia in controlled conditions, e.g. during the initial stabilisation. I doubt that this serves any useful purpose. The first hypoglycaemic attack at home may be years away, when anything learned will have been long forgotten. In addition, talking with parents it is clear that nothing prepares them for the panic of a first hypoglycaemic attack at home.

Treatment of hypoglycaemia in a child depends upon the clinical state. Rapidly absorbed carbohydrate is given provided the child can swallow; gels that contain glucose can be rubbed on to the inside of the cheek, where absorption will take place through the mucous membrane; intravenous glucose, or subcutaneous or intramuscular glucagon, may be necessary in the unconscious or uncooperative child. It seems impossible to persuade doctors treating hypoglycaemia with intravenous glucose to use a more sensible dose than 50 ml of 50% – 25 g of glucose intravenously is a huge dose and it would be entirely appropriate to use somewhere between one-fifth and one-half this dose, repeating it if the response was inadequate. It is also necessary to remember that glucagon will only raise blood glucose by 1–2 mmol/l (18–36 mg/dl) and therefore it may be ineffective or only partially effective. Its most useful function is to raise blood glucose concentration and hence cooperative state sufficiently for oral intake to occur.

LONG-TERM COMPLICATIONS AND PROGRESS

Children are prone to the short-term complications of diabetes to the same degree as their elders.

Long-term complications, as would be expected, are hardly ever seen in childhood. Klein, Klein and Moss (1992), in the Wisconsin epidemiologic study of diabetic retinopathy, found no evidence of proliferative retinopathy in the eyes of diabetic children below the age of 16 years but microaneurysms were noted by Burger *et al.* (1986) in children under the age of 15 and with diabetes for less than 5 years. The earliest retinopathy noted by Knowles *et al.* (1965) was at the age of 16. These workers found that the cumulative risk of developing retinopathy increased in almost linear fashion to a 70% risk of retinopathy in the 20th year of diabetes. The onset of retinopathy was later, in terms of diabetes duration, among those with an onset before the growth-spurt years than among those with an onset during the growth-spurt years. The time of appearance from the growth-spurt years was the same in both groups. This suggests that the years before puberty have little influence in determining the onset of retinopathy, and the same observation was made by Kostraba *et al.* (1989).

The evolution of renal disease is more difficult to study but may be assumed to run a parallel course to that of retinopathy. Changes in albumin excretion presumed to reflect underlying pathological change can be found in children and adolescents (Huttenen *et al.*, 1981). Rowe *et al.* (1984) found a relationship of diabetic control with microalbuminuria and also observed little contribution to the process from the years before puberty.

Neuropathy has attracted little attention but is probably just as frequent and of the same character as in the adult (Knowles *et al.*, 1965; Young, Ewing and Clarke, 1983).

Impaired ventricular performance detected on echocardiography has been demonstrated in diabetic children (Friedman *et al.*, 1982).

The mortality of diabetes in childhood has almost disappeared. First, ketoacidosis was conquered by the better understanding of fluid replacement, then infection yielded to antibiotics. Unhappily the survival of diabetic children into adult life has underlined our failure to prevent or treat the vascular complications which now cause the vast majority of deaths. Deckert, Poulsen and Larsen (1979) reported that 50% of patients who developed diabetes before the age of 30 died before reaching the age of 50 although, in order to follow patients up for a lengthy period, diabetics diagnosed before the year 1933 were studied.

GROWTH

The height of children at diagnosis has been a point of interest for many workers. Early reports were of children who were tall at diagnosis and a number of studies confirmed this finding. An equal number of studies found conflicting results and it seems likely that not enough attention was paid to matching of a control group, particularly with respect to social class, which led to the original claim.

Early reports also indicated that children on insulin grew poorly but it now seems likely that with reasonably controlled diabetes growth is normal. Many writers found the average height lower than that of a control group but this was usually due to the inclusion of 5–10% with markedly stunted growth (Knowles *et al.*, 1965). These patients with dwarfism were once quite common and

118 of them were reported by Wagner, White and Bogan (1942). The definition in this series was a height 4 or more inches below standard. There were 92 boys and most of them became diabetic before the age of 5. Initially thin, they often became obese later. The most interesting point about this condition is that it almost disappeared between 1935 and 1945 and is now rare if not unknown. It is, therefore, unlikely that uncontrolled diabetes was the cause, for the control did not show any definite improvement in this era. It seems more likely that malnutrition was the cause of dwarfism and the liver enlargement that so often went with it. Liberal attitudes to dieting in children were slow to follow the introduction of insulin but may have made their impact by 1940.

Savage, Lee and Stewart-Brown (1986), in a follow-up of 116 children in Bristol, found a deceleration in height velocity after diagnosis and instigation of insulin treatment in the prepubertal years. In individuals they suggested that well controlled children grew normally but those with poor control could grow very poorly. They also suggested that catch-up growth could occur if control was improved. These findings are similar to those of Rudolf *et al.* (1982), who introduced intensive insulin treatment to nine adolescent diabetics, improved blood glucose control markedly and produced a dramatic increase in growth velocity.

When pubertal growth was examined by Savage, Lee and Stewart-Brown (1986) it was found to be normal in boys but impaired in girls. Wise, Kolb and Sauder (1992) found that growth deceleration at puberty only occurred with extremely poor diabetic control.

PUBERTY

Puberty is an important time in a number of ways and has special importance for the diabetic both in how diabetes affects the onset and development of puberty and how puberty affects diabetes.

The menarche occurred normally in the patients of Danowski (1957) and Knowles *et al.* (1965), regardless of the age at onset of the diabetes, and this would seem to be the current view, although Kjaer *et al.* (1992) recently reported their large survey of Danish women with insulin-dependent diabetes suggesting a delay of menarche when diabetes developed before puberty. Any differences there might be between diabetic and non-diabetic girls would seem to be relatively minor. In a small group of diabetic girls Savage, Lee and Stewart-Brown (1986) confirmed a delay, with menarche at a mean age of 14 years compared with 13.2 years in a control group.

It is widely held that insulin resistance develops with puberty with a rise in circulating insulin in non-diabetic adolescents and an increase in insulin requirement around this time in diabetic adolescents. Direct experimental support for this concept was given by the demonstration of impaired insulin-stimulated glucose disposal in puberty by Amiel *et al.* (1986), who suggested that it might contribute to metabolic instability.

OBESITY

The problem of the stunted growth of diabetic children has largely disappeared in recent years. It has been replaced by difficulties of the adolescent, particularly female, to avoid weight gain. It is difficult to be sure that overweight or obesity is commoner in the diabetic than the non-diabetic population. What is self-evident, however, is the difficulties presented to the insulin-dependent patient of weight loss. Most realize that weight gain is less, or that weight can be lost, by adjusting insulin to allow poor control. It is also realized that this brings them into conflict with the health-care team. The combined resources of the dietician adjusting dietary recommendation and doctors adjusting insulin, with patient cooperation, can lead to weight loss without poor control. It is

a time-consuming process for all, demanding regular contact and encouragement. Spectacular success can be achieved but as in any age group trying to lose weight, failure or transient success only is the norm.

PSYCHOLOGICAL PROBLEMS

Take an incurable disease which can only be kept at bay by constant self-discipline and abstention from many pleasant foods; the daily confrontation of monitoring and the ritual of insulin injection; the prospect of a shortened life with the threat of blindness and other complications; for the parents, the feeling of guilt that they may be responsible for the disease in the child; the burden to them of constant vigilance and the attempt to achieve a childhood as near normal as possible: all this provides the perfect playground for the psychiatrist, amateur or professional. In general, diabetic children are surprisingly well adjusted if their parents are reasonably sensible. As would be expected the earlier the disease begins the more easily the adjustments are made. Davis, Shipp and Pattishall (1965) found that the great majority of children did not appreciate the seriousness of their condition and were able to deny many of its more frightening aspects. All of them thought it better to have diabetes than to be constipated and most preferred it to acne or obesity.

There is no doubt that the majority of diabetic children have a normal personality. All the same, major problems of behaviour do arise in some and the diabetes is used as a weapon in a variety of ways. Refusal of an insulin injection is one way of expressing rebellion. Hypoglycaemic attacks, often accompanied by erratic behaviour, are disturbing. Because an attack may upset the parents, the child may induce one at will or mimic an attack in order to get his or her way. Manipulation of insulin injections in order to reduce weight is a well recorded abuse almost always confined to adolescent girls.

Hospital admissions may be sought as an escape from family discord. At an early stage the feeling of being different and set apart can begin to weigh heavily on the child. Sooner or later the realization that the disease is lifelong and threatens early death calls for powerful adjustment. Depression can be severe when this happens and quasisuicidal or even frankly suicidal lapses of treatment occur.

There is nothing to suggest that the intelligence and school record of diabetic children is significantly different from the average. Problems of absenteeism and emotional difficulties in some are perhaps balanced by exceptional effort on the part of student and teacher in others.

CONGENITAL DIABETES

True congenital diabetes is excessively rare. There are a number of case reports in the literature but a common picture does not emerge. Some infants have a mother with insulin-dependent diabetes but this is not invariable. In some, congenital absence of the B cells is recorded; in others aplasia of pancreas or of the B cells; and in the remainder, the majority, the underlying defect may never be known as the infant survives with the help of insulin.

Congenital absence of the B cell may apparently be the only abnormality although it has also been reported as an accompaniment to methyl malonic CoA mutase deficiency (Blum *et al.*, 1993). It is difficult to argue that the B cells fail to develop since fetal insulin is clearly necessary for fetal development. Rather it is postulated that the B cells fail or are destroyed in the third trimester (Wong, Tse and Chan, 1988). This may result from autoimmune attack, intrauterine viral infection or unrecognized factors. It is clear that the first two explanations do not hold for all cases.

Temporary diabetes in the neonatal period is perhaps a separate entity. It is said to occur in small for gestational age infants and has been attributed to a delay in B-cell maturation. The infant, often postmature, is normal at birth but rapidly wastes and shows signs of dehydration without vomiting or diarrhoea. Glycosuria and hyperglycaemia are well marked but there is no ketonuria (it may be noted that normal infants do not show ketosis in response to stress or starvation). Onset is before the third week of life and insulin treatment is needed. The response to insulin is good and after a period which varies from a few days to 12 months it becomes unnecessary and a full diet is tolerated. Follow-up in a number of such children for 5–10 years, and in one case for 25 years, suggests complete recovery.

Whether it is strictly correct to say that insulin is needed is debatable; the biochemical abnormality of a raised blood glucose is not typically accompanied by ketonuria or markedly raised blood ketone bodies. At this stage, however, temporary diabetes is indistinguishable from true congenital diabetes and the temporary nature of the condition only becomes apparent with the passage of time. Usually insulin is not required for longer than 3 months.

MODY

Children or young adolescents should always be assumed to be insulin-dependent. There are few exceptions, of which the commonest is maturity-onset diabetes of youth (MODY) (see also Chapter 3). MODY is characterized by a strong family history, non-insulin-dependent diabetes and age of onset under 25 years.

It is clearly a heterogeneous condition, as evidenced by recent genetic studies (Froguel *et al.*, 1992), with some patients having a type of diabetes that can be called mild. Both the biochemical defect and the tissue complications in these patients and families are mild. Dietary treatment of the biochemical disorder may be sufficient to maintain normoglycaemia with, occasionally, a small dose of a sulphonylurea being necessary. Long-term follow-up has shown a dearth of complications developing in this group. Occasional microaneurysms may be found after 20–30 years of diabetes but little else appears.

In other families the diabetes cannot be labelled mild; long-term complications develop and insulin treatment may become necessary.

It is important to be clear that the syndrome is distinct. There is a strong family history and patients are not grossly overweight. Diagnosis often depends upon a glucose tolerance test and this will often reveal an abnormality in an exceptionally young child.

The differential diagnosis of MODY, non-insulin-dependent diabetes and slow-onset type 1 diabetes can be difficult. Particular care must be taken when extrapolating from MODY in caucasoids to other ethnic groups. It is clear that insulin-dependent diabetes is less common in certain ethnic groups. Distribution of obesity may also be different and age of onset. It is not acceptable to consider NIDDM in a youngster as synonymous with MODY.

DIDMOAD

In contrast to MODY, this syndrome (see also Chapter 3) is particularly unpleasant. The acronym derives from diabetes insipidus, diabetes mellitus, optic atrophy and deafness. Diabetes is insulin-dependent and difficult to control. Death at an early age is encountered and because of the extent of the disability life can be grossly impaired. Not all the defects appear at the same time and diabetes insipidus is always difficult to diagnose when diabetes mellitus is already present. It is unclear whether the occasional coexistence of diabetes mellitus and insipidus, or mellitus and optic atrophy, reflect partial emergence of this syndrome.

REFERENCES

Allen, F. M. (1917) The role of fat in diabetes. *Am. J. Med. Sci.*, **153**, 313–371.

Amiel, S. A., Sherwin, R. S., Simonson, D. C. *et al.* (1986) Impaired insulin action in puberty. *N. Engl. J. Med.*, **315**, 215–219.

Bergada, I., Suissa, S., Dufresne, J. and Schiffrin, A. (1989) Severe hypoglycemia in IDDM children. *Diabetes Care*, **12**, 239–244.

Bloom, A., Hayes, T. M. and Gamble, D. R. (1975) Register of newly diagnosed diabetic children. *Br. Med. J.*, **3**, 580–583.

Blum, D., Dorchy, H., Mouraux, T. *et al.* (1993) Congenital absence of insulin cells in a neonate with diabetes mellitus and mutase-deficient methylmalonic acidaemia. *Diabetologia*, **36**, 352–357.

Brush, J. M. (1944) Initial stabilization of the diabetic child. *Am. J. Dis. Child.*, **67**, 429–444.

Burger, W., Hovener, G., Dusterhus, R. *et al.* (1986) Prevalence and development of retinopathy in children and adolescents with type 1 (insulin-dependent) diabetes mellitus. A longitudinal study. *Diabetologia*, **29**, 17–22.

Canadian–European Randomized Control Trial Group (1988) Cyclosporin-induced remission of IDDM after early intervention. *Diabetes*, **37**, 1574–1582.

Cook, J. J., Hudson, I., Harrison, L. C. *et al.* (1989) Double-blind controlled trial of azathioprine in children with newly diagnosed type 1 diabetes. *Diabetes*, **38**, 779–783.

Dahlquist, G., Blom, L., Tuvemo, T. *et al.* (1989) The Swedish childhood diabetes study – results from a nine year case register and one-year case-referent study indicating that type 1 (insulin-dependent) diabetes mellitus is associated with both type 2 (non-insulin-dependent) diabetes mellitus and autoimmune disorders. *Diabetologia*, **32**, 2–6.

Daneman, D., Frank, M., Perlman, K. *et al.* (1989) Severe hypoglycemia in children with insulin-dependent diabetes mellitus: frequency and predisposing factors. *J. Pediatr.*, **115**, 681–685.

Danowski, T. S. (1957) *Diabetes Mellitus*, Williams & Wilkins, Baltimore, MD.

Davis, D. M., Shipp, J. C. and Pattishall, E. G. (1965) Attitudes of diabetic boys and girls towards diabetes. *Diabetes*, **14**, 106–109.

Deckert, T., Poulsen, J. E. and Larsen, M. (1979) Prognosis of diabetics with diabetes onset before the age of thirty-one. *Diabetologia*, **14**, 363–370.

Diabetes Epidemiology Research International

Group (1988) Geographic patterns of childhood insulin-dependent diabetes mellitus. *Diabetes*, **37**, 1113–1119.

Duck, S. C. and Wyatt, D. T. (1988) Factors associated with brain herniation in the treatment of diabetic ketoacidosis. *J. Pediatr.*, **113**, 10–14.

Elliott, R. B. and Chase, H. P. (1991) Prevention or delay of type 1 (insulin-dependent) diabetes mellitus in children using nicotinamide. *Diabetologia*, **34**, 362–365.

Friedman, N. E., Levitsky, L. L., Edidin, D. V. *et al.* (1982) Echocardiographic evidence for impaired myocardial performance in children with type 1 diabetes mellitus. *Am. J. Med.*, **73**, 846–850.

Froguel, P., Vaxillaire, M., Sun, F. *et al.* (1992) Close linkage of glucokinase locus on chromosome 7p to early-onset non-insulin-dependent diabetes mellitus. *Nature*, **356**, 162–164.

Gorsuch, A. N., Spencer, K. M. Lister, J. *et al.* (1981) Evidence for a long prediabetic period in type 1 (insulin-dependent) diabetes mellitus. *Lancet*, **ii**, 1363–1365.

Greene, S. A. (1991) Diabetes mellitus in childhood and adolescence, in *Textbook of Diabetes*, (eds J. C. Pickup and G. Williams), Blackwell Scientific Publications, Oxford, p. 866–883.

Gundersen, E. (1927) Is diabetes of infectious origin? *J. Infect. Dis.*, **41**, 197–202.

Harrison, L. C., Colman, P. G., Dean, B. *et al.* (1985) Increase in remission rate in newly diagnosed type 1 diabetic subjects treated with azathioprine. *Diabetes*, **34**, 1306–1308.

Hocking, M. D., Crase, J., Rayner, P. H. W. and Nattrass, M. (1986) Metabolic rhythms in adolescents with diabetes during treatment with porcine or human insulin. *Arch. Dis. Child.*, **61**, 341–345.

Hocking, M. D., Rayner, P. H. W. and Nattrass, M. (1986) Metabolic rhythms in adolescents with diabetes. *Arch. Dis. Child.*, **61**, 124–129.

Huttenen, N. P., Kaar, M. L., Puukka, R. and Akerblom, H. K. (1981) Exercise-induced proteinuria in children and adolescents with type 1 (insulin dependent) diabetes. *Diabetologia*, **21**, 495–497.

Jacobi, A. (1896) In *Therapeutics of Infancy and Childhood*, JB Lippincott, Philadelphia, PA, pp. 137–139.

Jones, T. W., Boulware, S. D., Kraemer, D. T. *et al.* (1991) Independent effects of youth and poor diabetes control on responses to hypoglycemia in children. *Diabetes*, **40**, 358–363.

Joslin, E. P., Root, H. F. and White, P. (1925) The growth, development and prognosis of diabetic children. *J. A. M. A.*, **85**, 420–422.

Keller, R. J., Eisenbarth, G. S. and Jackson, R. A. (1993) Insulin prophylaxis in individuals at high risk of type 1 diabetes. *Lancet*, **341**, 927–928.

Kjaer, K., Hagen, C., Sando, S. H. and Eshoj, O. (1992) Epidemiology of menarche and menstrual disturbances in an unselected group of women with insulin-dependent diabetes mellitus compared to controls. *J. Clin. Endocrinol. Metab.*, **75**, 524–529.

Klein, R., Klein, B. E. K. and Moss, S. E. (1992) Epidemiology of proliferative diabetic retinopathy. *Diabetes Care*, **15**, 1875–1891.

Knowles, H. C., Guest, G. M., Lampe, J. *et al.* (1965) The course of juvenile diabetes treated with unmeasured diet. *Diabetes*, **14**, 239–273.

Kostraba, J. N., Dorman, J. S., Orchard, T. J. *et al.* (1989) Contribution of diabetes duration before puberty to development of microvascular complications in IDDM subjects. *Diabetes Care*, **12**, 686–693.

Landin-Olsson, M., Karlsson, A. and Dahlquist, G. (1989) Islet cell and other organ-specific autoantibodies in all children developing type 1 (insulin-dependent) diabetes mellitus in Sweden during one year and in matched control children. *Diabetologia*, **32**, 387–395.

LaPorte, R. E., Tajima, N., Akerblom, H. *et al.* (1985) Geographic differences in the risk of insulin-dependent diabetes mellitus: the importance of registries. *Diabetes Care*, **8(suppl 1)**, 101–107.

Ludvigsson, J., Heding, L., Lieden, G. *et al.* (1983) Plasmapheresis in the initial treatment of insulin-dependent diabetes mellitus in children. *Br. Med. J.*, **286**, 176–178.

Mirouze, J., Selam, J. L., Pham, T. C. *et al.* (1978) Sustained insulin-induced remissions of juvenile diabetes by means of an external artificial pancreas. *Diabetologia*, **14**, 223–227.

Morton, R. (1689) *Phthisologia* (English translation 1694: second edition 1720), London, 1689.

Nattrass, M. and Hale, P. J. (1984) Clinical aspects of diabetic ketoacidosis, in *Recent Advances in Diabetes 1*, (eds M. Nattrass and J. V. Santiago), Churchill Livingstone, Edinburgh, p. 231–238.

Patterson, C. C., Smith, P. G., Webb, J. *et al.* (1988) Geographical variation in the incidence of diabetes mellitus in Scottish children during the period 1977–1983. *Diabetic Med.*, **5**, 160–165.

Pinkney, J. H., Bingley, P. J., Sawtell, P. A. *et al.* (1994) Presentation and progress of childhood diabetes mellitus: a prospective population-based study. *Diabetologia*, **37**, 70–74.

Rowe, D. J. F., Hayward, M., Bagga, H. and Betts, P. (1984) Effect of glycaemic control and duration of disease on overnight albumin excretion in diabetic children. *Br. Med. J.*, **289**, 957–959.

Rudolf, M. C. J., Sherwin, R. S., Markowitz, R. *et al.* (1982) Effect of intensive insulin treatment on linear growth in the young diabetic patient. *J. Pediatr.*, **101**, 333–339.

Savage, D. C. L., Lee, T. J. and Stewart-Brown, S. L. (1986) Growth in children with diabetes, in *Recent Advances in Diabetes 2*, (ed. M. Nattrass), Churchill Livingstone, Edinburgh, p. 119–125.

Schade, D. S., Eaton, R. P., Alberti, K. G. M. M. and Johnston, D. G. (1981) *Diabetic Coma*, University of New Mexico Press, Albuquerque, NM, p. 67.

Simell, T., Simell, O., Lammi, E. M. *et al.* (1993) Glucose profiles in children two years after the onset of type 1 diabetes. *Diabetic Med.*, **10**, 524–529.

Stewart-Brown, S., Haslum, M. and Butler, N. (1983) Evidence for increasing prevalence of diabetes mellitus in childhood. *Br. Med. J.*, **286**, 1855–1857.

Stiller, C. R., Dupre, J., Gent, M. *et al.* (1984) Effects of cyclosporine immunosuppression in insulin-dependent diabetes mellitus of recent onset. *Science*, **223**, 1362–1367.

Szopa, T. M., Titchener, P. A., Portwood, N. D. and Taylor, K. W. (1993) Diabetes mellitus due to viruses – some recent developments. *Diabetologia*, **36**, 687–695.

Tarn, A. C., Thomas, J. M., Dean, B. M. *et al.* (1988) Predicting insulin-dependent diabetes. *Lancet*, **i**, 845–850.

Underwood, M. (1799) *A Treatise on the Diseases of Childhood*, 4th ed, London.

Virtanen, S. M., Rasanen, L., Ylonen, K. *et al.* (1993) Early introduction of dairy products associated with increased risk of IDDM in Finnish children. *Diabetes*, **42**, 1786–1790.

Wagner, R., White, P. and Bogan, I. K. (1942) Diabetic dwarfism. *Am. J. Dis. Child.*, **63**, 667–727.

WHO (1985) Diabetes mellitus. Report of a WHO Study Group *Technical Report Series 646*, World Health Organization, Geneva.

Wise, J. E., Kolb, B. L. and Sauder, S. E. (1992) Effect of glycemic control on growth velocity in children with IDDM. *Diabetes Care*, **15**, 826–830.

Wong, K. C., Tse, K. and Chan, J. K. C. (1988) Congenital absence of insulin-secreting cells. *Histopathology* **12**, 541–545.

Young, R. J., Ewing, D. J. and Clarke, B. F. (1983) Nerve function and metabolic control in teenage diabetics. *Diabetes*, **32**, 142–147.

Characteristic changes in the retina of diabetic patients were described by Jaeger (1855) and microaneurysms were found in flat preparations of the retina by Mackenzie and Nettleship (1879). Nettleship (1888) gave a good description of the ophthalmoscopic appearances including those of new vessel formation. Waite and Beetham (1935) showed that the incidence of diabetic retinopathy was not related to the presence of arteriosclerosis or hypertension while Ballantyne and Loewenstein (1943) who revived the use of flat preparations, described the capillary changes and the characteristic microaneurysms and thereby gave a new impetus to research on this highly individual disorder. Ashton (1953), with injection of indian ink, was able to observe the capillary network in the flat preparation in great detail. He extended these studies with the technique of trypsin digestion introduced by Kuwabara and Cogan (1960). With the advent of electron microscopy attention shifted somewhat from the vessels to the retinal cells.

Retinopathy became a recognized problem of diabetes after insulin had kept alive for several years some patients who formerly would have died of ketosis. It must, in fact, have been quite common in middle-aged patients before the insulin era but was probably confused with arteriosclerotic disease. Indeed the distinction was not universally made until the time of Ballantyne's work, although by 1935 the individual nature of the retinopathy and its relation to the duration of diabetes was clearly indicated by Waite and Beetham.

Early attempts to treat retinopathy medically produced little improvement in prognosis. Hard exudates could be reduced in number and size by clofibrate although other features of retinopathy were largely unchanged. Furthermore, improvement in visual acuity by this treatment was not forthcoming. Surgical intervention in the form of pituitary ablation for advanced proliferative retinopathy resulted in such devastating side effects that it was always a treatment of last resort and its use is now strictly historical.

Meyer-Schwickerath (1959) realized the potential of xenon arc photocoagulation as a treatment of diabetic retinopathy and in the 1960s and early 1970s many groups reported beneficial results in the treatment of proliferative diabetic retinopathy. L'Esperance (1968) and Little, Zweng and Peabody (1970) introduced the argon laser. Early results were favourable using either the xenon or argon source but progression of diabetic retinopathy can be unpredictable and it was not until controlled trials were instigated and reported that the true nature of the benefit was recorded (Diabetic Retinopathy Study Research Group, 1976; British Multicentre Study Group, 1977).

PATHOLOGY

The earliest change in the retina, seen only with the electron microscope, is thickening of the capillary basement membrane. In the normal retina the basement membrane supports two cell types, endothelial cells and pericytes, in approximately a 1:1 ratio. Cogan, Toussaint and Kuwabara (1961) noted a change in this ratio, with the appearance of ghost cells within the capillary wall. They reported areas of retina where both endothelial cells and pericytes were lost, leaving tubes of basement membrane and other capillaries with selective loss of pericytes. Pericytes, with their close proximity to vessels, are probably obligatory for the maintenance of structural integrity of the vessels; indeed, there is a good correlation between the degree of pericyte loss and the number of microaneurysms.

Retinal vessels are relatively deficient in smooth muscle cells and Cogan, Toussaint and Kuwabara (1961) postulated that pericytes might exert some control over vascular tone. This remains a possibility working through two distinct mechanisms. Orlidge and D'Amore (1987) found that culture of endothelial cells and pericytes in close contact resulted in inhibition of endothelial cell proliferation. This inhibition was lost if contact was absent and appears to result from production by either pericytes or endothelial cells of a growth-inhibiting factor (Antonelli-Orlidge *et al.*, 1989). Alternatively, or perhaps additionally, control of vascular tone may be a function of the vasoconstrictor peptide, endothelin (Yanagisawa *et al.*, 1988). Takahashi *et al.* (1989) found production of endothelin by bovine endothelial cells with endothelin receptors, normally found on smooth muscle cells, present on pericytes.

The microaneurysm, the most striking of diabetic lesions, appears on the arterial and the venous side of the capillary network but more often on the latter. It arises commonly on one side of the capillary wall, often in kinks or loops of the vessel. The aneurysmal sac is often thin-walled but some are hyalinized, staining PAS-positive, while some contain fat. Dissecting and tubular forms are probably not separate. At this stage an increase in the number of endothelial cells is apparent, especially in the microaneurysms, while the pericytes are greatly reduced in number. Many of the capillaries, although patent, seem to carry no circulation and have no nuclei in their walls. This appearance in digested specimens correlates with areas that in injected specimens appear avascular. Micro-

aneurysms are mainly seen on capillaries that are patent. It may be that the absence of circulation leads to the appearance of fat in anoxic retinal tissue and to the formation of loops and new vessels, which are so prominent in the late stages of the retinopathy. In injected preparations the clusters of microaneurysms are seen to be widespread in the posterior pole of the retina and patches of capillary obliteration occur at an early stage, particularly in relation to the arteries.

None of the components of the picture of diabetic retinopathy is specific for diabetes. Microaneurysms may be seen in central retinal vein thrombosis, in Eales disease, in multiple myelomatosis and in great profusion in macroglobulinaemia. Their aggregation at the posterior pole of the eye, however, is characteristic of diabetes. With their observation of focal degeneration of pericytes in the capillary wall, Cogan and Kuwabara (1963) argued that this specific loss of cells would remove the tonic control which normally regulates blood flow. As a result rerouting of blood with bypassing of some capillaries and distension of others would occur, which could lead to microaneurysms and endothelial proliferation.

Progression of retinopathy leads to breakdown of the blood–retinal barrier, allowing the intraretinal development of hard exudates. The waxy hard exudates of diabetic retinopathy appear as hyaline structures, which stain with eosin and PAS. They consist of extracellular fluid, lipid and macrophages. Electron microscopy shows an amorphous structure with occasional areas having a finely fibrillar pattern. The origin of the exudate is unknown but it is generally thought to be serum.

Soft exudates result from interrupted axonal transport, which occurs in areas of under- or non-perfusion. Axonal swelling follows, with accumulation of cytoplasmic organelles due to loss of the normal bidirectional transport of organelles in the exoplasm of the ganglion cell.

Lesions of the arteries and arterioles, though of frequent occurrence in the diabetic, do not appear to play any part in the rather specific changes in the retina.

No theory has so far explained the venous engorgement which is often a striking feature clinically, before microaneurysms are visible with the ophthalmoscope. There is nothing to suggest an obstructive element in this distension; indeed, increased blood flow has been suggested.

While background retinopathy is an intra-retinal feature, proliferative retinopathy is largely preretinal. Initially, however, the budding of new vessels is within the retina, with perforation of the internal limiting membrane following.

A rich plexus of capillaries of friable permeable vessels develops on the retinal surface. Histology shows that tight junctions between endothelial cells are deficient, which presumably allows leakage from the new vessels. Most areas are surrounded by ischaemic sites, with dominant growth towards the area of ischaemia. Vessels may enter the vitreous and cause retraction of the vitreous. Rupture of the vessels can ensue or, with firm retinal–vitreous attachment, the retina may be put under such pressure that detachment results.

PATHOGENESIS

The nature of the distinct changes in the retina continues to defy elucidation. Early reports that diabetic retinopathy was related to arteriosclerosis were discounted after the careful study of Waite and Beetham (1935). While, in general, there is a close correlation of retinal changes and glomerular lesions, even this rule is not inviolate (Chavers *et al.*, 1994).

DIABETIC CONTROL

Anyone with experience of a diabetic population will have the impression that poorly controlled diabetes predisposes to the early onset of retinopathy and speeds its progress. This is especially true of young patients with repeated attacks of ketosis. Some authors have reported that none of their long-term cases with excellent control had significant retinopathy, surely an overstatement of the situation. In taking a less extreme view, Dunlop (1954) found that in patients with diabetes of 15 years duration retinopathy was present in 44% of those with good control and 79% of those with poor control. Pirart (1978), in his mammoth retrospective study, found a clear relationship between the degree of control and the severity of retinopathy. In prospective studies beneficial effects of improving control have been found by a number of groups (Job *et al.*, 1976; Lauritzen *et al.*, 1983; Kroc Collaborative Study, 1988; Brinchmann-Hansen *et al.*, 1985). These studies randomized patients to two levels of blood glucose control and, by nature of their labour-intensive design, they were performed in small numbers of patients with a relatively short (1–2 year) study period. This type of study has culminated recently in the Diabetic Control and Complications Trial in the US, which has clearly shown the benefit of good diabetic control in the development and progression of diabetic retinopathy (Diabetes Control and Complications Trial Research Group, 1993).

Retrospective studies of the relationship of diabetic control and retinopathy, and prospective studies, present a relatively unanimous view, but as often is the case it is the exceptions that make an impression. At one end of the scale is the feckless patient who is admitted repeatedly with ketosis and is never well controlled yet miraculously escapes retinopathy for 15 or more years; at the other end is the conscientious observer of the rules who has never needed hospital admission yet is blind from vitreous haemorrhage in 10–15 years from the onset. The problem is not simple. The conviction that control matters has obscured our asking: to what extent? Does poor control contribute 90% or 10% to the development of retinopathy? No one would dispute, surely, that other factors are in play.

If diabetic control plays a part in the development of retinopathy, how could this be mediated? As with the other specific diabetic complications, the two major mechanisms have revolved around haemodynamic change associated with less than optimal control, and a metabolic mechanism.

HAEMODYNAMIC CHANGE

Blood flow to the retina is increased in poorly controlled diabetes and normalization of blood glucose reduces flow (Grunwald *et al.*, 1986). This increase in blood flow is maintained in patients with early diabetic retinopathy (Fallon, Chowiencyzk and Kohner, 1986). It has been argued that increased flow and changes in flow with fluctuations in blood glucose will lead to damage of the capillary endothelium and capillary dilatation. Leakage from the damaged capillaries may be reversible at an early stage but when long-standing, retinopathy becomes irreversible.

Endothelial cell damage also reduces the efficacy of the fibrinolytic system, resulting in microthrombi and possible vascular occlusion. Controversy surrounds the extrapolation of *in vitro* tests of platelet function to the *in vivo* situation and indeed not all reports confirm abnormal platelet function in patients with diabetic retinopathy. Nevertheless the DAMAD Study Group (1989) reported a reduction in the number of microaneurysms in patients given aspirin with or without dipyridamole.

METABOLIC FACTORS

Much of the investigation of metabolic causes of retinopathy has been performed in animals, in endothelial cells from sites other than the retina, and in tissue culture, using galactose as substrate rather than glucose. How far the findings can be extrapolated to the human *in vivo* is unclear.

Summarizing these studies briefly, the polyol pathway has been identified in pericytes and basement membrane thickening in rats can be prevented by an aldose reductase inhibitor (Williamson *et al.*, 1987). This has led to intervention studies in diabetic patients with early diabetic retinopathy but, as yet, there is little evidence of a beneficial effect of aldose reductase inhibitors in slowing the progression or in reversing established change.

GENETIC FACTORS

Genetic factors have been sought but with little reward. An excess of DR_4 in patients with retinopathy has been reported but confirmation is lacking. The problem is enhanced by the lack of information on the specific genetic tendency to non-insulin-dependent diabetes. In twins with non-insulin-dependent diabetes the severity of retinopathy tends to be similar (Leslie and Pyke, 1982), although others have found that family history is not a predictor of the severity.

GROWTH HORMONE

Among recurrent themes of the pathogenesis of diabetic retinopathy, growth hormone occupies a special place. Poulsen (1953) reported:

A woman, diabetic from the age of 9 years, was found to have diffuse retinopathy at the age of 30; she was then pregnant and after delivery typical Simmonds' disease developed. Her insulin sensitivity greatly increased and her tendency to ketosis ceased. At the age of 34 her retinopathy was less and at the age of 36 it was no longer visible.

On the other hand, the growth-hormone-deficient dwarf (Kriefer, Sirota and Lieberman, 1970) displayed normal basement membrane thickness and absence of retinopathy after 10–12 years of follow-up. Growth hormone regulation is abnormal in diabetes:

higher levels, with highest in diabetic retinopathy; increased secretion in response to exercise; and abnormal responses to growth hormone releasing factors are all well documented. Yet despite the length of time since the first postulated connection, certainty still eludes us and we are left with the rather bland statement that growth hormone may not be essential to the development of retinopathy but elevated levels may enhance progression.

OTHER FACTORS

Other factors have been implicated with varying degrees of conviction. Some have implicated insulin-like growth factors and there is also evidence linking hypertension with the development of retinopathy. Most physicians are aware of the risk of rapid progression of retinopathy with pregnancy, although the evidential basis for this is rather thin.

PROTECTIVE FACTORS

There are also factors that appear to protect against the development of retinopathy. Myopia is probably the best recognized, but retinal–choroidal scarring, unilateral optic atrophy and raised intraocular pressure may protect against retinopathy, as may unilateral carotid artery stenosis.

NEW VESSEL FORMATION

New vessel formation is found in a variety of conditions in which vascular occlusion occurs. Michaelson (1948) suggested that it was a response to a secretory product from the ischaemic area. More recently such factors have been identified (D'Amore and Klagsbrun, 1984; Baird *et al.*, 1985). Retina-derived angiogenic factor or retina-derived growth factor are similar to fibroblast growth factor which stimulates cell proliferation (Schweigerer *et al.*, 1987).

PREVALENCE AND INCIDENCE OF DIABETIC RETINOPATHY

There is general agreement that retinopathy becomes commoner with advancing age but much more with the duration of diabetes. The incidence varies considerably with some claims of 100% in patients with diabetes of 15–25 years duration. Scott (1951) in his careful study of diabetics after 15–25 years found retinopathy in 80%. Others have reported having many patients of 30 years of diabetes without retinopathy. Many other cross-sectional and longitudinal studies have been reported with similar widely discrepant findings. These divergent findings suggest some degree of case selection and, particularly, poor separation between insulin-dependent patients where duration may be estimated with reasonable precision and non-insulin-dependent patients where duration since diagnosis gives only a poor estimate of duration of disease. In the population-based study in Wisconsin (Klein *et al.*, 1984) retinopathy was sought in young insulin-dependent patients and older (> 30 years!) diabetic patients either taking insulin or not taking insulin.

In the younger patients 2% had retinopathy within 2 years of diagnosis and 98% after 15 years of diabetes. Proliferative retinopathy did not occur before 5 years of diabetes; after 15 years 26% had evidence of it and after 20 years the figure was 56%. In the older group taking insulin 23% had retinopathy within 2 years, with 4% showing proliferative retinopathy. In the group not taking insulin the respective figures were 20% and 3%. A lesser prevalence in Europe has been reported (EURODIAB IDDM Complications Study Group, 1994), with 82% of patients having retinopathy after 20 years and the prevalence of proliferative change being 36% after 30 years.

Summarizing studies of duration in insulin-dependent patients leads to figures of 25–50% of patients showing some degree of retinopathy after 5–10 years of disease and 75–95% after 10–15 years. Proliferative change is unusual but not unknown before 10 years and after 20–25 years is between 20% and 40%. In non-insulin-dependent diabetes data from Yanko *et al.* (1983) indicate that 23% of patients are affected after 11–13 years, 43% after 14–16 years and 60% after 16 years. Diabetes in their patients was detected by screening of Israeli government employees throughout the 1960s and on more than one occasion. Thus duration could be calculated with a reasonable degree of certainty from the sequential follow-up. These data, because of the method of diagnosis, will not have a great application to the prevalence in the average diabetic clinic.

While the general relationship between duration of diabetes and incidence of retinopathy is certain it should not be forgotten that retinopathy is often present at diagnosis. To a large extent the precise incidence will depend upon the referral pattern to a particular clinic and the diligence with which the retinopathy is sought. Quoted figures are around 4–6%, although we found retinopathy present in 268 of 2775 newly diagnosed cases (9.7%). These patients were mostly elderly (Table 14.1).

It is difficult in many studies to separate the influence of duration from that of age. Thus, while numerous studies have reported increasing incidence of retinopathy with age, the Israeli study and Klein *et al.* (1984) reported a decreasing prevalence of retinopathy when duration was corrected for age.

In 1960 the 752 cases of diabetic retinopathy formed 7.5% of the total new blind registrations in England and Wales and this lesion was fifth in the diagnostic classification (Sorsby, 1963). In the age group 30–39 years diabetic patients formed 16% of the newly registered blind and diabetes was responsible for 13% of blindness in the age group 50–59 years. In 1963–1968 the figure had risen, with diabetic retinopathy responsible for 13% of new blind registrations in men and 18% in women (Sorsby, 1972). The most recent figures, for the year 1985/6 and in the age group 16–64 years, show diabetic retinopathy was responsible for 15.4% of blind and partially-sighted registrations (Table 14.2) (Department of Health and Social Security Statistical Bulletin, 3/8/88).

Although there are difficulties in comparing reporting rates from year to year, Figure 14.1 suggests a fall in diabetic retinopathy as a cause of blindness; nevertheless it continues to make a significant contribution despite improvements in treatment.

CLASSIFICATION

The most useful classification of retinal changes is dictated by prospects of treatment:

1. Background retinopathy
2. Background retinopathy with maculopathy
3. Preproliferative retinopathy
4. Proliferative retinopathy.

OPHTHALMOSCOPIC PICTURE

BACKGROUND RETINOPATHY (Plate 1)

Often the earliest suggestion of retinal involvement is enlargement of the veins. This may

Table 14.1   Retinopathy at diagnosis of diabetes by age

Age at diagnosis	Number with retinopathy	Percentage of total in age group
0–29	0	0
30–39	3	1.3
40–49	24	5.6
50–59	66	8.7
60–69	121	16.5
70–79	46	12.4
80–89	8	13.1
Total	268	9.7

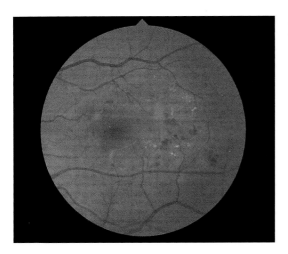

Plate 1 Background retinopathy with microaneurysms, haemorrhages and hard exudates.

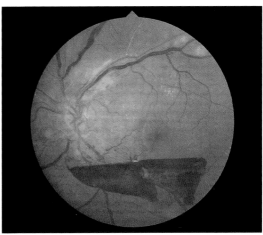

Plate 3 Extensive new vessels on and below the optic disc with preretinal haemorrhage.

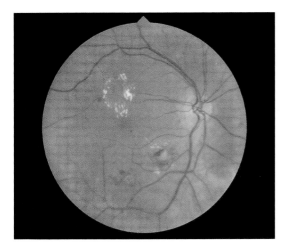

Plate 2 Background retinopathy of microaneurysms and haemorrhages with hard exudates at and above the macula.

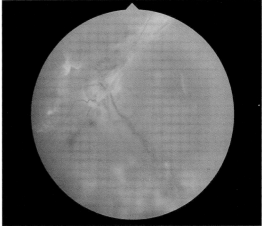

Plate 4 End-stage retinits proliferans with obliteration of the normal retinal architecture.

Table 14.2 Causes of blindness and partial sight among new registrations age 16–64 years for the year ended 31 March 1986 – no. of registrations (%) are given for major conditions only (Source: further details are contained in Department of Health and Social Security, 1988)

	Age groups		
	16–64	*16–54*	*55–64*
Blindness			
Diabetic retinopathy	141 (15.4)	64 (12.3)	77 (19.5)
Optic atrophy	130 (14.2)	99 (19.1)	31 (7.8)
Hereditary retinal dystrophies	110 (12.0)	83 (16.0)	27 (6.8)
Degeneration of macula and posterior pole	80 (8.8)	25 (4.8)	55 (13.9)
Others	453 (49.6)	248 (47.8)	205 (51.9)
Total	914	519	395
Partial sight			
Diabetic retinopathy	119 (12.5)	50 (9.3)	69 (16.7)
Degeneration of macula and posterior pole	88 (9.3)	42 (7.9)	46 (11.1)
Hereditary retinal dystrophies	76 (8.0)	63 (11.8)	13 (3.1)
Optic atrophy	73 (7.6)	56 (10.5)	17 (4.1)
Myopia	64 (6.7)	31 (5.8)	33 (8.0)
Visual field defects	51 (5.4)	22 (4.1)	29 (7.0)
Others	478 (50.4)	271 (50.7)	207 (50.0)
Total	949	535	414

be apparent at the disc or start a disc's breadth or so from it, but does not extend to the peripheral branches, being at times fusiform. The affected veins look darker than normal. In a well developed example the segmental swelling of veins is very characteristic but lesser degrees of enlargement are hard to assess and most physicians would not regard this change alone, in the absence of microaneurysms, as sufficiently diagnostic of diabetic retinopathy.

Microaneurysms are the earliest diagnostic manifestation. While they are usually described as appearing first around the macula it is common to see one or two single dots close to a main vein one or two discs' breadth from the disc, with no lesions at the posterior pole. They are tiny rounded dots 20–50 μm in diameter, dark red and deep in the retina.

During the next stage larger dots and blots – haemorrhages of less regular outline – appear. The blots have been well described as resembling the impression made by a minute sponge soaked in blood. They probably represent haemorrhages from microaneurysms and are situated in the deeper layers of the retina. Like the microaneurysms they tend to be most profuse around the macula but at times are very numerous and distributed all over the retina except the periphery. Exudates occur in the same distribution as the haemorrhages but not in relation to their number. Sometimes exudate is scanty when haemorrhages are very profuse, at others exudate may be widespread with very few haemorrhages. Initially appearing as white specks these exudates later enlarge and coalesce to from masses of varying size which assume a yellowish colour and are described as waxy. Quite often exudates form a ring round the macula, or circinate pattern.

The changes so far described make up the characteristic picture of diabetic retinopathy. The microaneurysms and haemorrhages, aggregated between the main temporal veins, which themselves show characteristic disten-

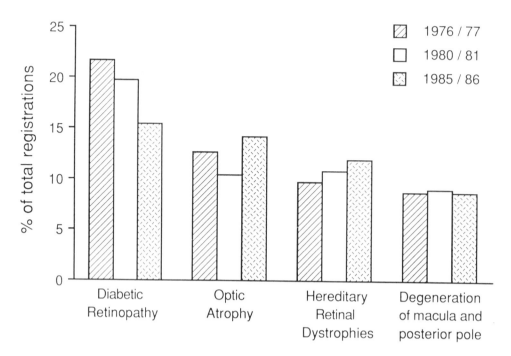

Fig. 14.1 Percentage distribution of the causes of blindness among new registrations of adults aged 16–64 for 12-month periods ending 31 March 1977, 1981 and 1986. (Source: data obtained from Department of Health and Social Security, 1988.)

sion, make a diagnosis of diabetes almost certain. At times a picture of combined hypertensive and diabetic retinopathy may be distinguished. In hypertension there are obvious arterial changes and haemorrhages, which are in the nerve fibre layer, are striate or flame-shaped and bright red.

MACULOPATHY (Plate 2)

Concentration of microaneurysms, haemorrhages and hard exudates around the macula warrants the separate term of maculopathy. As distinct from background changes elsewhere in the retina, which merit careful monitoring but not intervention, maculopathy has important prognostic considerations. A large exudate at the macula may decrease visual acuity gradually or acutely but even when lesser abnormalities occur the patient

is at risk of macular oedema. Hypoxic or damaged vessels are sources of oedema and fluorescein angiography can aid detection of the site of leakage.

RETINITIS PROLIFERANS

An intermediate stage between background retinopathy and proliferation is now well recognized. The warning signs are due to areas of ischaemia in the retina and the manifestations most easily recognized are soft exudates and intraretinal microvascular abnormalities (IRMA). Soft exudates are caused by obstructed arterioles resulting in infarction of the nerve fibre layer. Their appearance is characteristic. Occasionally, profusion of these cotton wool spots is seen, heralding a poor prognosis with a high risk of proliferative change in 1 year. Intraretinal microvascular abnormalities are arteriovenous shunts appearing as dilated capillaries. Distinction between them and neo-vascularization may be difficult at times.

NEOVASCULARIZATION (Plate 3)

New vessel formation takes place quite apart from the typical changes just described and may even be seen rarely when no micro-aneurysms or haemorrhages are visible. The ophthalmoscopic picture is often hard to define because vitreous haemorrhage may well be the first indication that new vessels have formed, and nothing but a haze can be seen. Even when the vitreous is clear some skill is needed in constant changes of the ophthalmoscope lens because the vessels are not all flush with the surface of the retina but often extend forwards at an angle. One may see a simple vein anastomosis, a rete mirabile, horse tails or fans. Fine new vessels appear often at the disc itself. After repeated vitreous haemorrhage fibrous tissue in dense white strands appears along the course of the vessels, often coming forward into the vitreous (Plate 4). When it contracts detachment of the retina may occur.

THE COURSE OF UNTREATED RETINOPATHY

Simple retinopathy with changes in the deep layers of the retina may be visible for as long as 10–15 years before any serious extension interferes with vision but the general rule is for the condition to progress. Undoubtedly the lesions come and go in an inexplicable manner without relation to diabetic control. A florid picture with many microaneurysms and blot haemorrhages may sometimes be replaced a year later by that of minimal disease. Regression of microaneurysms is comparatively common and an annual rate of regression of about 15% in the first year and 3% in the fifth year has been calculated. In the case of haemorrhages and exudate the mean annual regression rate for a 5-year period is about 6%.

Thus a finding of microaneurysms, haemor-rhages and exudates, while of concern, is not necessarily a threat of early disturbance of vision. In fact the visual prognosis is very hard to estimate at this stage. Perhaps the appearance of the veins is the best guide. If they look nearly normal the outlook is good; if they are grossly distended there is a probability of vitreous haemorrhage in the near future. Once new vessel formation has been followed by vitreous haemorrhage the rule is for bleeding to recur. At first the vitreous clears but later a permanent opacity remains. Fibrous tissue appears along the vessels and true retinitis proliferans may occur. Retinal detachment and glaucoma are often the immediate cause of blindness and rubeosis of the iris may give a clue to the gravity of the situation.

Even after repeated vitreous haemorrhage regression to an inactive phase may occur; Beetham (1963) reported that 35 out of 351 patients with proliferative diabetic retino-pathy showed spontaneous arrest over a period of a year or longer. In general he thought the prognosis of the lesions was better than most people believed and the average rate of deterioration was 1.5 years per degree of change (as seen with the ophthalmoscope) dividing the appearances into five degrees from slight to extreme. The prospects were worse in 'mature-onset' than in 'growth-onset' diabetes.

Caird and Garrett (1963) reported serial measurements of visual acuity in patients with and without retinopathy. After 5 years 14.5% of eyes with retinopathy and visual acuity of 6/18 or better had become 'blind' (visual acuity below 6/60) and 34% had a visual acuity of 6/24 or less; 50% of eyes that began at 6/24 or less had become 'blind'. The chances of deterioration were greater the older the patient at the time of diagnosis – in contrast to opinions expressed with less evidence. Curiously there was an insignificant difference between the outlook for eyes with haemorrhages and exudates and those with microaneurysms alone.

PREVENTION AND TREATMENT

Retinopathy is an almost inevitable consequence of long-standing diabetes. Delay of the onset may be achieved by good control of the diabetes (Diabetes Control and Complications Trial Research Group, 1993) and once it has begun delay in progression can be obtained by improvements in diabetic control (Job *et al.*, 1976; Diabetes Control and Complications Trial Research Group, 1993). There is no evidence that the microvascular changes can be reversed by improvement in diabetic control. Assessment of the effect of control has been made difficult by the fluctuation which occurs in diabetic retinopathy. Even repeated vitreous haemorrhage may cease and be followed by a quiet phase, while there are a significant number of people who after active treatment have retinopathy that is quiescent for years. Controlled studies of rapid lowering of blood glucose levels in patients with retinopathy reported a disturbing development of retinal change. Initially thought to be worsening of retinopathy it now appears to be accentuation of ischaemic areas, with gradual recovery even if good control is maintained (Brinchmann-Hansen *et al.*, 1985).

Hypophysectomy in cases of juvenile diabetes was first reported by Luft, Olivecrona and Sjogren (1952). The aim was to eliminate pituitary factors which were known to aggravate the diabetic state. The report by Poulsen (1953) of remarkable remission of retinopathy coinciding with the development of post-partum hypopituitarism stimulated other workers and in 1962 a total of 134 cases were collected in a symposium published in the journal *Diabetes*. The postoperative mortality was 15 (11.2%). Subsequent deaths at intervals up to 6 years from operation numbered 39, of which 20 were due to renal disease, 11 to hypoglycaemia and six to coronary or other vascular disease. The effect upon insulin dosage when ablation was complete was striking. The need for insulin was reduced by half to one-quarter although without an effect upon the ease of diabetic control. Ketoacidosis was rare and ketogenesis impaired, as in the Houssay animal model. Patients unstable before the operation remained so and the problem of hypoglycaemia was aggravated, as the substantial mortality from this cause bears witness. Fortunately such drastic remedies for diabetic retinopathy can be mentioned in the past tense with the advent of photocoagulation.

PHOTOCOAGULATION

Meyer-Schwickerath (1959) pioneered photocoagulation for the treatment of diabetic retinopathy. The discovery of this use for photocoagulation is instructive. The xenon arc lamp was the first source to be used, followed by the ruby laser (Beetham *et al.*, 1970) and the argon laser (L'Esperance, 1968). The argon laser is now most widely used. It produces short flashes of blue-green light at wavelengths of 488 nm (blue) and 514 nm (green). These wavelengths are better absorbed by haemoglobin than the red light (694 nm) of the ruby laser. The burn area of the argon laser is considerably smaller than that of the xenon arc lamp. The latter therefore tends to be painful, often necessitating local anaesthetic during its use. After the introduction of photocoagulation there was a rush to use it, particularly in retinal neovascularization. Since the likely course of new vessels was so poor there was a tendency to treat anyone without evidence of its beneficial value having been obtained from controlled trials.

TREATMENT OF NEW VESSELS

In the initial phase of use of photocoagulation for treatment of new vessels a majority of studies reported beneficial results. This view was not unanimous, however, and some studies reported that the untreated eye fared as well as the treated eye. The need for a controlled trial clearly existed and was finally filled by a number of well-designed and well-executed studies. First among these was the Diabetic Retinopathy Study Research Group (1976). More than 1700 patients with either unilateral or bilateral proliferative retinopathy (or severe non-proliferative retinopathy in both) received treatment to one eye with either the argon laser or the xenon arc lamp. In addition to the panretinal photocoagulation employed, new vessels in the periphery or disc new vessels were treated directly in the patients who received treatment with the argon laser. The endpoint taken was deterioration to blindness (a visual acuity of 5/200 or less) on two visits separated by 4 months. After 3 years of follow-up 26% of untreated eyes were blind and only 8% of those treated with the xenon source and 13% treated with the argon laser. A number of analyses were undertaken to determine which eyes had shown the most favourable outcome with treatment. The most striking difference that emerged was the influence of macular oedema on outcome. When macular oedema was present before treatment 27% of untreated eyes deteriorated to blindness compared with 11% when it was absent at the start of the study. In treated eyes 15% with macular oedema and 7% without deteriorated to blindness over the 3 years.

Hercules *et al.* (1977) followed a similar protocol for treatment in 94 patients with retinal neovascularization. Using panretinal photocoagulation with the argon laser they found that neither eye went blind in 57 patients, both eyes became blind in six and the untreated eye only went blind in 30 patients. In only one patient did the treated eye become blind without blindness being reached in the untreated eye. Similar results were reported by the British Multicentre Study Group (1977). They also found an average loss of only one line in visual acuity

in treated eyes compared with an average loss of four lines in untreated eyes.

TREATMENT OF MACULOPATHY

While blindness most often results from neovascularization it is macular oedema that is responsible for the majority of patients with mild or moderate decreases in visual acuity. Patz *et al.* (1973) showed the improved prognosis for visual acuity in treated eyes and this was subsequently confirmed by Townsend, Bailey and Kohner (1979). They followed patients for 5 years, showing an average visual acuity in treated eyes that was two lines better than untreated eyes. The Early Treatment Diabetic Retinopathy Study Research Group (1985) (ETDRS) treated patients in whom macular oedema was either reducing vision or threatening to do so. They found reduced visual loss with focal argon laser photocoagulation. An important finding of nearly all the studies is that treatment is likely to be most beneficial if given before the visual acuity has deteriorated too far, and conversely prognosis is poor if visual acuity is poor before treatment. Macular oedema is the end result of a number of different lesions at the macula and considerable work has gone into identifying which lesions respond best to treatment. Briefly, focal areas of leakage respond well while poor prognostic findings are diffuse leakage, cystoid macular oedema and hard exudates in the foveal zone.

COMPLICATIONS OF PHOTOCOAGULATION (TABLE 14.3)

The majority of complications of photocoagulation occur after panretinal ablation following intensive treatment with many hundreds of burns.

Occasionally, structures anterior to the retina may be damaged, particularly the ciliary nerves, leading to pupillary abnormalities. Resulting chronic dilatation produces a Holmes–Adie pupil. Transient glaucoma may follow treat-

Table 14.3 Complications of photocoagulation

Anterior
- Non-progressive lens opacities
- Ciliary nerve damage
- Raised intraocular pressure and transient glaucoma
- Transient myopia

Posterior
- Choriovitreal proliferations
- Decreased visual field
- Decreased colour vision
- Decreased dark adaptation
- Foveal burn
- Interruption of macula blood supply
- Ischaemic papillitis

ment, which usually resolves within 7 days. Bruch's membrane may be ruptured leading to chorio-vitreal proliferations, which are difficult to treat.

Some degree of visual field constriction may follow panretinal photocoagulation depending upon the type of laser used and the intensity of treatment. Russell, Sekuler and Fetkenhour (1985) observed that 50% of patients reported visual field abnormality, which can be extensive – up to 50% of field. Repeated treatments are likely to worsen field loss.

Both dark adaptation and colour discrimination may be impaired in untreated patients and both show a tendency to worsen after treatment. Loss of dark adaptation is particularly hazardous when driving at night. Colour loss is a blue–yellow defect. Bleeding from new vessels following rupture may occur with direct attempts to treat peripheral new vessels. Macular oedema with a decline in visual acuity may be a result of panretinal treatment. Fortunately, this usually resolves. Inadvertent treatment of the fovea is a serious complication, while intensive treatment around the macula may occlude the blood supply to the macula and intensive treatment around the disc may occlude the choroidal supply leading to an ischaemic papillitis.

It is not appropriate to conclude this section on a note of treatment difficulties and dangers. Photocoagulation has revolutionized the treatment of diabetic retinopathy. Senior physicians recall the days when the detection of diabetic retinopathy was of interest only – a demonstration of clinical skills to be shown to the junior doctors or medical students. It was no more than that and early detection was of moderate importance. The advent of a treatment has changed the situation such that, with detection and appropriate treatment, diabetic retinopathy is no longer the major cause of morbidity of the previous generation.

DETECTION OF DIABETIC RETINOPATHY

With the advent of successful treatment for diabetic retinopathy has come the responsibility for early detection and careful follow-up. Much has been written on how and by whom this should be done. I should say at the outset that I am unimpressed by the suggestion that the diabetologist is too busy to visualize the fundi of his or her patients. In any list of the duties and responsibilities of a diabetologist fundal examination would be near to, or at, the top. How is the time being spent if ophthalmoscopy is not being performed? Thus alternatives to ophthalmoscopy by the physician are only justified to my mind if they increase the detection rates of retinopathy of moderate degree or more severe, where treatment is indicated.

Suggested methods of screening for diabetic retinopathy have included training nurse practitioners, schemes involving the use of ophthalmic opticians and the use of photography. The use of non-mydriatic retinal photography has been assessed by a number of groups (Ryder *et al.*, 1985; Taylor *et al.*, 1990). It is as good as fundoscopy with mydriasis in routine clinics in detecting new vessel formation but is superior in detecting maculopathy (Taylor *et al.*, 1990). It must be borne in mind, however, that at the moment the photographs are reviewed by a trained

Table 14.4 Indications and contraindications for vitrectomy

Indications	Contraindications
Recurrent vitreous haemorrhage	No light perception
Bilateral vitreous haemorrhage	Neovascularization of iris
Disabling vitreous haemorrhage	Severe glaucoma
Tractional retinal detachment, particularly if recent or involving macula	Ischaemic optic neuritis
Inactive neovascularization	Active neovascularization

operator, i.e. a person trained through ophthalmoscopy, and results might be less impressive if the skill of ophthalmoscopy in the diabetic clinic is allowed to atrophy.

VITRECTOMY

Severe vitreous haemorrhage with retinal detachment may necessitate vitrectomy (Table 14.4). Where this is indicated early treatment is advisable since retinal function declines with duration of detachment. Good results are reported, about two-thirds of patients showing improvement, although further retinal detachment and neovascular glaucoma are acknowledged side effects.

OTHER DISORDERS OF THE EYE

TRANSITORY CHANGES IN REFRACTION

At the onset of major diabetic symptoms a change in refraction is common and nearly always predicts severe diabetes which will need more than dietary restriction. It was noted by Horner in 1873 and is often the presenting symptom of diabetes. Like the thirst it may pass spontaneously without treatment and return months later. Typically the change is myopic (2–3 dioptres), but rarely can be hypermetropic.

When treatment is begun the myopic change is quickly corrected. Rarely, under treatment the reverse effect is seen, the patient becoming less hypermetropic or even myopic. Those who have not previously noticed any disturbance of vision may, within a day or two of starting treatment, become hypermetropic and find that vision loses definition at all distances. This phase lasts 2–3 weeks, never long, and corrects itself completely. Patients can be reassured (and often need to be), while they must obviously not be tested for new glasses until it is over, though temporary glasses can be provided.

The mechanism of the refractive change is unknown. The suggestion that variations in hydration of the lens are responsible hardly explains the persistence of the refractive error long after the blood glucose is corrected. It is possible that changes in the ciliary processes or the vitreous are involved.

CHANGES IN VISION DURING HYPOGLYCAEMIA

Difficulty in focusing, mistiness, visual field defects, diplopia and flashing lights are described by patients at the onset of a hypoglycaemic attack and are a common warning symptom. They are presumably central in origin, nuclear and cortical.

The pattern of symptoms is fairly constant for each individual patient. Some recognize this form of onset as the warning of a severe rather than a mild hypoglycaemic attack.

WEAKNESS OF ACCOMMODATION

Paresis of accommodation was found in 21% of 759 diabetic eyes studied by Waite and Beetham (1935). It is most often seen in young patents and is usually sudden in onset. The weakness, which is bilateral, may be of the order of 3–4 dioptres or at times complete. The pupil reaction remains normal. Glycogen deposits, which occur frequently in this area and certainly in the ciliary body, have been suggested as the cause.

PUPIL CHANGES

Irregularity, sluggish light reflex and the true Argyll Robertson pupil have been recorded in diabetic patients, but nearly always in association with gross neuropathy. A miotic pupil that reacts sluggishly to light and better to accommodation is probably the most common change. Sometimes glycogen is deposited in the muscles of the sphincter and may then be the cause of an absent or sluggish pupil response. Loss of pupillary oscillation (hippus) is also a common manifestation of autonomic neuropathy.

IRITIS

The incidence of iritis in diabetics does not exceed that of the general population (Waite and Beetham, 1935) although at times it has been suggested that a true autoimmune iritis may occur.

DEPIGMENTATION OF THE IRIS

There is cystic degeneration of the pigment layer on the posterior surface of the iris, and pigment may be deposited on the posterior surface of the cornea. Waite and Beetham (1935) found this change in 6% of diabetic eyes but in only 2% of non-diabetic eyes. The appearance, also called lacy vacuolization, which can be seen as pinhole defects with a slit lamp, results from deposits of glycogen in vacuoles.

RUBEOSIS IRIDIS DIABETICA

The name was given by Salus (1928) to an appearance of blood-red discoloration of the central part of the iris. Close examination shows that this is due to a network of small vessels forming a ring just outside the margin of the pupil but not passing over it. New vessels may be seen, using the ophthalmoscope, at the periphery of the iris spreading over the angle to form vascular synechiae. The neovascularization seems to be an extension of changes in the retina and always occurs in association with advanced retinopathy, being therefore rather more common than earlier writers suggested. There is a great risk of congestive glaucoma and recognition of rubeosis is of some importance as a warning of this disaster. It would preclude holidays or travel away from facilities for emergency ophthalmic treatment. Rubeotic glaucoma should always be suspected in a patient with a painful eye and a history of proliferative retinopathy.

THE DIABETIC CATARACT

The first description of specific changes in the diabetic lens was by Schnyder (1923). 'Diabetic' cataracts are becoming less common as the incidence of very poor control of diabetes diminishes. They were always rare, occurring mainly in young patients below the age of 25. The highest reported incidence was 16% but others found a more realistic incidence of around 4–5%.

The lens changes start with small greyish-white snowflake opacities immediately under the capsules of the lens, especially the posterior. Subcapsular vacuoles, which are seen with the slit-lamp to contain iridescent jewels, and clefts are a feature. Gradually a diffuse grey mistiness develops and the white opacities coalesce. Sometimes a saucer-like posterior subcapsular cataract forms. Finally the whole lens looks greyish-white. This total opacity may be reached rapidly, within 2–3 weeks, in young children even in a few days. Treatment of the diabetes may arrest the process at any stage, but does not necessarily do so. Temporary cataract, in which lens opacities clear completely, is a rare condition. It probably occurs when clefts in a hazy lens are the cause of the opacity and may occur at any position of the lens. The clearing occurs in a few days. Temporary cataracts occur also in cholera, presumably associated with dehydration.

Pathogenesis

True diabetic cataract is indistinguishable from those of hypoparathyroidism, dystrophia myotonica, galactose intolerance or neutron irradiation. Experimentally the changes can be produced by extirpation of the pancreas. Animals develop cataracts when kept on a diet deficient in tryptophan or when fed monosaccharides such as galactose.

No doubt diabetic cataract is metabolic but its nature is not fully explained. Uptake of glucose by the lens is enhanced in the presence of hyperglycaemia and the sorbitol pathway has been implicated in the development of this type of cataract. The evidence is somewhat circumstantial. The development of cataract is closely related to the level of the blood glucose and if that is lowered, for example by phlorizin, which does not improve metabolism, the onset of cataract is delayed. Morphologically, these cataracts are similar to those produced by feeding experimental animals diets high in galactose. As far as diabetic cataract in man is concerned there is no question that the lens opacities appear only during a period of very poor control.

Treatment

Strict control of the diabetes is vital. Surgical removal of the cataract at the appropriate time yields admirable results.

SENILE CATARACT

It has usually been held that senile cataract is no more common in diabetic than non-diabetic populations. It is obviously difficult

to avoid selection in either instance. Caird, Hutchinson and Pirie (1964) tried to overcome this difficulty by studying a compact population served by only one ophthalmic hospital. It seemed that extraction of senile cataract was between four and six times as common in diabetic than non-diabetic patients of both sexes, taking into account all the difficulties of comparison. These workers could not show that senile cataract appears at an earlier age in diabetics. In view of the apparent relation of diabetic control to lens opacity in the young, one would expect an increased incidence of senile cataract in older patients, especially those with poor control. There is some evidence for this in the figures of Caird, Hutchinson and Pirie (1964) and the cataract was the presenting feature in as many as one-third.

The appearance of the lens in the diabetic with senile cataract has no distinguishing features, with the possible exception of the diabetic 'needle' or 'Roman numeral', which appears as a linear opacity at the periphery of the lens, arranged like the figures on a clock. This can be distinguished from the ordinary cuneiform cataract because it is not thicker at the peripheral than at the central end. 'Needles' are suggestive, perhaps diagnostic, of diabetes.

Treatment

There is no reason to withhold surgical treatment from the diabetic with cataract. The results of lens extraction are not significantly worse than in the non-diabetic. The specific problem is that of retinopathy. The lens opacity often makes the diagnosis of retinal disease a matter of guesswork based on the duration of diabetes and the record of proteinuria. The result of operation can therefore be predicted with less confidence in a diabetic but this should not influence too strongly the decision to operate.

GLAUCOMA

A number of studies suggest that the intra-ocular pressures of a diabetic population are higher than those in non-diabetic control subjects. Pressure is affected by changes in blood glucose concentration and by the presence of background diabetic retinopathy. Proliferative retinopathy does not seem to have an effect upon intraocular pressure except in the presence of advanced retinopathy and rubeosis iridis.

There has been a suggestion abroad for many years that glaucoma or raised intra-ocular pressure may protect against diabetic retinopathy. It is based mainly upon the finding in patients with unilateral elevated intraocular pressure that this eye shows less diabetic retinopathy than the normal-pressure eye.

DISC LESIONS

Lubow and Makley (1971) described a condition they labelled pseudopapilloedema, which occurred in young diabetics. Others have confirmed an acute disc oedema which may be unilateral or bilateral. Clinically there is deterioration in visual acuity, visual field loss, which may be an enlarged blind spot or other scotoma, or the patient may be asymptomatic. The appearance of the disc may show severe swelling or mild oedema. The former may be accompanied by hard and soft exudates. Prognosis for full recovery is excellent.

In middle-aged individuals unilateral swelling of the disc may result from ischaemic optic neuritis, a condition found also in non-diabetic people. Prognosis for retaining useful vision in the affected eye is poor.

REFERENCES

Antonelli-Orlidge, A., Saunders, K. B., Smith, S. R. and D'Amore, P. A. (1989) An activated form of transforming growth factor Beta is produced by cocultures of endothelial cells and pericytes. *Proc. Nat. Acad. Sci. USA*, **86**, 4544–4548.

Ashton, N. (1953) Arteriolar involvement in diabetic retinopathy. *Br. J. Ophthalmol.*, **37**, 282–292.

Baird, A., Esch, F., Gospodarowicz, D. and Guillemin, R. (1985) Retina- and eye-derived endothelial cell growth factors: partial molecular characterization and identity with acidic and basic fibroblast growth factors. *Biochemistry*, **24**, 7855–7860.

Ballantyne, A. J. and Loewenstein, A. (1943) The pathology of the retina in diabetes mellitus. *Trans. Ophthalmol. Soc. UK*, **63**, 95–115.

Beetham, W. P. (1963) Visual prognosis of proliferating diabetic retinopathy. *Br. J. Ophthalmol.*, **47**, 611–619.

Beetham, W. P., Aiello, L. M., Balodimos, M. C. and Koncz, L. (1970) Ruby laser photocoagulation of early diabetic neovascular retinopathy. *Arch. Ophthalmol.*, **83**, 261–272.

Brinchmann-Hansen, O., Dahl-Jorgensen, K., Hanssen, K. F. *et al.* (1985) Effects of intensified insulin treatment on various lesions of diabetic retinopathy. *Am. J. Ophthalmol.*, **100**, 644–653.

British Multicentre Study Group (1977) Proliferative diabetic retinopathy: treatment with xenon-arc photocoagulation. *Br. Med. J.*, **i**, 739–741.

Caird, F. I. and Garrett, C. J. (1962) Progression and regression of diabetic retinopathy. *Proc. Roy. Soc. Med.*, **55**, 477–479.

Caird, F. I., Hutchinson, M. and Pirie, A. (1964) Cataract and diabetes. *Br. Med. J.*, **ii**, 665–668.

Chavers, B. M., Mauer, S. M., Ramsay, R. C. and Steffes, M. W. (1994) Relationship between retinal and glomerular lesions in IDDM patients. *Diabetes*, **43**, 441–446.

Cogan, D. G. and Kuwabara, T. (1963) Capillary shunts in the pathogenesis of diabetic retinopathy. *Diabetes*, **12**, 293–300.

Cogan, D. G., Toussaint, D. and Kuwabara, T. (1961) Retinal vascular patterns. IV Diabetic retinopathy. *Arch. Ophthalmol.*, **66**, 366–378.

DAMAD Study Group (1989) Effect of aspirin alone and aspirin plus dipyridamole in early diabetic retinopathy. *Diabetes*, **38**, 491–498.

D'Amore, P. A. and Klagsbrun, M. (1984) Endothelial cell mitogens derived from retina and hypothalamus: biochemical and biological similarities. *J. Cell Biol.*, **99**, 1545–1549.

Department of Health and Social Security Statistical Bulletin, (1988) Issued 3/8/88, DHSS, London.

Diabetes Control and Complications Trial Research Group (1993) The effect of intensive treatment of diabetes on the development and progression of long-term complications in insulin-dependent diabetes mellitus. *N. Engl. J. Med.*, **329**, 977–986.

Diabetic Retinopathy Study Research Group (1976) Preliminary report on effects of photocoagulation therapy. *Am. J. Ophthalmol.*, **81**, 383–396.

Dunlop, D. M. (1954) Are diabetic degenerative complications preventable? *Br. Med. J.*, **2**, 383–385.

Early Treatment Diabetic Retinopathy Study Research Group (1985) Photocoagulation for diabetic macular oedema. *Arch. Ophthalmol.*, **103**, 1796–1806.

EURODIAB Complications Study Group (1994) Microvascular and acute complications in IDDM patients: the EURODIAB IDDM Complications Study. *Diabetologia*, **37** 278–285.

Fallon, T. J., Chowiencyzk, P. and Kohner, E. (1986) Measurement of retinal blood flow in diabetes by the blue-light entoptic phenomenon. *Br. J. Ophthalmol.*, **70**, 43–46.

Grunwald, J. E. Riva, C. E. Sinclair, S. H. *et al.* (1986) Laser doppler velocimetry study of retinal circulation in diabetes mellitus. *Arch. Ophthalmol.*, **104** 991–996.

Hercules, B. L. Gayed, I. I., Lucas, S. B. and Jeacock, J. (1977) Peripheral retinal ablation in the treatment of proliferative diabetic retinopathy: a three-year interim report of a randomised, controlled study using the argon laser. *Br. J. Ophthalmol.*, **61**, 555–563.

Horner, J. F. (1873) Refractionsänderungen. *Klin. Mbl. Augenheilk.*, **11**, 488–489.

Jaeger, E. (1855) *Beitrage zu Pathologie des Auges* KK Hof und Staatsdruckerei, Vienna, p. 33.

Job, D., Eschwege, E., Guyot-Argenton, C. *et al.* (1976) Effect of multiple daily insulin injections on the course of diabetic retinopathy. *Diabetes*, **25**, 463–469.

Klein, R., Klein, B. E. K., Moss, S. E. *et al.* (1984) The Wisconsin epidemiologic study of diabetic retinopathy. *Arch. Ophthalmol.*, **102**, 520–526; 527–532.

Krieger, D. T., Sirota, D. K. and Lieberman, T. (1970) Cryohypophysectomy for diabetic retinopathy. *Ann. Intern. Med.*, **72**, 309–316.

Kroc Collaborative Study Group (1988) Diabetic retinopathy after two years of intensified insulin treatment. *J.A.M.A.*, **260**, 37–41.

Kuwabara, T. and Cogan, D. G. (1960) Studies of retinal vascular patterns. I Normal architecture. *Arch. Ophthalmol.*, **64**, 904–911.

Lauritzen, T., Frost-Larsen, K., Larsen H. W. *et al.* (1983) Effect of one year of near-normal blood glucose levels on retinopathy in insulin-dependent diabetics. *Lancet*, **i**, 200–204.

Leslie, R. D. G. and Pyke, D. A. (1982) Diabetic retinopathy in identical twins. *Diabetes*, **31**, 19–21.

L'Esperance, F. A. (1968) An ophthalmic argon laser photocoagulation system; design, construction and laboratory investigations. *Trans. Am. Ophthalmol. Soc.*, **66**, 827–904.

Little, H. L., Zweng, H. C. and Peabody, R. R. (1970) Argon laser slit-lamp retinal photocoagulation. *Trans. Am. Acad. Ophthalmol. Otolaryngol.*, **74**, 85–89.

Lubow, M. and Makley, T. A. (1971) Pseudo-papilledema of juvenile diabetes mellitus. *Arch. Ophthalmol.*, **85**, 417–422.

Luft, R., Olivecrona, H. and Sjogren, B. (1952) Hypopysectomi på manniska. *Nord. Med.*, **47**, 351–354.

Mackenzie S. and Nettleship E (1879) A case of glycosuric retinitis with comments: microscopical examination of the eyes. *Ophth. Hosp. Rep. Lond.*, **9**, 134–137.

Meyer-Schwickerath, G. (1959) *Lichtcoagulation*, Enke Verlag, Stuttgart.

Michaelson, I. C. (1948) The mode of development of the vascular system of the retina. *Trans. Ophthalmol. Soc. UK*, **68**, 137–180.

Nettleship, E. (1888) Chronic retinitis in diabetes. *Trans. Ophthalmol. Soc. UK.*, **8**, 159–162.

Orlidge, A. and D'Amore, P. A. (1987) Inhibition of capillary endothelial cell growth by pericyte and smooth muscle cells. *J. Cell Biol.*, **105**, 1455–1462.

Patz, A., Schatz, H., Berkow, J. W. *et al.* (1973) Macular edema – an overlooked complication of diabetic retinopathy. *Trans. Am. Acad. Ophthalmol. Otolaryngol.*, **77**, 34–42.

Pirart, J. (1978) Diabetes mellitus and its degenerative complications: a prospective study of 4400 patients observed between 1947 and 1973. *Diabetes Care*, **1**, 168–188; 252–263.

Poulsen, J. E. (1953) The Houssay phenomenon in man: recovery from diabetic retinopathy in a case of diabetes with Simmonds' disease. *Diabetes*, **2**, 7–12.

Russell, P. W., Sekuler, R. and Fetkenhour, C. (1985) Visual function after pan-retinal photocoagulation: a survey. *Diabetes Care*, **8**, 57–63.

Ryder, R. E. J., Vora, J. P., Atiea, J. A. *et al.* (1985) Possible new method to improve detection of diabetic retinopathy: Polaroid non-mydriatic retinal photography. *Br. Med. J.*, **291**, 1256–1257.

Salus, R. (1928) Rubeosis iridis diabetica, eine bisher unbekannte diabetische Irisveränderung. *Med. Klin.*, **24**, 256–258.

Schnyder, W. F. (1923) Untersuchungen über Vorkommmen und Morphologie der Cataracta diabetica. *Klin. Mbl. Augenheilk.*, **70**, 45–78.

Schwelgerer, L. Neufeld, G., Friedman, J. *et al.* (1987) Capillary endothelial cells express basic fibroblast growth factor, a mitogen that promotes their own growth. *Nature*, **325**, 257–259.

Scott, G. I. (1951) Diabetic retinopathy. *Proc. Roy. Soc. Med.*, **44**, 744–747.

Sorsby, A. (1963) *Modern Ophthalmology*, vol. 1, Butterworth, London, p. 505.

Sorsby, A. (1972) *The Incidence and Causes of Blindness in England and Wales 1963–1968*, Reports on Public Health and Medical Subjects No. 28, Her Majesty's Stationery Office, London.

Takahashi, K., Brooks, R. A., Kanse, S. M. *et al.* (1989) Production of endothelin 1 by cultured bovine retinal endothelial cells and presence of endothelin receptors on associated pericytes. *Diabetes*, **38**, 1200–1202.

Taylor, R. Lovelock, L. Tunbridge, W. M. G. *et al.* (1990) Comparison of non-mydriatic retinal photography with ophthalmoscopy in 2159 patients: mobile retinal camera study. *Br. Med. J.*, **301**, 1243–1247.

Townsend, C., Bailey, J. and Kohner, E. M. (1979) Xenon arc photocoagulation in the treatment of diabetic maculopathy. *Trans. Ophthalmol. Soc. UK*, **99**, 13–16.

Waite, J. H. and Beetham, W. P. (1935) The visual mechanism in diabetes mellitus. *N. Engl. J. Med.*, **212**, 367–37; 429–443.

Williamson, J. R., Chang, K., Tilton, R. G. *et al.* (1987) Increased vascular permeability in spontaneously diabetic BB/W rats and in rats with mild versus severe streptozocin-induced diabetes. *Diabetes*, **36**, 813–821.

Yanagisawa, M., Kurihara, H., Kimura, S. *et al.* (1988) A novel potent vasoconstrictor peptide produced by vascular endothelial cells. *Nature*, **332**, 411–415.

Yanko, L., Goldbourt, U., Michaelson, I. C. *et al.* (1983) Prevalence and 15-year incidence of retinopathy and associated characteristics in middle-aged and elderly diabetic men. *Br. J. Ophthalmol.* **67**, 759–765.

Erasmus Darwin (1801) was the first to recognize a form of diabetes in which the urine could be coagulated by heat and he associated this combination with the appearance of dropsy. Armanni (1875) described hyaline vacuolization of the tubular epithelium of the kidney (later shown to be due to the presence of glycogen), which for many years was regarded as the most valuable evidence of diabetes available at postmortem. Changes in the glomeruli of the diabetic kidney were first observed by Bell and Clawson (1928), who published a photograph of a nodular lesion, but it was not until Kimmelstiel and Wilson (1936) emphasized the distinctive character of the nodular changes in the glomeruli of eight patients, of whom seven had definite diabetes, that the idea of a specific diabetic renal disease (diabetic nephropathy) was born.

Laipply, Eitzen and Dutra (1944) reported that a diffuse type of glomerulosclerosis also occurred, but this was not generally accepted as an essential and specific part of the diabetic lesion until the same changes were fully described by Bell (1950). Many writers have claimed that the nodular lesion is always accompanied by diffuse glomerulosclerosis (Gellman et al., 1959) and have assumed that it is merely an advanced manifestation of the same process. Kimmelstiel (1966) believed, however, that the nodular and diffuse changes were separate, the former being highly specific for diabetes and the latter non-specific, but that both types of change resulted from altered metabolism in the 'mesangial' cells lying between the glomerular capillaries.

When Kimmelstiel and Wilson (1936) first described nodular intercapillary glomerulo-sclerosis they pointed out that most of their patients had renal failure, proteinuria and oedema and clinicians have tended to use the term 'Kimmelstiel–Wilson kidney' to designate not a histological lesion but a clinical syndrome. Yet even the early reports that followed the paper of Kimmelstiel and Wilson made it clear that this was misleading, since by no means all the patients with the nodular lesion had the clinical syndrome.

The advent of percutaneous renal biopsy confirmed this observation and clarified the position, since studies could now be made on living patients and the analysis of clinical detail was no longer based on retrospective reading of case notes following the study of post-mortem material. It is now apparent that a considerable proportion of diabetic patients show diffuse glomerular changes without evidence of renal failure or proteinuria. Indeed, the greater resolution that can be obtained with the electron microscope has suggested that even when light microscopy appears to show normal appearances there may be considerable thickening of the basement membrane.

While diabetic nephropathy leading to renal failure has been the focus of attention for many years it has also become apparent that diabetes influences the kidney throughout the life of the diabetic patient – from diagnosis to death. Diabetic nephropathy is part of this spectrum, sadly often the terminal part, but it also includes alterations in form and function before nephropathy is present and the influence upon the kidney of associated diseases such as infection, atherosclerosis and tubular lesions. Some earlier writers allowed diabetic nephropathy to include changes due to atheroma and pyelonephritis but this is no longer admissible and the term nephropathy should be confined to the glomerular lesion.

CHANGES IN STRUCTURE AND FUNCTION OF THE KIDNEY EARLY IN THE DISEASE

STRUCTURAL CHANGE

At diagnosis of insulin-dependent diabetes a number of changes in kidney structure can be detected. Of particular interest, since it is reflected in function, is the finding that the kidney is larger than in control non-diabetic subjects (Mogensen and Anderson, 1972; Mogensen, Osterby and Gundersen, 1979). This is a generalized renal hypertrophy rather than an infiltrative or osmotic condition, which extends to an increase in glomerular volume and size (Osterby and Gundersen, 1975). That it is a relatively acute change has been confirmed in the rat when increased glomerular volume occurs after induction of diabetes. Osterby and Gundersen (1980) observed a 30% increase after only 4 days of diabetes. The renal tubules also participate in kidney expansion, albeit at a slower rate (Seyer-Hansen, Hansen and Gundersen, 1980). The underlying mechanism for these changes remains elusive, although at moderate degrees of hyperglycemia there is a close relationship between kidney growth and hyperglycaemia, which can be prevented by insulin (Seyer-Hansen, 1977).

Microscopy at this stage reveals some accumulation of basement membrane material in the glomeruli, which is not reversible with 4 weeks of diabetic control. The subsequent course of these early abnormalities is unclear although the kidney remains large (Ellis *et al.*, 1985). When sequential biopsies have been performed they reveal a 15% thickening of basement membrane after 2–3 years of diabetes and a 25% thickening after 5 years (Osterby, 1986).

FUNCTIONAL CHANGE

Alterations in function mirror structural change. Cambier (1934) proposed that diabetic patients had an elevated glomerular filtration rate and this has been repeatedly confirmed. The mechanism by which it comes about remains obscure, although a contribution from hyperglycaemia, insulin lack and other hormonal factors seems likely (Viberti and Wiseman, 1986). The elevated glomerular filtration rate corresponds to the enhanced filtration surface, which has been estimated to show an increase of 80% (Kroustrup, Gundersen and Osterby, 1977). In the later stages of diabetic nephropathy there is a strong relationship between loss of filtration surface and declining renal function with proteinuria. In the early phase the situation is less clear although glomerular leak of protein may occur.

THE DEVELOPMENT OF DIABETIC NEPHROPATHY

The first clinical manifestation of nephropathy is proteinuria. It is difficult therefore to overestimate the importance of a finding of proteinuria at any stage of diabetes. Yet the detection of proteinuria is somewhat arbitrary, resulting from the skill of the industrial chemist in devising a simple test. This has been highlighted by recent interest in microalbuminuria or microproteinuria. These terms refer to a small concentration of albumin in the urine measured by radioimmunoassay or similar sensitive technique. When measured in this way it is clear that proteinuria (microalbuminuria) can be detected long before it is found using the routine but less sensitive tests based on colour change or precipitation with sulphasalicylic acid.

MICROALBUMINURIA

It was Keen and Chlouverakis who in 1963 reported a sensitive radioimmunoassay for albumin in urine capable of detecting low concentrations. Subsequent studies showed that small yet abnormal amounts of albumin could be detected in this way which were not detected by less specific methods particularly the routine tests of clinical practice. Viberti *et al.* (1982) introduced the term 'microalbuminuria' to describe the presence of small amounts of protein in the urine not detectable by Albustix or precipitation with sulphasalicylic acid. Although the term leaves a lot to be desired in the use of the English language, referring to small amounts rather than small proteins, it has passed into common usage.

Normal healthy subjects excrete small amounts of albumin – approximately 5 μg/min although it may be up to 12.5 μg/min. Excretion over 24 hours varies somewhat between investigators, more as a result of the conditions under which the 24-hour collection is made rather than for technical reasons. About 92% of healthy individuals excrete less than 18 mg/24 hours. (Viberti, Wiseman and Redmond, 1984). At the other end of the scale clinical proteinuria, that is Albustix-detectable proteinuria, corresponds to a 24-hour excretion rate greater than 250 mg/24 hours. The interval between normal albumin excretion and clinical proteinuria (an unsatisfactory term but preferable to the ugly and totally incorrect term 'macroproteinuria', which some people persist in using) is assigned to microalbuminuria.

Urinary albumin excretion in healthy individuals is affected by posture and exercise. In diabetic patients it has been shown to be abnormal in newly diagnosed insulin-dependent diabetics (Mogensen, 1971), in insulin-dependent patients after insulin withdrawal (Parving *et al.*, 1976) and in newly-detected non-insulin-dependent patients (Keen *et al.*, 1969). In established insulin-dependent diabetic patients it correlates with hyperglycaemia (Viberti, Mackintosh and Keen, 1983) and blood pressure (Wiseman *et al.*, 1984).

It is clear, therefore, that microalbuminuria may occur at an early stage of diabetes or at a time of poor blood glucose control and that the abnormality may be reversible at this stage. The question arises as to whether it is anything more than an epiphenomenon; i.e. does it have any prognostic meaning?

In longitudinal studies it is reported that urinary albumin excretion will increase slowly with duration of disease. In cohort studies there appears to be a threshold above which progression to clinical proteinuria is likely (Viberti *et al.*, 1982; Mathiesen *et al.*, 1984; Mogensen and Christensen, 1984). There is a lack of uniformity about the actual level. The range is from 15 μg/min (Mogensen and Christensen, 1984) to 70 μg/min (Mathiesen *et al.*, 1984). This latter value is based on 24-hour urine collections, which tend to give higher results because of the effect upon protein excretion of exercise.

Much has been made of this phase of incipient diabetic nephropathy. About 80% of diabetics with albumin excretion in the risk range develop overt nephropathy (Viberti *et al.*, 1982). The relative risk of developing overt nephropathy is increased 20-fold when albumin excretion rate exceeds the threshold. But it must be remembered that microalbuminuria is not a distinct entity – all that is being measured is proteinuria, albeit by sensitive methodology. The fundamental question is whether the detection of microalbuminuria signals anything other than diabetic nephropathy detected earlier. That is, is it a stage in the development of diabetic nephropathy at which change is reversible, progression can be slowed or deterioration halted?

There is no clear answer to this question and perhaps it will prove impossible to answer. In any group of patients for study a contribution to the microalbuminuria will come from poor diabetic control, hypertension and diabetic nephropathy. Thus improvement in blood glucose control and treatment of hypertension could lower albumin excretion without having any effect upon diabetic nephropathy.

Even the instigation of tight blood glucose control does not universally lower albumin excretion (Feldt-Rasmussen *et al.*, 1986). Low protein diets will lower albumin excretion (Viberti and Wiseman, 1986) but their effect upon nephropathy is unknown. Treatment of hypertension early has been the focus of attack yet the ability of antihypertensive agents to postpone nephropathy remains unconvincing (Mathiesen *et al.*, 1991).

It might have been better if the term microalbuminuria had not been invented. Linguistically abhorrent, it purports to define a specific phase in a continuum – yet the phase has no individualistic meaning because it is defined only by the sensitivity of laboratory tests. It has led to exaggerated claims and hijacking of resources (can you really have a 20th century diabetic clinic without microalbuminuria measurement?), yet the interpretation remains illusory.

CLINICAL PROTEINURIA

After the stage of microalbuminuria comes that of proteinuria detected by more conventional tests. Proteinuria heralding diabetic nephropathy has a typical pattern which, while inconclusive in solitary samples of urine, becomes readily apparent from careful records of urine tests for protein during the years of diabetes.

At first proteinuria is slight and intermittent and may remain so for 5–10 years but there is generally a steady increase in both frequency and amount. Retinopathy is apparent a few years earlier or later than the first record of proteinuria and in the later stages runs roughly parallel with the degree of renal functional impairment, although there are notable and obvious exceptions to this. An occasional case of hopelessly destructive retinopathy retains adequate renal function for 10 or more years after the patient has become blind. Less often, a diabetic reaches the final stage of renal failure with retinopathy of only moderate degree.

The period of time when intermittent proteinuria is detected may last months or a few years. Eventually proteinuria becomes constant and heavier, such that the maximum amount detectable by routine tests is found in the urine on each attendance in the clinic. During the period of constant, heavy proteinuria serum creatinine remains within the normal range or just above it.

As with the previous phase this one also lasts a variable length of time. Eventually it is superseded by an accelerated phase leading to end-stage renal failure. A progressive rise in serum creatinine marks the beginning of this decline in renal function.

About 15% of patients attending a diabetic clinic will have shown proteinuria more than once in their last 2 years of clinic attendance. In the main these patients are women whose diabetes is diagnosed in middle or later life but it is not uncommon to find it in young males. In patients under the age of 30 it is unusual for proteinuria to be recorded within the first 10 years of diagnosed diabetes but in later life the interval is much shorter and over the age of 70 the mean duration is only just above 2 years, while many have proteinuria at the time of diagnosis of diabetes (Figure 15.1). Experience has indicated that isolated finding of a trace of proteinuria may occur commonly in the first 5 years of diabetes in young subjects, but it can be many years before the next positive clinic specimen is obtained.

Table 15.1 shows the cause of proteinuria in a random sample of a hundred patients from the diabetic clinic. In men nephropathy seems to be virtually the only cause and the same is true for all patients under the age of 40. It is only in middle-aged and elderly women that causes other than nephropathy become significant, but even then nephropathy is nearly always a contributory factor. In no case was infection thought to be the sole cause of proteinuria. Indeed it was sur-

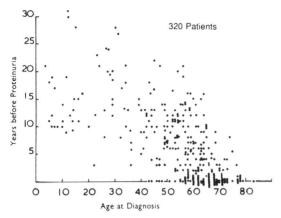

Fig. 15.1 The relationship of age at diagnosis to the appearance of proteinuria. (Source: from O'Sullivan, 1961.)

PATHOLOGY OF DIABETIC NEPHROPATHY

LIGHT MICROSCOPY

A variety of glomerular appearances can be found in the diabetic kidney by light microscopy. The unifying end point is glomerulosclerosis with extensive hyalinization. This may be preceded by nodular (Figure 15.2) or diffuse (Figure 15.3) lesions.

Nodular lesions (Figure 15.2) may affect the centre of single or multiple peripheral glomerular lobules. As the nodules become larger the deposits come to resemble more and more the Kimmelsteil–Wilson nodules. The fully developed lesion may be round or spherical, homogeneous or vacuolated, and fibrillar or lamellar. The nodules are pathognomic of diabetes.

A diffuse glomerular lesion (Figure 15.3) is also recognized. It is twice as common as the nodular lesion and correlates to a greater extent with the degree of renal impairment (Gellmann *et al.*, 1959). The lesion begins with thickening of the wall of peripheral capillaries of the glomerular tuft. As it progresses the lesion becomes diffuse within the glomerulus and generalized within the kidney. Narrowing of the capillary lumen occurs, with eventual hyalinization. Gellman *et al.* (1959) emphasized that the nodular lesions only occur in glomeruli displaying diffuse lesions (Figure 15.4), although they regarded the two as distinct entities.

prising to find that the incidence of urinary tract infection is no greater in diabetics with proteinuria than in the diabetic or non-diabetic populations as a whole. This contradicts the experience of others, but both proteinuria and infection are most often found in middle-aged women and if age and sex are taken into account the direct relationship between the two findings disappears.

Renal biopsy studies have made it clear that diabetic patients with proteinuria almost invariably have moderate or severe diffuse glomerular lesions although changes of comparable severity may also be seen in biopsies taken from patients without proteinuria.

Table 15.1 Causes of proteinuria in 100 diabetic patients

Age	Sex	Total	Diabetic nephropathy	Other causes	Not known
0–19	Males	7	7	0	0
	Females	5	3	0	2
20–39	Males	7	7	0	0
	Females	9	8	0	1
40–59	Males	11	10	0	1
	Females	30	24	4	2
> 60	Males	8	7	0	1
	Females	23	17	3	3
Total		100	83	7	10

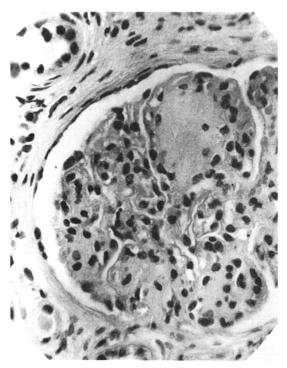

Fig. 15.2   Glomerulus from a diabetic patient showing the characteristic nodular lesion (H&E stain; × 450).

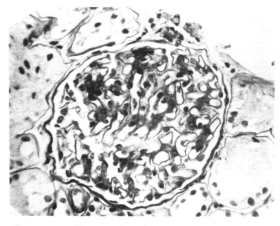

Fig. 15.3   Glomerulus from a diabetic patient showing an early diffuse lesion (PAS stain; × 450).

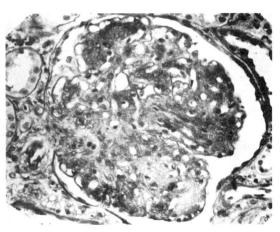

Fig. 15.4   Glomerulus from a 38-year-old diabetic patient after 18 years of diabetes. An advanced diffuse lesion is present with early nodule formation (PAS stain; × 375).

Others have concluded that the diffuse lesion is a precursor of the nodular lesion. Histologists also distinguish another form of glomerular lesion, resulting from an accumulation of protein and appearing as a small PAS-positive brightly eosinophilic mass. This may be found either at the periphery of the glomerular tuft, forming a little curved cap at the outer surface of a capillary loop (Figure 15.5) or on the inner surface of Bowman's capsule (Figure 15.6). This 'fibrin cap' or 'capsular drop' is composed of fibrinogen, lipoproteins and other circulating proteins and, while it was originally termed an exudative lesion, it is more appropriately referred to as an insudative lesion.

Specificity

While nodules are pathognomic of diabetes the diffuse lesion may be found in membranous glomerulonephritis and amyloidosis. The exudative lesion occurs in other glomerular disorders associated with renal failure. Early reports that the nodule also occurred in exudative non-diabetic glomerular lesions or lobular nephritis are accepted as incorrect,

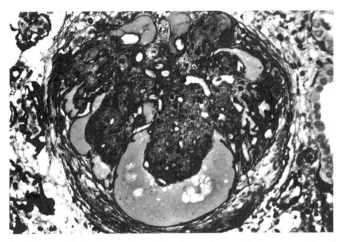

Fig. 15.5 Glomerulus from a diabetic patient showing a large fibrin cap with a few smaller ones to the side. The glomerulus shows nodular and diffuse glomerulosclerosis while both afferent and efferent arteriosclerosis is well demonstrated (Periodic–methenamine stain; × 500). (Source: courtesy of Dr Susan Lee, Department of Pathology, University of Birmingham.)

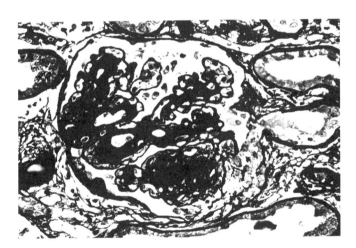

Fig. 15.6 Glomerulus from a diabetic patient showing a capsular drop (Periodic–methenamine stain; × 500). (Source: courtesy of Dr Susan Lee, Department of Pathology, University of Birmingham.)

because of confusion of the lesions or failure to detect carbohydrate disturbance.

ELECTRON MICROSCOPY

Examination of renal biopsy material under the electron microscope shows that the earliest manifestation of diabetic glomerulosclerosis consists of thickening of the glomerular basement membrane. At first this is an irregular expansion of the normally accepted upper limit of 3000 Å (Figure 15.7). In more advanced cases thickening up to four or even six times normal is found (Figure 15.8) and the thickened membrane is homogeneous in appearance (Osterby, 1992).

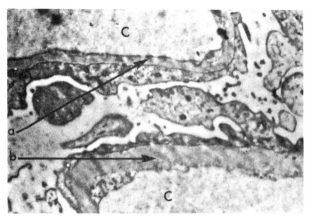

Fig. 15.7 Electron micrograph from a renal biopsy. Adjacent capillary loops are shown (C). Capillary basement membrane (a) is 2600 Å thick while (b) is 6100 Å ($\times$ 15 000).

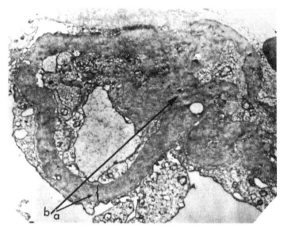

Fig. 15.8 Electron micrograph from a renal biopsy. Capillary basement membrane (a) is 10 000 Å thick. Basement-membrane-like material is also deposited in the axial zone (b) ($\times$ 10 000).

In addition, focal deposits of basement-membrane-like material are occasionally noted on the endothelial side of the membrane, sometimes forming small nodules or spans, or a meshwork in advanced cases. These changes are particularly apparent in the axial or centrilobular zones. The foot processes frequently show areas of fusion and in the most advanced cases have practically disappeared. Bowman's capsule also shows a similar thickening. The early appearances have suggested to many observers that the primary site of the glomerular change lies in the capillary basement membrane but it has also been suggested that the mesangial cells, lying between the capillaries, are covered by a basement membrane continuous with that of the capillaries and that basement-membrane-like material progressively encroaches on the capillary, producing the appearance of increased thickness.

It is important to realize that basement-membrane change has now been found in every type of diabetes, including that due to pancreatitis, haemochromatosis and after total pancreatectomy. It has also been found in kidneys from normal people transplanted into diabetic patients (Mauer *et al.*, 1976).

NATURE OF THE BASEMENT MEMBRANE CHANGE

The abnormality of basement membrane in the diabetic kidney lies mainly in quantity rather than quality. Nevertheless, there are some differences in the chemical composition of glomerular basement membrane. Normal basement membrane is composed of collagen, numerous non-collagenous compounds and carbohydrate moeties (Brownlee and Cerami, 1981). The non-collagenous components include proteoglycans, glycosaminoglycan and laminin. About 10% (dry weight) of basement membrane is carbohydrate. Many sugars are present predominantly in disaccharide or polysaccharide forms, and within glycosaminoglycans. They include glucose, galactose, mannose and fucose. In diabetic basement membrane most agree that collagen is increased. Results for sugar and amino acid content have given conflicting results in comparisons with normal basement membrane.

PREVALENCE OF HISTOLOGICAL LESIONS

Early studies of electron microscopic examination of biopsy specimens from young patients with symptoms of acute diabetes of only a few weeks duration and in whom there was no suspicion of renal disease were in many instances reported to be abnormal. The changes were slight and almost certainly the result of inadequate methodology. Unfortunately, many fruitless hours of argument have followed these observations. The implication was clear – if basement membrane thickening was present at diagnosis of diabetes then prolonged exposure to hyperglycaemia was unnecessary for diabetic complications. This erroneous view was finally corrected by publication of the meticulous study by Osterby-Hansen (1965), in which the basement-membrane thickness was measured at constant intervals on montages of glomerular cross-sections with about 1000 measurements for each glomerulus. There were no differences in basement membrane thickness in three groups of subjects: young diabetics before treatment (needle biopsy); the same patients after control of their diabetes (needle biopsy); non-diabetics (open biopsy). The modal value for basement-membrane thickness was 2140–2860 Å in the diabetics and 2500–2860 Å in the non-diabetics; the mean values were somewhat higher.

Kimmelstiel (1966) reported that the mean width of peripheral basement membrane in the glomeruli of diabetics was within normal limits except for those in whom nodules were present. He claimed that his measurements were confined strictly to those areas of basement membrane in which a perpendicular plane of section could be assured, and that he had excluded from measurement areas in which the basement membrane covered the mesangium.

All reports from post-mortem work and from biopsy series stress the close correlation that normally exists between the severity of the lesions and diabetes duration. The biopsy series also comment on the very large proportion who show some degree of diffuse change even when there is no suggestion of renal disease. Thus in a series of 29 biopsies done in our clinic on diabetics of varying duration and severity light microscopy was normal in only three cases. All the patients with diabetes of more than 15 years duration were considered to have histological changes of either moderate or severe degree. Well established changes were also present at diagnosis in a number of middle-aged and elderly patients. This was attributed to delay in diagnosis owing to the insidious nature of diabetic symptoms at this age (O'Sullivan, 1961) and is comparable to the finding of retinopathy at diagnosis with which it is often associated. Gellman *et al.* (1959) also emphasized the very high rate of abnormal histology, for in their series of 53 biopsies only 16 (25%) were considered normal on light microscopy, and Honey, Pryse-Davies and Roberts (1962) found much the same in a series of 24 biopsies done on young patients who had been receiving insulin for at least 10 years. However, all these series are made up of selected cases and the true prevalence of demonstrable glomerular lesions is unknown, since it is hardly possible to subject a random sample of the diabetic population to renal biopsy.

FROM NEPHROPATHY TO END-STAGE RENAL FAILURE

OEDEMA

The first symptom of nephropathy is swelling of the ankles from peripheral oedema. There is a tendency to immediately assume that the cause of the oedema is a marked reduction in circulating albumin concentration. In truth the underlying reason for the accumulation of fluid is often more complex. Cardiac failure and neuropathic lesions of the feet account for oedema in some patients but in a significant number no obvious cause can be found. Increased capillary fragility can be demonstrated in the majority of patients and it is possible that oedema is related to abnormal capillary permeability. Whatever the immediate cause of the oedema in these cases, any considerable degree of swelling in diabetic nephropathy suggests long-standing renal disease and there is a correlation between the presence and degree of oedema and the duration of proteinuria.

HYPERTENSION

The early and moderate degrees of the diffuse glomerular lesion are not a cause of hypertension. This can be stated with some degree of certainty since lesions of this severity are common yet hypertension is less widely distributed in this population. In the later stages of diabetic nephropathy hypertension most certainly is a feature and there is a significant relationship between the height of the blood pressure and the duration of proteinuria.

Somewhat paradoxically, the weight of evidence suggests that the decline in glomerular filtration rate and hypertension are not related (Parving *et al.*, 1981; Viberti *et al.*, 1983), yet treatment of hypertension slows the decline in glomerular filtration rate (Mogensen, 1976; Parving *et al.*, 1983). In advanced nephropathy, when renal failure threatens, a considerable proportion of patients, if not all, develop significant hypertension. It complicates the clinical picture and may cause congestive heart failure.

SERUM CREATININE

In the phase of intermittent proteinuria the serum creatinine is usually within the normal range and it may remain so, or just above the upper limit of the reference range, even when proteinuria becomes constant and heavy. It is not until the final accelerated phase of deterioration that creatinine rises and continues to rise until intervention or death.

URINARY PROTEIN

The quantity of protein that may be excreted in 24 hours by patients with nephropathy can vary from very small amounts to more than 20 g/24 hours. The average excretion is around 2.5 g/24 hours. In about 20% of patients the amount excreted is less than 1 g/24 hours and in only 15% is the amount in excess of 5 g/24 hours. Thus proteinuria, although varying widely in amount, is usually moderate and only rarely of the degree found in the nephrotic syndrome. Although patients with proteinuria of considerable duration pass larger amounts than those in whom it had only just been noticed the quantity often remains slight and even in some of those who die from renal failure it is never found to exceed 5 g/24 hours.

CIRCULATING PROTEINS

A number of changes in serum proteins have been recorded in patients with diabetic nephropathy. A majority have found raised alpha-2 globulins but the only constant abnormality is a low serum albumin. Similarly, extensive abnormalities in serum lipoproteins have been reported but can also be found in uncontrolled diabetes, non-diabetic renal failure, obesity and atheroma.

URINARY DEPOSIT

If we put on one side the important question of the diagnosis of urinary tract infection, the urinary deposit is not a helpful investigation in the diagnosis of diabetic nephropathy. Red blood cells may be present at an early stage and this finding is underappreciated, leading to numerous wasted investigations of, and referrals for, haematuria. Casts may be identified if the lesion is advanced.

RENAL FUNCTION

Detailed studies of renal function in diabetic nephropathy at an advanced stage have been reported. The pattern of equally decreased glomerular and tubular function without a corresponding fall in renal blood flow was not different from that found in glomerulonephritis. Gellman *et al.* (1959) found some agreement between the severity of histological change and loss of renal function, but the degree of nodular change did not fit into this correlation.

In those patients with early or moderate histological change renal function does not differ significantly from diabetics with normal kidneys. It is only when diffuse lesions are gross that there is a consistent elevation of serum creatinine and reduction in creatinine clearance. The preservation of renal function in spite of widespread glomerular change can be very striking.

COURSE AND PROGNOSIS OF DIABETIC NEPHROPATHY

The physician does not have to be of advanced years in order to recall the course of diabetic nephropathy when untreated. Until recently effective treatment did not exist and even when dialysis and transplantation became successful treatments of renal failure, the diabetic population was severely underrepresented in the treatment group compared with their non-diabetic counterparts. Only in the last few years has acceptance on to a dialysis and transplant programme become the norm for the diabetic rather than the exception.

It is now established that renal lesions appear at an early stage of diabetes and that proteinuria, which indicates that these lesions are significant, may be recorded within the first few years, even in young patients. Obviously, therefore, the general prognosis of nephropathy is comparatively favourable. Caird (1961) followed 134 of our diabetics for up to 10 years from the onset of proteinuria and compared their survival with that expected in the general population and among the diabetic population. It was found that 65% survived 5 years and 28% 10 years from the onset of proteinuria. This represented 77% of the natural expected rate for 5 years and 44% for 10 years in the general population and 89% and 59% respectively for the diabetic population in general. Individual variations are striking. In some the lesion hardly seems to progress over a period of many years; in others a malignant phase develops after as little as 10–15 years and we see the melancholy picture of a young patient who is anaemic, oedematous, half-blind and probably crippled by neuropathy as well – the diabetic triopathy of Root, Pote and Frehner (1954). Yet as a rule the progress of renal disease is so slow that death from other degenerative complications anticipates renal failure. Even in our 12 patients with advanced nephropathy only six died of uraemia, and this experience agrees with that of others (Deckert, Poulsen and Larsen, 1978).

The factors that determine the progress of nephropathy are unknown. There is little evidence that the lesions are reversible with control of blood glucose yet the degree of hyperglycaemia must remain a putative factor determining the rate of progression, as evidenced by studies of diabetic control and complications including the DCCT (Diabetes Control and Complications Trial Research Group, 1993). Clearly it cannot be held responsible to any great degree in the later stage, when the rate of deterioration far exceeds the prodromal time with proteinuria. Hypertension finds more support as a determinant of rate of decline of renal function, based largely on the work of Mogensen (1976, 1982). It has to be said that Mogensen (1982) studied only a small group of patients and his findings require confirmation. They have been read and accepted all too quickly by those who spend hours and detail minutiae about which antihypertensive agent should be used.

Fortunately for the worker but unfortunately for the patient there is a ready model upon which changes in therapy can be tested. Once the accelerated phase of declining renal function is reached the progression is inexorable and subsequent events can be predicted. A plot of the reciprocal of the serum creatinine concentration against time reveals a linear relationship that correlates closely with the decline in glomerular filtration rate once the serum creatinine exceeds 200 μmol/l (Viberti *et al.*, 1983). The slope is constant, although varying widely in the angle of descent between patients. The object of intervention is to produce a dog-leg effect upon this slope, i.e. to convert the slope from steep to shallow. Mogensen (1982) suggests that this can be done by treating hypertension, with successful treatment slowing the rate of decline.

In the later stages the management is the same as in other forms of chronic renal disease. Fluid intake should be kept rather above normal. As the serum creatinine and blood urea rise the protein content of the diet may be reduced to 40–60 g daily but not lower. As losses of protein in the urine are seldom great this is usually the indication,

but in the uncommon case of nephrotic syndrome a balance must be struck between the deficiency of protein and the tendency of the circulating urea and creatinine to rise, and this usually means an average intake of protein in the diet. Acid–base balance can seldom be corrected without disadvantages that outweigh any benefit achieved. The blood pressure tends to rise and may be lowered by drugs if due regard is paid to their effect on renal blood flow and the levels of potassium and creatinine. Vomiting may be controlled by an antiemetic orally or by injection. As renal failure develops the need for insulin gets less, but the risk of ketosis does not entirely disappear. There is a tendency for the blood glucose to swing from very high to very low levels and hypoglycaemic attacks are rather common. The urine may be sugar-free when the blood glucose is well above 15 mmol/l (270 mg/dl). All this makes the management of the diabetes a delicate matter. In particular, a single high blood glucose reading should not be regarded too seriously and the insulin dose should be kept down to the level required to avoid symptoms and ketonuria.

TREATMENT OF THE PATIENT WITH DIABETIC NEPHROPATHY

BLOOD GLUCOSE CONTROL

While the lesion cannot be considered to be reversible, all the available evidence is for a slowing of progression of diabetic complications with good diabetic control. There is a certain air of too little, too late in the introduction of good control at this stage and the approach must be to attempt tight control early in the disease, especially in those at high risk of the development of nephropathy. Currently much work is being done to identify markers which would delineate a high risk group and it may be that this function is the most appropriate use of microalbuminuria measurements. The alternative view is to regard all as equally at risk.

HYPERTENSION

By the time the patient reaches the stage of advanced nephropathy most, if not all, will have hypertension and be receiving treatment. The goal of treatment must be to lower blood pressure rather than to simply administer a particular drug. Having said that, the undoubted vogue is for the use of angiotensin converting enzyme (ACE) inhibitors and for them to be used early in the course of the disease. In practice this means that there is a tendency to introduce treatment with an ACE-inhibitor as soon as diabetic nephropathy is suspected. At this stage the introduction has more to do with potential renoprotective effects than with the antihypertensive effect. The consequence of this way of thinking is that the antihypertensive agents are being given to normotensive patients.

There is clear evidence of the damaging effect upon glomerular structure of arterial hypertension and therefore little room for doubt that hypertension should be enthusiastically treated (Rossing *et al.*, 1993). As to the question of which agent should be used, studies in streptozotocin-induced diabetic animals show a beneficial effect with ACE-inhibition over and above the antihypertensive effect. Similar results have been reported in insulin-dependent diabetic patients with impaired renal function from diabetic nephropathy (Lewis *et al.*, 1993).

In non-insulin-dependent patients Nielsen *et al.* (1994) compared lisinopril with atenolol and found that, with similar falls in blood pressure, the ACE-inhibitor lowered albumin excretion and fractional albumin clearance while the beta-blocker did not. Importantly, however, over the 12-month period of study glomerular filtration rates fell to the same extent in the two groups. The authors discuss whether it is possible to draw meaningful conclusions on glomerular filtration rate in

12-month studies, which begs the question of why the design of such studies is not better, since there seems to be an initial decline in the rate in patients given ACE-inhibitors following which there may be a better effect than other antihypertensive regimens. Whether this decline is confined to the ACE-inhibitor, or more severe than that which occurs with the introduction of any hypertensive agent, is, to my mind, not proven.

In a 2-year study of insulin-dependent diabetic patients with nephropathy Elving *et al.* (1994) found similar reductions in blood pressure, proteinuria and glomerular filtration rate when captopril was compared with atenolol.

TREATMENT OF THE PATIENT WITH END-STAGE RENAL FAILURE

RENAL DIALYSIS

Initial experience with dialysis in diabetic patients was discouraging. Mortality was high, blindness frequent and adjustment poor. Major improvements have been noted during recent years and diabetics now make up 25–33% of patients entering programmes in the USA.

Yet the patients presenting to the dialysis programme may be markedly more ill than their non-diabetic counterparts. Hypertension is invariably present which becomes more difficult to control in the later stages. Often evidence of widespread macrovascular disease is present including a history of myocardial infarction. Congestive cardiac failure exacerbated by fluid retention from hypoproteinuria may be almost terminal. Diabetic retinopathy is invariable, although by no means are all patients blind. Painful neuropathy and disabling autonomic neuropathy may also be in evidence. Postural hypotension and neurogenic bladder may exacerbate the decline in renal function.

Nor can the diabetes of the patient be disregarded. Although insulin sensitivity is decreased in uraemia this is offset against a tendency to hypoglycaemia presumed to result from altered clearance of injected insulin and decreased renal gluconeogenesis. Decreasing insulin requirement is the rule.

Haemodialysis

Haemodialysis may present a problem in gaining vascular access because of extensive atheromatous disease. Experience suggests that maintaining this access is also difficult. About 50% of patients may be successful with a simple fistula but others require alternative access such as a graft or a different type of dialysis. The presence of other diabetic complications confounds treatment. Diabetic retinopathy leading to blindness was a major problem in early reported series but more recent figures show a marked reduction in blindness, in line with improved treatment of eye disease (Whitley and Shapiro, 1985). Peripheral vascular disease leading to amputation occurs in about 5% of patients, although this figure may be higher in non-insulin-dependent patients. Autonomic neuropathy presents probably the major difficulty. While hypertension is an invariable accompaniment of end-stage renal failure, postural fall in blood pressure resulting from autonomic neuropathy may coexist. This presents particular problems in fluid and electrolyte management.

Survival rates have improved in recent years. First-year survival is of the order of 80%, with a 3-year survival of 50–55%. Young patients do better than the elderly. The major causes of death are cardiac and cerebrovascular disease, sepsis and discontinuation of dialysis (Whitney and Shapiro, 1985).

Peritoneal dialysis

In the UK peritoneal dialysis is the favoured method of management, as a prelude to transplantation. The technique has the distinct advantages that it can be carried out in

Table 15.2 Advantages and disadvantages of chronic ambulatory peritoneal diaylsis (CAPD) in diabetic patients

The advantages of CAPD are:
1. Some patients are still alive when they would have been dead without treatment.
2. The quality of life while on this treatment is reasonable.
3. Diabetes (i.e. blood glucose) can be controlled relatively easily.

The disadvantages are:
1. Total blindness or partial sight can make the technique too difficult to learn and relatives may then have to accept the task.
2. Ultrafiltration may decrease with time.
3. Loss of protein and amino acids in the dialysate may lead to protein malnutrition.

the home and that intraperitoneal insulin can be used to control blood glucose (Table 15.2).

There appears to be a small but negative effect upon diabetic retinopathy for, although 85% of eyes remain unchanged, 15% show some deterioration (Khanna *et al.*, 1985). Patients whose eyes fare worst had either advanced proliferative retinopathy or other eye disease. Approximately 7.5% of patients require an amputation with progression of peripheral vascular disease (Khanna *et al.*, 1985). Survival rates are good, with a number of centres reporting 1-year survival rates ranging from 70% to 90%. Causes of death are similar to haemodialysis.

Blood glucose control

During haemodialysis twice-daily subcutaneous insulin may be used to control blood glucose. With continuous ambulatory peritoneal dialysis (CAPD) insulin added to the dialysate and therefore administered intraperitoneally is preferable to subcutaneous insulin, producing better control of blood glucose.

The amount of insulin required per day

depends not only upon oral feeding but also on the amount of glucose in the dialysis fluid. Many of the solutions that can be obtained are markedly hypertonic, with glucose concentrations of 25–250 mmol/l (0.45–4.5%). A typical regimen would be of 4×2 litres exchanges per day. Most long-term reports indicate that about 100–120 units insulin per day is necessary, using a type of sliding scale based upon dialysate glucose concentration. No figure is inviolate, however, and a patient may require as little as 10 units/day or as much as 200 units/day. Home blood glucose monitoring is essential to assess progress.

There is a great tendency among patients to see dialysis as the answer to all their problems. To a large extent this view is shared by diabetologists and nephrologists and it acknowledges that without some form of intervention death is a certainty.

The language of science, however, is necessarily different to the language of communicating with patients. To talk of encouraging results is all right for a patient but is rarely necessary for the scientific community when real numbers or percentages are available. After all, a reduction in mortality from 100% to 99% is encouraging but hardly comforting to the patient. Survival rates from different centres are difficult to compare, because of different criteria for acceptance on to dialysis/ transplantation programmes, small numbers, a non-homogeneous population of insulin-dependent and non-insulin-dependent patients and clearly different forms of behaviour between patient groups (in one report (Lameire *et al.*, 1983), 16 of 19 patients on dialysis could not be persuaded to do home blood glucose monitoring). In one centre CAPD may be the short-term tool prior to transplantation in young insulin-dependent diabetics. In another centre it may be used predominantly in older non-insulin-dependent diabetics where extensive vascular disease precludes haemodialysis. Considerable differences in approach exist (Raine, 1993). If a centre starts with small

numbers of patients, the early mortality reduces the groups to a negligible number.

TRANSPLANTATION

Transplantation in Europe is undoubtedly handicapped by reliance upon cadaveric donors. For ethical reasons (either real or imaginary) living related donors have rarely been used in Europe, but experience in centres where such practice is readily accepted reveals excellent results for diabetics. In young insulin-dependent patients, 2-year survival is of the order of 95% (Goetz *et al.*, 1986). With cadaveric donors the survival rate is less (about 81% at 2 years). Patients who do worst are over the age of 40 years with evidence of vascular disease and such patients should be proposed only very cautiously for transplantation.

MANAGEMENT

By the time dialysis or transplantation is necessary the diabetologist will know the patient well. It is advisable some time before this to introduce the nephrologist and have a clear plan for the patient. Individual care and clinic policy probably emerges best in joint clinics between the diabetologist and the nephrologist. While this type of clinic works well across disciplines, for example between the physician and obstetrician or between a paediatrician and a physician, it is much more difficult to get two physicians working jointly! At an appropriate time a decision is taken to intervene. Quite what is the optimum time for intervention is debatable but recent moves are towards earlier intervention in diabetic patients compared with non-diabetic patients. Deterioration may be rapid when serum creatinine reaches 500 μmol/l and dialysis may be needed when it reaches 600–800 μmol/l. Usually this will mean CAPD while a suitable kidney is awaited.

DISEASE OF THE KIDNEYS AND URINARY TRACT OTHER THAN DIABETIC NEPHROPATHY

URINARY TRACT INFECTION

Pyelonephritis

This is a non-specific bacterial infection involving the renal pelvis and parenchyma. In the acute form the kidneys are usually enlarged with multiple small abscesses and inflammatory exudate in the pelvis. The tubules show degenerative lesions and are filled with leucocyte casts.

In the chronic form there may be contraction of the kidney. The surface is irregular, with obvious scars and nodular areas of normal tissue. The cortex is of varying thickness and the boundary between cortex and medulla is ill-defined. The microscopical picture is complex. Areas in which glomeruli and tubules are completely replaced by scar tissue alternate with normal zones, but in some areas the glomeruli are crowded together by shrinking of the cortex and periglomerular fibrosis may be seen. Atrophic tubules filled with colloid casts appear here and there. Vascular lesions are of variable extent but are most evident in the fibrotic areas. Endarteritis obliterans is common but hyaline change in the arterioles is rather rare. Hypertensive lesions up to the most severe may be found.

The diagnosis by renal biopsy is fraught with difficulty because of the small specimens obtained and the difficulty in distinguishing scars due to infection from those that result from arterial disease. No single lesion is pathognomonic of chronic pyelonephritis.

Pyelonephritis in the diabetic patient

Prevalence

Although there can be no doubt about the importance of urinary tract infections to the individual diabetic patient, the usual care is required before accepting the widespread clinical impression that they occur with greater frequency among diabetics than in the non-diabetic population. Since both diabetes and urinary infections occur most commonly in middle-aged and elderly women it is not surprising that the number of diabetics with such infections should seem large and the age/sex distribution has not always been considered in comparative studies. Moreover, the hazards of pyelonephritis to the diabetic are likely to lead to hospital admission.

The majority of reports that claim a greater incidence of urinary infection in diabetics base their conclusions either on autopsies or on the follow-up of hospital inpatients. Some evidence of renal infection is common in patients dying in hospital, but Robbins and Tucker (1944) reported it in 19.5% of diabetic autopsies, nearly five times more often than in the non-diabetic. It is quite possible that a terminal infection is more common in the presence of diabetes, but the importance of pyelonephritis as a cause of death is undetermined.

Clinical studies of urinary tract infection have usually suggested a significantly higher prevalence in the diabetic. Lundbaek (1953) recorded it in as many as 30% of men and 64% of women with long-term diabetes. O'Sullivan *et al.* (1961) collected 150 ambulant diabetic patients drawn at random from a clinic population but corresponding in age and sex with the clinic population as a whole. A total of 150 control patients of the same age and sex were drawn from the patients attending the casualty department with minor trauma and their friends and relatives. Midstream specimens of urine were taken for culture and counts above 100 000ml were considered to be significant. Such counts were obtained in 20 (13.3%) of the diabetics and in 18 (12.0%) of the controls, the difference not being significant. A total of 18 of the diabetics and 17 of the controls were women and infection became much more common with age. An interesting finding was the greater height of the bacterial count in the infected diabetics than in the infected controls, for 15 of the former had counts of more than 1 000 000/ml, whereas only seven of the latter had counts in this range. This might indicate that diabetics have more severe infection but it is possible that glucose in the specimens from diabetic patients created a more favourable medium for the multiplication of organisms.

If it is difficult to demonstrate any excess of urinary infection in ambulant diabetics without symptoms, it is likely that the incidence of acute and chronic pyelonephritis with symptoms is not much beyond that of the non-diabetic population, but one cannot be certain of this. Evidence from renal biopsy is inconclusive but supports the view that chronic pyelonephritis is not an important element in diabetic kidney disease.

Clinical effects

Typical acute pyelonephritis with high fever, pain in the loin and dysuria is easily recognized but in the elderly a presentation with persistent vomiting and no other definite symptom is quite common. In some cases the picture of diabetic ketosis predominates and may conceal the infection that has precipitated it. Urinary infection once established tends to be more severe than in the non-diabetic and often requires more intensive and prolonged antibiotic treatment. The results have to be checked by examination of repeated specimens. Catheterization, if at all possible, should be avoided.

PAPILLITIS NECROTICANS (RENAL MEDULLARY NECROSIS)

This lesion was first described by von Friedreich in 1877 and Gunther (1937) recognized the association with diabetes, which was present in eight of his 10 cases. The lesion is an ischaemic necrosis of the renal papilla and sometimes the renal medulla also. Both kidneys are involved as a rule, but not necessarily. It is usually associated with pyelonephritis but, although this may be present throughout the cortex, the necrosis is anatomically limited to the medulla (Lauler, Schreiner and David, 1960). The pathogenesis, as far as diabetes is concerned, has not been established but most writers have suggested a combination of infection and vascular sclerosis.

In the full review of Lauler, Schreiner and David (1960) 250 cases are collected of which 57% had diabetes. Of the diabetics 86% had the disease for less than 15 years and 32% for less than 5 years. The vast majority seem to have been poorly controlled.

Clinical features in the diabetic

The great majority of patients are women and most of them elderly. Although few are under the age of 40 it is possible that the condition is overlooked in younger patients, who recover.

The illness usually begins with symptoms of urinary infection and high fever, but lumbar and abdominal pain are unduly prominent. Typical renal colic may indicate the passage of a sequestered papilla. In the worst cases there is acute and profound prostration so that localizing features are impossible to elicit.

A subacute form with recurrent urinary infection runs a course of several months, while a chronic and asymptomatic variety is occasionally recorded in which the diagnosis is made by pyelography and the patient survives for several years. At post-mortem the lesions are found to be healed.

Diagnosis

Only a minority of cases are diagnosed in life, but the condition should be suspected in any very severe pyelonephritis, especially if there is frank haematuria or evidence of oliguria. The appearance of fragments of renal papilla in the urine is diagnostic. When intravenous pyelography is possible the findings are

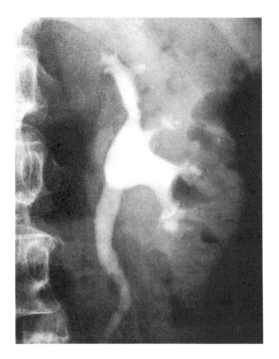

Fig. 15.9 Intravenous urography in a diabetic patient showing features of papillitis necroticans (see Table 15.3).

Table 15.3 Characteristic features on intravenous urography in a patient with papillitis necroticans

1. Delay or lack of function, usually unilateral
2. Mild to moderate dilatation of the collecting system
3. Mottled, motheaten appearance of the fornices
4. Gross filling defects throughout the calcyes and pelvis (due to slough and clots)

and

5. Ring shadows – radiolucent halos, the paths of contrast media from opposite fornices uniting as necrosis becomes complete

characteristic (Figure 15.9), as first described by Gunther (1937). The appearances have been listed by Evans and Ross (1956) (Table 15.3). Retrograde pyelography is hardly ever indicated and could well be a provoking cause of this lesion in a patient with active infection.

Treatment

Massive and prolonged antibiotic therapy offers the only hope. Dialysis may be needed to tide a patient over a period of acute renal failure. Nephrectomy is very rarely to be entertained as the remaining kidney is nearly always grossly diseased even when pyelography is encouraging.

Prognosis

The mortality is generally regarded as very high but one can only guess at the number of unrecognized cases that recover. Recovery is well documented and the unexpected finding of healed lesions at autopsy confirms the belief that the disease is not rare.

PNEUMATURIA

Gas formation within the renal tract is sometimes encountered as the result of urinary infection. It results from the common organisms of pyelonephritis, or yeasts fermenting glucose if there is any residual urine. This usually produces pneumaturia but the gas may find its way into the bladder walls, producing a curious radiological appearance (Figure 15.10). It may be recognized within the renal substance (Figure 15.11) or even escape into the tissue planes and produce subcutaneous emphysema.

RENAL ARTERY STENOSIS

The widespread atheroma of diabetes would be expected to increase the incidence of renal artery stenosis as a cause of hypertension. Indeed such a finding has been reported from post-mortem studies (Hall, 1952). In over 5000 autopsies a greater than 50% narrowing of at least one renal artery was found in 4.3%. The clinical records showed that dia-

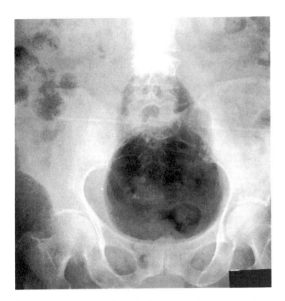

Fig. 15.10 Gas in the bladder of a diabetic patient.

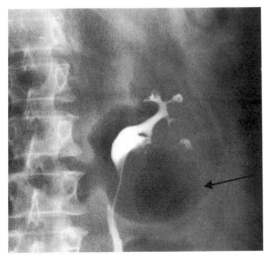

Fig. 15.11 Acute pyelonephritis in a diabetic patient with abscess formation causing distortion of the pelvis and calyces. There is a large gas shadow in the area of the abscess (arrow).

betes was present in 52% of those with renal artery stenosis and in 34% it was bilateral (Sawicki *et al.*, 1991). Detection rates in life are not reported and it is unusual to search

for unilateral impairment. Isotope uptake scans as well as aortic arteriography provide sensible methods for investigating the possibility although sometimes the unilateral appearance of the intravenous pyelogram is an important clue. The importance of its detection lies in the potential disastrous impact of ACE-inhibitors in patients with renal artery stenosis.

CARBOHYDRATE INTOLERANCE IN RENAL FAILURE

Disturbance of carbohydrate metabolism in renal failure was first reported by Hamman and Hirschman (1917), who found an abnormal oral glucose tolerance curve in all of six patients with uraemia. Perkoff *et al.* (1958) showed that both the oral and the intravenous glucose tolerance test were mildly diabetic in uraemic patients and demonstrated a decreased insulin action, suggesting the presence of resistance to insulin. This has been confirmed in 24-hour studies of hormones and intermediary metabolites (Heaton *et al.*, 1985). In the diabetic with renal failure insulin resistance does not dominate the picture. It is usual to see a decrease in insulin requirements. This may be due to reduced intake as malaise supervenes, a decreased contribution by the kidney to gluconeogenesis, or impaired insulin clearance.

REFERENCES

Armanni (1875) Cantanni A. Pathoologia e terapia del ricambio materiale. *Milan* 1, 352.
Bell, E. T. (1950) *Renal Diseases*, 2nd edn, Lea & Febiger, Philadelphia, PA.
Bell, E. T. and Clawson, B. J. (1928) Primary (essential) hypertension. A study of four hundred and twenty cases. *Arch. Path.*, **5**, 939–1002.
Brownlee, M. and Cerami, A. (1981) The biochemistry of the complications of diabetes mellitus. *Ann. Rev. Biochem.*, **50**, 385–432.
Caird, F. I. (1961) Survival of diabetics with proteinuria. *Diabetes*, **10**, 178–181.
Cambier, P. (1934) Application de la theorie de

Remberg a l'étude clinique des affections renales et du diabete. *Ann. Med.* **35**, 273–299.

Darwin, E. (1801) *Zoonomia or the Laws of Organic Liffe*, vol 1, 3rd edn, Johnson, London.

Deckert, T., Poulsen, J. E. and Larsen, M. (1978) Prognosis of diabetics with diabetes onset before the age of thirty-one. *Diabetologia*, **14**, 363–370.

Diabetes Control and Complications Trial Research Group (1993) The effect of intensive treatment of diabetes on the development and progression of long-term complications in insulin-dependent diabetes mellitus. *N. Engl. J. Med.*, **329**, 977–986.

Ellis, E. N., Steffes, M. W., Goetz, F. C. *et al.* (1985) Relationship of renal size to nephropathy in type 1 (insulin-dependent) diabetes. *Diabetologia*, **28**, 12–15.

Elving, L. D., Wetzels, J. F. M., van Lier, H. J. J. *et al.* (1994) Captopril and atenolol are equally effective in retarding progression of diabetic nephropathy. *Diabetologia*, **37**, 604–609.

Evans, J. A. and Ross, W. D. (1956) Renal papillary necrosis. *Radiology*, **66**, 502–508.

Feldt-Rasmussen, B., Mathiesen, E. R., Hegedus, L. and Deckert, T. (1986) Kidney function during 12 months of strict metabolic control in insulin-dependent diabetic patients with incipient nephropathy. *N. Engl. J. Med.* **314**, 665–670.

von Friedreich, N. (1877) Ueber Necrose der Nierenpapillen bei Hydronephrose. *Virchows Arch. Path. Anat. Physiol.*, **69**, 308–312.

Gellman, D. D., Pirani, C. L., Soothill, J. F. *et al.* (1959) Diabetic nephropathy: a clinical and pathologic study based on renal biopsies. *Medicine*, **38**, 321–367.

Goetz, F. C., Elick, B., Fryd, D. and Sutherland, D. E. R. (1986) Renal transplantation in diabetes. *Clin. Endocrinol. Metab.*, **15**, 807–821.

Gunther, G. W. (1937) Die Papillennekrosen der Niere bei Diabetes. *Münch. Med. Wschr.*, **84**, 1695–1699.

Hall, G. F. M. (1952) The significance of atheroma of the renal arteries in Kimmelstiel–Wilson's syndrome. *J. Path. Bact.*, **64**, 103–120.

Hamman, L. and Hirschman, I. I. (1917) Studies on blood sugar. *Arch. Intern. Med.*, **20**, 761–808.

Heaton, A., Johnston, D. G., Haigh, J. W. *et al.* (1985) Twenty-four hour hormonal and metabolic profiles in uraemic patients before and during treatment with continuous ambulatory peritoneal dialysis. *Clin. Sci.*, **69**, 449–457.

Honey, G. E., Pryse-Davies, J. and Roberts, D. M. (1962) A survey of nephropathy in young diabetics. *Q. J. Med.*, **31**, 473–483.

Keen, H. and Chlouverakis, C. (1963) An immunoassay method for urinary albumin at low concentrations. *Lancet*, **ii**, 913–914.

Keen, H., Chlouverakis, C., Fuller, J. H. and Jarrett, R. J. (1969) The concomitants of raised blood sugar: studies in newly detected hyperglycaemics. II. Urinary albumin excretion, blood pressure and their relation to blood sugar levels. *Guy's Hosp. Rep.*, **118**, 247–254.

Khanna, R., Wu, G., Prowant, B. *et al.* (1985) Continuous ambulatory peritoneal dialysis in diabetics with ESRD: a combined experience of two North American centers, in *Diabetic Renal–Retinal Syndrome*, (eds E. A. Freidman and F. A. L'Esperance) Grune & Stratton, Orlando, FL, pp. 363–381.

Kimmelstiel, P. (1966) Basement membrane in diabetic glomerulosclerosis. *Diabetes*, **15**, 61–63.

Kimmelstiel, P. and Wilson, C. (1936) Intercapillary lesions in the glomeruli of the kidney. *Am. J. Path.*, **12**, 83–97.

Kroustrup, J. P. Gundersen, H. J. G. and Osterby, R. (1977) Glomerular size and structure in diabetes mellitus. III. Early enlargement of the capillary surface. *Diabetologia*, **13**, 207–210.

Laipply, T. C. Eitzen, O. and Dutra, F. R. (1944) Intercapillary glomerulosclerosis. *Arch. Intern. Med.*, **74**, 354–364.

Lameire, N., Dhaene, M., Matthijs, E. *et al.* (1983) Experience with Capd in diabetic patients, in *Prevention and Treatment of Diabetic Nephropathy*, (eds H. Keen and M. Legrain), MTP Press, Boston, MA, p. 289–297.

Lauler, D. P., Schreiner, G. E. and David, A. (1960) Renal medullary necrosis. *Am. J. Med.*, **29**, 132–156.

Lewis, E. J., Hunsicker, L. G., Bain, R. P. and Rohde, R. D. (1993) The effect of angiotensin-converting-enzyme inhibition on diabetic nephropathy. *N. Engl. J. Med.*, **329**, 1456–1462.

Lundbaek, K. (1953) *Long-term Diabetes*, E. Munksgaard, Copenhagen, p. 73.

Mathiesen E. R., Oxenboll, B., Johansen, K. *et al.* (1984) Incipient nephropathy in Type 1 (insulin-dependent) diabetes. *Diabetologia*, **26**, 406–410.

Mathiesen, E. R., Hommel, E., Giese, J. and Parving, H. H. (1991) Efficacy of captopril in postponing nephropathy in normotensive insulin dependent diabetic patients with microalbuminuria. *Br. Med. J.*, **303**, 81–87.

Mauer, S. M., Barbosa, J., Vernier, R. L. *et al.* (1976) Development of diabetic vascular lesions in normal kidneys transplanted into patients with diabetes mellitus. *N. Engl. J. Med.*, **295**, 916–920.

Mogensen, C. E. (1971) Urinary albumin excretion in early and long-term juvenile diabetes. *Scand. J. Clin. Lab. Invest.*, **28**, 183–193.

Mogensen, C. E. (1976) Progression of nephropathy in long term diabetics with proteinuria and effect of initial anti-hypertensive treatment. *Scand. J. Clin. Lab. Invest.*, **36**, 383–388.

Mogensen, C. E. (1982) Long-term antihypertensive treatment inhibiting progression of diabetic nephropathy. *Br. Med. J.*, **285**, 685–688.

Mogensen, C. E. and Andersen, M. J. F. (1972) Increased kidney size and glomerular filtration rate in early juvenile diabetes. *Diabetes*, **22**, 706–712.

Mogensen, C. E. and Christensen, C. K. (1984) Predicting diabetic nephropathy in insulin-dependent patients. *N. Engl. J. Med.*, **311**, 89–93.

Mogensen, C. E., Osterby, R. and Gundersen, H. J. G. (1979) Early functional and morphologic vascular renal consequences of the diabetic state. *Diabetologia*, **17**, 71–76.

Nielsen, F. S., Rossing, P., Gall, M. A. *et al.* (1994) Impact of lisinopril and atenolol on kidney function in hypertensive NIDDM subjects with diabetic nephropathy. *Diabetes*, **43**, 1108–1113.

Osterby, R. (1986) Structural changes in the diabetic kidney. *Clin. Endocrinol. Metab.* **15**, 733–751.

Osterby, R. (1992) Glomerular structural changes in type 1 (insulin-dependent) diabetes mellitus: causes, consequences, and prevention. *Diabetologia*, **35**, 803–812.

Osterby, R. and Gundersen, H. J. G. (1975) Glomerular size and structure in diabetes mellitus 1. Early abnormalities. *Diabetologia*, **11**, 225–229.

Osterby, R. and Gundersen, H. J. G. (1980) Fast accumulation of basement membrane material and the rate of morphological changes in acute experimental diabetic glomerular hypertrophy. *Diabetologia*, **18**, 493–500.

Osterby Hansen, R. (1965) A quantitative estimate of the peripheral glomerular basement membrane in recent juvenile diabetes. *Diabetologia*, **1**, 97–100.

O'Sullivan, D. J. (1961) Proteinuria in diabetes. MD thesis, University of Birmingham.

O'Sullivan, D. J., FitzGerald, M. G. Meynell, M. J. and Malins, J. M. (1961) Urinary tract infection. *Br. Med. J.*, **1**, 786–788.

Parving, H. H., Smidt, U. M., Friisberg, B. *et al.* (1981) A prospective study of glomerular filtration rate and arterial blood pressure in insulin-dependent diabetics with diabetic nephropathy. *Diabetologia* **20**, 457–461.

Parving, H. H., Andersen, A. R., Smidt, U. M. and Svendsen, P. A. (1983) Early aggressive antihypertensive treatment reduces rate of decline in kidney function in diabetic nephropathy. *Lancet*, **i**, 1175–1178.

Parving, H. H. Noer, I., Deckert, T. *et al.* (1976) The effect of metabolic regulation on microvascular permeability to small and large molecules in short-term juvenile diabetics. *Diabetologia*, **12**, 161–166.

Perkoff, G. T., Thomas, C. L., Newton, J. D. *et al.* (1958) Mechanism of impaired glucose tolerance in uremia and experimental hyperazotemia. *Diabetes*, **7**, 375–383.

Raine, A. E. G. (1993) Epidemiology, development and treatment of end-stage renal failure in type 2 (non-insulin-dependent)diabetic patients in Europe. *Diabetologia*, **36**, 1099–1104.

Robbins, S. L. and Tucker, A. W. (1944) The cause of death in diabetes. A report of 307 autopsied cases. *N. Engl. J. Med.*, **231**, 865–868.

Rossing, P., Hommel, E., Smidt, U. M. and Parving, H. H. (1993) Impact of arterial blood pressure and albuminuria on the progression of diabetic nephropathy in IDDM patients. *Diabetes*, **42**, 715–719.

Root, H. F., Pote, W. H., and Frehner, H. (1954) Triopathy of diabetes. Sequence of neuropathy, retinopathy, and nephropathy in one hundred fifty-five patients. *Arch. Intern. Med.*, **94**, 931–941.

Sawicki, P. T., Kaiser, S., Heinemann, L. *et al.* (1991) Prevalence of renal artery stenosis in diabetes mellitus – an autopsy study. *J. Intern. Med.*, **229**, 489–492.

Seyer-Hansen, K. (1977) Renal hypertrophy in experimental diabetes: relation to severity of diabetes. *Diabetologia*, **13**, 141–143.

Seyer-Hansen, K., Hansen, J. and Gundersen, H. J. G. (1980) Renal hypertrophy in experimental diabetes. *Diabetologia*, **18**, 501–505.

Viberti, G. C. and Wiseman, M. J. (1986) The kidney in diabetes: significance of the early abnormalities. *Clin. Endocrinol. Metab.*. **15**, 753–782.

Viberti, G. C., Hill, R. D., Jarrett, R. T. *et al.* (1982) Microalbuminuria as a predictor of clinical nephropathy in insulin-dependent diabetes mellitus. *Lancet*, **i**, 1430–1432.

Viberti, G. C., Bilous, R. W., Mackintosh, D. and Keen, H. (1983) Monitoring glomerular function in diabetic nephropathy. *Am. J. Med.*, **74**, 256–264.

Viberti, G. C., Mackintosh, D. and Keen, H. (1983) Determinants of the penetration of proteins through the glomerular barrier in insulin-dependent diabetes mellitus. *Diabetes*, **32**(suppl. 2), 92–95.

Viberti, G. C., Wiseman, M. and Redmond, S. (1984) Microalbuminuria: its history and potential for prevention of clinical nephropathy in diabetes mellitus. *Diabetic Nephropathy*, **3**, 79–82.

Whitley, K. Y. and Shapiro, F. L. (1985) Hemodialysis for the uremic diabetic, in *Diabetic Nephropathy*, (eds E. A. Friedman and C. M. Peterson), Martinus Nijhoff, Boston, MA, p. 85–103.

Wiseman, M., Viberti, G., Mackintosh, D. *et al.* (1984) Glycaemia, arterial pressure and microalbuminuria in type 1 (insulin-dependent) diabetes mellitus. *Diabetologia*, **26**, 401–405.

Symptoms which could be those of neuro-pathy appear in diabetic case reports from the end of the 18th and the beginning of the 19th century (Rollo, 1798) but credit for the first clear recognition of the condition is given to Marchal de Calvi, the Corsican, who wrote in 1864:

> ever since experimental physiology has shown that various lesions of the central nervous system may produce diabetes or at least glycosuria the problem has been looked at from this point of view. When-ever neurological phenomena have been observed in diabetics they have been con-sidered primary. It has not occurred to anybody to wonder whether they could be secondary to the diabetes rather than the cause of it . . . evidently experimental cerebral lesions producing diabetes have prevented doctors from recognizing ner-vous lesions produced by diabetes.

Marchal described paraesthesiae and shoot-ing pain in the legs and recognized that sciatica could be the presenting symptom of diabetes.

Bouchardat (1883) recognized pain in the limbs at night and paraesthesiae: he found impotence to be a common complication in neglectful patients while Pavy (1885) reported cases of disordered sweating in a paper which described the clinical picture well. Auche (1890), in an excellent review, gave a detailed account of the symptoms and added perforating ulcer and cranial nerve palsy to the list of neurological complications.

The effect of the introduction of insulin on the incidence and character of neuropathy was not documented and the next major paper is that of Jordan (1936), whose pain-staking review was influential; the clinical descriptions were admirable and the prognosis with treatment of the diabetes was analysed for the first time. Arteriosclerosis was thought to be the cause in most cases.

Rundles (1945) studied 125 patients with symptoms either of neuropathy or of newly diagnosed diabetes and noted frequent occur-rence of gastrointestinal symptoms. In addi-tion difficulties of micturition, impotence, abnormal sweating and postural hypotension were not rare. These manifestations of auto-nomic damage have been extensively studied since that time.

PREVALENCE

There is no definition of diabetic neuropathy and therefore estimates of the incidence vary greatly. Joslin found it in only 0.1% of his 6000 diabetics up to 1928, while Rundles (1950), who required objective signs in the nervous system persisting beyond the acute stage of diabetes, made the diagnosis in 4% of 3000 cases.

While the attribution of pain, paraesthesiae, weakness and abnormal neurological signs to diabetes must always be speculative the problem becomes more difficult still when the patient is elderly. Sensory complaints are common in old age, including stabbing or aching pains in the lower limbs and dysaesthesiae. Loss of vibration sense is also common, and disappearance of ankle jerks not rare. These changes have been attributed to a kind of senile polyneuritis.

Mayne (1965) made a careful comparison between a random sample of 222 diabetic patients and 110 control subjects (not patients) drawn from the lists of general practitioners. The diagnosis of neuropathy was made if two definite abnormal signs, compatible with the diagnosis and otherwise unexplained, were present or one such sign and a definite history. Peripheral neuropathy was definitely present in 29% of control subjects and 64% of diabetic patients. The overall prevalence of 64% agrees closely with results from other studies, the 67% of Jordan (1936) and the 62% of Goodman *et al.* (1953). These figures are dramatically higher than those obtained in more recent studies, for example those of Walters *et al.* (1992). They ascertained the prevalence of distal sensory neuropathy, diagnosed in a similar way, i.e. symptoms plus one abnormal sign or two abnormal signs, in over 1000 diabetics and 480 age- and sex-matched controls. In non-diabetic subjects the prevalence was 2.9% while in the diabetic patients it was 16.3%. These figures more closely approximate recent studies and the lower prevalence figures are undoubtedly due to choosing not to include propriocep-tion as a modality for examination and using a dichotamous classification; i.e. the options for recording symptoms or signs are 'present' or 'absent' and impaired cannot be concluded.

In a large sample in the United States, Harris, Eastman and Cowie (1993) identified symptoms of sensory neuropathy by ques-tionnaire and found a prevalence of 36% in men and 40% in women with non-insulin-dependent diabetes. Among people with insulin-dependent diabetes the prevalence was 30%. These figures contrast with those in the control group of 10% for men and 12% for women.

In a clinic survey Young *et al.* (1993) found of 6487 diabetic patients that the overall pre-valence of neuropathy was 28.5% (23% in type 1 patients and 32% in type 2) using a definition based on a scoring system for symp-toms and signs. Symptoms and signs could be mild, moderate or severe and neuropathy was defined as mild signs with moderate symptoms or moderate signs (with or with-out symptoms). They found it was more than 50% in non-insulin-dependent patients over the age of 60 years.

As would be expected there is a steady increase in the incidence of neuropathy with advancing age (Figure 16.1), but the changes in the diabetic are more frequent and occur at an earlier age. Mayne concluded that the neuropathy of ageing, presenting with minor symptoms and certain signs, especially im-paired ankle jerks and vibration sense at the ankle, is degenerative and probably ischaemic. This condition is fairly common in a control group and no doubt at least as common in diabetic patients of the same age.

Neuropathy is uncommon in children being found in less than 2%. Nevertheless when duration of diabetes exceeds 5 years evidence of neuropathy increases (Eng *et al.*, 1976). This relationship with duration persists in adulthood. In the long-term study of Pirart (1978) neuropathy was found in less than 10% of patients at diagnosis but more than 50% after 25 years of diabetes

CLASSIFICATION

Neuropathy resists attempts to classify it in any logical manner. The nature of the manifestations is so variable while the cause can rarely be demonstrated with certainty. The situation is further complicated by an imprecise definition of neuropathy, which to one physician may be simply absent ankle jerks while to another symptoms will be re-quired. As investigational tests become more refined it is possible to recognize 'subclinical' stages of both peripheral and autonomic neuropathy.

Nevertheless it is clearly inadequate to label a constellation of symptoms and signs as dia-betic neuropathy and some attempt at classi-fication can be made on probable pathogenesis, likely outcome or simply predominant nerves affected. This provides endless scope for different classifications but the one I prefer is

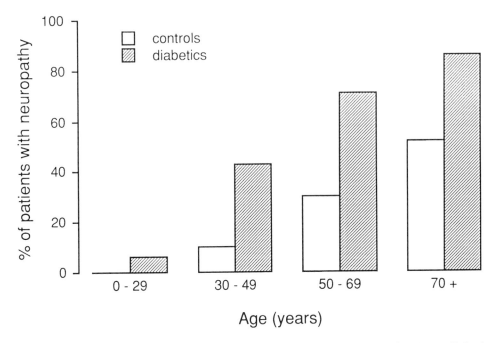

Fig. 16.1 Incidence of neuropathy by age group in 222 diabetic patients and 110 non-diabetic control subjects. (Souce: adapted from Mayne, 1965.)

Table 16.1 Classification of diabetic neuropathy

A. Somatic neuropathy
  1. Distal symmetrical sensory polyneuropathy
  2. Proximal painful neuropathy (synonyms: diabetic amyotrophy; femoral amyotrophy; asymmetrical motor neuropathy)
  3. Mononeuropathy and mononeuritis multiplex

B. Autonomic neuropathy

that of Ward and his colleagues (Scarpello and Ward, 1984) (Table 16.1).

CLINICAL FEATURES

DISTAL SENSORY POLYNEUROPATHY

Paraesthesiae

These take the form of pins and needles, tingling, numbness and a sensation of dead-ness or coldness. They occur in the upper limbs as well as the lower limbs although there is a tendency towards underdiagnosis in the upper limbs since they may be hard to distinguish from other common conditions such as carpal tunnel syndrome.

Pain

Paraesthesiae merge into a burning sensation and pain. Burning is characteristically worse at night on getting into bed and with the bedclothes on the affected area. Some relief is obtained with exercise although whether this is simply distraction is unclear. Pain is usually felt symmetrically and distally and can affect upper as well as lower limbs. When it affects one thigh it may be difficult to distinguish from other types of diabetic neuropathy. An almost characteristic feature of the pain is its unremitting nature and a failure to achieve relief with simple analgesics.

Table 16.2 Findings on examination in a group of 220 unselected diabetic patients and 110 matched control subjects (%) (Source: from Mayne, 1965)

Age (years)	Absent/impaired vibration sense		Absent/impaired proprioception		Absent/impaired ankle jerk		Absent/impaired knee jerk	
	Control	Diabetic	Control	Diabetic	Control	Diabetic	Control	Diabetic
0–29	0	6	0	19	0	44	0	31
30–49	0	30	10	19	5	61	10	40
50–69	16	5	36	41	33	83	11	24
70+	67	6	52	68	40	84	16	42

Motor weakness

Motor weakness is not a dominant feature of this type of neuropathy although it should be acknowledged that any painful neuropathy may lead to wasting and weakness.

Sensory loss

This is often difficult to assess in elderly patients. It may be comparatively slight in cases with pain and paraesthesiae. It is more marked in the legs than in the arms and tends to be peripheral, occasionally in the distribution of one nerve or one of its branches. In order of frequency the modalities lost are vibration sense, position sense, pain, touch and deep pain sensation. Vibration sense is seldom impaired in the arms, but frequently in the legs, and the defect may be unilateral. While complete absence of position sense is unusual, impairment is quite common in the big toes; it is uncommon in the thumbs. Pain is more often affected than touch sensation, which is not lost unless pain feeling is absent. Deep pain sensation in the calves is occasionally absent. The findings of Mayne (1965) in his unselected groups of diabetics and matched controls are summarized in Table 16.2. Impairment of co-ordination was not a feature in either group.

Tendon reflexes

Abnormalities of the tendon reflexes have been noted since the time of Pavy (1885) and loss of the ankle jerk has been particularly stressed by a number of writers.

Plantar reflexes

Extensor plantar reflexes certainly occur in patients with diabetic peripheral neuropathy; in 11% of unselected diabetic patients (Mayne 1965); but they were also found in non-diabetic control subjects (7%) so that the significance of this finding is doubtful.

ACUTE PROXIMAL NEUROPATHY

Acute proximal neuropathy is characterized by severe pain in one or both thighs, mainly at the front, with a varying degree of weakness of the muscles. Contact paraesthesiae and hyperaesthesia over the anterior thigh are the rule. The weakness of the thighs may be sufficiently severe for the legs to give way. On examination the weakness and wasting are obvious; the knee-jerk is impaired or absent, often on both sides, the plantar reflexes are sometimes extensor, the skin over the quadriceps is extremely tender to light touch and the muscle itself to pressure. Vibration and position sense are sometimes impaired.

This picture is usually seen in patients of middle age at least, whose diabetes is never trivial but seldom very severe. Pain is gradually relieved when control has been established, but weakness may persist for months or even years. Deep reflexes may or may not return, but plantar responses revert to normal. Coppack and Watkins (1991) reviewed 27 patients diagnosed with this condition, of whom 24 had non-insulin-dependent diabetes. Only 10 patients had bilateral symptoms. The natural history was recorded as a gradual improvement in symptoms after about 3 months with complete recovery after 16 months (range 6–42 months). Six patients had recurrent attacks, often affecting the other side. Interestingly, there was no obvious relationship between recovery and insulin treatment or glycaemic control.

The occurrence of proximal muscle wasting and weakness with pain in these muscles but without objective sensory loss was described in the 19th century. It closely resembles the picture just presented and the cases of Garland and Taverner (1953), who introduced the term 'myelopathy'. Garland, in a later paper (1955), described the most usual features as diffuse pain, weakness, wasting and areflexia, usually asymmetrical and limited to the legs. Less constant were extensor plantar responses and raised cerebrospinal fluid protein concentration. Electromyography often suggested a cord lesion, but sometimes peripheral nerve damage. He suggested 'amyotrophy' as a more suitable title than 'myelopathy'. Garland wrote in a lively and aggressive style, attributing failure to recognize this syndrome to the fact that physicians who look after diabetic patients are not trained neurologists! Nevertheless the features he described, other than the extensor plantars, are a commonplace of diabetic practice and some physicians must have realized how often they had seen 'myelopathy'. An interesting feature of Garland's patients was the mild character of the diabetes. Yet with good control recovery was the rule after months or even years.

Whether the cord is involved or not in such cases has not been settled. Pathological findings are indefinite but not exclusive of such a possibility. The completeness of recovery is perhaps a point against major cord damage while the diffuse pain must surely be peripheral in origin.

MONONEURITIS AND MONONEURITIS MULTIPLEX

It will be apparent that if distal sensory polyneuropathy and acute proximal neuropathy are to be considered the major types of somatic neuropathy then many presentations will not fit either category. This is particularly true when the predominant lesion appears to be in one nerve or root and these will be considered as a mononeuritis.

Foot drop

This occurs not infrequently and the weakness may be the presenting feature of diabetes. It can be acute in onset and an isolated symptom or may form part of a more diffuse weakness, in which case it usually persists after recovery has taken place elsewhere. Pain is not a feature and sensory loss is usually slight. The prognosis in acute cases is good, but when there has been a longstanding and widespread weakness some degree of foot drop may persist indefinitely. It is recognized that foot drop, often unexplained, is not rare in the normal population, but the incidence in diabetics is probably greater.

Cranial nerve lesions

Oculomotor palsy

This has been attributed to diabetes since Saundby (1891) recorded third and sixth nerve paralysis, ptosis and pupillary disturbances. Transient oculomotor palsy is by no means rare in the elderly who have no diabetes but it is thought to be more common among diabetic patients. It is seen in our clinic five or six times a year. The patients are nearly always over the age of 50, usually over 60 and may have evidence of arterial disease with hypertension but not necessarily of active neuropathy. Diplopia is noticed at a time when the patient is well and is usually painless, although headache and facial neuralgia occasionally precede it. The signs are those of single third, fourth or sixth nerve weakness and the pupil is spared. Recovery always occurs and is usually complete in 3 months regardless of diabetic control. Second attacks may occur even after many years. The relation of this condition to diabetes is uncertain and pathological evidence is lacking, but the most probable cause is a localized vascular lesion.

Trigeminal neuralgia

This is not recognizable as a feature of diabetic neuropathy distinct from the common, unexplained disorder.

Facial palsy

This condition likewise occurs but with a frequency which is not definitely beyond that seen in the non-diabetic population.

Auditory nerve involvement

Although difficult to identify as a manifestation of neuropathy, auditory nerve involvement may be suspected when perceptive deafness begins rather acutely and is otherwise unexplained. At present it cannot be distinguished by any form of investigation.

Radiculopathy

Trunk pain occurs and may present enormous problems in diagnosis. It may involve any nerve root but the lower thoracic and lumbar nerve roots are more commonly affected. If around the chest it may mimic ischaemic heart disease in its severity. About half of the patients have unilateral involvement, when it may resemble an attack of herpes zoster with pronounced hyperaesthesiae of the skin. When round the abdomen it can be confused with pancreatitis and other intra-abdominal lesions.

Mononeuritis multiplex

This condition is underdiagnosed but readily recognizable. It is probably at its worst in what Ellenberg (1974) termed diabetic neuropathic cachexia. Pain is the dominant feature, affecting the arms and hands as often as the legs. Pain is intractable and may require immobilization as a temporary measure. Young women seem more affected than men and often have a history of poorly controlled diabetes with multiple episodes of diabetic ketoacidosis.

OTHER SOMATIC NEUROPATHIES RELATED TO DIABETES

It is stating the obvious to say that diabetic patients are also prone to peripheral neuropathies unrelated to diabetes. This is dealt with below but here should be mentioned some other types of neuropathy which do not fit easily into the classification outlined above (Table 16.1). A more extensive classification of neuropathy to accommodate these conditions is set out in Table 16.3.

First on the list would be the impairment of motor nerve conduction velocities which may be identified at diagnosis of diabetes. Except where diabetes was long-standing but undia-

Table 16.3 Classification of diabetic neuropathy

A. Somatic neuropathy
  1. Distal symmetrical sensory polyneuropathy
  2. Proximal painful neuropathy (synonyms: diabetic amyotrophy; femoral amyotrophy; asymmetrical motor neuropathy)
  3. Mononeuropathy and mononeuritis multiplex

B. Neuropathies related to control
  4. Neuropathy at diagnosis
  5. Neuropathy of poor control
  6. Neuropathy of improved control
  7. Chronic hypoglycaemic neuropathy

C. Ischaemic neuropathy

D. Autonomic neuropathy

gnosed the impairment improves with treatment of the high blood glucose levels. There have been attempts in the past to suggest that a particular agent is best at reversing the process but it seems clear that any treatment leads to an improvement. The significance of this finding at diagnosis is uncertain. To my mind it represents nothing more than deranged metabolism with probable accumulation of sorbitol in the apparently damaged nerves. Others have suggested, however, that impaired function at diagnosis may be of prognostic significance in the development of a true diabetic neuropathy.

Occasionally one sees a neuropathy develop at a time of imperfect diabetic control. It is not always easy to ascribe any causative role to the poor control but there is a temptation to invoke the same explanation as in the preceding paragraph. A note of caution must be sounded, however, since the reversibility of this form of neuropathy does not follow the same pattern as the neuropathy at diagnosis. Reversible it usually is, but only over a rather longer time scale of 3–12 months. Because it is often indistinguishable from the true diabetic peripheral neuropathy, recovery cannot be promised.

It is well recognized that rapid improvements in diabetic control can lead to a reversible deterioration in diabetic retinopathy, but a similar effect upon the nervous system seems less well appreciated. Nevertheless such a condition clearly exists when improved control is quickly followed by the appearance of peripheral neuropathy which is often extremely painful. It would appear that this form of neuropathy, like retinopathy which develops in identical circumstances, is reversible over a period of 6–12 months.

It is also well accepted that a severe peripheral neuropathy may be present in patients with hypoglycaemia from an insulin-secreting tumour. In the diabetic patient too there may be an association. It is difficult to be precise in attributing the development of a peripheral neuropathy solely to hypoglycaemia in a diabetic patient since so much else is usually happening, and in particular, episodes of hyperglycaemia may alternate with the hypoglycaemia. Where I think this type of neuropathy may be seen is in the fortunately uncommon patient whom treatment has rendered chronically hypoglycaemic. This type of neuropathy often affects the hands, with wasting of the small muscles of the hands. While other aspects of the hypoglycaemia, particularly the chronic neuroglycopenia, are reversible I am less sure that the neuropathic change is reversible.

Ischaemic neuropathy borders on neuropathy from causes other than diabetes but it is so common and characteristic in the diabetic patient that I would include it in any classification of diabetic neuropathies. It is almost always in the leg which, on examination, is revealed to be ischaemic. The predominant feature is pain which follows a classical description of neuropathic pain rather than ischaemic pain. It is often difficult to distinguish this type of neuropathy from the more classical distal symmetrical polyneuropathy and indeed it is possible that with our tendency to compartmentalize symptoms and diseases that the contribution of ischaemia to the symptoms of neuropathy is underestimated.

AUTONOMIC NEUROPATHY (TABLE 16.4)

Although sweating disturbances were mentioned by Pavy (1885) the first clear description of autonomic defects in neuropathy was that of Rundles (1945) and since then autonomic neuropathy has been rather too freely diagnosed. Convincing evidence of this lesion is best derived from vasomotor and sweating responses in the skin and defects of blood pressure regulation. Visceral disorders resemble so closely those that result from proved autonomic interference that their origin may reasonably be assumed. Pathological data are unsatisfactory and no lesion has been demonstrated by biopsy or at post-mortem.

Table 16.4 Clinical features of autonomic neuropathy

Vasomotor	Tachycardia
	Postural hypotension
	Abnormal sweating
	Gustatory sweating
	Peripheral oedema
Gastro-intestinal	Delayed gastric emptying
	Vomiting
	Diarrhoea
	Constipation
Genito-urinary	Neurogenic bladder
	Impotence
Pupillary	Loss of hippus
	Miosis
	Sluggish response to light
	Argyll Robertson pupil

The incidence of autonomic involvement in neuropathy depends entirely upon definition and has been estimated at 40% based upon abnormal cardiovascular responses (Ewing and Clarke, 1986).

Vasomotor changes

These are probably a good deal more common than we suspect. Tachycardia unaffected by carotid pressure or respiration may be unrecognized. Postural hypotension is the most striking manifestation, found in 6–16% of patients with neuropathy. A difference of 30 mmHg between the standing and lying figures is taken as indicative of postural hypotension, but it should be noted that abnormal findings in a patient who is ill or fluid-depleted may have disappeared if the examination is repeated after recovery. It is probably at its commonest in diabetics of long duration of disease.

Oedema of the feet may be attributed to vasomotor changes but the mechanism is unknown. Oedema certainly occurs frequently in patients with severe neuropathy and does not seem to be renal in most cases.

Unexpected cardiorespiratory arrest has been reported in patients with severe autonomic neuropathy undergoing anaesthesia or with bronchopneumonia (Page and Watkins, 1978).

Abnormal sweating

Night sweats are certainly a common symptom in patients with neuropathy but they are also reported by newly discovered patients in whom no signs to suggest the causation are apparent.

Decrease or absence of sweating in the legs or feet was found by Mayne (1965) in 32% of diabetics and 8% of controls, although it must be pointed out that about one-third of all the patients questioned apparently had feet that had never sweated. Barany and Cooper (1956) made a study of sweating induced by heating the body in diabetic men and controls. The sweating pattern was abnormal in nine of the diabetics, four of whom had signs of marked neuropathy. The upper and lower limbs were affected but the trunk was not examined. In addition the application of a faradic current or the injection of acetylcholine into the skin of areas that did not sweat failed to produce an area of sweating and vasodilatation. This axon reflex disappears after section of postganglionic fibres but is retained when preganglionic fibres only are cut, so that there was evidence of a lesion of the postganglionic fibres.

Patchy sweating may be seen in patients with neuropathy when they are hypoglycaemic. If large areas fail to sweat, excessive sweating may occur over the unaffected areas in the maintenance of normal temperature. Abnormal sweating may be related to ingestion of food (Watkins, 1973). It usually affects the face and neck and begins a few minutes after starting to eat.

Gastrointestinal disturbances

Gastrointestinal disturbances include severe constipation, chronic diarrhoea, anorexia and nausea.

Gastroparesis

Impaired motility of the stomach is the major feature of autonomic neuropathy affecting the upper gastrointestinal tract. The barium meal shows delayed emptying of the stomach, the pylorus being patulous with failure of propulsion waves in the stomach wall. The appearance closely resembles that seen after vagotomy. It is present in about one-third of patients with diabetic diarrhoea, but is not rare in diabetic patients with no gastro-intestinal symptoms. This being so it is not easy to be sure whether anorexia or occasional vomiting can be attributed to gastroparesis, but at least the response to the general run of gastric disturbances may be considerably modified by it.

There is little doubt that episodes of intractable vomiting, suggestive of high intestinal obstruction, occur in diabetic patients, and that no organic cause for the vomiting is found if a surgeon is persuaded to open the abdomen. These attacks begin very acutely in a patient who was previously well and the first symptom is nausea, soon followed by repeated vomiting. Abdominal discomfort is slight and constipation is usual, although rarely there is diarrhoea. After a few days the vomiting subsides but attacks may recur over a number of years.

Recent studies have shown an impact of diabetic control upon gastric motility. A high blood glucose may delay gastric emptying, particularly in insulin-dependent patients (Fraser *et al.*, 1990). This finding is of some importance, since it implies that not all delays in gastric emptying are from autonomic neuropathy and therefore irreversible.

Diabetic diarrhoea

In 1936, Bargen, Bollman and Kepler referred to a characteristic diarrhoea seen in severe diabetes. The stools were numerous and watery but not particularly fatty, unlike those of pancreatic diarrhoea, and pancreatic enzymes were present in normal quantity in the duodenal juice. It is a most disabling complication of diabetes, since the diarrhoea is usually explosive with little warning of impending evacuation. Although classically it is described as nocturnal it may only be confined to evenings and nights when relatively mild. Later it is not confined to any particular part of the day and the lack of warning may result in the patient being reluctant to leave the home, with its proximity to a toilet.

The diagnosis of diabetic diarrhoea is at all times made after exclusion of other causes. There is nothing wholly characteristic about the clinical features but their presence in a diabetic with evidence of neuropathy and no sign of pancreatic insufficiency or organic disease of the gut makes the diagnosis likely.

Constipation

This is probably a more frequent disturbance than diarrhoea in the diabetic but escapes detection because it is thought to be 'just normal'. At times constipation may be very severe with complete loss of sphincter tone and practically no expulsive force. Faecal retention may require regular enemata. In general, treatment is ineffective but substances that increase the bulk of the stools may be helpful and, as with diarrhoea, spontaneous improvement may occur.

Neurogenic bladder disturbance

Disturbance of micturition is an infrequent finding, but lesser symptoms may be comparatively common, being difficult to distinguish from other causes of middle and later life. The name 'cord bladder' has been used but there is no evidence that the lesion is central rather than peripheral.

The earliest symptom is difficulty in emptying the bladder completely, which at first may only be apparent when the patient is confined to bed, followed by hesitation, a poor stream, a feeling that emptying is incomplete and finally incontinence. Sometimes a greatly distended bladder is found at routine examination and I have seen this at the time diabetes was diagnosed. There were no symptoms of neuropathy but signs were present. Rarely, the patient her/himself notices the distension. On cystoscopy the bladder capacity is increased, sensation of filling is diminished and there is fine trabeculation of the bladder wall. On cystometry the tone is poor and only a few contractions (not noticed by the patient) are recorded.

The lesion is dangerous because the threat of infection is great and it may be impossible to eradicate.

Instrumentation should be avoided as long as possible. The patient should be allowed to stand or sit in order to pass urine. Transurethral resection of the bladder neck designed to overcome the resistance to the impaired expulsive force may be very successful, but in women the sphincter is more difficult to identify and there is a risk of permanent incontinence.

Sex disorders

Impotence is usually assumed to be a result of autonomic neuropathy. It is known that erection is a parasympathetic and ejaculation a sympathetic function. The frequency of impotence as a symptom varies with the relationship between doctor and patient. It is surely one of the most common symptoms of male diabetics when ascertained by direct questioning rather than waiting for the complaint to be volunteered. Rubin and Babbott (1958) found it two to five times as common as in the normal population; 25% of diabetic men aged 30–34 were impotent, increasing to 54% at age 50–54. There was no unusual incidence before the diagnosis of diabetes but 30% of those who became impotent did so within 1 year of the diagnosis being made. They found no relation between age at onset, duration, severity or the presence of complications including neuropathy. This is surprising because there is a strong impression

that patients with severe neuropathy are very likely to be impotent, but Rundles recorded it in no more than 27.5% of his male patients who had neuropathy.

Perhaps therefore the nature of impotence in diabetes should not be too readily assumed to be neurogenic. Few series have attempted to assess the prevalence of non-diabetic causes of impotence in the diabetic male. Thus in most series a few cases are reported that show spontaneous improvement. McCulloch *et al.* (1984) reported an incidence of 35% – 5 years later 28% of potent men had become impotent and 9% of those originally impotent had become potent.

At the onset of acute diabetes in younger patients impotence may occur but usually recovers with the establishment of control. The impotence that begins insidiously in the treated case and where diabetes seems the probable cause very rarely improves. I would say never, but for one patient who, after 5 years of impotence, recovered his sex function completely although already suffering from renal failure.

Diabetic men also suffer in other aspects of their sex-life. In a carefully controlled study they were shown to have significant decreases in sexual desire, subjective arousal, erectile capacity, coital frequency and sexual satisfaction (Schiavi *et al.*, 1993).

Pupil changes

The commonest pupillary abnormality is a sluggish reaction to light with a normal response to accommodation. Less often irregular and unequal pupils and miosis are seen. The true Argyll Robertson pupil is probably rare but certainly does occur. Loss of hippus, pupillary oscillation, is a well documented feature of autonomic neuropathy.

PATHOGENESIS

The cause of diabetic neuropathy is unknown. There is nothing specific in any of its manifestations; nothing that could not occur in other forms of neuropathy. This means that description of typical cases of diabetic neuropathy must be carefully scrutinized. Proximal neuropathy and the combination of somatic with autonomic changes are rather characteristic but night cramps are as common in a control population as in diabetic patients.

Early writers associated neuropathy with uncontrolled diabetes, which was no doubt common enough before the introduction of insulin. A belief that vitamin B_1 deficiency was the cause arose naturally from increasing knowledge of the effects of thiamine deficiency and the essential role of this vitamin in maintaining the function of nervous tissue. There was also experimental evidence that thiamine is important in the intermediary metabolism of carbohydrate. Deficiency of thiamine disturbs the normal breakdown sequence of carbohydrate and there is an accumulation particularly of pyruvate in the tissues. There is, however, no evidence that the diet of diabetic patients is commonly deficient in thiamine and investigations of urinary excretion in patients with neuropathy have given negative results. In addition the response to treatment with thiamine has been far from obvious. Improvement has been described after 12 months whereas the change in true thiamine deficiency is apparent within a week or two, at least as far as the motor changes are concerned. Enthusiasm for this cause of neuropathy has entirely evaporated.

VASCULAR CHANGES

The vascular theory began with the description of ischaemic nerve lesions in 10 cases by Woltman and Wilder (1929) from which evidence it has often been supposed that disease of small arteries is a sufficient cause for all neuropathy. Jordan (1936) thought that about one-third of his cases were associated with arteriosclerosis. Many have been sceptical of ischaemia as the cause of more than a small minority of cases, because if the

lesion were the result of structural change in the vessel walls, they could not envisage the degree and duration of recovery that often occurs in severe cases. In addition they have not found evidence of peripheral vascular disease unduly often in their patients. The features of neuropathy associated with severe peripheral vascular disease are very different from those that commonly arise in diabetes. In the atherosclerotic patient the neuropathic symptoms are overshadowed by those of ischaemia, so that they nearly always have to be enquired for specifically. Absent tendon reflexes are relatively infrequent, sensory symptoms vague and sensory loss slight.

In recent time the vascular theory has revived with the idea that neuropathy, like retinopathy and nephropathy, is related to the specific capillary angiopathy of diabetes. Fagerberg (1959), was more impressed with lesions of the intraneural arterioles, which he found to be closely associated with the incidence of neuropathy. Endoneurial capillaries from 20 patients with diabetic neuropathy showed increased basement membrane compared to epineurial capillaries, in contrast to non-diabetic non-neuropathic controls where epineurial and endoneurial capillaries are similar. Other abnormalities found were an increase in endothelial cell area and a decrease in luminal area, and furthermore these abnormalities correlated with myelinated fibre density and reduced nerve conduction velocities (Malik *et al.*, 1993).

Peripheral blood flow in diabetic patients with neuropathy is far from normal. Arteriovenous shunting has been well demonstrated by a variety of techniques (Tesfaye, Malik and Ward, 1994) and results from sympathetic denervation of blood vessels. Sural nerve oxygen tension is decreased but P_{O_2} in foot veins is elevated.

There is a decent amount of evidence that isolated nerve palsies may be of vascular origin. The clinical course of such lesions suggests this view, with sudden onset, a patient without evidence of distal polyneuropathy, and complete recovery. Asbury *et al.* (1970) were able to examine nerves from patients who died shortly after experiencing an isolated palsy. They concluded that vascular lesions were responsible although vascular thrombosis was not directly identified. Asbury's patient was all the more remarkable because the same lesion had occurred on the opposite side of the body 3 years earlier. No residual pathological lesion could be identified.

The vascular theory has recently undergone a revival promulgated with evangelical zeal by a group in Sheffield. Could polyneuropathy be the result of multiple infarcts of the nerves? This would seem to stretch belief too far and indeed there is little to support the view. While platelet plugs can be demonstrated in phases of acute metabolic decompensation, trials of antiplatelet drugs fail to show any beneficial effect. Slightly stronger evidence links vascular change and proximal neuropathies (Sugimura and Dyck, 1982).

METABOLIC THEORIES

Meanwhile, there have always been those who have adhered to the view that neuropathy is essentially the result of a metabolic disturbance associated with uncontrolled diabetes. Support for this view is given by many studies of the relationship of diabetic control to the development of complications which culminated in the DCCT (Diabetes Control and Complications Trial Research Group, 1993). The biochemical/metabolic theory of the causation of diabetic neuropathy has at its core the sugar alcohol of glucose, sorbitol (Figure 16.2). Nerve tissue, like other tissues damaged in long-term diabetes is independent of insulin for glucose uptake. Thus hyperglycaemia *per se* regulates nerve glucose uptake, although it is suggested that increased intracellular glucose does not accelerate glycolysis. Faced with excess availability of glucose, nerve has an alternative pathway for metabolism involving aldose reductase and sorbitol dehydrogenase.

Aldose reductase

$$Glucose + NADPH + H^+ \rightleftharpoons Sorbitol + NADP^+$$

Sorbitol dehydrogenase

$$Sorbitol + NAD^+ \rightleftharpoons Fructose + NADH + H^+$$

Fig. 16.2   The sorbitol pathway.

Sorbitol dehydrogenase is rate-limiting and, combined with the inability of sorbitol to diffuse across plasma membranes, inevitably leads to sorbitol accumulation. The latter is suggested as an osmotic cause of functional and morphological change.

A second sugar alcohol, myo-inositol, has strong support as a causative agent from Greene and his colleagues, but few others. It is argued that the reduced levels of myo-inositol found in diabetic nerves by some but not by us (Hale *et al.*, 1981) are linked with Na–K ATPase activity and parallel decreases are found with motor nerve conduction velocity. This argument can be followed in Greene, Lattimer and Sima (1987), where it remains unconvincing.

In recent years a further mechanism has evolved whereby diabetic complications may be caused. Glycation of proteins, identified mainly for haemoglobin originally but with broader application, alters the properties of the specific protein and may, for example with haemoglobin, increase its affinity for oxygen with the potential for exacerbation of tissue hypoxia. In other cases condensation or pleating of the protein may occur. Peripheral nerve protein is glycated in experimental diabetes, including peripheral nerve myelin. In turn this may alter metabolism or turnover of these proteins.

Considerable interest in recent years has focussed upon axonal transport systems. Two major systems exist: anterograde, moving proteins and neurotransmitters from the site of synthesis in the cell body down the axon; and retrograde, returning degradative products.

In experimental diabetes changes occur in these transport systems (Sidenius and Jakobsen, 1987).

Pathogenesis remains as elusive as ever and this must be due partly to the ethical difficulties of study but also to the difficulties of recognition of the natural history. It is likely that by the time of presentation of 'diabetic neuropathy' an end-stage destruction has been reached which is both non-specific and non-contributory from the investigational standpoint.

PATHOLOGY OF DIABETIC NEUROPATHY

Early reports of histological examination of the nervous system are not informative. Auche (1890) found normal nerve tissue proximal to diseased peripheral nerve and thought the lesion in neuropathy could not therefore be in the spinal cord. Jordan, Randall and Bloor (1935) confirmed that the distal part of the nerve was more damaged than the proximal. The greater the amount of vascular disease the more marked were the changes in the nerves but the specimens were taken at amputation or post-mortem. A famous paper of this period was that of Woltman and Wilder (1929), who reported the findings in six amputated legs from autopsies. The patients had complained of mild pain or paraesthesiae. There was extensive degeneration of the peripheral nerves, usually diffuse but sometimes patchy, while changes in the spinal cord were very slight. The most important finding was a marked thickening of the walls of the intraneural vessels, more pronounced towards the periphery, and the conclusion was that atherosclerosis was the most significant factor in the lesions of the nerves. This work has been freely quoted by protagonists of the vascular theory of the aetiology of diabetic neuropathy, presumably because it supports their beliefs rather than because of any merit in the general application of these findings, in a small and highly selected group, to the problem of neuropathy.

Further support for the vascular theory came with the publication of a series of articles examining the small vessels from Fagerberg (1959) in which arteriolar narrowing with thickening of endothelium from deposition of PAS staining material was described. There was myelin sheath degeneration, which correlated with symptoms of neuropathy, as did neuropathy with changes in the arterioles.

The predominant pathological lesion in the patient with neuropathy depends upon the severity or duration of peripheral neuropathy. Axonal degeneration and fibre loss is the major finding in long-standing peripheral neuropathy and this is preceded by segmental demyelination with remyelination. Lesions in the autonomic system have not been found.

Examination of the cord in early studies showed indefinite changes and interest in it waned after Woltman and Wilder's report. Suggestions that the cord could be involved as in Garland and Taverner's 'myelopathy' revived the question but there are few informative studies.

ELECTROPHYSIOLOGY

Many studies have been performed using electrophysiological techniques in diabetic neuropathy. Findings to some extent depend upon the type of neuropathy present. Even when clinical symptoms are absent, abnormalities of sensory conduction may be found (Lamontagne and Buchthal, 1970). Reduced sensory conduction velocity and amplitude of the action potential, with increase in time-spread of the action potential, have been observed. Motor nerve conduction velocity may also be reduced, although this is more marked when neuropathy is clinically detectable. Lamontagne and Buchthal (1970) related the clinical severity of neuropathy with the degree of reduction in motor nerve conduction velocities. In a biopsy study of sural nerves from insulin-dependent diabetic patients with early peripheral neuropathy good correlations were found between sensory and motor nerve conduction velocities and myelinated fibre density, a reliable criterion for the diagnosis of neuropathy (Veves *et al.*, 1991).

In acute proximal neuropathy Garland and Taverner (1953) found fewer complexes than normal while in focal lesions the abnormality may be confined to the affected nerve. Entrapment syndromes, particularly carpal tunnel syndrome, are said to be commoner in the diabetic population and can be demonstrated with electrophysiology.

At diagnosis of diabetes or in times of poor diabetic control electro-physiological tests may demonstrate abnormalities which correct with treatment of diabetes. This is hardly true diabetic neuropathy and the significance of the finding awaits elucidation. Another unusual finding is the resistance to ischaemia of the evoked sensory action potential in the diabetic patient (Seneviratne and Peiris, 1968). This anomaly is also found clinically, with an ability of the patient to perceive vibration, touch and pain for a longer time during ischaemia.

Electromyography in patients with neuropathy shows denervation of affected muscles, and fibrillation potentials may be observed.

The findings with electrophysiological tests, particularly in distal sensory polyneuropathy, are by no means specific for diabetes. They can be found in other peripheral neuropathies. In addition, the relationship of some findings to the age of the patient may obscure a clear view. For these reasons and with the exception of entrapment syndromes, their clinical use is limited. Of course, for studies of natural history, or putative treatments, they form part of the assessment, although there is growing awareness that severely reduced conduction velocities may reflect end-stage, irreversible nerve damage.

THE CEREBROSPINAL FLUID

The only abnormal finding is an increase in the protein content found in about half the patients with neuropathy. It is, of course, a common accompaniment of every form of neuropathy if the nerve roots are involved.

Root and Kenny (1952) recorded the CSF protein in 157 cases of diabetic neuropathy and found it to be 15–50 mg/dl in 28%, 51–70 mg/dl in 27%, 71–120 mg/dl in 34% and 121–440 mg/dl in 11%.

DIFFERENTIAL DIAGNOSIS

Other potential causes of peripheral neuropathy occur in patients with diabetes. Often it is not possible to state with certainty that a distal sensory polyneuropathy originates in the patient's diabetes or in an accompanying disease such as hypothyroidism or uraemia. When we were recruiting patients for a study of diabetic neuropathy we found that only 105 out of 200 patients with polyneuropathy had no other potential cause (Table 16.5) (Krentz, Honigsberger and Nattrass, 1989).

Vascular disease is the biggest confounding factor and it may be difficult to evaluate the respective roles of ischaemic and diabetic neuropathy. Patients are encountered with features of both. Other than this combination

Table 16.5 Potential causes of neuropathic symptoms in 200 diabetic patients (Source: from Krentz, Honigsberger and Nattrass, 1989)

	No.	(%)
Peripheral vascular disease	22	(11.0)
Chronic excessive alcohol intake	13	(6.5)
Chronic renal failure	10	(5.0)
Primary hypothyroidism	8	(4.0)
Malignant disease	4	(2.0)
Pernicious anaemia	3	(1.5)
Rheumatoid arthritis	1	(0.5)
Demyelinating disease	1	(0.5)
Positive syphilis serology	1	(0.5)
Diabetes		
Asymmetrical sensory neuropathy	15	(7.5)
Amyotrophy	8	(4.0)
Entrapment syndromes	9	(4.5)
Distal symmetrical polyneuropathy	105	(52.5)
Total	200	(100.0)

it is seldom of great clinical import to separate out potential causes. Far more important is the potential pitfall of labelling a patient as having proximal neuropathy when the true cause of the pain and wasting is a spinal cord lesion. It is a fortunate physician who is not caught out at least once in his professional life by a cauda equina tumour presenting with the features of femoral amyotrophy.

AUTONOMIC FUNCTION TESTS

A vast array of autonomic function tests have become available in the past few years. They are based upon loss of reflex arcs and the most useful focus upon the cardiovascular system. The simplest test is the change in heart rate in response to deep breathing. Deep breathing accentuates the normal sinus arrythmia – an increase in heart rate during inspiration and a decrease in expiration – and these changes can be recorded on an electrocardiograph. Measurement of the R–R interval allows calculation of the expiration/inspiration ratio, the maximum–minimum heart rate, or some other index of variability. Loss of variability indicates autonomic dysfunction. In practice, if a sinus arrhythmia can be detected at the bedside by palpation then severe autonomic dysfunction is extremely unlikely.

A second test utilizes the reflex changes in heart rate and/or blood pressure on standing. Normally heart rate increases with standing to a maximum 15 beats after standing and then slows with the nadir at 30 beats after standing. The 30/15 ratio of R–R intervals is a measure of these changes.

Blood pressure also goes through a range of changes with standing and may be measured lying and after standing. There is a tendency only to measure standing blood pressure within the first minute of standing as was done for ganglion-blocking drugs used in the treatment of hypertension. This is inadequate in postural hypotension from diabetic autonomic neuropathy, when the fall after standing may be gradual and continue for 10–15

minutes (Horrocks *et al.*, 1987). Thus measurement on standing or within the first minute only may miss the diagnosis or underestimate the severity of the lesion.

The Valsalva manoeuvre – forced expiration against a closed glottis – leads to a fall in the heart rate and blood pressure followed by a rise in both to greater than resting levels. The longest R–R interval/shortest R–R interval is a measure of variation. Blood pressure changes during sustained handgrip have also been used.

In practical terms deep breathing (6 breaths/ min) over 1 minute during electrocardiograph recording is the simplest test. The Valsalva manoeuvre also requires little in the way of specialized equipment since a simple pressure gauge can be improvised. Using a sphygmomanometer the patient blows at 40 mmHg for 15 seconds through a suitable mouthpiece while the electrocardiograph is recorded. The tests should always be interpreted in the light of the clinical situation; atrial fibrillation, multiple atrial ectopics, some drugs and coincident disease such as heart failure obscure the results.

Other tests of autonomic function are rarely needed in the clinic although they may be useful in occasional patients. Cine-radiography, oesophageal manometry or gastric emptying times may be used to investigate the upper gastrointestinal tract. Specialized bladder function tests such as cystometry are available and acetylcholine sweat tests and measures of pupillary oscillation can also be performed.

The assessment of impotence may include measurement of nocturnal penile tumescence in an attempt to differentiate loss of erection from organic cause from psychogenic impotence.

PROGNOSIS

Generally the prognosis for symptoms of neuropathy is good (Watkins, 1992), but for sensory loss and reflexes uncertain and usually incomplete. Recovery of motor function is typically complete, although improvement is slow and may take 12–18 months. The prognosis for autonomic manifestations is poor, although the disability is often surprisingly slight.

TREATMENT

Current treatment is directed on two fronts. Attempts to slow progression of the neuropathy involve optimizing diabetic control. A number of patients will show improvement in symptoms with improved control, although this is rarely miraculous. Paradoxically, some patients may show worsening of symptoms with improved control.

Other treatment is aimed at relief of symptoms perceived as pain. It is surprising how many patients suffer needlessly through inadequate prescription of analgesia. Certainly it is logical to start with simple analgesia but in many patients this is inadequate to relieve symptoms. Without hesitation, stronger analgesics should be introduced, often approaching the potency of opiates, although these remain a last resort. Occasional success may be achieved through the use of phenytoin or carbamazepine. Stronger support in recent years has come for imipramine or similar tricyclic antidepressant (Davis *et al.*, 1977; Young and Clarke, 1985). There is a general feeling that this is the treatment of choice if simple analgesia is insufficient for symptom relief.

Aldose reductase inhibitors have been undergoing clinical trials. So far results have been mixed and are far from convincing. It may be that they have had unfair trials in established diabetic neuropathy when damage is irreversible but prevention studies raise organizational and financial difficulties. The alternative view, that aldose reductase is in no way causal in diabetic neuropathy, has received less attention.

Treatment of autonomic neuropathy is a depressing experience because of a barren therapeutic armamentarium. 9-alpha-fludrocortisone in high doses (0.9 mg/day) may be effective in relieving the symptoms of postural hypotension but resting hypertension may be the penalty of success. Nevertheless it is clearly worthy of use (Campbell, Ewing and Clarke, 1975) when the only alternative is elastic tights or antigravity suit. Gastrointestinal symptoms also respond poorly to treatment, although metaclopromide may be tried for upper gastrointestinal problems. Other drugs that can promote gastric emptying include domperidone, cisapride and erythromycin. If diabetic diarrhoea does not respond to codeine phosphate or imodium a small dose of tetracycline will, in the occasional patient, produce a dramatic remission. Sweating may be helped or even abolished by poldine methylsulphate or propantheline, although anticholinergic side effects may exacerbate problems with a neurogenic bladder.

Impotence in men has finally become treatable. Smooth muscle relaxants such as papaverine or vasodilators, the alpha-blockers phentolamine or phenoxybenzamine, can be given by intracavernous injection in order to achieve an erection. A specific drug may not be licensed for this particular use and this should be checked locally. Patients can be taught to self-inject. The dose of papaverine is increased gradually following a test dose until a satisfactory erection is achieved. Complications of this method are few, although occasional cases of infection or fibrosis are recorded (Wiles, 1992). The major risk is priapism and if the erection lasts more than a few hours help should be sought. Blood can be removed from the corpus cavernosus by syringe and an alpha-adrenergic agent injected.

Dislike or failure of this method seems to be quite common and leads to a consideration of mechanical devices. Vacuum condom devices draw blood into the penis and the erection is maintained by a ligature round the base of the penis. Side-effects are few and limited to bruising and subjective comments from the man or his partner. Despite the apparent 'clumsiness' of the procedure a significant proportion of couples have satisfactory intercourse using these devices (Price *et al.*, 1991) and vacuum devices and self-injection tend to be equally acceptable.

A more permanent solution is offered by implantable rigid rods or inflatable rods. Good results can be achieved but the selection of patients is probably crucial.

REFERENCES

Asbury, A. K., Aldredge, H., Herschberg, R. and Fisher, O. M. (1970) Oculomotor palsy in diabetes mellitus: a clinico-pathological study. *Brain*, **93**, 555–566.

Auche, B. (1890) Des altérations des nerfs periphérique chez les diabetiques. *Arch. Med. Exp.*, **2**, 635–676.

Barany, F. R. and Cooper, E. H. (1956) Pilomotor and sudomotor innervation in diabetes. *Clin. Sci.*, **15**, 533–540.

Bargen, J. A., Bollman, J. L. and Kepler, E. J. (1936) The diarrhoea of diabetes and steatorrhoea of pancreatic insufficiency. *Proc. Mayo. Clin.*, **11**, 737–742.

Bouchardat, A. (1883) *De la Glycosurie ou Diabete Sucré*, vol. 1, Germer-Baillière, Paris.

Campbell, I. W., Ewing, D. J. and Clarke, B. F. (1975) 9-alpha-fluorohydrocortisone in the treatment of postural hypotension in diabetic autonomic neuropathy. *Diabetes*, **24**, 381–384.

Coppack, S. W. and Watkins, P. J. (1991) The natural history of diabetic femoral neuropathy. *Q. J. Med.*, **79**, 307–313.

Davis, J. L., Lewis, S. B., Gerich, J. E. *et al.* (1977) Peripheral diabetic neuropathy treated with amitryptyline and fluphenazine. *J.A.M.A.*, **238**, 2291–2292.

Diabetes Control and Complications Trial Research Group (1993) The effect of intensive treatment of diabetes on the development and progression of long-term complications in insulin-dependent diabetes mellitus. *N. Engl. J. Med.*, **329**, 977–986.

Ellenberg, M. (1974) Diabetic neuropathic cachexia. *Diabetes*, **23**, 418–423.

Eng, G. D., Hung, W., August, G. *et al.* (1976) Nerve conduction velocity determinants in juvenile diabetes: continuing study of 190 patients. *Arch. Phys. Med. Rehab.*, **57**, 1–5.

Ewing, D. J. and Clarke, B. F. (1986) Autonomic neuropathy: diagnosis and prognosis. *Clin. Endocrinol. Metab.*, **15**, 855–888.

Fagerberg, S. E. (1959) Diabetics neuropathy. A clinical and histological study on the significance of vascular affections. *Acta. Med. Scand. Suppl.* **345**.

Fraser, R. J., Horowitz, M., Maddox, A. F. *et al.* (1990) Hyperglycaemia slows gastric emptying in type 1 (insulin-dependent) diabetes mellitus. *Diabetologia*, **33**, 675–680.

Garland, H. (1955) Diabetic amyotrophy. *Br. Med. J.*, **ii**, 1287–1290.

Garland, H. and Taverner, D. (1953) Diabetic myelopathy. *Br. Med. J.*, **i**, 1405–1408.

Goodman, J. I., Baumoel, S., Frankel, L. *et al.* (1953) *The Diabetic Neuropathies*, Charles C. Thomas, Springfield, IL.

Greene, D. A., Lattimer, S. A. and Sima, A. A. F. (1987) Sorbitol, phosphoinositides, and sodium-potassium-ATPase in the pathogenesis of diabetic complications. *N. Engl. J. Med.*, **316**, 599–606.

Hale, P. J., Nattrass, M., Silverman, S. H. *et al.* (1981) Peripheral nerve concentrations of glucose, fructose, sorbitol and myoinositol in diabetic and non-diabetic patients. *Diabetologia*, **30**, 464–467.

Harris, M., Eastman, R. and Cowie, C. (1993) Symptoms of sensory neuropathy in adults with NIDDM in the US population. *Diabetes Care*, **16**, 1446–1452.

Horrocks, P. M., FitzGerald, M. G., Wright, A. D. and Nattrass, M. (1987) The time course and diurnal variation of postural hypotension in diabetic autonomic neuropathy. *Diabetic Med.*, **4**, 307–310.

Jordan, W. R. (1936) Neuritic manifestations in diabetes mellitus. *Arch. Intern. Med.*, **57**, 307–366.

Jordan, W. R., Randall, L. O. and Bloor, W. R. (1935) Neuropathy in diabetes mellitus. Lipid constituents of the nerves correlated with the clinical data. *Arch. Intern. Med.*, **55**, 26–41.

Joslin, E. P. (1928) *The Treatment of Diabetes Mellitus*, 4th edn, Lea & Febiger, Philadelphia, PA.

Krentz, A. J., Honigsberger, L. and Nattrass, M. (1989) Selection of patients with symptomatic diabetic neuropathy for clinical trials. *Diabete Metab.*, **15**, 416–419.

Lamontagne, A. and Buchthal, F. (1970) Electrophysiological studies in diabetic neuropathy. *J. Neurol. Neurosurg. Psychiat.*, **33**, 442–452.

McCulloch, D. K., Young, R. J., Prescott, R. J., *et al.* (1984) The natural history of impotence in diabetic men. *Diabetologia*, **26**, 437–440.

Malik, R. A. Tesfaye, S., Thompson, S. D. *et al.* (1993) Endoneurial localisation of microvascular damage in human diabetic neuropathy. *Diabetologia*, **36**, 454–459.

Marchal de Calvi (1864) *Recherches sur les Accidents Diabetiques*, P. Asselin, Paris.

Mayne, N. (1965) Neuropathy in the diabetic and non-diabetic populations. *Lancet*, **ii**, 1313–1316.

Page, M. McB. and Watkins, P. J. (1978) Cardiorespiratory arrest and diabetic autonomic neuropathy. *Lancet*, **i**, 14–16.

Pavy, F. W. (1885) Introductory address to the discussion on the clinical aspect of glycosuria, *Lancet*, **ii**, 1033–1035.

Pirart, J. (1978) Diabetes mellitus and its degenerative complications: a prospective study of 4400 patients observed between 1947 and 1973. *Diabetes Care* **1**, 168–188; 252–263.

Price, D. E., Cooksey, G., Jehu, D. *et al.* (1991) The management of impotence in diabetic men by vacuum tumescence therapy. *Diabetic Med.*, **8**, 964–967.

Rollo, J. (1798) *An Account of Two Cases of the Diabetes Mellitus; to Which are Added a General View of the Nature of the Disease and Its Appropriate Treatment*, T. Dilly at the Poultry, London.

Root, H. F. and Kenny, A. J. (1952) The nervous system and diabetes, in *The Treatment of Diabetes Mellitus*, (eds E. P. Joslin, H. F. Root, P. White and A. Marble), Henry Kimpton, London, pp. 476–477.

Rubin, A. and Babbott, D. (1958) Impotence and diabetes mellitus. *J. A. M. A.*, **168**, 498–500.

Rundles, R. W. (1945) Diabetic neuropathy. General review with report of 125 cases. *Medicine*, **24**, 111–160.

Rundles, R. W. (1950) Diabetic neuropathy. *Bull. N. Y. Acad. Med.*, **26**, 598.

Saundby, R. (1891) *Lectures on Diabetes*, John Wright, Bristol.

Scarpello, J. H. B. and Ward, J. D. (1984) Diabetic neuropathy, in *Recent Advances in Diabetes 1*, (eds M. Nattrass and J. V. Santiago), Churchill Livingstone, Edinburgh, p. 207–221.

Schiavi, R. C., Stimmel, B. B. Mandeli, J. and Rayfield, E. J. (1993) Diabetes mellitus and male sexual function: a controlled study. *Diabetologia*, **36**, 745–751.

Seneviratne, K. N. and Peiris, O. A. (1968) The effect of ischaemia on the excitability of sensory nerves in diabetes mellitus. *J. Neurol. Neurosurg. Psychiat.*, **31**, 348–353.

Sidenius, P. and Jakobsen, J. (1987) Axonal transport in human and experimental diabetes, in *Diabetic Neuropathy*, (eds P. J. Dyck, P. K. Thomas, A. K. Asbury *et al.*), W. B. Saunders, Philadelphia, PA, p. 206–265.

Sugimura, K. and Dyck, P. J. (1982) Multifocal fiber loss in proximal sciatic nerve in symmetric distal diabetic neuropathy. *J. Neurol. Sci.*, **53**, 501–509.

Tesfaye, S., Malik, R. and Ward, J. D. (1994) Vascular factors in diabetic neuropathy. *Diabetologia*, **37**, 847–854.

Veves, A., Malik, R. A., Lye, R. H. *et al.* (1991) The relationship between sural nerve morphometric findings and measures of peripheral nerve function in mild diabetic neuropathy. *Diabetic Med.*, **8**, 917–921.

Walters, D. P., Gatling, W., Mullee, M. A. and Hill, R. D. (1992) The prevalence of diabetic distal sensory neuropathy in an English community. *Diabetic Med.*, **9**, 349–353.

Watkins, P. J. (1973) Facial sweating after food: a new sign of diabetic autonomic neuropathy. *Br. Med. J.*, **1**, 583–587.

Watkins, P. J. (1992) Clinical observations and experiments in diabetic neuropathy. *Diabetologia*, **35**, 2–11.

Wiles, P. G. (1992) Erectile impotence in diabetic men: aetiology, investigation and management. *Diabetic Med.*, **9**, 888–892.

Woltman, H. W. and Wilder, R. M. (1929) Diabetes mellitus. Pathologic changes in the spinal cord and peripheral nerves. *Arch. Intern. Med.*, **44**, 576–603.

Young, R. J. and Clarke, B. F. (1985) Pain relief in diabetic neuropathy: the effectiveness of imipramine and related drugs. *Diabetic Med.*, **2**, 363–366

Young, M. J., Boulton, A. J. M., Macleod, A. F. *et al.* (1993) A multicentre study of the prevalence of diabetic peripheral neuropathy in the United Kingdom hospital clinic population. *Diabetologia*, **36**, 150–154.

Atherosclerosis of large vessels is the major cause of mortality and morbidity in diabetes. Although some have argued that macrovascular disease has a specificity in diabetes, within the framework of diabetic angiopathy (Lundbaek, 1954), or that atherosclerosis and a second macrovascular disease may coexist in diabetes (Heickendorff, Ledet and Rasmussen, 1994), the majority view the process as identical to atherosclerosis in the non-diabetic population. While the histopathology may prove identical the end-result is dissimilar. The manifestation tends to occur at an earlier age, there is no sex difference at any age in the diabetic in contrast to the male preponderance at earlier ages in the general population, and the distribution focusses on coronary arteries and distal peripheral arteries.

The pathogenesis remains uncertain. The concept of an inherited tendency to atherosclerosis alongside or linked to the inherited contribution to diabetes cannot be ruled out; risk factors, well identified for the non-diabetic population, may be additive in diabetes, or as yet unidentified risk factors may play a role; and hyperglycaemia, hyperinsulinism or their interaction could contribute.

What is clear from numerous studies is the lack of a relationship between diabetic control and macrovascular disease, in direct contrast to that which exists for microvascular disease. No studies that I know of can demonstrate prevention or amelioration of atherosclerosis simply by manipulation of blood glucose control. Thus the major killer remains probably the least well understood complication of diabetes and the least amenable to treatment.

ATHEROSCLEROTIC LESIONS

Atherosclerosis is characterized by focal thickening of the intima, in which stainable lipids can readily be demonstrated in and between the cellular elements. Fatty streaks and plaques are readily found at autopsy. The damage probably begins with injury to endothelial cells. One suggestion for the mechanism of this lies with alterations in blood flow changing stress and shear factors. The evidence for this is more hypothetical than real but somehow endothelial damage happens. There follows a sequence of events in non-diabetic and diabetic alike which appears to have a certain inevitability. Platelets adhere and aggregate to the endothelium and subendothelial collagen and elastic fibres. Clotting factors are released, as is a substance capable of promoting smooth muscle proliferation. Accumulation of cholesterol and lipoproteins with collagen and elastic tissue lead to a patch of atheroma. Ulceration with further clot can lead to arterial occlusion. There are many areas in this progression where diabetes would be expected to exert an effect over and above that which is found in the general population.

RISK FACTORS FOR ATHEROSCLEROSIS

Several large population studies have clarified views on risk factors for atherosclerosis. The forerunner in the general population was the Framingham Study (Kannel and McGee, 1979). The important findings from this study and many others are for obesity, hypertension, hyperlipidaemia, cigarette smoking and finally diabetes. The immediate and obvious problem is the interrelationship of these factors.

OBESITY

In the non-diabetic population obesity has been identified as a risk factor for atherosclerosis (Keys *et al.*, 1972) although recently this role has come under review. Establishing a clear link is confounded by the interrelationship of risk factors, in that obesity is linked with hypertension and lipids and with diabetes.

If obesity and diabetes are separate risk factors for arterial disease it would be reasonable to assume that obese diabetics would fare badly. Confirmation of this is lacking if not contradictory. In our clinic survey of a cohort of diabetics there was no evidence of an adverse effect of overweight at diagnosis (Hayward and Lucena, 1965). The relative mortality of those > 20% overweight was similar to those of normal weight compared to the West Midlands conurbation mortality. Similar results were reported by Pell and D'Alonzo (1970). In the University Group Diabetes Program Study cardiovascular death rates were less in placebo, tolbutamide and both insulin groups for patients greater than 1.25 ideal body weight in comparison with patients less than 1.25 ideal body weight.

Angina pectoris has been used as an endpoint denoting coronary atherosclerotic disease. When this is examined there is no doubt that obese diabetics are more likely to develop angina. Keen, Jarrett and Fuller (1974) confirmed this in the Bedford Survey of borderline diabetes. More surprisingly, however, they found that if electrocardiographic change was examined there was no difference between groups divided on the basis of their ponderal index. They have suggested that symptoms may be more marked in the obese group because increased demands upon the heart unmask coronary insufficiency.

It cannot be concluded that the case for obesity in diabetes as atherogenic is by any means proved. Nevertheless it would be incautious to conclude the opposite. While we wait for clarification it might be appropriate to relax our blinkered obsession with weight loss in the diabetic clinic. There does seem to be a feeling that a person who becomes obese is deserving of some form of retribution, be that in excess mortality or morbidity or simply in being bullied in the diabetic clinic. Disappointed that obesity cannot explain the difference in mortality between diabetic and non-diabetic populations, and rather similar to the approach used for the failure of lipids to explain the increased risk in the diabetic population, attention has switched to a qualitative change in fat, i.e. in its distribution, rather than a simple effect of quantity. Thus it is argued that the 'apple' distribution of body fat, i.e. a predominantly central or abdominal distribution, carries a risk greater than the 'pear' shape or mainly buttock preponderance of fat distribution (Larsson *et al.*, 1984).

HYPERTENSION

Ascertaining the role of hypertension in promoting atherosclerosis in diabetic patients is equally difficult. It has long been thought that diabetics were more likely to be hypertensive but a critical evaluation of this concept is difficult to find. True, when diabetic nephropathy supervenes a link is established, as is the case in the hypokalaemic hypertension of Conn's syndrome or Cushing's syndrome. These are comparatively rare occasions in the diabetic clinic and our major concern is with the more typical patient in the clinic.

Records of hypertension in the diabetic clinic are prone to bias. Firstly, blood pressure is often recorded on the first visit at a time of maximum stress. Most physicians are aware of the unrepresentative nature of this measurement and would now seek confirmation of the elevated reading. Not so in the past and studies have been published on data analysed from this instance. Secondly, and this reservation must apply to all 'associated' diseases, the diabetic population is a well screened population and an increased prevalence might well be expected solely on this basis. Thirdly, patients attending hypertension clinics are a similarly well screened population where diabetes, if present, should be diagnosed. Fourthly there is the role of drug therapy. Corticosteroids will produce both hypertension and diabetes while the thiazide diuretics, so often used in the treatment of hypertension, will precipitate or unmask diabetes. In addition to these specific problems the basic ground rules of hypertensive studies – elimination of observer bias, standardization of conditions under which the pressure is measured and selection of appropriate age, sex- and weight-matched non-diabetic control subjects – must be taken into account.

Pyke (1968) compared blood pressure at presentation of diabetes with a second group who had diabetes for up to 16 years. There was a rise in mean pressure with age and women had higher values than men over the age of 40 years. Freedman, Moulton and Spencer (1958) found some increase in elevated levels but only in elderly diabetics while Jarrett and Keen (1975) found no differences in systolic or diastolic pressures between a diabetic population, or a hospital or community series of non-diabetic controls.

In contrast the Framingham Study (Garcia *et al.*, 1974) and the DuPont employees study (Pell and D'Alonzo, 1967) concluded the opposite. Mean systolic pressure of the diabetics was significantly higher than non-diabetics, with the excess being contributed by women (Garcia *et al.*, 1974). Pell and D'Alonzo (1967) reported that the prevalence of hypertension in the Du Pont employees was 54% higher in the diabetics. Furthermore, this relationship was independent of obesity. Perhaps even more convincing was the observation that borderline or hypertensive levels of blood pressure could be found more often in the period before diagnosis of diabetes.

Table 17.1 Mean systolic and diastolic (± s.d.) pressures in normal (control) subjects, borderline diabetic patients and newly diagnosed diabetic patients aged 20–79 years. (Source: adapted from Jarrett, Keen and Chakrabarti, 1982)

	Normal	*Borderline*	*Diabetic*
Systolic			
Male	143.7 ± 25.0	157.5 ± 29.7	161.7 ± 31.1
Female	156.3 ± 28.4	169.7 ± 35.4	175.0 ± 35.4
Diastolic			
Male	85.3 ± 14.9	91.1 ± 15.8	90.4 ± 12.2
Female	88.2 ± 14.8	90.1 ± 22.4	92.5 ± 13.3

In the Bedford Survey diabetes was diagnosed from a 2-hour after 50 g glucose concentration of > 11.1 mmol/l (200 mg/dl). A value of 6.7–11.1 mmol/l (120–200 mg/dl) categorized a patient as borderline, and < 6.7 mmol/l (< 120 mg/dl) was normal. There is a rough correspondence between these categories and the WHO diagnostic classes of normal, impaired glucose tolerance and diabetic, although substantial differences in methodology cannot entirely be ignored. The mean systolic and diastolic pressures for the three groups are given in Table 17.1 and, subdivided by decade, these pressures are presented in Jarrett, Keen and Chakrabarti (1982).

A second large survey from the same group screened male civil servants aged 45–64. Previously diagnosed diabetics were included and some newly diagnosed and borderline diabetics were identified. Values for known diabetics closely approximated those for the group (> 19 000) overall while borderline and newly diagnosed subjects were higher.

CIGARETTE SMOKING

Few comparisons of cigarette smoking in non-diabetic and diabetic populations have been made. In the Whitehall Survey 37% of diabetics were ex-smokers and a similar

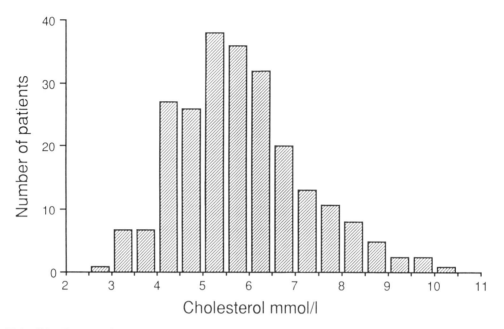

Fig. 17.1 Distribution of non-fasting plasma cholesterol concentration in diabetic patients attending an annual review clinic.

percentage continued to smoke, which was broadly similar to the non-diabetic population. More recently Horsley, Barrett and MacFarlane (1987) reported 22% ex-smokers and 31% continuing to smoke of a sample of over a thousand diabetic patients while Rosengren *et al.* (1989) found 41% who smoked in both non-diabetic and diabetic populations.

These counting-of-heads studies are difficult to interpret but they do not present a case for substantial differences in smoking habits between the non-diabetic and diabetic populations.

HYPERLIPIDAEMIA

It is well recognized that disturbances of circulating lipids occur in diabetic patients. The main abnormality is gross hypertriglyceridaemia secondary to poor blood glucose control. Difficulties in improving control, sufficient to maintain euglycaemia, often

preclude certainty that this is a secondary phenomenon.

This biochemical abnormality may have been exaggerated as a risk factor for atherosclerosis in the diabetic population. The status of triglycerides as a risk factor for coronary heart disease has waned in recent years and the focus has shifted emphatically toward cholesterol. Cholesterol is less susceptible to manipulation by attention to blood glucose control and indeed the prevalence of raised cholesterol concentrations in our diabetic clinic appears similar to the non-diabetic population (Figure 17.1).

Measurement of total cholesterol concentration may not reveal the full story, however, with more subtle alterations in the component cholesterol fractions which go to make up the total cholesterol concentrations.

Hypertriglyceridaemia, an excess of very low density lipoprotein (VLDL), results predominantly from an inability to clear triglyceride from the plasma. Lipoprotein

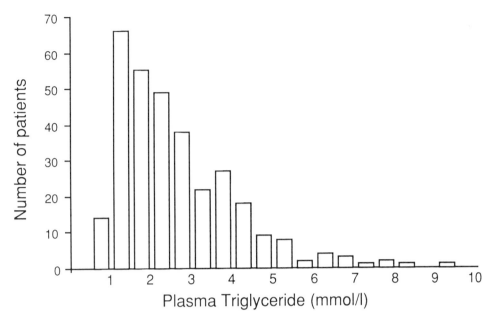

Fig. 17.2 Distribution of non-fasting plasma triglyceride concentration in diabetic patients attending an annual review clinic.

lipase, which clears triglyceride, is an insulin-sensitive enzyme and inadequate insuliniza-tion decreases activity and allows triglyceride accumulation. Thus hypertriglyceridaemia is common at times of poor metabolic control and responds to treatment of diabetes. Over-production of triglyceride may also play a part due to increased substrate supply of non-esterified fatty acids from insulin deficiency or insulin resistance in the periphery. There is no doubt that a substantial proportion of diabetic patients have raised triglyceride concentrations (Figure 17.2).

Clearance of low density lipoprotein (LDL) is also impaired in diabetes through a dual mechanism. Non-enzymic glycation of the apoprotein reduces affinity for the LDL receptor (Steinbrecher and Witztum, 1984) while LDL receptor activity is also sensitive to insulin (Chait, Bierman and Albers, 1979). High density lipoprotein (HDL), which appears to have a protective effect against atheroma, is reduced in non-insulin-dependent diabetes (Harno, Nikkila and Kuusi, 1980), whereas in insulin-dependent diabetic patients concentrations may be normal or raised.

The findings for lipoproteins in diabetic patients have proved somewhat disappointing for lipidologists. Quantitatively the differences between diabetic and non-diabetic patients are small and cannot explain all, or even much, of the increased mortality in the diabetic population. Not daunted, however, our erstwhile colleagues have altered their story and would now suggest that the difference between the two populations may lie in a qualitative difference in the lipids of the diabetic population rather than in a quantitative change.

PROTEINURIA

I find it difficult to accept that proteinuria or microalbuminuria are risk factors for macro-vascular disease as has been suggested (Jarrett *et al.*, 1984; Schmitz and Vaeth, 1988). It would seem to be much easier to regard them as risk predictors on the basis of the evidence to date. After all, it has been known for many years that severe heart disease is accompanied by proteinuria and it seems more likely to me that, when present, proteinuria is a marker for the presence of macrovascular disease. It then becomes tautologous to claim that proteinuria is a risk factor.

This may be a rather idiosyncratic view in that there is ample opportunity for proteinuria in particular to alter risk. Firstly it is associated with hypertension although the risk remains when hypertension is taken out of the equation. Secondly, proteinuria is accompanied by a more atherogenic look to the lipid profile, and thirdly, proteinuria aggravates the clotting profile, being associated with higher fibrinogen and greater platelet stickiness. The question of altered vascular permeability as a risk factor is unresolved.

DIABETES

These risk factors are common to both the non-diabetic and diabetic populations. Indeed the question arises whether, having considered the clustering of risk factors in the diabetic population, there is any excess atherosclerosis unaccounted for; in other words is 'diabetes' a separate risk factor?

In the Framingham study it was acknowledged that established risk factors were increased in frequency in the diabetic population yet this increased frequency did not entirely account for the increased incidence of coronary artery disease. Using multivariate analysis, and the majority of studies utilize this technique, they concluded that a unique effect of diabetes was operating.

The findings of the Du Pont employees study were similar. Using mortality as the endpoint, Pell and D'Alonzo (1970) found that 25% of diabetics died compared with only 10% of the non-diabetic population. While some of this excess could be attributed to known risk factors, particularly hypertension, it did not account for all. For the

moment we should conclude that diabetes *per se* confers an increased risk of atherosclerosis.

MECHANISM IN DIABETES

If it is accepted that diabetes increases the risk of atherosclerosis the possible underlying explanations are legion. Multiple biochemical abnormalities occur in untreated or inadequately treated diabetes which could be implicated. Indeed, it is not necessary to postulate a specific risk factor since it may well be the result of interaction between one of the biochemical abnormalities and a known risk factor. The two most likely biochemical abnormalities, however, must be hyperglycaemia and insulin levels. The third explanation, an interaction of glucose and insulin, is virtually unconsidered.

GLUCOSE

The most telling implication of glucose comes from the Whitehall Study of borderline diabetics. They found that when 2-hour blood glucose concentration after 50 g glucose exceeded the 95th centile for glucose concentration there was an increase in arterial disease (Jarrett, Keen and Chakrabarti, 1982). Other studies have reported similar findings.

INSULIN

The idea that hyperinsulinaemia and atherosclerosis are related has been around since the studies of Stout (1975) and the situation remains unresolved and unsatisfactory. To my mind it is one of the most pertinent questions in diabetes and urgently requires an answer. The concentration upon diabetic control and the prevention of microvascular disease has led to tacit acceptance of peripheral hyperinsulinaemia. The thought that prevention of morbidity is being achieved at the expense of mortality is too horrible to contemplate.

The suggestion of hyperinsulinaemia promoting atherosclerosis stems from animal experiments and circumstantial evidence. In pieces of rat aorta Stout (1975) observed enhanced lipid deposition with medium containing insulin.

In human studies the picture is one of confusion. Early studies suggested strongly that non-diabetic patients with coronary, cerebral or peripheral vascular disease have higher insulin levels than control patients; and that diabetic patients with macrovascular disease also have higher insulin levels than controls. To examine this three large prospective studies were carried out and they have reported their results for the relationship of cardiovascular risk and hyperinsulinaemia in the normal population. In each of the three studies there was a clear relationship of risk to insulin levels when a simple relationship was sought. When the contribution of a number of factors was examined simultaneously, however – obesity, hypertension, lipids – the picture was much more complicated. In the study of Paris policemen, only fasting insulin levels remained predictive (Ducimetiere *et al.*, 1980); in Helsinki there was a relationship between 1- and 2-hour post-glucose plasma insulin levels, but not fasting levels, and atherosclerosis (Pyorala, 1979); while in the Busselton study in Western Australia an initial relationship disappeared (Welborn and Wearne, 1979).

For hyperinsulinaemia to be a major risk factor in diabetes we would have to have firm evidence of its existence. It is clear that in insulin-dependent patients adequate exposure of the liver to insulin must be associated with the loss of the normal portal/peripheral ratio. Thus hyperinsulinaemia in the periphery is a logical consequence of attempts to obtain normoglycaemia.

In non-insulin-dependent diabetes the situation is less clear. It is generally accepted that non-insulin-dependent diabetes is a disease of insulinopenia and insulin resistance. It would appear that the natural history of the disorder is that insulin resistance with minor abnormality of glucose metabolism is followed by loss of insulin secretion and greater abnormality of blood glucose.

This progression presents difficulties in demonstrating a relationship between hyperinsulinaemia and atherosclerosis. In particular the phase of hyperinsulinaemia may precede diagnosis in a large number of patients. Thus when diagnosis of diabetes or presentation of atherosclerosis occurs the patient may be insulinopenic and the degree of or length of exposure to hyperinsulinism is never known. The argument is further complicated by the concept of hyperinsulinism in non-insulin-dependent diabetes. Glucose tolerance test responses invariably show postprandial hyperinsulinism but this is a consequence of a decreased early insulin response allowing hyperglycaemia. Clarification of these factors awaits careful study.

It seems paradoxical that as we begin to discard obesity as a risk factor for atherosclerosis so hyperinsulinism rears its ugly head. Few relationships are as clear-cut as the hyperinsulinaemia of obese non-diabetic subjects. To substantiate hyperinsulinism we could at least expect a significant increase in atherosclerosis in this group. I find this argument against hyperinsulinism telling although I would reserve judgement upon the combination of hyperinsulinism and hyperglycaemia. Perhaps the latter is necessary for manifestation of the effects of the former.

INSULIN RESISTANCE

Reaven (1988) has drawn attention to the clustering of risk factors in certain populations. Non-insulin-dependent diabetes, impaired glucose tolerance and obesity are linked by resistance to insulin-stimulated glucose uptake and hyperinsulinaemia. Furthermore, insulin resistance can be identified in patients with hypertension, as can a degree of glucose intolerance. These patients may also manifest disturbances of lipoprotein metabolism, particularly hypertriglyceridaemia, which cor-

Table 17.2 Syndrome X of diabetes

- Glucose intolerance
- Hyperinsulinaemia
- Impaired insulin-stimulated glucose uptake
- Increased VLDL
- Reduced HDL cholesterol
- Hypertension
- Obesity

relates with the degree of hyperglycaemia and hyperinsulinaemia. In addition there is an inverse correlation with high density lipoprotein cholesterol. This combination of risk factors in the population may well go some distance toward explaining the development of atherosclerosis and has been labelled syndrome X or the metabolic syndrome (Table 17.2). It is unclear just how many diabetic patients manifest the full-blown syndrome. It is also unclear whether certain other considerations that hover on the periphery of the syndrome should be included, such as a raised urate and a raised gamma glutamyl transpeptidase.

DIABETES AND HEART DISEASE

Heart disease is the principal cause of deaths in patients whose diabetes begins in adult life. Even among those who have advanced renal disease the final illness is often coronary thrombosis rather than renal failure. The effect of the increased incidence of coronary disease in later life is clearly shown in the death rates of diabetics. The specific problem is coronary heart disease although microvascular disease of the heart continues to be debated.

PHYSIOLOGY

Under normal circumstances the heart derives its energy from a range of substrates. About 60% is obtained from non-esterified fatty acids, 30% from glucose and the remaining 10% from other substrates such as lactate, pyruvate and ketone bodies. Ischaemia pro-

foundly alters this arrangement. Oxidation of non-esterified fatty acids is almost totally inhibited, with accumulation of long-chain fatty acyl CoA and non-esterified fatty acids. In turn these inhibit pyruvate dehydrogenase (Randle, 1984) leaving an almost total dependency upon anaerobic glycolysis. This, too, is slowed by ischaemia through inhibition of phosphofructokinase and glyceraldehyde-3-phosphate dehydrogenase.

CORONARY HEART DISEASE

Reports in the literature, while almost unanimous in reporting an increased frequency of coronary artery diseases in diabetes, vary greatly in the figures they give. In some instances this is due to a failure to take into account the age and sex distribution of a diabetic population, in others to ignoring the local factors that determine the admission of diabetics to one hospital or another and in a few to disregard of the criteria for the diagnosis of diabetes.

Clawson and Bell (1949), in a review of 50 000 autopsies, found fatal coronary disease to be about twice as frequent in males and three times as frequent in females with diabetes compared with non-diabetics. The incidence of disease of the coronary arteries was almost as high in diabetic women as in diabetic men; 4% of deaths from coronary disease in men and 14% of those in women were associated with diabetes. Liebow, Hellerstein and Miller (1955), in a cardiac survey of 383 living outpatient diabetics with a average age of 58.1 years, found 42% with atherosclerotic heart disease, 10.2% with angina and 6.8% with myocardial infarction.

More recent studies have not indicated a need to revise these figures. Crall and Roberts (1978) sectioned coronary arteries at 0.25 cm intervals from young diabetics and non-diabetics. The diabetic patients had a greater incidence of severe stenosis of a major coronary artery (75%) and a greater length of artery was narrowed by 50% or more. Vigorita,

Moore and Hutchins (1980) found more myocardial infarcts, more collaterals and more diffuse disease in a larger number of diabetic patients at autopsy than non-diabetic patients.

MYOCARDIAL INFARCTION

Somewhat surprisingly there has been some confusion in the literature about whether the diabetic patient is more likely to die after a myocardial infarction. Some of the studies recording negative results were too small and if these are omitted from further consideration the case becomes stronger. Gwilt and Pentecost (1984) reanalysed 19 trials where they considered numbers of patients were large enough to allow an answer. Of 19 studies, there was an increase in mortality in the diabetic in 15 and in 4 rates were similar. Even if the rejected studies are included 29 of 32 studies show a diabetic mortality ratio greater than any which has a probability of arising by chance of less than one in a million.

We have never shared the view of similar mortality rates. Our experience of mortality rates since 1970 and before the introduction of thrombolytic agents has been 18% in non-diabetics and 33% in diabetics. We are convinced that this is a real difference. As with any mortality rate in hospital it is influenced by many other factors than the presenting disease. Diabetic patients admitted to hospital with myocardial infarction show significant differences from non-diabetics for age, sex, atypical symptoms, pre-existing ischaemia and hypertension. In our own population we find age as the only different factor which might account for an increased mortality. When the age-corrected rate for non-diabetics is calculated, however, the non-diabetic mortality only rises to 19%. A further factor that can influence mortality rates is duration of symptoms on admission. We wondered whether diabetic patients were gaining admission quicker than non-diabetics and we were including some early mortality. In fact, the reverse was true. The median time for the diabetics to reach hospital was 5 hours compared with the lesser time of 3.5 hours in non-diabetics.

In recent years mortality rates have fallen in both the non-diabetic and diabetic populations immediately after myocardial infarction. This has been ascribed to the introduction of thrombolytic therapy. Currently our rates are approximately 8.5% in non-diabetic patients and 17.0% in diabetic patients (Lynch *et al.*, 1993).

Why do diabetics have an increased mortality?

There are many possible answers to this question. We have looked closely at two of them. Firstly, does the answer lie in the metabolic and hormonal response to a myocardial infarction, which assumes increased importance in a patient whose counteraction of this is impaired?

A brief consideration of the intracellular effects of ischaemia is given above. Hormonal responses are also important, since they exacerbate the problem. Myocardial infarction results in high circulating concentrations of catecholamines. Not only does adrenalin impair glucose uptake into cells, thus decreasing substrate availability, but there is a potent effect upon insulin secretion. The inhibition of insulin secretion in the non-insulin-dependent diabetic patient fails to provide the adequate stimulus for insulin-mediated glucose uptake into muscle. In addition the enhanced catecholamine effect and decreased action of insulin allow increased rates of lipolysis, further increasing non-esterified fatty acid levels. Glucose entry into cells is further moderated by elevated circulating concentrations of glucagon, cortisol and growth hormone. Even in normal patients glucose intolerance after myocardial infarction is observed, indicating an inability, even with considerable insulin secretory reserve, to overcome the catabolic drive. With fixed insulin availability as in insulin-dependent patients or limited secretory reserve as in non-insulin-dependent patients the catabolic effects of the counter-insulin hormones are enhanced.

The toxic nature of high fatty acid levels is well documented. Oxidative phosphorylation is uncoupled, myocardial membrane ATPase is inhibited and oxygen consumption is increased. At the organ level this results in a shorter action potential, reduced cardiac function and increased infarct size (de Leiris, Opie and Lubbe, 1975).

There is no doubt that post-infarction arrythmias correlate with circulating fatty acid levels and this has been proposed as an explanation of the increased mortality in diabetic patients (Oliver, Kurien and Greenwood, 1968). Unfortunately, on closer inspection this theory does not explain the finding. The majority of diabetic patients die of pump failure and only about 5–10% from dysrhythmias. This figure is similar to the non-diabetic population.

Experimental work in animals has indicated the importance of reduced glycolysis. It has been argued that increasing the supply of glucose and insulin reduces the effect of ischaemia (Dalby, Bricknell and Opie, 1981). Although there are strong protagonists of this view, its value is denied (Medical Research Council Working-Party Report, 1968).

A complication of the argument can be found in publications from our clinic in Birmingham. Soler *et al.* (1975) and Gwilt *et al.* (1984) have clearly shown a rise in mortality with admission blood glucose level. Yet this can be interpreted in many ways. The higher blood glucose level may simply reflect a bigger infarct with a greater catabolic response. It may simply indicate the 'worst' diabetics. Or it could be that poor metabolic control at the time of the infarct influences outcome.

We have devised an insulin infusion regime (Gwilt, Nattrass and Pentecost, 1982) designed to lower blood glucose smoothly and safely to relatively normal blood glucose levels. Although we may not achieve this aim

totally, and in any case are handicapped by the concept of normal blood glucose post-myocardial infarct, the regimen has produced better control than we obtained historically. Despite this improved control we have had no effect upon mortality. The Dundee Group (Clark *et al.*, 1985), using our regimen, reported a reduction in mortality. The numbers of patients studied, however, was very small and may well have produced an artefactual group. It is well known that when counting mortality in ketoacidosis or myocardial infarction it is possible to have periods of mortality approaching zero until the next group of patients emerges with a very high mortality.

The second possibility we have considered is that diabetic patients have larger infarcts than non-diabetics. If traditional teaching is correct the infarct in the diabetic patient must be set against the backcloth of earlier, more extensive, distal disease. Infarct size is the major predictor of death following coronary thrombosis. We attacked his hypothesis in a three-pronged manner. In a retrospective study of 456 diabetics and 1951 non-diabetics we found no difference in the distribution of peak aspartate transaminase levels. What was apparent, however, was that at every level of aspartate transaminase the mortality in the diabetics was greater than in the non-diabetics (Figure 17.3).

Prospectively, in 120 diabetics and 120 age- and sex-matched non-diabetics, aspartate transaminase levels were identical yet the increased mortality and incidence of pump failure in the diabetics remained (Figure 17.4).

Finally and in a smaller study, 30 patients in matched pairs had creatine kinase MB measured at intervals over 72 hours. This reliable way of sizing infarcts in the non-diabetic population did not reveal any differences in infarct size between diabetics and non-diabetics. None of these studies are without flaw and in particular the CK-MB mapping study makes the assumption that the kinetics of this enzyme are similar in

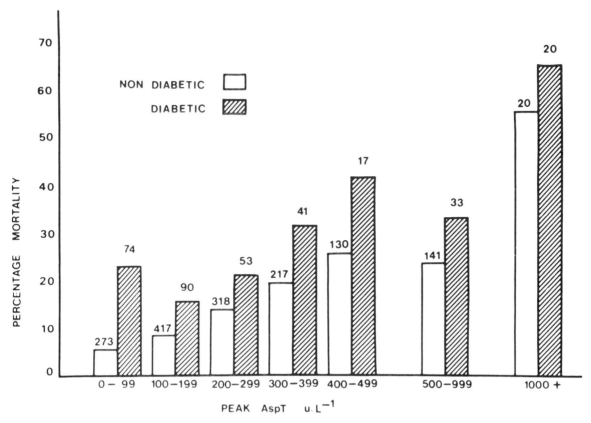

Fig. 17.3 Mortality in relation to peak aspartate transaminase concentration in 456 diabetic patients and 1951 non-diabetic patients following myocardial infarction. (Source: reproduced with permission from Gwilt *et al.*, 1984.)

diabetics to non-diabetics. Yet in concert they appear to make a strong case against the idea of bigger infarcts in diabetics.

Weitzman *et al.* (1984) used a QRS scoring method of measuring infarct size and did find support for larger infarcts in diabetics. Jaffe *et al.* (1984), using enzyme release methods, found that while cardiac failure and post-discharge mortality was increased in the diabetic group infarct size was assessed as smaller. And in the Corpus Christi Heart Project (Orlander *et al.*, 1994) infarct size was the same in diabetic and non-diabetic Mexican Americans and non-Hispanic whites.

A number of other reasons for the increased mortality have been proposed. Of these the fatty acid/dysrhythmia story is the oldest. As previously discussed, the theoretical nature of this is justifiable – that fatty acids promote dysrhythmias, and that diabetics, with an inability to compensate the stress response, have higher fatty acids and are more prone to sudden death from dysrhythmia following myocardial infarction. In practice the theory cannot entirely be discounted. From our own experience it is not the explanation of the greater hospital mortality since the majority of deaths in the diabetics are from pump failure and not from dysrhythmia. Indeed the overwhelming finding is of a similar manner of death in the diabetic and non-diabetic group and a major increase in cardiac failure

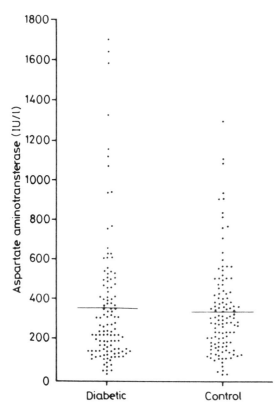

Fig. 17.4 Peak aspartate transaminase concentration in 120 diabetic patients and 120 matched non-diabetic patients following myocardial infarction. (Source: reproduced with permission from Gwilt *et al.*, 1984.)

even without death. Still, we must consider the temporal nature of the hospital mortality. If deaths from dysrhythmia are increased this may well be in the pre-hospitalization phase. In turn this implies an even greater early mortality in the diabetic group.

The multitude of endocrine and metabolic effects of a myocardial infarction increase the propensity of the diabetic to abnormal haemostasis. A number of authors have called attention to increased platelet stickiness and aggregation in diabetes, which has led to the suggestion that platelet plugging of small vessels could enhance ischaemia and lead to more severe effects. Indeed platelet plugs

have been demonstrated in human diabetic heart at autopsy, lending some support to this hypothesis.

Other abnormalities of the microcirculation may occur. Blood flow through capillaries may be impaired from increased viscosity or from decreased red-cell deformability. Poor diabetic control leads to an increase in capillary leakiness (Parving *et al.*, 1976), which may explain pulmonary oedema. Glycation of haemoglobin reduces the delivery of oxygen to the tissues (Ditzel, 1976).

For many years there has been a suggestion that diabetics may have a specific cardiopathy or cardiomyopathy. This is discussed in more detail below but briefly it is argued that microvascular disease can affect the arteries and capillaries of heart muscle as it does in other tissues. If this occurs then clearly it would reduce the ability of the diabetic heart to open a collateral circulation, which in turn could contribute to death.

Perhaps the most attractive suggestion is derived from the high incidence of heart failure and pump failure deaths. Is there reason to think that the compliance of heart muscle is abnormal? The stiff ventricles could result from platelet plugging or microvascular disease but a third possibility must be considered. It is well recognized that hyperglycaemia can lead to post-translational glycation of proteins. This has been used to advantage in assessing diabetic control using circulating proteins, but intracellular glycation can also occur. If heart muscle protein was glycated this could lead to decreased compliance and go a long way to explaining the frequency of heart failure.

Presentation of myocardial infarction

The manifestations of coronary artery disease in the diabetic are not obviously different from those in the non-diabetic. Perhaps painless coronary artery occlusion is more common, due to loss of afferent painful impulses as a result of autonomic neuropathy, although our own figures do not support this view, with similar rates (approximately 15%) of silent infarction in diabetics and non-diabetics. There is inevitably a selective process in patients sent to hospital and those admitted to the general wards or coronary care units so accurate quantification is almost impossible. It could be argued however, that the effect of an infarct upon diabetic control results in silent infarcts being detected more commonly in the diabetic than the non-diabetic population.

There are special problems in relation to the diabetes. Vomiting may be the outstanding symptom in coronary occlusion and if praecordial pain is not severe the finding of heavy glycosuria and ketonuria may be diagnosed incorrectly as diabetic ketoacidosis.

In our experience of ketoacidosis, concurrent myocardial infarction is rare but when the two conditions co-exist the mortality is greater than 50%. It is wise to perform an ECG on all patients over the age of 40 with diabetic ketoacidosis.

Management

Management of the thrombosis is similar in the non-diabetic and the diabetic. Thrombolytic agents and aspirin are used in both groups of patients. Currently there is a reluctance to use this treatment in diabetic patients with proliferative retinopathy although evidence that it is harmful is not available.

Management of diabetes demands flexibility in regimen. Apart from a few patients whose normal treatment is diet and in whom the diabetes is little upset by the infarct, diabetic patients are best managed with insulin after a myocardial infarction. Many regimens have been devised using twice-daily or more frequent subcutaneous injections of short- or intermediate-acting insulin. It is nigh on impossible to show a benefit for one regimen over the next and indeed perhaps it is of little import in the final outcome. Nevertheless it would be inappropriate to assign a patient to poor control and most physicians attempt to obtain near-normal blood glucose levels. I am a firm believer in the regimen that creates least anxiety. Intermittent subcutaneous injections present difficulties when vomiting occurs or in matching the dose to the degree of response to the infarct. We developed an intravenous insulin infusion regimen with the rate of infusion dependent upon blood glucose level and have used this method in more than 200 diabetic patients (Table 17.3). Initially we hoped to see a reduction in mortality, which remains unconvincing. We have decided to use the regimen latterly because our original judgement of it has been borne out. It is 'simple, safe, and effective'. The nursing staff on the coronary care unit like it because it creates a degree of uniformity in management between firms in the hospital. They are actively involved in the treatment, and they can gain considerable expertise in its use. Despite this we still have the occasional junior registrar who attempts to enforce his previous (often minimal) experience of management upon us.

Briefly, quick-acting insulin is diluted in normal saline to which albumin is added to prevent adsorption of insulin to the plastic surfaces of the equipment. The infusion is given by a syringe pump at a rate that depends upon, and is adjusted according to, hourly blood glucose measurement. A steady fall in blood glucose concentration is obtained and the decreasing dose as normoglycaemia approaches helps to level out blood glucose. Neither hypoglycaemia nor hypokalaemia have proved to be problems.

Other workers have used similar insulin infusion regimens but accompanied by infusions of 10% glucose. This is a hybrid approach based partly on the glucose/insulin/potassium regimen and partly on the idea that more insulin and hence more glucose will drive glucose into cells and provide substrate. It seems to me an unnecessarily complicated regimen.

It is simple to keep our insulin infusion running for 48–72 hours. Then a decision has to be made on the further management of

Table 17.3 Management of diabetes following myocardial infarction

1. Patients

All known diabetics on diet only, oral hypoglycaemic agents or insulin who experience an episode of myocardial ischaemia (ischaemic pain of at least 30 min duration)

2. Indications for insulin infusion

Blood glucose on admission greater than 10 mmol/l (180 mg/dl) or if treatment is normally with insulin

3. Regimen

50 ml syringe containing 47 ml saline (154 mmol/l)
　　　　　　　　　　　　 2.5 ml human albumin (10%)
　　　　　　　　　　　　 50 units quick-acting insulin

If Blood Glucose*	infuse insulin	at flow rate
< 8 mmol/l	1 u/h	1 ml/h
8–11.9 mmol/l	2 u/l	2 ml/h
12–15.9 mmol/l	3 u/h	3 ml/h
16–24 mmol/l	4 u/h	4 ml/h
> 24 mmol/l	6 u/h	6 ml/h

NB   It is preferable to infuse 0.5 u/h rather than stopping insulin infusion when blood glucose is low. Careful monitoring is necessary to avoid hypoglycaemia.

4. Monitoring

On admission measure blood glucose and test urine for ketones thereafter:

First 24 h – measure blood glucose hourly for first 4 h then 4-hourly

Subsequently – measure blood glucose 6-hourly or more frequently if infusion rate is 4 u/h or more.

5. Subsequent progress

Continue insulin infusion for 48 h then change to Actrapid, 6 u hourly before meals. Some patients treated by diet only may be able to return to diet only treatment at this stage. Insulin infusion should be discontinued 30 min after first subcutaneous injection (i.e. just before the following meal)

*Conversion factor: mmol/l × 18 = mg/dl.

the diabetes. At this time patients may be returned to their original therapy or may continue on insulin. I think there are certain advantages in continuing insulin subcutaneously.

At 48 or 72 hours it is often difficult to predict whether the patient will respond to oral agents. A poor response at this time may commit the patient to insulin for the rest of his/her life. Continuing insulin for 2–3 months it is usually very apparent who can be returned to insulin successfully. Good blood glucose control, normal glycated protein levels and a small dose of insulin indicate a high chance of success with oral agents. It is necessary, however, to make a clear and conscious note that this aspect of management will be reviewed. Metformin, because of effects upon lactate metabolism, should be stopped on admission, never given in the acute phase of an infarct and, rather more debatable, should not be used in a patient with a history of ischaemic heart disease.

The excess mortality for the diabetic in the hospital phase of treatment continues after discharge. Figures from studies before the introduction of thrombolytic treatment show that 12 months after discharge the mortality is 18% in diabetics and 6% in non-diabetics (Ulvenstam *et al.*, 1985). Orlander *et al.* (1994) found a cumulative mortality over 44 months of follow-up after myocardial infarction of 37.4% in diabetic and 23.3% in non-diabetic patients.

ANGINA

With the increase in atheroma in the diabetic population angina is a common problem in the diabetic clinic. The antianginal agents used in the non-diabetic may all be used in the diabetic although most have side effects, usually marginal, upon aspects of diabetic management.

Of the commonly used drugs, beta-blockers have probably received the worst reviews although whether justified is difficult to decide. In insulin-treated patients they are said to block the warning of hypoglycaemia. Presumably what is meant is that symptoms of the adrenergic response to hypoglycaemia are modified or obliterated although neuro-glycopenic symptoms persist. Whether this is a feature of all beta-blockers or only non-selective agents may be debated. I have never been very impressed by this argument, neither by the evidence from systematic study nor from the evidence of the diabetic clinic. I find the evidence that beta-blockers delay recovery from hypoglycaemia more pertinent, presumably from the effects upon glycogen mobilization. A second argument against their use lies in the effect upon the lipid profile. It is not clear whether this is more of a problem with non-selective agents which raise triglycerides (Wright *et al.*, 1979). The changes produced are of minor degree but in an at-risk population are clearly of some import. Perhaps the most telling arguments against their use in the male diabetic is the side effect of impotence, likely to be a sizeable problem in the treated population. In addition it is surprising how many patients we see with peripheral vascular disease who have been prescribed a beta-blocker inappropriately.

Nitrates do not seem to have any major side effects specific to the diabetic population, while the effects of calcium-channel antagonists are also relatively free from specific problems. In careful studies minor effects upon plasma glucose can be found but it is doubtful if this finding is of major clinical significance (Chellingsworth, Kendall and Wright, 1989).

The problems of choosing a suitable anti-anginal regimen are considerably less than deciding upon antihypertensive treatment and many patients can be well controlled with currently available regimens. Nevertheless,

and as in the non-diabetic population, control of angina is difficult in some patients and further investigations with a view to surgery may be indicated. In the past there has been a reluctance to investigate diabetics with a view to further treatment. This view is based upon the illusionary argument that if only the other problems of diabetes were treated adequately, particularly hyperlipidaemia, the problem would somehow diminish. When this argument fails a second rears its head – that if atheroma is more diffuse and extensive in the diabetic the benefits of surgery are likely to be lessened. These arguments are similar to those produced to deny diabetic patients renal dialysis and transplantation and penalize the diabetic patient by ill-informed bias rather than securely grounded opinion. The cost in mortality to the diabetic population of macrovascular disease is of such magnitude that it is unjustifiable to deny them the benefits of surgical advances.

Coronary angioplasty is of uncertain value in the battle against mortality in the non-diabetic population and likewise in the diabetic population. There would be grounds for believing that it would be a less successful treatment for morbidity in diabetic patents since it is likely to be most successful in dealing with one or two discrete lesions rather than diffuse disease.

Coronary artery bypass surgery may be preferable to angioplasty as treatment in diabetic patients. Results do not seem as good in the diabetic population. There is a suggestion of a higher early mortality and a reduced long-term survival. Lawrie, Morris and Glaeser (1986) found 15-year survival rates of 43% in diabetic patients on diet only, 33% in diabetics taking oral hypoglycaemic agents and only 19% in those on insulin.

DIABETIC CARDIOPATHY

The suggestion that diabetics may have a specific cardiomyopathy was made in the 1970s. In the Framingham Study Kannel,

Hjortland and Castelli (1974) indicated that the high incidence of heart failure could not be explained by ischaemic heart disease. Hamby, Zoneraich and Sherman (1974) found a high incidence of diabetes in a series of patients with congestive cardiomyopathy which could be explained by a specific effect.

HISTOLOGY

A number of studies have demonstrated histological change in small blood vessels of the myocardium. Endothelial cell proliferation, PAS-positive deposit and colloidal fibrils in the vessel wall were noted by Blumenthal, Alex and Goldenberg (1960) in two-thirds of hearts from diabetic patients. These changes, which produced vascular obstruction, were also present in non-diabetics but in less than one third of patients. Endothelial proliferation has been the main finding in autopsy studies and in endomyocardial biopsy specimens. The opposite view has also been advanced since endothelial cell proliferation was not found in hearts from diabetic animals or humans by Shirey, Proudfit and Hawk (1980) or Ledet (1976). Crall and Roberts (1978) found endothelial cell proliferation and increased PAS formation but concluded that it was rare, affecting about 1% of the vessels examined.

Microaneurysms have been seen in the diabetic heart (Factor, Okun and Minase, 1980) using a post-mortem injection technique and electron microscopy has revealed capillary basement membrane thickening (Fischer, Barner and Leskiw, 1979). These changes collectively point to a specific microangiopathy in the diabetic heart.

FUNCTIONAL STUDIES

Non-invasive studies of cardiac function have focussed upon measurement of systolic time intervals and echocardiography. In many diabetics the pre-ejection period is increased and the left ventricular ejection time is shortened, indicating reduced left ventricular function. Furthermore these abnormalities are accen-

tuated in the presence of microvascular disease (Seneviratne, 1977). In other diabetic patients systolic time intervals are normal.

Echocardiography has been used to measure peak rate of left ventricular filling. This tends to be normal in diabetics without microvascular complications, reduced in patients with background retinopathy or moderate proteinuria and markedly reduced when severe complications are present. These findings were associated with delayed mitral valve opening. These findings lend support to the idea of a specific small-vessel disease affecting the heart. Nevertheless it is impossible to dispel doubt totally that the changes observed were due to minor degrees of atherosclerosis, or to alterations in ventricular compliance.

INVASIVE STUDIES

Regan *et al.* (1974) observed reduced left ventricular compliance in alloxan diabetic dogs and found higher left ventricular and diastolic pressure with lower end diastolic volume in diabetic humans (Regan *et al.*, 1977). Importantly these patients had normal coronary angiography and a normal lactate response to atrial pacing, making significant atherosclerosis unlikely.

MECHANISMS

The area is difficult to assess and it may be that a clear-cut answer will not be obtained. There appears to be sufficient evidence of a functional defect over and above that which is produced by atherosclerosis. Whether this can be or should be construed as a cardiopathy along the lines of retinopathy or nephropathy must remain non-proven for the moment and the term cardiomyopathy is preferred with connotation of muscle abnormality rather than small-blood-vessel abnormality. Deposition of PAS-positive material or collagen would result in stiff ventricles and cardiac contractile protein may be abnormal. In animal studies a reduction in actinomyosin and myosin ATPase has been demonstrated

(Dillmann, 1980). Thus there are a variety of mechanisms by which myocardial function may be altered even without invoking asymptomatic coronary artery disease and ischaemic cardiomyopathy.

DIABETES AND PERIPHERAL VASCULAR DISEASE

Peripheral vascular disease is a major cause of morbidity in the diabetic population. The major end-point is gangrene and amputation and it is considered in more detail in the chapter on the diabetic foot (chapter 18). It is about five times as common in the diabetic population as in the non-diabetic population and is more diffuse and distal. It has been estimated that 1 in 10 newly diagnosed diabetic patients has peripheral vascular disease and the cumulative incidence of lower extremity arterial disease is 45% with a 20-year duration of diabetes (Orchard and Strandness, 1993). There is a strong relationship between the presence of peripheral vascular disease and cardiovascular mortality (Janka, Standl and Mehnert, 1980).

The clinical presentation can be with symptoms which are typical of intermittent claudication with or without rest pain of the calves, thighs or buttocks. These may be altered dramatically by coexistent peripheral neuropathy. An important group of patients present with distal gangrene, often with little in the way of a previous history of claudication.

Medical treatment is depressingly unsuccessful. Vasodilators and drugs that enhance red cell deformability have been recommended but results in our hands are disappointing. From the patient's point of view the best solution is to have in hand something that can be given up. Smoking may well have contributed to the disease but its abolition may still save a limb, albeit one that is impaired. Similarly, to be able to discontinue propranolol or other beta-blockers may extend the useful life of the limb.

When arteriography is performed in a patient with distal gangrene it usually reveals bilateral diffuse disease which is not amenable to simple reconstructive surgery. Distal disease is also present in the diabetic patient with claudication but in these patients there may also be proximal narrowing or block which could benefit from angioplasty or proximal arterial grafting. In attempting limb salvage there is surely no longer a place for sympathectomy, especially since it can be demonstrated that many of these patients already have an auto-sympathectomy! Amputation, though a radical solution, can restore health quickly, although the fate of the second leg is a source of concern.

When contemplating surgical intervention careful clinical and radiological assessment is of paramount importance. Arterial surgeons quickly forget that diabetic physicians see many more diabetic foot lesions than the surgeons ever do and both physician and surgeon have a contribution to make to the management plan. The success of proximal grafts as assessed by graft patency is as good in the diabetic population as the non-diabetic population. Distal arterial grafting, which would seem more useful in the diabetic with predominantly distal disease, is demanding of technique and resource. Spectacular success can be obtained but it is not without cost in mortality (Rhodes *et al.*, 1987). Angioplasty, which is best suited to discrete proximal narrowing or blockage, is less successful in diabetics because of the distal nature of the macrovascular disease (Johnston *et al.*, 1987). Even with angioplasty, follow-up reveals the greater mortality in diabetic patients than in non-diabetic patients and there is also a greater requirement for surgery after angioplasty in the diabetic patients (Davies *et al.*, 1992).

DIABETES AND CEREBROVASCULAR DISEASE

Cerebrovascular disease is approximately one-and-a-half times to twice as common in diabetic patients. It is indistinguishable from atherosclerotic cerebral disease in the non-diabetic although the suggestion has been made that it carries a higher mortality.

Yamasaki *et al.* (1994) undertook high resolution ultrasound imaging of over 100 young insulin-dependent and more than 500 non-insulin-dependent diabetic patients. The intimal plus medial thickness in the young patients was significantly greater than in age-matched non-diabetic controls and in the diabetic patients it was related both to age and duration of diabetes.

An apparent clinical presentation of stroke may be a manifestation of other conditions within diabetes. For example, it is well recognized that hypoglycaemia may present as a hemiparesis and this should not be overlooked in the Casualty Department. Transient ischaemic attacks may also present from postural hypotension while neurological presentation of ketoacidosis and hyperosmolar coma is well reported.

In non-diabetic patients transient diabetes or hyperglycaemia may follow a cerebrovascular accident (the piqûre diabetes of Claude Bernard).

REFERENCES

Blumenthal, H. T., Alex, M. and Goldenberg, S. (1960) A study of lesions of the intramural coronary artery branches in diabetes mellitus. *Arch. Pathol.*, **70**, 13–28.

Chait, A., Bierman, E. L. and Albers, J. J. (1979) Low-density lipoprotein receptor activity in cultured human skin fibroblasts. *J. Clin. Invest.*, **64**, 1309–1319

Chellingsworth, M. C., Kendall, M. J. and Wright, A. D. (1989) The effects of calcium antagonists on glycaemic control in non-insulin-dependent diabetes mellitus. *Human Hypertension*, **3**, 35–39.

Clark, R. S., English, M., McNeill, G. P. and Newton, R. W. (1985) Effect of intravenous infusion of insulin in diabetics with acute myocardial infarction. *Br. Med. J.*, **291**, 303–305.

Clawson, B. J. and Bell, E. T. (1949) Incidence of fatal coronary disease in non diabetic and in diabetic persons. *Arch. Pathol.* **48**, 105–106.

Crall, F. V. and Roberts, W. C. (1978) The extramural and intramural coronary arteries in juvenile diabetes mellitus. *Am. J. Med.*, **64**, 221–230.

Dalby, A. J., Bricknell, O. L. and Opie, L. H. (1981) Effect of glucose-insulin-potassium infusions on epicardial ECG changes and on myocardial metabolic changes after coronary artery ligation in dogs. *Cardiovascular Res.* **15**, 588–598.

Davies, A. H., Cole, S. E., Magee, T. R. *et al.* (1992) The effect of diabetes mellitus on the outcome of angioplasty for lower limb ischaemia. *Diabetic Med.* **9**, 480–481.

Dillmann, W. H. (1980) Diabetes mellitus induces changes in cardiac myosin of the rat. *Diabetes*, **29**, 579–582.

Ditzel, J. (1976) Oxygen transport impairment in diabetes. *Diabetes*, **25(suppl 2)**, 832–838.

Ducimetiere, P., Eschwege, E., Papoz, L. *et al.* (1980) Relationship of plasma insulin levels to the incidence of myocardial infarction and coronary heart disease mortality in a middle-aged population. *Diabetologia*, **19**, 205–210.

Factor, S. M., Okun, E. M. and Minase, T. (1980) Capillary microaneurysms in the human diabetic heart. *N. Engl. J. Med.*, **302**, 384–388.

Fischer, V. W., Barner, H. B. and Leskiw, M. L. (1979) Capillary basal laminar thickness in diabetic human myocardium. *Diabetes*, **28**, 713–719.

Freedman, P., Moulton, R. and Spencer, A. G. (1958) Hypertension and diabetes mellitus. *Q. J. Med.*, **27**, 293–305.

Garcia, M. J. McNamara, P. M., Gordon, T. and Kannell, W. B. (1974) Morbidity and mortality in diabetics in the Framingham population. Sixteen year follow up study. *Diabetes*, **23**, 105–111.

Gwilt, D. J. and Pentecost, B. L. (1984) The heart in diabetes, in *Recent Advances in Diabetes 2*, (ed. M. Nattrass), Churchill Livingstone, Edinburgh, p. 177–194.

Gwilt, D. J., Petri, M., Lamb, P. *et al.* (1984) Effect of intravenous insulin infusion on mortality among diabetic patients after myocardial infarction. *Br. Heart J.* **51**, 626–630

Gwilt, D. J., Nattrass, M. and Pentecost, B. L. (1982) Use of low-dose insulin infusions in diabetics after myocardial infarction. *Br. Med. J.*, **285**, 1402–1404.

Hamby, R. I., Zoneraich, S. and Sherman, L. (1974) Diabetic cardiomyopathy. *J.A.M.A.*, **229**, 1749–1754.

Harno, K., Nikkila, E. A. and Kuusi, T. (1980) Plasma HDL-cholesterol and postheparin plasma hepatic endothelial lipase (HL) activity:

relationship to obesity and non-insulin dependent diabetes (NIDDM). *Diabetologia*, **19**, 281.

Hayward, R. E. and Lucena, B. C. (1965) An investigation into the mortality of diabetics. *J. Inst. Actuaries*, **91**, 286–336.

Heickendorff, L., Ledet, T. and Rasmussen, L. M. (1994) Glycosaminoglycans in the human aorta in diabetes mellitus: a study of tunica media from areas with and without atherosclerotic plaque. *Diabetologia*, **37**, 286–292.

Horsley, J. R., Barrett, J. A. and MacFarlane, I. A. (1987) Diabetic patients: smoking habits and beliefs. *Health Trends*, **19**, 13–15.

Jaffe, A. S., Spadaro, J. J., Schechtman, K. *et al.* (1984) Increased congestive heart failure after myocardial infarction of modest extent in patients with diabetes mellitus. *Am. Heart J.*, **108**, 31–37.

Janka, H. U., Standl, E. and Mehnert, H. (1980) Peripheral vascular disease in diabetes mellitus and its relation to cardiovascular risk factors: screening with the Doppler ultrasonic technique. *Diabetes Care*, **3**, 207–213.

Jarrett, R. J. and Keen, H. (1975) Diabetes and atherosclerosis, in *Complications of Diabetes*, 1st edn, (eds H. Keen and R. J. Jarrett), Edward Arnold, London, p. 179–203.

Jarrett, R., J. Keen, H. and Chakrabarti, R. (1982) Diabetes, hyperglycaemia and arterial disease, in *Complications of Diabetes*, 2nd edn, (eds H. Keen and R. J. Jarrett), Edward Arnold, London, p. 179–203.

Jarrett, R. J., Viberti, G. C., Argyropolous, A. *et al.* (1984) Microalbuminuria predicts mortality in non-insulin-dependent diabetes. *Diabetic Med.*, **1**, 17–19.

Johnston, K. W., Rae, M., Hogg-Johnston, S. A. *et al.* (1987) 5-year results of a prospective study of percutaneous transluminal angioplasty. *Ann. Surg.*, **206**, 403–412.

Kannel W. B. and McGee, D. L. (1979) Diabetes and glucose tolerance as risk factors for cardiovascular disease: the Framingham study. *Diabetes Care*, **2**, 120–126.

Kannel, W. B., Hjortland, M. and Castelli, W. P. (1974) Role of diabetes in congestive heart failure: the Framingham study. *Am. J. Cardiol.*, **34**, 29–34.

Keen, H., Jarrett, R. J. and Fuller, J. H. (1974) Tolbutamide and arterial disease in borderline diabetics, in *Proceedings of the 8th Congress of the International Diabetes Federation*, (eds W. J. Malaisse and J. Pirart), Excerpta Medica, Amsterdam, p. 588.

Keys, A., Aravanis, C., Blackburn, H. *et al.* (1972) Coronary heart disease: overweight and obesity as risk factors. *Ann. Intern. Med.*, **77**, 15–27.

Lawrie, G. M., Morris, G. C. and Glaeser, D. H. (1986) Influence of diabetes mellitus on the results of coronary bypass surgery. *J.A.M.A.*, **256**, 2967–2971.

Larsson, B., Svardsudd, K., Welin, L. *et al.* (1984) Abdominal adipose tissue distribution, obesity and risk of cardiovascular disease and death: 13-year follow up of participants in the study of men born in 1913. *Br. Med. J.*, **288**, 1401–1404.

Ledet, T. (1976) Diabetic cardiopathy. Quantitative histological studies of the heart from young juvenile diabetics. *Acta Path. Microbiol. Scand. (Sect. A)*, **84**, 421–428.

de Leiris, J., Opie, L. H. and Lubbe, W. F. (1975) Effects of free fatty acid and enzyme release in experimental glucose on myocardial infarction. *Nature*, **253**, 746–747.

Liebow, I. M., Hellerstein, H. K. and Miller, M. (1955) Arteriosclerotic heart disease in diabetes mellitus. A clinical study of 383 patients. *Am. J. Med.*, **18**, 438–447.

Lundbaek, K. (1954) Diabetic angiopathy. *Lancet*, **i**, 377–379.

Lynch, M., Gammage, M. D., Lamb, P. *et al.* (1993) Acute myocardial infarction in diabetic patients in the thrombolytic era. *Diabetic Med.*, **11**, 162–165.

Medical Research Council Working-Party Report (1968) Potassium, glucose, and insulin treatment for acute myocardial infarction. *Lancet*, **ii**, 1355–1360.

Oliver, M. F., Kurien, V. A. and Greenwood, T. W. (1968) Relation between serum-free-fatty-acids and arrhythmias and death after acute myocardial infarction. *Lancet*, **i**, 710–715.

Orchard, T. J., and Strandness, D. E. (1993) Assessment of peripheral vascular disease in diabetes. *Circulation*, **88**, 819–828.

Orlander, P. R., Goff, D. C., Morrissey, M. *et al.* (1994) The relation of diabetes to the severity of acute myocardial infarction and post-myocardial infarction survival in Mexican-Americans and non-Hispanic whites. *Diabetes*, **43**, 897–902.

Parving, H. H., Noer, T., Deckert, T. *et al.* (1976) The effect of metabolic regulation on microvascular permeability to small and large molecules in short-term juvenile diabetics. *Diabetologia*, **12**, 161–166.

Pell, S. and D'Alonzo, C. A. (1967) Sickness absenteeism in employed diabetics. *Am. J. Pub. Health*, **57**, 253–260.

Pell, S. and D'Alonzo, C. A. (1970) Factors associated with long-term survival of diabetics. *J.A.M.A.*, **214**, 1833–1840.

Pyke, D. A. (1968) In *Clinical Diabetes and its Biochemical Basis*, (eds W. G. Oakley, D. A. Pyke, and K. W. Taylor), Blackwell, Oxford, p. 530.

Pyorala, K. (1979) Relationship of glucose tolerance and plasma insulin to the incidence of coronary heart disease: results from two population studies in Finland. *Diabetes Care*, **2**, 131–141.

Randle, P. J. (1984) Regulatory devices in metabolism and medicine. *J. Roy. Coll. Phys. (Lond.)*, **18**, 211–218.

Reaven, G. M. (1988) Role of insulin resistance in human disease. *Diabetes*, **37**, 1595–1607.

Regan, T. J., Ettingen, P. O., Khan, M. I. *et al.* (1974) Altered myocardial function and metabolism in chronic diabetes mellitus without ischaemia in dogs. *Circulation Res.*, **35**, 222–237.

Regan, T. J., Lyons, M. M., Ahmed, S. S. *et al.* (1977) Evidence for cardiomyopathy in familial diabetes mellitus. *J. Clin. Invest.*, **60**, 885–899.

Rhodes, G. R., Rollins, D., Sidawy, A. N. *et al.* (1987) Popliteal-to-tibial in situ saphenous vein bypass for limb salvage in diabetic patients. *Am. J. Surg.*, **154**, 245–247.

Rosengren, A., Welin, L., Tsipogianni, A. and Wilhelmsen, L. (1989) Impact of cardiovascular risk factors on coronary heart disease and mortality among middle age diabetic men: a general population study. *Br. Med. J.*, **299**, 1127–1131.

Schmitz, A. and Vaeth, M. (1988) Microalbuminuria: a major risk factor in non-insulin-dependent diabetes. A 10-year follow-up study of 503 patients. *Diabetic Med.*, **5**, 126–134.

Seneviratne, B. I. B. (1977) Diabetic cardiomyopathy: the preclinical phase. *Br. Med. J.*, **1**, 1444–1446.

Shirey, E. K., Proudfit, W. L. and Hawk, W. A. (1980) Primary myocardial disease. Correlation with clinical findings, angiographic and biopsy diagnosis. *Am. Heart J.*, **99**, 198–207.

Soler, N. G., Bennett, M. A., Pentecost, B. L. *et al.* (1975) Myocardial infarction in diabetics. *Q. J. Med.*, **44**, 125–132.

Steinbrecher, U. P. and Witztum, J. L. (1984) Glucosylation of low-density lipoproteins to an extent comparable to that seen in diabetes slows their catabolism. *Diabetes*, **33**, 130–134.

Stout, R. W. (1975) The effect of insulin on the incorporation of D-glucose-U ^{14}C into the lipids of the rat aorta in vivo. *Hormone Metab. Res.*, **7**, 31–34.

Ulvenstam, G., Aberg, A., Bergstrand, R. *et al.* (1985) Long-term prognosis after myocardial infarction in men with diabetes. *Diabetes*, **34**, 787–792.

Vigorita, V. J., Moore, G. W. and Hutchins, G. M. (1980) Absence of correlation between coronary arterial atherosclerosis and severity or duration of diabetes mellitus of adult onset. *Am. J. Cardiol.*, **46**, 535–542.

Weitzman, S., Rennert, G., Saltz, H. and Wanderman, K. (1984) Myocardial infarction size in diabetes. *Diabetologia*, **27**, 345A.

Welborn, T. A. and Wearne, K. (1979) Coronary heart disease incidence and cardiovascular mortality in Busselton with reference to glucose and insulin concentrations. *Diabetes Care*, **2**, 154–160.

Wright, A. D., Barber, S. G., Kendall, M. J. and Poole, P. H. (1979) Beta-adrenoceptor-blocking drugs and blood sugar control in diabetes mellitus. *Br. Med. J.*, **1**, 159–161.

Yamasaki, Y., Kawamori, R., Matsushima, H. *et al.* (1994) Atherosclerosis in carotid artery of young IDDM patients monitored by ultrasound high-resolution B-mode imaging. *Diabetes*, **43**, 634–639.

Devoting a chapter specifically to the diabetic foot is justified by the tremendous clinical importance of foot lesions and the fact that, in Britain at least, more hospital beds are occupied by patients with bad feet than all other complications of diabetes put together. The loss of a limb or even a digit, or the debilitating effect of chronic foot sepsis, is rightly considered a disaster by both patient and doctor. The drain upon financial and valuable hospital resources is anathema to society. In his review of hospital admissions of diabetic patients in the East Anglian region Williams (1985) found that peripheral vascular disorders were the cause of the greatest proportion of both admissions and daily bed occupancy.

The lesions are usually complex in nature and can be considered only rarely as pure manifestations of vascular disease. Ischaemia is probably the most important factor in ulceration and gangrene of the foot but neuropathy is not far behind as it contributes diminished sensation, trophic defects and impaired shape and position of the foot. Infection is the third member of the triad and the spread of even minor infections is encouraged by a number of factors, including poorly controlled diabetes. Examples of these three contributors to the pathogenesis of the diabetic foot sometimes occur clinically in an almost pure form but more often it is difficult to assess the degree to which each one is operating.

In a surveillance programme to identify all foot ulceration within a defined community Walters *et al.* (1992) found that 7.4% of diabetics had past or present foot ulceration compared with 2.5% of non-diabetic controls.

Of the ulcers found on examination 39% were held to be neuropathic, 24% vascular and the remaining 36% were mixed.

GANGRENE

Descriptions of the incidence of gangrene and its treatment in the diabetic patient show wide variations because the elements of neuropathy and infection are not always realized. The vascular surgeon will have a different experience of the frequency in the diabetic population from the experience of the diabetologist. The largest comparative survey of the incidence of gangrene in the diabetic and non-diabetic is that of Bell (1957) in which he reviewed the post-mortem records of the University of Minnesota from 1911–1955. Cases of trauma, frost-bite, acute arteritis and embolism were excluded. Of those with atherosclerosis and no diabetes half had no recorded urine test. He noted that gangrene did not occur below the age of 40 and was uncommon under the age of 60 in non-diabetics, who showed a 3:2 preponderance of males due principally to men over the age of 80. In the diabetic there were a few cases of gangrene under the age of 40 and it was present in 14% of those who died between the ages of 40 and 60, and 29% of those who died between 60 and 80. The sex incidence was equal, but diabetes was twice as frequent, in the series as a whole, in women than in men. Bell calculated that atherosclerotic gangrene was 53 times as frequent in diabetic as in non-diabetic men over the age of 40 and 71 times as frequent in diabetic women as in non-diabetic women. Two-thirds of episodes of atherosclerotic gangrene in men under the age of 80 and one-quarter of those in men over the age of 80 were due to diabetes, while 80% of those in women were associated with diabetes. The development of gangrene was not related to insulin requirement or to the duration of diabetes.

Semple (1953) also found no relationship between arterial disease and the severity or duration of diabetes but he did find a relationship to increasing age. In his 100 diabetics aged over 50 there were signs of arterial disease in 42%. In the diabetic this presented more often with gangrene than claudication. Janka, Standl and Mehnert (1980) compared rates of isolated proximal occlusive lesions in diabetics and non-diabetics, finding a similar figure (5.8%) in both populations and clearly indicating that the excess of atherosclerotic disease is distal disease.

From evidence in many clinical and pathological studies it may be concluded that arterial disease in the lower limb of the diabetic patient differs from that of the non-diabetic patient in a specific manner. It occurs at a younger age, is more extensive and tends to affect the more distal vessels so that occlusions occur at a lower level – in the popliteal and tibial rather than the femoral. In addition, diabetes clearly removes any protective effect that being female has in the non-diabetic population for peripheral vascular disease.

CLINICAL FEATURES

THE ISCHAEMIC LIMB

Intermittent claudication preceding the foot lesion is comparatively uncommon, but a sudden pain associated with arterial occlusion may continue as rest pain in the foot, which has an ominous significance and indicates that amputation will probably be necessary within 6 months without intervention. Ulcerated or necrotic lesions may quickly follow an arterial occlusion or be precipitated by minor injuries. Injury probably determines the site of the lesion, except in massive gangrene from major arterial blocks. Gangrene of individual toes or of the heel is commonly due to the pressure of shoes or of resting the limb (Plate 5), although at times extensive blocks of digital or rather larger arteries seem to be responsible for local gangrene without an element of trauma. A gangrenous area is commonly dry and black, the demarcation zone showing little evidence of repair by granulation tissue.

Palpable pulsation in the dorsalis pedis and posterior tibial arteries virtually excludes ischaemia, although, rarely, digital artery occlusion may cause gangrene of one toe with preservation of distal pulses. Absence of these pulses does not necessarily mean that ischaemia is severe and oedema of the foot may make it difficult to feel pulsation. There are other useful signs, however, of poor blood supply: coldness of the foot, especially if there is a sharply defined change of temperature at one level; blanching on elevation and congestion on dependence, with a delay in venous filling beyond 20 seconds; a thin, shiny, atrophic skin; and radiological evidence of osteoporosis of the bones of the foot.

An X-ray may show calcification of the vessels, which is not in itself evidence of ischaemia.

THE NEUROPATHIC LIMB

The role of neuropathy in ulceration and gangrene is well established. Many of the manifestations resemble those of other peripheral nerve lesions such as leprosy and tabes, although the combination with arterial disease gives a specific character to some diabetic feet. Apart from the loss of painful sensations, which allows trauma that would not normally be tolerated, there is a tendency to flatfoot and to prominence of the metatarsal heads as a result of retraction of the toes. Conventional signs of neuropathy – sensory disturbance and altered reflexes – are of limited value as they are common in elderly

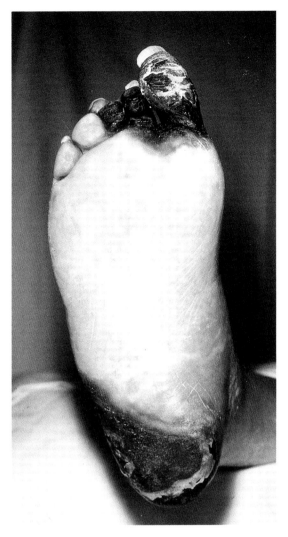

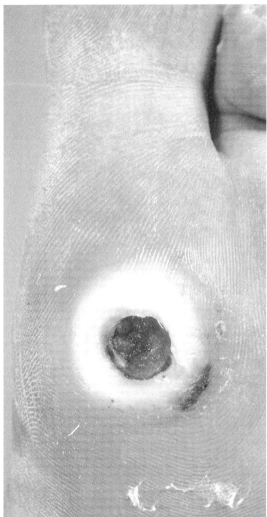

Plate 5 Extensive gangrene of the foot.

Plate 6 Typical neuropathic ulcer.

patients. Lesions on the toes commonly present as blisters, which appear without recognized trauma. Though sensory loss may not be very obvious, these are assumed to be neuropathic. Some writers have regarded arterial disease as a necessary accompaniment but there is no clinical evidence of ischaemia in most cases. The bullae rupture and usually a black area of superficial gangrene appears, then the necrotic skin slowly separates and leaves a shallow granulating ulcer. The alarming appearance may be distinguished from that of ischaemia by the healthy appearance of the surrounding skin and the presence of foot pulses.

Another common presentation is the perforating ulcer below the first, less often other, metatarso-phalangeal joints (Plate 6). Retraction of the toes from neuropathy throws weight on the metatarsal heads, a callus forms and ulceration often follows. The lesion may extend into the bone or joint and becomes extremely chronic. Healing with rest is followed by relapse when walking is resumed and the sequence may be repeated many times.

Pressure ulceration of the heel occurs after prolonged bed rest and has to be distinguished, by the general appearance of the foot, from the much more serious ischaemic lesion. Trauma produces ulceration at other sites. Burns from hot water bottles or sitting close to a fire occur because pain sensation is lost, and damage from ill-fitting shoes or nails projecting from the sole of the shoe are common. The initial appearance of the foot may be lurid but with appropriate treatment the end result is often surprisingly good.

All these neuropathic lesions are painless or almost so, but if infection spreads into the foot an abscess commonly forms and pain may then be severe and persistent. The presence of such pain in a neuropathic foot strongly suggests than an abscess is present, even if clinical signs of it are absent, and justifies surgery with drainage.

MIXED LESIONS

A particularly difficult presentation is that of the ischaemic limb with symptoms and signs of neuropathy. All peripheral neuropathy in the diabetic tends to be labelled 'diabetic' but paraesthesiae from ischaemic neuropathy can and do occur. The correct approach is aimed at the ischaemia rather than the more conservative approach to diabetic peripheral neuropathy.

INFECTIVE LESIONS

Most infective lesions are associated with trauma to an insensitive neuropathic foot. The infective element in ischaemia is often over-rated, that in neuropathy underrated. The controlled diabetic has no undue tendency to infection, but in the presence of poor control infection may develop and spread rapidly.

PATHOGENESIS

Atherosclerosis in the arteries of the diabetic patient is histologically identical to that in the non-diabetic. Quite why the distribution of atherosclerotic plaques, favouring distal sites, should be dissimilar is unclear. Reduction in perfusion, either by narrowing of arteries or by occlusion, leaves the ischaemic limb at risk of tissue necrosis should a further insult such as trauma or infection occur. There is uncertainty over the contribution to the pathogenesis that is made by occlusive lesions of small arterioles or capillaries (Logerfo and Coffman, 1984).

In the neuropathic foot small and large sensory fibres and motor fibres are damaged. Loss pain and temperature sensation through affected small fibres may precede large fibre damage with loss of vibration and light touch sensation (Guy *et al.*, 1985). Damaged motor fibres result in weakness and wasting of the small muscles of the foot, leading to deformity. There is also evidence of sympathetic denervation (Fagius, 1982).

Sympathetic denervation alters peripheral blood flow in the neuropathic foot. Increased blood flow with an altered pattern (Scarpello, Martin and Ward, 1980) leads to an increase in skin temperature in the limb (Ward *et al.*, 1983). Measurements of venous P_aO_2 confirm the finding from contrast radiology and Doppler sonograms that there is considerable arteriovenous shunting (Boulton, Scarpello and Ward, 1982). Denervation of vascular smooth muscle not only induces functional change but also structural change (Bevan and Tsuru, 1979).

INVESTIGATION

Clinical examination of the diabetic foot remains of paramount importance and should be performed at least annually; more frequently in the at-risk foot. When an ulcer is found an early decision should be made on the probable nature of origin of the lesion, whether ischaemic or neuropathic. This is not simply an intellectual exercise but is done in anticipation of likely treatment. In general terms neuropathic ulceration may respond to conservative treatment or may involve relatively conservative amputation. This is not so for ischaemic lesions, where surgery, if performed, is more likely to be radical. The effects of potentially radical surgery upon the patient should never be underestimated and any way of breaking this news to the patient in a gradual manner is beneficial. Thus the answer to the question neuropathic or ischaemic will allow the doctor to start preparing the patient for the likely outcome. It is sad to see patients with ischaemic lesions treated conservatively, with little likelihood of success, yet with increasing hope because the dreaded words gangrene and amputation are never mentioned, having to be told of the imminence of radical surgery in a bold and seemingly heartless way. Better that the time had been used to greater effect in preparation and reconciliation of the patient to the likely outcome.

Diabetic neuropathy as the underlying cause of ulceration of the foot is essentially a clinical diagnosis. Absent vibration sense at the ankles with deformity of shape and ulceration of pressure areas point the way notwithstanding the natural loss of sensation and reflexes which tends to occur with age. If, in addition, pedal pulses are present then the diagnosis is certain. Further investigation from a diagnostic standpoint is unnecessary. Nerve conduction times will only add extra weight at best and at worst may serve to confuse. Assessment of abnormal pressure areas may be of value if healing can be achieved, giving warning of other areas of the foot that may be at risk, although these may often be detected by naked eye examination.

In the clinical examination of the ischaemic foot the important questions are which peripheral pulses are absent, that is to what level are they absent and whether the finding is unilateral or bilateral. Again this has prognostic relevance. Unilateral absence of foot or leg pulses may suggest a localised block amenable to reconstructive arterial surgery. Bilateral absence has a more severe implication raising doubts of whether reconstructive surgery will be feasible.

X-RAY CHANGES IN THE DIABETIC FOOT

X-rays of the foot are useful only to a limited extent, since it is difficult to ascribe specific causation to most of the appearances seen. In about half the patients over 50 years of age with foot symptoms calcification in the vessels, especially the digital arteries (Figure 18.1), is seen but is of uncertain significance as the medial lesion which it denotes is not directly associated with narrowing of the lumen. Decalcification of bone (Figure 18.2) is common in ischaemic lesions and may be extensive. It is then a rough measure of ischaemia. Bone necrosis is more characteristic of neuropathic than ischaemic lesions.

Unsuspected fractures of the metatarsals (Figure 18.3) are a feature, albeit rare, of

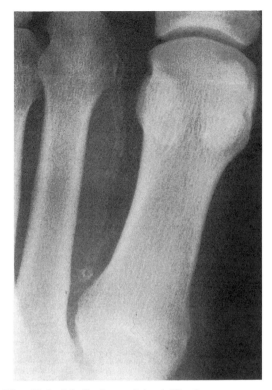

Fig. 18.1 Medical arterial calcification.

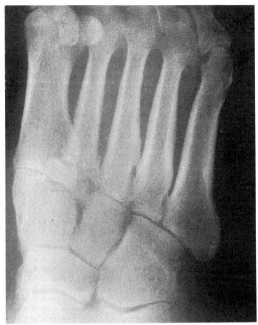

Fig. 18.3 Fracture through the base of the second metatarsal in a diabetic man. There was no history of trauma to the area.

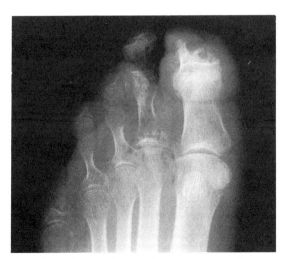

Fig. 18.2 Destruction of the terminal phalanx of the great toe of an infected foot. Further evidence of infection can be seen in the gas shadows over the second toe.

neuropathy (Krentz *et al.*, 1989) as is the more common tapering or sucked-candy appearance of the metatarsal heads.

ARTERIOGRAPHY

Femoral arteriography has been widely used in the last few years both as a guide to the level for amputation and as a means of identifying segmental blocks which would be suitable for arterial repair. The occlusive patterns were well described and classified by Haimovici, Shapiro and Jacobson (1960).

Arteriography seeks to answer questions on occlusion patterns, collateral groups and their efficiency, and the degree of run-off, that is to say the filling of the patent major artery below a segmental occlusion. The main collateral groups are: (1) the profunda femoris–geniculate; (2) the geniculo-tibial; and (3)

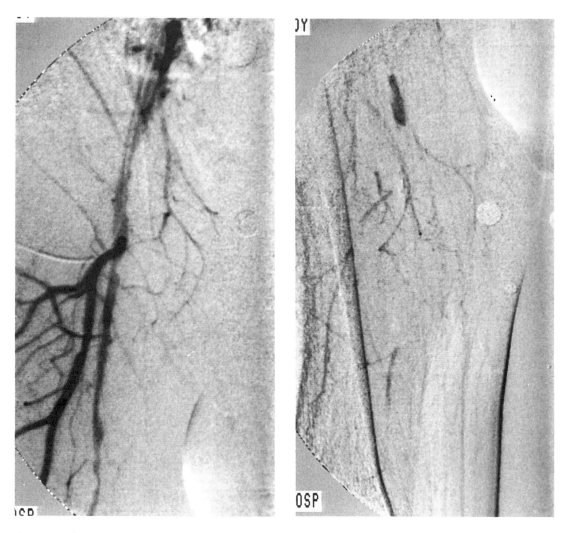

Fig. 18.4 Subtraction angiogram of the right femoral artery. **(a)** The right iliac artery contains a catheter but the outline is clearly irregular because of atheroma. The profunda femosis is well outlined with only moderate irregularity. The superficial femoral artery shows a tight stenosis just distal to its origin and then shows marked irregularity from atheroma, being virtually occluded towards the bottom of the picture. **(b)** Subsequent films more distally show poor 'run-off' through vessels of small calibre.

the profunda femoris–geniculate–tibial anastomoses. The efficiency of collateral circulation is judged from the number, size and outline of the collaterals, the extent of major artery block and the presence of re-entry into the main artery below the block. The degree of 'run-off' is assessed from the outline of the artery and its size and rate of filling.

The evidence from arteriograms is that diffuse atherosclerosis is more severe in the diabetic and occlusions occur at a somewhat lower level than in the non-diabetic. The involvement of the major leg arteries is especially striking (Figure 18.4).

Haimovici, Shapiro and Jacobson (1960) and Baddeley and Fulford (1964) classified the occlusion patterns which they found. In both series the incidence of obstruction in the major leg arteries was high. In the series of Haimovici, Shapiro and Jacobson (1960) nearly a quarter of the patients had a distal superficial femoral artery occlusion only; 17% had a proximal popliteal artery occlusion; and 15% had a total popliteal artery block. Baddeley and Fulford (1964) also found the proximal popliteal artery occluded in a significant number of patients (24%) but the major occlusive pattern in their series was diffuse atherosclerosis with multiple stenotic areas (39%). More recently, Mansell, Gregson and Allison (1992) found that half of their patients had proximal lesions that were potentially amenable to angioplasty. They also re-emphasized the importance of remembering that if diffuse distal disease is present in the presenting leg it is usually if not invariably present in the other leg.

Differences in the distribution of occlusion patterns in the two series are probably the result of case selection, our patients being all at the stage of amputation (Baddeley and Fulford, 1964). Bearing in mind the fact that necrotic lesions are accelerated by neuropathy and infection it is likely that amputation will be necessary at an earlier stage of ischaemia in the diabetic than in the non-diabetic.

Arteriography is useful as a guide to the level of amputation and goes some way to providing an estimate of the blood supply, an exercise which has been described as 'often a combination of clinical experience and guess-work' (Rosenberg and London, 1956).

Radiographs of the arterial tree in normal people will show good filling and peripheral perfusion. This may be the picture in those with neuropathic lesions of the toes and indicates that healing will occur readily. For toe amputations to heal the blood flow into the foot should appear good, while the dorsalis pedis, plantar and digital vessels should be well outlined. Midtarsal amputations require foot arteries that are clearly filled but the digital vessels need not be seen. Below-knee amputations require at least a fair degree of popliteal 'run-off' and are unlikely to succeed when the collateral supply is from a profunda–geniculate–tibial anastomosis. When the vessels below the level of the knee joint are inadequate an above-knee amputation is clearly indicated.

Occasionally a femoro-popliteal block with good 'run-off' suggests the possibility of end-arterectomy or bypass of the block. Ideally the lower aorta and common iliacs should be outlined.

NON-INVASIVE INVESTIGATIONS

Investigation of arterial blood supply

Systolic pressures at the ankle can be measured using a small blood pressure cuff and Doppler ultrasound. By dividing the reading obtained by the brachial systolic pressure a pressure ratio is derived, which in normal people is 1. Values of less than 0.5 indicate severe disease and between 0.5 and 0.9 mild to moderate disease. With values greater than 0.9 peripheral vascular disease is unlikely. Edmonds *et al.* (1985) found that 102 of 121 ulcers (84%) healed satisfactorily when the pressure ratio was greater than 0.6 but only 27 of 68 (40%) healed when the ratio was less than 0.6. Sometimes it is not possible to compress the ankle arteries and readings that are higher than the brachial pressure are obtained. This almost certainly indicates medial wall calcification and as an alternative toe systolic pressure can be measured. A toe systolic pressure of > 30 mmHg suggests that healing will occur.

Duplex scanning

Duplex scanning combines Doppler signals and ultrasound to give information on the anatomy from the echography and function from the Doppler spectrum. Thus the haemodynamic consequences of lesions can be assessed.

Pressure studies

The hallmark of the neuropathic foot is a change in shape such that the normal distribution of weight through the sole of the foot is lost. Pressure areas develop as weight is transmitted through a few small areas of the foot. Repeated use leads to callus formation. Often the distorted shape of the foot can be seen on observation, classically described as a clawing of the foot. Recent investigative techniques show the pressure areas and thus identify parts of the sole at risk of ulceration (Boulton *et al.*, 1983). The pedobarograph consists of pressure-sensitive plates along a walkway over which the patient attempts their normal gait. A pictorial impression is obtained of areas of the foot subjected to abnormal pressure. Similar results may be obtained by pressure transducers fitted in footwear.

TREATMENT

PROPHYLAXIS

General advice aimed at prophylaxis is always appropriate. Smoking should be adamantly discouraged and attempts to maintain patency of vessels and develop collaterals through exercise should be recommended. Specific instructions, often repeated, in the care of the feet amply repay a somewhat uninteresting exercise. The reward – feet saved from ulceration and gangrene – is invisible and often unappreciated. The striking rarity of lesions of the feet seen in private practice compared with the incidence in hospital practice in this country shows the importance of hygiene, proper footwear and the control of temperature.

Patients should be advised to wash the feet every day using warm, not hot, water and dry carefully between the toes. This is the best safeguard against epidermophytosis, a common starting-point for the entry of infection. If it occurs fungicidal powders are moderately effective. It used to be recommended often that if the feet were unduly moist spirit applications should be used, or that lanolin should be rubbed into dry skin every week. Beyond following the ancient ritual of dermatology that if it's wet, dry it, and if it's dry, wet it, I doubt that particular benefit is to be gained in this way.

Advice on nail cutting should be given. While it is often suggested that the toenails should be cut straight across after washing the feet it is eminently more sensible that the nails be cut to the shape of the digit. It should be stressed that if sight is not good there should not be attempts to use scissors on the feet but the patient should go to a chiropodist regularly, making it clear to the chiropodist that they have diabetes.

Common sense decrees that the diabetic should not walk about barefoot, especially on wooden floors; should wear good fitting shoes; and should not wear new shoes for more than an hour at a time. Shoes should be inspected regularly both inside and outside for areas that may damage feet, while open-toed shoes or sandals are best avoided.

A main source of injury is loss of temperature sense and the diabetic patient is well advised to avoid excessive heat and cold, particularly from fires, hot water bottles, electric blankets and particularly the temperature of the bath water.

DIY (do-it-yourself) chiropody for corns or callus should be forbidden and proprietary corn cures avoided.

Finally, all sore places, blisters or discoloured areas should be reported, however trivial they may seem.

Well directed chiropody is especially important in patients with peripheral neuropathy. Often areas of the foot exposed to increased amounts of pressure can be seen with the hallmark of extensive callus formation. This should be removed periodically by a chiropodist and before excessive shear forces lead to ulceration below the callus.

FOOTWEAR

Ill fitting shoes contribute all too easily to damage of the foot. When combined with a dulling of sensation the patient may be unaware of the harm being done. Appropriate footwear is therefore of paramount importance in prophylaxis. Many different types of ready-made shoes are available or footwear can be custom-made for the individual patient. Often expensive, the cost diminishes if they are successful in reducing hospital admission and amputation. Sadly it remains difficult to dissuade patients from wearing fashion shoes and to persuade them to change to something more 'sensible'.

TREATMENT OF NECROTIC LESIONS

Control of the diabetes should be strict in patients with infection and may help in the healing of neuropathic ulcers although it will not affect the neuropathy. In the aged with purely ischaemic lesions over-rigid control is unnecessary and hypoglycaemia may be dangerous.

TREATMENT OF ISCHAEMIC LESIONS

Vasodilator drugs

These are at best harmless and at worst may divert circulation into the areas with normal vessels at the expense of those with arterial occlusion, so that an ischaemic lesion may be aggravated. They have little to offer the ischaemic limb with the one, and fairly major, exception of intravenous praxilene which may be effective in relieving rest pain in the short term.

Low molecular weight dextran with a mean molecular weight of 40 000 has been used to reduce the viscosity of the blood and so increase capillary blood flow. During the intravenous infusion the effect seems to be demonstrable and it has a place in the treatment of acute arterial block before the collateral sup-

ply is established. The risk from expansion of plasma volume in a patient with widespread atherosclerosis presumed to involve the heart has to be taken into account.

Sympathectomy

The place of lumbar sympathectomy in the treatment of arterial disease in the lower limb remains uncertain. Interruption of the vasomotor impulses may have some effect in stabilizing blood flow and decreasing collateral resistance, while the removal of afferent fibres which conduct heat and cold impulses may ease pain but the results are not sufficiently striking to maintain enthusiasm for this operation. It is useless for intermittent claudication. In cases of primarily neuropathic origin the autonomic disturbance is commonly so extensive that sympathetic activity is reduced and sympathectomy a work of supererogation.

Arterial surgery

Aorta-to-femoral and femoral-to-popliteal grafts have become standard procedures for segmental arterial occlusion. Unfortunately, experience of these procedures for the ischaemic diabetic foot has not been happy and failure is normally attributed to the diffuse nature of the arterial disease. In particular the distal involvement of lower leg and foot arteries does not suggest a widespread role for by-pass grafts in treatment. Nevertheless there will always be a small group of patients in whom arterial grafts will produce a beneficial effect and consideration should always be given to the possibility, particularly if there is obvious asymmetrical involvement of the arterial tree. Where diffuse and bilateral distal disease coexist the role of arterial grafting of the aorta or femoral vessels remains unclear. At least in theory there is a possibility that increasing flow higher up the leg would aid perfusion of the distal vessels.

Angioplasty for peripheral atherosclerosis is a relatively new option in management.

Early results are mixed, as is to be expected until clearer indications for angioplasty emerge. Mansell, Gregson and Allison (1992), in 83 patients with peripheral vascular disease, found lesions in 42 patients that were amenable to angioplasty. In the main these were localized stenoses or short occlusions of iliac, femoral or popliteal arteries. Interestingly, although technical success was reported in 31 of the 42 patients, clinical improvement was only obtained in 15 patients by angioplasty alone. As always, results will tend to reflect the careful selection of patients who have lesions suitable for intervention by angioplasty. Among the patients of Mansell, Gregson and Allison (1992) the group that benefited most were those with intermittent claudication as their presentation. Others have obtained good results with carefully selected lesions. The procedure should probably be avoided when there is poor run-off, diffuse stenoses and peripheral ischaemia.

Other developments in the field of arterial microsurgery should also find a place eventually for treatment of an appropriately demarcated population. Proximal-to-distal arterial grafts and vascular reconstruction below the popliteal trifurcation are technically possible.

Amputation

There is still a tendency for younger surgeons to underestimate the seriousness of ischaemic lesions of the foot. There will always be a laudable desire to act as conservatively as possible but this is not always justified. More often than not the ischaemic lesion is a port of entry for sepsis with major effects upon diabetic control while the piecemeal nibbling of digit, forefoot then lower leg has a debilitating effect upon the patient both physiologically and psychologically.

The decision to amputate is forced upon the surgeon by persistent pain, gangrene or recurrent infection not completely eradicated. In the ischaemic foot pain at rest, steady and unrelieved, leaves no alternative and it is often the patient's decision that they would rather be without the offending limb. Criteria for the level of amputation have been described by Silbert and Haimovici (1954) and by Baddeley and Fulford (1964).

Clinical examination remains the most important guide. The appearance of the skin adjacent to necrotic lesions is very valuable. If it looks normal the circulation is probably adequate even if observations of the pulses suggest otherwise. If it is atrophic, scaly and cold, ischaemia is probably severe. The clinical signs with an arteriogram should give an accurate forecast of the prospects for healing of the amputation. No less important is the consideration of general health and social background of the individual patient. As a general rule the surgeon will seek the lowest level for amputation that will give viable skin flaps for healing. This decision may be modified if there is extensive vascular disease elsewhere, coronary or cerebral, or if retinopathy has seriously impaired vision when the future function of the stump may be of minor consideration. Similar reservations would apply if the patient was having a second amputation, although as always such prognostication would be taken in the light of the individual patent's morale and determination. In all cases a strong motive to get back to normal life and a family who will strengthen this impulse are vital factors in the end result.

Once the decision has been taken surgery should be promptly performed. This is especially true in the occasional instance of rapidly spreading gangrene, sometimes described as wet gangrene, which may be seen, which is life-threatening.

Toe or forefoot amputation

This may be considered in the ischaemic foot but is rarely successful. For success ischaemia should be limited and this is often difficult to judge. It should never be undertaken as a delaying measure but only when there is a good reason to anticipate good healing. Few of us are blessed with such foresight. More often a lower leg amputation will be necessary for ischaemia.

Below-knee amputation

This is often necessary in severe ischaemia of the foot and should succeed if the popliteal run-off on the arteriogram is adequate. It is generally agreed that the function of the stump is much better than with the above-knee procedure and when function is an important consideration some risk is justified. Healing and rehabilitation tend to be slower than with the above-knee operation (Hoar and Torres, 1962).

Above-knee amputation

This is reserved for the most severe cases of diffuse arterial disease when gangrene is extending well up the calf, when gas-forming infection is spreading upwards or when primary disease of the knee-joint makes its preservation useless. Certainty and rapidity of healing with the prospect of earlier limb fitting are advantages that incline some surgeons to prefer the above- to the below-knee operation in doubtful cases.

Outcome

Deerochanawong, Home and Alberti (1992) audited the lower limb amputations in one centre in the UK. They found that diabetic patients made up 39% of patients undergoing amputation and 42% of all operations. In 15% the diabetes was only diagnosed during the admission for amputation. Nearly half of the patients underwent below knee amputation and about one-third had amputation of a toe. The remainder had either above knee (17%) of forefoot (6%) amputations. The mortality within 30 days of operation was 10%; during 1–36 months of follow-up 19% had a further operation; and median life expectancy following amputation was 22 months.

TREATMENT OF NEUROPATHIC LESIONS

Local treatment

Rest is necessary for necrotic lesions. Neuropathic ulcers will usually heal if pressure is completely removed from the affected area and will not do so otherwise. The extent to which patents will comply with this advice is governed more by social circumstances than truculence and enforcement of bed rest by hospital admission is expensive.

In dressing the lesion a balance must be kept between the degree of wetness and that of dryness. The old adage of if dry, wet dressings and if wet, dry dressings is too simple an approach. The first consideration is eradication of infection. Lotions for the dressings should be of the simplest antiseptic character least likely to cause sensitization of the skin. Antibiotics in lotion or cream form are of dubious value and should not be used. Sensitization is extremely common and may be recognized by the sodden and unhealthy appearance of the surrounding skin, which rapidly improves when the drugs are withdrawn. Moreover antibiotics are more effective when given systemically and may be used almost routinely whether infection is obvious or not. The infecting organisms are mainly Gram-positive cocci and coliforms and anaerobes although more often the results of swabs are inconclusive. Hunt (1992), in a survey of infected foot ulcers in diabetic patients, found that from 52 ulcers 177 bacterial strains were isolated, a mean of 3.4 organisms per lesion. *Staphylococcus aureus* was isolated from 58% of ulcers and anaerobes were also found in 58%. A broad spectrum penicillin with a second antibiotic against staphylococcal infection is appropriate with the use of metronidazole if anaerobes predominate. Attempts to clean the area locally should be made with hydrogen peroxide or chlorhexidine. Eusol, which was an effective agent, seems to be out of favour with those who study *in vitro* evidence of problems with its use.

Healing may be slow, particularly when a rim of necrotic tissue surrounds the crater. With this appearance debridement, repeated as necessary to healthy looking tissue, will allow granulation from the edges as well as the slow granulation from the base. Where bony infection is apparent from X-rays of the foot it is doubtful whether this can be eradicated even by systemic antibiotics and it is an indication for amputation.

A novel way to relieve pressure on the ulcerated area is to enclose the lower limb in a lightweight plaster cast. A window is left in the cast through which the area can be seen and dressed. By using the cast a patient can remain mobile with downward pressure spread through the base of the cast.

Amputation

A decision to amputate may be based upon non-healing, bony involvement or recurrent lesions at the same site. Necrotic tissue, especially in bones or tendons, maintains chronic infection and disability with the constant threat of an acute spreading cellulitis. Toe amputation is often sufficient for neuropathic lesions. The toe is removed through the metatarsal head and the skin is brought loosely together. Trans-metatarsal amputation or mid-tarsal amputation is currently out of favour but a ray amputation can be most useful. This is best performed for lesions of the second, third or fourth toes with deep-seated or backward spreading infection. The phalanges are removed with the metatarsal down to the base. The wound is then packed for a few days before being left to granulate. An initial horrific appearance may take time to heal but leaves a cosmetically appealing and useful appendage.

CHARCOT FOOT

The Charcot foot may be regarded as the end-point of neuropathic damage to the diabetic foot. The architecture of the foot is completely destroyed and the patient may be left with an ugly-looking appendage. It can be precipitated by relatively minor trauma or begin with a spontaneous fracture (Krentz *et al.*, 1989) and in the early stages deformity is not apparent and radiographs are normal. Over the ensuing weeks and months the shape of the foot changes markedly to a point of maximum distortion (Figure 18.5). Radiographs show subluxation and disorganiza-

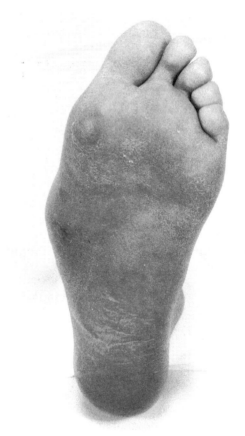

Fig. 18.5 Charcot foot of a male diabetic. The photograph was taken 4 months after the X-ray shown in Fig. 18.5.

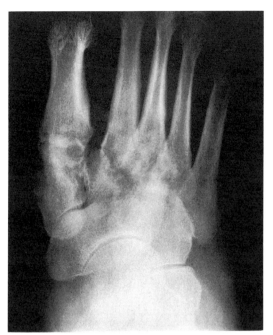

Fig. 18.6 Typical bony disorganization of X-ray of a Charcot foot. Although a different patient from Figures 18.3 and 18.5, the earliest manifestation in this diabetic woman was also a fracture through the base of the second metatarsal, which can still be seen.

tion of joints, osteolysis and new bone formation and occasionally fractures (Figure 18.6). The destructive process can be categorized into five stages on CT scanning with a consistent finding of changes in the medial tarsometatarsal joints. Later and more severe change involves the medial and, less commonly, lateral arches (Griffith *et al.*, 1995).

The foot is initially warm and if altered shape is not readily apparent the appearance may suggest infection. It is important to appreciate that destruction of the foot is an active inflammatory process. The old idea that bony destruction comes about by deformity brought about by exaggerated movement in a painless foot is no longer tenable. As destruction proceeds it is accompanied by warmth apparent to the observer.

There is a general acceptance that the early stages should be treated with rest or immobil-

ization using some form of plaster cast. A difficulty of this approach is that the process may last many months. Immobilization in a cast for 6 months or more is unlikely to be practised and the benefits of mobilization or rest for the first 6 weeks only are probably slim. Whether it leads to less deformity of the foot in the final analysis is doubtful and some might argue that continued use of the limb will mould the collapsing foot to a more useful shape. Made-to-measure footwear is necessary while the deformity is progressing and for the final result. Selby, Young and Boulton (1994) have reported preliminary results of the use of a biphosphonate in the treatment of Charcot foot. A decrease in skin temperature and a fall in alkaline phosphatase were taken to indicate a significant reduction in bone turnover. Care of the unaffected foot is vital yet three-quarters of patients show bilateral change (Griffith *et al.*, 1995).

NEUROPATHIC OEDEMA

Occasionally, oedema of the ankles is seen in patients with peripheral neuropathy but no obvious cause for the oedema. The association of neuropathy and peripheral oedema has been recognized since the last century but the pathogenesis remains obscure. It is usually a diagnosis of exclusion, nephropathy or other hypoalbuminaemic state having been excluded. Edmonds, Archer and Watkins (1983) report some success in treatment using ephedrine.

REFERENCES

Baddeley, R. M. and Fulford, J. C. (1964) The use of arteriography in conservative amputations for lesions of the feet in diabetes mellitus. *Br. J. Surg.*, **51**, 658–663.

Bell, E. T. (1957) Atherosclerotic gangrene of the lower extremities in diabetic and non diabetic persons. *Am. J. Clin. Pathol.*, **28**, 27–36.

Bevan, R. D. and Tsuru, H. (1979) Long term denervation of vascular smooth muscle causes not only functional but structural change. *Blood Vessels*, **16**, 109–112.

Boulton, A. J. M., Hardisty, C. A., Betts, R. P. *et al.* (1983) Dynamic foot pressure and other studies as diagnostic and management aids in diabetic neuropathy. *Diabetes Care*, **6**, 26–33.

Boulton, A. J. M., Scarpello, J. H. and Ward, J. D. (1982) Venous oxygenation in the diabetic neuropathic foot: evidence of arteriovenous shunting? *Diabetologia*, **22**, 6–8.

Deerochanawong, C., Home, P. D. and Alberti, K. G. M. M. (1992) A survey of lower limb amputation in diabetic patients. *Diabetic Med.*, **9**, 942–946.

Edmonds, M. E., Archer, A. G. and Watkins, P. J. (1983) Ephedrine: a new treatment for diabetic neuropathic oedema. *Lancet*, **i**, 548–551.

Edmonds, M. E., Gilbey, S., Walters, H. *et al.* (1985) Improved survival of the diabetic ischaemic foot. *Diabetic Med.*, **2**, 506A.

Fagius, J. (1982) Microneurographic findings in diabetic polyneuropathy with special reference to sympathetic nerve activity. *Diabetologia*, **23**, 415–420.

Guy, R. J. C., Clark, C. A., Malcolm, P. N. and Watkins, P. J. (1985) Evaluation of thermal and vibration sensation in diabetic neuropathy. *Diabetologia*, **28**, 131–137.

Griffith, J., Davies, A. M., Close, C. F. and Nattrass, M. (1995) Organized chaos? Computed tomographic evaluation of the neuropathic diabetic foot. *Br. J. Radiol.*, **68**, 27–33.

Haimovici, H., Shapiro, J. H. and Jacobson, H. G. (1960) Serial femoral arteriography in occlusive disease. *Am. J. Roentgenol.*, **83**, 1042–1062.

Hoar, C. S. and Torres, J. (1962) Evaluation of below-the-knee amputation in the treatment of diabetic gangrene. *N. Engl. J. Med.*, **266**, 440–443.

Hunt, J. A. (1992) Foot infections in diabetes are rarely due to a single microorganism. *Diabetic Med.*, **9**, 749–752.

Janka, H. J., Standl, E. and Mehnert, H. (1980) Peripheral vascular disease in diabetes mellitus and its relation to cardiovascular risk factors: screening with the Doppler ultrasonic technique. *Diabetes Care*, **3**, 207–213.

Krentz, A. J., FitzGerald, M. F., Wright, A. D. and Nattrass, M. (1989) Spontaneous fractures in patients with diabetic neuropathy. *J. Roy. Col. Phys. (Lond.)*, **23**, 111–113.

LoGerfo, F. W. and Coffman, J. D. (1984) Vascular and microvascular disease of the foot in diabetes. *N. Engl. J. Med.*, **311**, 1615–1619.

Mansell, P. J., Gregson, R. and Allison, S. P. (1992) An audit of lower limb arteriography in diabetic patients. *Diabetic Med.*, **9**, 84–90.

Rosenberg, N. and London, I. M. (1956) Excision and drainage for infections of the foot with gangrene in the diabetic. *Arch. Surg.*, **72** 160–165.

Scarpello, J. H. B., Martin, T. R. P. and Ward, J. D. (1980) Ultrasound measurements of pulse-wave velocity in the peripheral arteries of diabetic subjects. *Clin. Sci.*, **58**, 53–57.

Selby, P. L., Young, M. J. and Boulton, A. J. M. (1994) Bisphosphonates: a new treatment for diabetic Charcot neuroarthropathy. *Diabetic Med.*, **11**, 28–31.

Semple, R. (1953) Diabetes and peripheral arterial disease. *Lancet*, **i**, 1064–1068.

Silbert, S. and Haimovici, H. (1954) Criteria for the selection of the level of amputation for ischemic gangrene. *J.A.M.A.*, **155**, 1554–1558.

Walters, D. P., Gatling, W., Mullee, M. A. and Hill, R. D. (1992) The distribution and severity of diabetic foot disease: a community study with comparison to a non-diabetic group. *Diabetic Med.*, **9**, 354–358.

Ward, J. D., Simms, J. M., Knight, G. *et al.* (1983) Venous distension in the diabetic neuropathic foot (physical sign of arteriovenous shunting). *J. Roy. Soc. Med.*, **76**, 1011–1014.

Williams, D. R. R. (1985) Hospital admissions of diabetic patients: information from hospital activity analysis. *Diabetic Med.*, **2**, 27–32.

THE LIVER

The liver occupies a central place in carbohydrate metabolism and is the principal source of glucose production in the fasting state. After an overnight fast 75% of glucose released from the liver is from glycogen breakdown (Felig, 1973) while the remaining 25% comes from gluconeogenesis. Quantitatively, gluconeogenesis becomes more important in prolonged starvation.

Many tissues synthesize and degrade glycogen, of which muscle is probably the most important. The liver is unique, however, in having the enzyme glucose-6-phosphatase, which converts glucose-6-phosphate on the glycogen degrading pathway to glucose for subsequent release into the blood. It can be determined that the liver of an adult will produce glucose at a rate of 0.06 mol/h (10 g/h) in the fasting state. Liver glycogen is under continuous turnover, with replenishment of stores upon feeding. Part of the replacement of glycogen derives from dietary glucose supply but it is now held that some comes from gluconeogenesis. There appears to be a delay in shutting off gluconeogenesis when feeding begins but the fate of the gluconeogenic precursors changes at this time from glucose to glycogen.

Carbohydrate metabolism within the liver is regulated both hormonally and by substrate supply. Glycogen storage is promoted by insulin and glucose concentration. Gluconeogenesis is promoted by supply of gluconeogenic precursors lactate, pyruvate, alanine and glycerol but inhibited by a rise in insulin concentration. It is probable that the interplay between glucose concentration and circulating insulin level is important in regulating hepatic glucose output. Unfortunately the precise contribution of each is difficult to estimate because of technical difficulties. Infusion of insulin to raise the circulating concentration will serve to lower blood glucose. An ingenious solution to this problem is to clamp blood glucose during an insulin infusion with a simultaneously adjusted glucose infusion. Using this technique of euglycaemic clamping very high circulating concentrations of insulin will stop hepatic glucose output even giving negative figures at times, presumed to reflect glucose uptake, although there is some evidence that such figures may be a consequence of technical difficulties with the isotope. While splendid results can be achieved in glucose clamp studies it must constantly be borne in mind that insulin does not work *in vivo* in this manner. Blood glucose is lowered by insulin and insulin deficiency leads to raised blood glucose levels. Probably one of the few statements which can be made with certainty is that given insulin deficiency the removal of restraint upon hepatic glucose production cannot be compensated for by a rise in blood glucose concentration. Thus in the presence of hyperglycaemia in the diabetic patient hepatic glucose output remains inappropriately high.

Glucagon and adrenalin act in opposition to insulin, both promoting glycogen breakdown in liver. Glucagon also stimulates gluconeogenesis. These opposing actions of glucagon along with regulation of glucagon secretion by insulin have led some to postulate diabetes as a bihormonal disease (Unger and Orci, 1975).

At other times different hormones become important in regulating hepatic carbohydrate metabolism. Corticosteroids increase supply of lactate and pyruvate to the liver (Johnston *et al.*, 1979), increase alanine release from muscle (Wise, Hendler and Felig, 1973) and induce key gluconeogenic enzymes (Lecocq, Mebane and Madison, 1964). The time-scale of these effects is slower than the acute changes produced by glucagon and adrenalin. Large doses of thyroid hormone induce glycogen breakdown, as do high circulating levels of vasopressin such as are found in shocked patients.

EFFECTS OF LIVER DISEASE UPON NORMAL METABOLISM

Since the liver plays such an important part in the regulation of blood glucose, diffuse hepatic disease might be expected to disturb this mechanism profoundly. The dominant effect of liver disease is related to the extent of the underlying disease and appears to be upon the storage capacity of the liver in severe disease. In lesser degrees of disease there are effects upon the ability of the liver to remove a glucose load from the circulation and insulin resistance in peripheral tissues.

The major result, particularly of severe liver disease, is to produce hypoglycaemia. Rarely is this a clinical problem, which is fortunate since when it does occur it is often overlooked.

The oral glucose tolerance test in liver disease is usually normal but a few patients show an alternative picture of a low–normal fasting blood glucose, rising to 12–15 mmol/l (220–270 mg/dl) at 1–2 hours and falling after 3–4 hours to hypoglycaemic levels. The reduced ability of the liver to extract a glucose load is reflected in the high peak and some of this is attributable to shunting within the liver. The subsequent fall to hypoglycaemic levels is a consequence of shunting of insu-

lin leading to inappropriately elevated peripheral levels (Johnston *et al.*, 1977). These elevated peripheral insulin levels have been taken as reflecting insulin resistance as an accompaniment of liver disease.

EFFECT OF LIVER DISEASE ON DIABETES

In view of the preceding paragraphs it will not be surprising to find that when liver disease is superimposed on existing diabetes the need for insulin may be increased or, less often, diminished. Clearly, if the storage capacity of the liver is impaired then the risk of hypoglycaemia will necessitate the reduction of insulin dose. On the other hand, insulin resistance as a result of hepatic cirrhosis has been described many times (Kruszynska *et al.*, 1993).

LIVER FUNCTION IN DIABETES

There is no evidence that liver function is abnormal in diabetics under reasonable control. Normal liver function tests and liver biopsy have been fairly consistent findings although occasional reports of some fatty change in up to 50% of patients with well controlled diabetes and no clinical liver disease have appeared.

Mild abnormalities of liver function and occasional cholestatic jaundice were noted in the early days of treatment with the sulphonylurea drugs, especially chlorpropamide, but since the dosage has been reduced from the somewhat excessive levels of that period these complications have ceased to be a problem.

More recently, disturbances of liver function tests have been reported after hypoglycaemia (Soler and Khardori, 1985). Some investigators have failed to find support for this notion and even if it occurs the significance of it remains doubtful.

ENLARGEMENT OF THE LIVER IN DIABETES

Fatty infiltration of the liver has long been recognized in diabetes. Before insulin and during the early years of its use gross enlargement of the liver was commonly found in young patients. Marble *et al.* (1938) reported 60 cases in 1077 patients whose diabetes started before the age of 15. Those with big livers were notable for the frequency of ketosis, hypoglycaemia, dwarfism, neuropathy, tuberculosis and other infections. They believed that the deposition of fat rather than glycogen was responsible for the size of the liver. Treatment with raw pancreas and betain hydrochloride was ineffective, but control of diabetes with insulin was followed by a reduction in the size of the liver to normal.

Though the introduction of long-acting insulin was given the credit for lowering the incidence of this complication the possibility of a nutritional factor has to be considered. The frequent occurrence of dwarfism in association with the liver enlargement suggests the possibility of excessive dietary restriction, for dwarfism was once common in diabetic children in this country and has been eliminated more by liberal dieting rather than by better insulin control.

Certainly hepatic enlargement is no longer common. It is occasionally seen in adult patients whose diabetes is rather poorly controlled and can present with bouts of abdominal pain. Liver function tests show little abnormality apart from a slight increase in transaminase enzymes and occasionally a modest reduction in the serum albumin. Biopsy findings are variable, some showing pronounced fatty infiltration, some mainly glycogen and some a hydrops of the liver cells. The patients I have seen with this condition have not been conspicuous for their poor control or general care of their health. The liver enlargement usually subsides gradually over a period of months but whether in response to good diabetic control, or just spontaneously, is hard to tell. I am not aware that cirrhosis has ever followed this liver enlargement.

CIRRHOSIS OF THE LIVER

Most writers agree that cirrhosis of the liver is not unduly frequent in diabetes. If a patient presents with features of cirrhosis and diabetes the diagnosis of haemochromatosis must be carefully considered. The reverse, however, that glucose intolerance and diabetes is common in cirrhosis is widely accepted.

GALL STONES

There seems general acceptance of an increased risk of gall stones in the diabetic population. This was put at two- to eightfold by Leiber (1985). Inadequate emptying of the gall bladder was found by Stone *et al.* (1988) using radionuclide cholescintography but only in patients with autonomic neuropathy. Other reports have suggested that gall bladder motility is impaired by hyperglycaemia (de Boer *et al.*, 1994) and that diabetic patients have altered profiles of bile acids. Disease of the gall bladder is associated with the rare endocrine tumour somatostatinoma.

THE GASTROINTESTINAL TRACT

THE MOUTH

There is no evidence that oral disease is unduly common in controlled diabetic patients and dentition of children is normal. Loosening of the teeth, hypertrophied and inflamed gingivae and sometimes polypoid proliferation from under the free margin of the gum have been described but they must be exceptionally rare or almost always overlooked. The condition is said to improve remarkably when diabetes is brought under control.

A number of other conditions affecting the mouth are reportedly increased in diabetic patients: xerostomia, sialosis and impairment of taste have been described (Lamey, Darwazeh and Frier, 1992).

At times of poor control oral candidiasis may occur with oesophageal involvement. Inspection of the mouth is a useful exercise in patients with ketoacidosis.

THE STOMACH

The effects of insulin and glucagon on gastric secretion are well established. Insulin produces an initial inhibitory effect on basal gastric secretion followed by a stimulatory effect mediated through the vagus nerve. Acutely induced hypoglycaemia stimulates gastric secretion, probably via the vagus nerve, while glucagon enhances this effect. Glucagon has an inhibiting action when given alone, which is unexplained. The secretory responses do not consistently relate to the changes induced in blood glucose concentration.

Achlorhydria or hypochlorhydria has been a common finding in studies of diabetic clinic patients. Traditionally, peptic ulcer has been considered a rarity in diabetes although gastric ulcers are as common as in the general population and the deficiency therefore lies in the incidence of duodenal ulcer. Initial symptoms are often vague but the other clinical features unremarkable.

The observation that hyperglycaemia retards gastric emptying in the absence of autonomic neuropathy is rather underappreciated (Horowitz and Fraser, 1994).

DISORDERS OF THE SMALL AND LARGE INTESTINE

Walsh *et al.* (1978) reported 14 cases of diabetes mellitus coexisting with coeliac disease from our clinic. Despite many anecdotal reports the coincidence rates are not known. Of the 14, 10 were on insulin treatment and diabetes was first to be diagnosed in 13 patients. A variety of symptoms and signs initiated investigation for coeliac disease. Introduction of a gluten-free diet led to a rise in insulin requirement in the majority of patients.

Children with diabetes and coeliac disease have also been recorded and it has been postulated as a greater coincidence than by chance. Troublesome diarrhoea or hypoglycaemia in children is a common presentation. The former may account for delay in diagnosis due to similarities with diabetic diarrhoea and four of the 14 patients of Walsh *et al.* (1978) had been treated incorrectly for diabetic diarrhoea.

A possible link for the two diseases is supplied by the increased incidence of HLA B_8 in coeliac disease: 80% of patients with coeliac disease were HLA-B_8-positive compared with 30% of controls (Stokes *et al.*, 1972). Since HLA-B_8 is in linkage disequilibrium with DR_3 a predisposition to both diseases might be presumed.

DIABETES AND THE SKIN

There are certain peculiarities of metabolism in the skin – an absence of enzymes required for the Krebs cycle and for the synthesis of carbohydrate from pyruvate – but there is no evidence that any specific disturbance occurs as a result of diabetes. For instance, glycogen, which is not available for conversion to glucose, is present in normal amounts. In normal subjects glucose given parenterally or by mouth is said to cause a rise in skin glucose by, on average, 3.2 mmol/l (58 mg/dl) while a figure above 3.8 mmol/l (68 mg/dl) is pathological. In some patients with dermatitis, furunculosis and pruritus the skin glucose may be high although the oral glucose tolerance test is normal. It is, of course, an old tradition (or should it be superstition?) that skin infections are related to a high carbohydrate intake and can be relieved by restriction of sugar in the diet.

There is little evidence that increased glucose, in the blood at least, favours the growth of pyogenic organisms. Addition of glucose to blood cultures does not speed the growth of bacterial organisms. *In vivo*, dehydration seems to be as, or more, important than the excess glucose and skin infections in the diabetic patient do not seem to be unduly frequent unless control is very significantly disturbed. The finding of a minor abnormality of glucose tolerance in a patient with recurrent boils is probably coincidental.

Changes in the skin capillaries of the diabetic similar to those in the kidney and retina have been reported, as has endothelial proliferation in the small vessels of diabetics without complications. As in other organs the clinical significance of early lesions in the vessels is not apparent and there is nothing to suggest that the skin of patients with average control of their blood glucose, who do not have peripheral neuropathy, is unduly vulnerable to injuries and infections or that it heals slowly. Changes in the vessels of the skin must be interpreted with caution.

PYOGENIC SKIN INFECTIONS

The cause of furunculosis is obscure and diabetics are subject to sporadic attacks of boils no less than normal people, but their occurrence should suggest the possibility of poor diabetic control, which will certainly encourage the spread of infection with the risk of a carbuncle. Carbuncles still occur but are almost entirely confined to patients who neglect treatment and keep away from the doctor until the last moment. They were once a dreaded complication and a considerable cause of diabetic mortality before the introduction of penicillin.

Normal cleanliness is the preventive treatment of skin infections. Excessive washing and the use of antiseptics may actually diminish the resistance of the skin to infection. Antibiotics usually fail to prevent the full development of a boil even if taken at the earliest symptom but do limit the extent of infection. Local antibiotics, if used at all, should not be continued for more than a few days because the skin readily becomes sensitized to them. Carbuncles require full systemic treatment,

with culture of the organisms and tests of sensitivity to antibiotics if there is any doubt about the response to treatment. Surgery is often needed to promote drainage.

EPIDERMOPHYTOSIS

Fungal infections of the feet are probably no more common in the diabetic than the normal population – they hardly could be – but they have special significance in the diabetic foot, which is often vulnerable because of neuropathy or ischaemia and in which they provide a means of entry for other organisms. In the chronic case the distribution, particularly between the fourth and fifth toes, of hyperkeratotic macerated skin covered by a white membrane is easily recognized, but lesions on the heel and sole may only be detectable by culture. In more acute cases vesicles and pustules may be widespread and eczema superimposed to make a confusing picture. The most important treatment is to keep the feet dry, especially between the toes; socks should be changed daily. Fungicidal powders are generally disappointing but occasionally valuable.

MONILIASIS

Pruritus vulvae is very commonly associated with moniliasis in diabetic women; more frequently than in the pruritus of the non-diabetic. *Candida albicans* is nearly always present and when other yeasts occur they are saprophytic and do not cause symptoms. The localization of the eruption on and around the vulva strongly suggests that the sugar in the urine promotes the condition. Moreover the amount of glycosuria seems to be important, since pruritus and vulvitis often subside when glycosuria is reduced but not abolished, and patients with renal glycosuria, which is not as abundant as that of diabetes, rarely complain of vulval irritation. The treatment, therefore, in the majority is simply the abolition of glycosuria, which brings rapid relief. Certainly, without diminution of the glycosuria the infection will not clear even if local treatment with vaginal tablets and antifungal creams are used.

Occasionally, *Candida* infection of the fingers causes paronychia and rarely a generalized infection includes stomatitis and a papular eruption.

GENERAL PRURITUS

In spite of statements to the contrary, this is not a feature of diabetes (Neilly *et al.*, 1986).

SKIN GANGRENE

This is an occasional complication when diabetes is accompanied by severe prostration and dehydration, usually the result of severe ketosis. At pressure points, especially the buttocks and heels, the skin quickly becomes necrotic and black, ultimately sloughing to leave a shallow ulcer. This presentation of gangrene is not related to peripheral vascular disease, but neuropathy is usually manifest.

FOURNIER'S GANGRENE

This is perhaps a special case of gangrene associated with diabetes. It may accompany diabetic ketoacidosis, involving the skin of the scrotum and perineum. I favour enthusiastic treatment. Debridement is usually necessary, often exposing subcutaneous tissue over a wide area. Although healing may be slow it tends to be complete.

XANTHOMA DIABETICORUM

The lesions were first described by Addison and Gull (1851). One of their patients was a diabetic man of 27 with an eruption on the arms, legs, trunk and face. Curiously enough, the eruption began to subside during the few weeks of observation.

The condition is now recognized as a mani-

festation of hyperlipaemia not essentially different from other forms of xanthomatosis. The lesions occur mainly on the outer side of the forearms, the elbows, knees, buttocks and less often on the trunk and face. They are papules and nodules, discrete, single or in groups, of an orange, pink or yellow hue, the diameter being 2–5 mm. Each may be surrounded by a hyperaemic zone which is said to distinguish it from the xanthoma of primary hypercholesterolaemia. Yellow streaks appear in the creases of the palms and soles. The liver is often enlarged and infiltrated with fat while the appearance of lipaemia retinalis may be very striking. The whole retina has the colour of peaches and cream while the arteries are extremely pale.

The histological picture, of collections of histiocytes containing lipid, is like that of other xanthomata.

The diabetes is always severe enough to need insulin and is always out of control at the time when xanthoma appear. Insulin deficiency leading to mobilization of fat depots and an inability to clear fat from the blood is an adequate explanation of the hyperlipaemia but it is not so easy to see why xanthoma is such an uncommon disorder or what distinguishes the few patients who get it. The diagnosis is usually simple. The diabetes must be out of control and unless this is so other causes of xanthoma have to be considered particularly myxoedema and biliary cirrhosis although each has characteristic features apart from the skin eruption.

Treatment consists of vigorous treatment with insulin which leads to a rapid fall in blood lipids and an early regression of the lesions which disappear in about a month leaving no trace.

XANTHELASMA

This is the xanthomatous eruption on the lids associated with degeneration of the tarsal plates. It is unrelated to xanthomatosis and is not unduly frequent in diabetics.

VITILIGO

There is a strong feeling that the incidence of vitiligo is increased in diabetic patients although firm evidence is lacking. Perhaps it is the temptation of the immunological basis of the condition, or the link with pernicious anaemia which proves too strong to resist. Logic is not on our side, however, since a cursory glance into the diabetic clinic shows as many non-insulin-dependent diabetic patients with vitiligo, or at the very least, that vitiligo is not confined to insulin-dependent patients.

NECROBIOSIS LIPOIDICA DIABETICORUM

Necrobiosis lipoidica diabeticorum is a skin disorder occurring in diabetics before or after the diabetes has been recognized; perhaps in non-diabetics occasionally. About three-quarters of the patients are women and the lesions appear as a rule in early life, mostly before the age of 40. The name was suggested by Urbach in 1932, although cases had been described a few years earlier. The peculiar ingenuity of dermatologists has added other variants – necrobiosis maculosa and sclerodermiform, syphiloid and angiodermatitis-like forms – which are probably not distinct. The eruption starts with well-defined papules gradually enlarging to form oval or irregular plaques with a clear-cut margin. The colour is pink, often mixed with yellow from the presence of fat. The overlying epidermis is tightly stretched over the plaque and through it may be seen a fine network of vessels. This is the typical and instantly recognizable picture. Later atrophy of the epidermis may lead to scaling and ulceration, and in a late stage there may be a resemblance to varicose eczema. A more nodular form resembles sarcoid. The commonest site for the lesions is pretibial but they may also occur on the arms

and hands, and on the trunk. Occasional plaques may be seen on the female breast.

Histology

Unsurprisingly, the most constant histological change is scattered necrobiosis, a homogenization and degeneration rather than necrosis of the connective tissue, the elastic tissue often being intact in these areas. Deposits of lipid, mainly phospholipid and cholesterol, are usually, but not invariably seen, mostly extracellular and towards the centre of the lesion. Obliterative changes in small blood vessels are common and a peripheral perivascular reaction with histiocytes and lymphocytes is the rule. Glycogen can be found in the histiocytes and tissue spaces. The precise nature of the lesion is unknown. It seems unlikely that the obliterative vessel changes are primarily responsible; there is no disturbance of blood lipids.

When lesions appear in an established diabetic they bear no relationship to the degree of control, but in the vast majority of cases the diabetes has required insulin. Necrobiosis lipoidica is particularly interesting because it may appear some years before clinical diabetes is manifest.

Some dermatologists believe that necrobiosis lipoidica is not necessarily associated with diabetes because after several years of observation the skin lesion has not been followed by diabetes. There is, however, no evidence that serious attempts at follow-up have been made and the subject is still open. If in fact there is always an association between the two disorders, as seems to me more probable, then necrobiosis lipoidica is at times a truly prediabetic manifestation and deserves more study than it has received.

Treatment

In many instances the skin plaques are symptomless and call for no treatment. A number of proprietary make-ups are available which will disguise the lesions to a certain extent.

When ulceration occurs healing may be slow. A favourable response to injections of hydrocortisone into the lesions has been reported. Marten and Dulake (1957) used injections of 2 ml of 25 mg/ml hydrocortisone in 18 lesions, 17 of which showed improvement or complete resolution, though the time of follow-up is not stated. Ulceration in three cases and cellulitis in two were attributed to the injections and it seems that the indications for interfering at all must be quite clear before embarking on this form of treatment. I must confess that the long-term benefits of injecting the lesions with steroid preparations has singularly failed to impress me and I am resistant to this line of treatment.

In severe cases, which often means cosmetically severe, skin grafting may be considered. Success is limited by recurrence within or around the graft.

DIABETIC DERMOPATHY

The name has been given to well circumscribed brown patches on the lower legs. The initial appearance is of small plaques or papules which are red fading to brown. Histologically the lesions are non-specific and eventually the appearance is of depressed brown scars.

DIABETIC BULLAE

Rarely, non traumatic blistering of the skin, particularly affecting the lower legs, may occur in diabetic patients. Lesions may be single or multiple and there is often underlying peripheral neuropathy. Complete healing over weeks or months is the likely outcome (Toonstra, 1985).

OTHER SKIN LESIONS

Numerous attempts have been made to link specific dermatological diseases to diabetes, particularly granuloma annulare and lichen planus. The reservations voiced elsewhere in this volume on the association of common diseases in well screened populations apply. Some diseases, like haemochromotosis and glucagonoma, which have diabetes as part of their manifestation also have particular skin lesions. For the rest and with the exception of acanthosis nigricans (Chapter 3) and the thickened skin of cheiroarthropathy, the evidence is unconvincing.

DIABETES AND CONNECTIVE TISSUE DISORDERS

The major connective tissue disorders have no increased frequency in diabetes. Minor features such as Dupytren's contracture and frozen shoulder occur but a positive association is difficult to show. Indeed it is highly probable that Dupytren's contracture is overdiagnosed in early literature and that some of these patients have the association of limited joint mobility and diabetes. This was redescribed by Rosenbloom *et al.* (1981), who showed the association of cheiroarthopathy with diabetes. It can be demonstrated by the prayer sign, where the patient finds opposing the hands palm to palm impossible for the third, fourth and fifth fingers. In similar manner the hand cannot be placed flush with a level surface palm down. There is a clear relationship between duration of diabetes and the development of cheiroarthropathy and it has been suggested that cheiroarthropathy may precede diabetic microvascular disease and therefore serves as a warning. This is always a safe bet in diabetes in view of the numbers of patients developing complications and difficult to prove one way or another. Instinctively more attractive is the suggestion of a pathogenesis through abnormal glycation of collagen, which alters structural and functional properties.

GOUT AND DIABETES

The association of gout with diabetes mellitus was regarded as a significant combination throughout the 19th century. Both diseases have been considered as related to super-alimentation and therefore as pathological results of modern civilization.

There are theoretical reasons for associating uric acid metabolism with diabetes, for alloxan can be produced from uric acid by oxidation *in vitro*.

Clinical impression suggests that there is no undue prevalence of gout in a diabetic population in England. Mohan *et al.* (1984) found no difference in uric acid levels between diabetic patients and controls but in the offspring of conjugal diabetics uric acid levels were greater than controls. Similarly, serum uric acid levels were higher than normal in prediabetic individuals when reported by Herman, Medalie and Goldbourt (1976). Others have reported the converse, a high incidence of diabetes in patients with gout.

Recently there has been increased interest in the occurrence of hyperinsulinaemia in patients with gout. It is unclear whether this is part of a multifactorial risk group including obesity–hypertension–hypercholesterolaemia–hypertriglyceridaemia. Certainly the association of glucose intolerance, gout and hypertriglyceridaemia (type IV hyperlipoproteinaemia) has been documented for some time.

DIABETES AND CYSTIC FIBROSIS

The association of glucose intolerance and frank diabetes mellitus with the multisystem disorder cystic fibrosis has been reported. In the presence of severe exocrine disease the disordered carbohydrate metabolism is brought about by low insulin responses to a carbohydrate load. The endocrine effects are closely linked to the exocrine function (Geffner *et al.*, 1984) and some patients with exocrine deficiency and normal glucose tolerance have increased muscle insulin sensitivity (Moran *et al.*, 1994).

DIABETES AND NEUROLOGICAL DISEASE

The relationship of diabetes and neurological disease is of interest. Genetic factors would suggest that disseminated sclerosis should be uncommon or rare in association with insulin-dependent diabetes since the genetic marker of this disease, DR_2, is decreased in insulin-dependent diabetes. It is difficult to be dogmatic on this point since the disorder occurs infrequently but certainly we have insulin-dependent diabetics with disseminated sclerosis attending our clinic.

In contrast, there are grounds for anticipating a link between diabetes and myotonic dystrophy. The glucose intolerance of this disorder has long been regarded as due to end-organ unresponsiveness to insulin. The gene for myotonic dystrophy appears to lie in close proximity to the insulin receptor gene, and while insulin responses to oral glucose are heterogeneous, some patients show massive insulin rises following glucose (Krentz *et al.*, 1990). Resistance to insulin action has also been demonstrated using a variety of techniques (Krentz, Williams and Nattrass, 1991). Friedreich's ataxia also shows an association with diabetes. Patients have hyperglycaemia and hyperinsulinaemia in response to oral glucose, although the mechanism of this insulin resistance is unclear (Khan, Andermann and Fantus, 1986). Interestingly this finding extends to first degree relatives of patients with Friedreich's ataxia (Fantus *et al.*, 1991).

Optic atrophy may occur in diabetic patients for a number of reasons. In the absence of glaucoma or an alternative cause of optic atrophy it is often difficult to know whether the association is a partial expression of the DIDMOAD syndrome. Nowhere is caution over assuming an association more necessary than in linking eye disease with diabetes. Few populations get such extensive monitoring of their eyes and other abnormalities are bound to be detected. Whether their frequency of association is more common often remains in doubt.

PERNICIOUS ANAEMIA AND DIABETES

The combination of pernicious anaemia and diabetes has been regarded as significant by most writers since the beginning of the 20th century. The incidence of pernicious anaemia in diabetic patients in published studies ranges from 0.2% to 1% whereas the incidence of pernicious anaemia in the general population of several European countries is reckoned to be between 0.1% and 0.15%. The incidence of diabetes in recorded cases of pernicious anaemia is also variable, from 1.3% to 2.1%.

There are difficulties in assessing these results. The collection of examples of this combination must depend to some extent on the emphasis in the hospital on diabetic and haematological services. Very few writers allow for the somewhat different age incidence of the two diseases and a comparison of the prevalence of pernicious anaemia in a predominantly elderly population of diabetics with that in the general population would not be valid. Further, the frequency of the diagnosis of both diseases has changed over the years. In the case of pernicious anaemia screening methods have increased the chance of recognizing early disease, although the numbers have in the same period been considerably eroded by the more accurate methods for assessing the mechanism of vitamin B_{12} deficiency. No doubt many of the earlier recorded patients with pernicious anaemia, particularly when it occurred under the age of 30, would now be diagnosed differently.

A number of studies have shown antibodies to thyroid and gastric mucosa occur to a significantly greater extent in the diabetic population compared with the non-diabetic population.

DIABETES AND INFECTION

The frequency and enhanced severity of infections in uncontrolled diabetes were well known in the days before insulin. Even when insulin became available death was commonly due to overwhelming infections in the poorly controlled patient. In the Joslin Clinic deaths from infection reached their highest proportion, 13.6% of the total, in the era 1922–1936. With the introduction of antibiotics infection as a cause of death is no more common in the diabetic than in the general population, but the lowered resistance is still seen in a few patients who are grossly careless in their diabetic treatment or whose diabetes has escaped diagnosis.

There is no evidence that a well controlled diabetic is abnormal in his response to infection. Attempts have been made to demonstrate a defective mechanism of resistance to infection in experimental or human diabetes but with little success. Other writers have been impressed by the effect of dehydration following the observation that in dehydrated animals the extent of experimental skin infection is enhanced.

Staphylococcal infection and mucocutaneous candidiasis are reportedly more common in the diabetic population (Robertson and Polk, 1974). Disordered and deficient neutrophil movement has been proposed for a role. Abnormal neutrophil movement in diabetic patients has been reported with a similar observation in first-degree relatives of diabetic patients (Molenaar *et al.*, 1976). While the authors have suggested a relationship with poor control these results argue against this and for an intrinsic defect. Lawley *et al.* (1981) showed poor macrophage function in people who were HLA-B_8/DR_3 positive.

There is little to suggest an impairment of phagocytosis in diabetic patients, although organism killing may be affected (Wilson and Reeves, 1986).

The association of diabetes and some specific infections is worthy of further comment.

No-one who has seen a patient with muco-cutaneous candidiasis will forget the sight nor fail to regret that the diagnosis took so long and that the treatment was insufficiently aggressive.

Of bacterial infections tuberculosis is of historical interest in the Western world but continues to be important in certain sub-groups of the population and in other lands. The association with diabetes may have been noted by Avicenna nearly 1000 years ago. Bouchardat (1883) found that every case of diabetes which came to autopsy had tubercles in the lungs, at a time when nearly half the patients in the public hospitals of Europe were found to have phthisis at post-mortem. In this century first the tuberculous and later the diabetic populations have been segregated to an increasing degree so that it is almost impossible to judge the true incidence of the combination of diseases. In the early part of the 20th century an incidence three times that of the normal population was recorded while as the cause of death in the diabetic population estimates ranged from 18% to 40%.

Recently tuberculosis has not been a serious problem but new cases still occur, mostly over the age of 50. In Britain there is a new element in the immigrant population from Asia, which has a higher incidence of tuberculosis and an increased incidence of diabetes.

DIABETES AND LIPIDS

It is difficult to find a middle-ground on the topic of lipids and diabetes. Physicians either love the subject, devoting long hours to applying the fruits of lipid research to their patients, or they loath it, ignoring it whenever possible. The latter group, into which I fall, tend to know little of the subject, which increases at an alarming rate.

A number of situations where disordered lipid metabolism in diabetes is important can be identified; firstly, the diabetic lipaemic syndrome of lipaemia retinalis, eruptive xanthomata and hepatosplenomegaly resulting from insulin deficiency. This syndrome, which may accompany diabetic ketoacidosis, is characterized by massive accumulation of chylomicrons and VLDL. Perhaps the major risk from its occurrence is the development of acute pancreatitis. The clinical features and biochemical findings quickly revert to normal with the institution of insulin therapy in the majority of patients, although some show an underlying familial form of hypertriglyceridaemia in addition to diabetes (Brunzell and Bierman, 1982).

Secondly, more moderate degrees of hypertriglyceridaemia are common in diabetes. Pfeifer *et al.* (1983) demonstrated a linear relationship between hypertriglyceridaemia and hyperglycaemia before treatment and showed a similar relationship between the change in triglyceride and glycosylated haemoglobin concentration after treatment was commenced. Further improvements in diabetic control resulted in greater lowering of triglyceride levels. Many other studies testify to the response of raised VLDL to improvements in diabetic control in insulin-dependent diabetes and in non-insulin-dependent patients. The underlying problem appears to be low activity of lipoprotein lipase, which is restored by appropriate hypoglycaemic therapy (Pfeifer *et al.*, 1983). Failure to improve with instigation of treatment suggests an underlying primary hypertriglyceridaemia or other cause of secondary hypertriglyceridaemia. The message that emerges from these observations is clear. An alternative cause for lipoprotein disorder cannot be identified until optimum diabetic control has been achieved and this should remain the major aim of treatment.

With regard to cholesterol and LDL-cholesterol the situation is less clear. Improvements in control which improve VLDL abnormalities may not result in change in cholesterol and LDL-cholesterol. The consensus that emerges from a number of studies indicates that major improvements in control leading to tight diabetic control are needed for correction of cholesterol and LDL-cholesterol abnormalities (Pietri, Dunn and Raskin, 1980). Even when VLDL and LDL abnormalities are corrected by tight control there may be little or no improvement in HDL concentration. This appears to reflect the slow turnover time of this fraction and persistence with tight diabetic control leads to an increase in the HDL fraction (Dunn, Pietri and Raskin, 1981).

Thus the case for tight metabolic control is overwhelming in attempting to correct lipoprotein abnormalities secondary to diabetes. Only if abnormalities persist when this has been achieved and maintained is further investigation and possible intervention indicated.

In the real world, however, diabetic control for a majority of patients continues to be suboptimal, while cardiovascular disease extracts a high price in morbidity and mortality. The question of intervention in patients with suboptimal diabetic control remains unanswered.

Superimposed upon this background is the debate about treatment of lipid abnormalities in the general population. It is not my intention to enter this area here but two thoughts spring to mind. Firstly, there are an inordinate number of measurements of lipids being done in both the non-diabetic and the diabetic populations. I belong to a school that says that results of tests which are requested must be acted upon and therefore I would urge that clear protocols are in place detailing action based upon specific results before any systematic measurement of lipids is done in the diabetic clinic or, indeed, elsewhere.

Secondly, the scale of the problem should not be underestimated. About 25% of diabetic patients who attend our annual review clinic have lipid results that would be considered by many authorities to require treatment. To undertake this treatment would generate one new clinic for every four annual review clinics done. This is not put forward

as a reason for complete inertia but simply to indicate that problems must be anticipated.

THYROID DISEASE AND DIABETES

THYROTOXICOSIS

Glycosuria is said to be common in thyrotoxicosis although the finding has never struck me. Some have found an incidence in excess of one-third. In most instances the glycosuria is related to a mild abnormality of the glucose tolerance test. Fasting levels are normal or slightly raised, there is a considerable peak at a half to 1 hour and at 2 hours the blood glucose is not quite back to normal. This abnormality may be attributed to an increased rate of absorption of glucose from the gut and perhaps to impairment of liver function in relation to glycogen storage. That it is not truly diabetic is suggested by the lower incidence of abnormality found when the intravenous glucose tolerance test is used. Nevertheless, the incidence of true diabetes in thyrotoxic patients is considerable. This is not surprising, as thyrotoxicosis affects particularly women in middle and later life, who also show a high incidence of diabetes, often revealed when the thyroid abnormality is diagnosed.

Naturally the diagnosis may be difficult. When there are clinical symptoms of a specifically diabetic character – thirst with polyuria – and the blood glucose is persistently above 11.1 mmol/l (200 mg/dl) it is certain that permanent diabetes is present that will not be abolished by treating the thyrotoxicosis. When the only abnormality is an abnormal glucose tolerance test it is probable but not certain that normal tolerance will be restored when thyroid function becomes normal. In my experience most cases of glycosuria discovered at the time that thyrotoxicosis is diagnosed have diabetes that persists after the patient has been rendered euthyroid.

Thyrotoxicosis may arise in a patient with known diabetes and there is nothing to suggest that the incidence is more or less than in a non-diabetic population. In a known diabetic the diagnosis may be suspected from minor changes in appearance or behaviour (such as an unusual intolerance to being kept waiting), from weight loss unexplained by the control of the diabetes, or from other toxic symptoms. As in the non-diabetic population in elderly patients atrial fibrillation may be the only manifestation.

The effects of thyrotoxicosis in aggravating diabetes may be very serious. The tendency to ketosis in those who are insulin-dependent is much increased and the onset of ketosis can be very rapid. Occasionally an elderly woman is admitted in diabetic ketosis of such severity that the presence of thyrotoxicosis is not suspected until, if she is fortunate, the diabetes has been brought under control.

MYXOEDEMA

The effect of thyroid deficiency is essentially the opposite of that of thyrotoxicosis. The rate of absorption of glucose is decreased and the glucose tolerance curve tends to be flat, the 2-hour figure sometimes lying just above the accepted upper limit of normal. The effect of hypothyroidism is to make diabetes somewhat easier to control and to lessen the need for insulin, though not greatly. Hypoglycaemia in myxoedematous patients seems to change its character with the loss of some of the warning symptoms in accord with the relationship between thyroid hormones and adrenal medullary function.

THYROID DISEASE AND DIABETIC CONTROL

There is dispute about whether change in thyroid function affects diabetic control. Older physicians were dubious about a relationship although there are grounds for expecting some modification of control. There is some evidence of increased glucose recycling in thyrotoxic patients (McCulloch *et al.*, 1983) with consequent turning of calories into heat.

Despite this, thyrotoxic patients have fasting hyperinsulinaemia with the corollary of insulin resistance. An increased appetite and insulin resistance would favour an increased requirement of insulin in thyrotoxic diabetic patients offset to some extent by the change in glucose metabolism which would favour a decreased requirement. The effect of thyroid disease upon insulin clearance has received less attention but could be potentially the most important influence upon diabetic control. In practice, in the insulin-dependent patient any change tends to be to a reduction in insulin dose with myxoedema and an increase with thyrotoxicosis.

HYPERPARATHYROIDISM

It is unclear whether an association exists between hyperparathyroidism and diabetes mellitus. Walsh, Soler and Malins (1975) reported eight patients with both disorders attending our clinic and drew attention to the similarity in symptoms between the two diseases. Not only are thirst and polyuria common to both conditions; fatigue and weight loss may also be features of both. An obvious association could exist through pancreatitis, although insulin resistance has also been reported in hyperparathyroidism (Kim *et al.*, 1971).

THE ADRENAL CORTEX

The influence of the adrenal cortex on carbohydrate metabolism has been a subject of constant study since the turn of the last century. Even before insulin was discovered it was known that hypoglycaemia occurred in adrenalectomized dogs. Later it was shown that the severity of experimental pancreatic diabetes was lessened by total adrenalectomy, while at the same time the hypoglycaemic effect of insulin was enhanced.

The effects of glucocorticoids upon carbohydrate metabolism are to increase the rate of hepatic glucose production through an enhancement of gluconeogenesis. This comes about through increased substrate supply, particularly of alanine from muscle; increased activity of hepatic aminotransferases; and increased activity of gluconeogenic enzymes; while at the same time effecting an inhibition of glucose uptake in the periphery.

ADDISON'S DISEASE

In Addison's disease the blood glucose is low, particularly in the fasting state, and sensitivity to insulin is increased, though these defects do not as a rule cause any prominent symptoms. When the two diseases co-exist in the one patient the daily requirement of insulin tends to be low although replacement corticosteroids increase the dose somewhat. When diabetes precedes Addison's disease then the presentation is usually with frequent and persistent hypoglycaemia. The onset of both diseases may be simultaneous although when presented with a newly diagnosed diabetic patient with an acute history and typical Addisonian pigmentation the diagnosis is probably more likely to be an ectopic ACTH-secreting tumour.

THE ANTERIOR PITUITARY GLAND

Houssay and Biasotti (1930) first showed the importance of the anterior pituitary in experimental diabetes, when they produced by hypophysectomy a marked improvement in the diabetes which followed removal of the pancreas. Experience of hypophysectomy in diabetic patients has fully confirmed the Houssay effect in man. In spite of full substitution treatment with cortisone the need for insulin is much decreased and insulin sensitivity is greatly enhanced. Ketone formation is much reduced and ketosis rarely develops even when insulin is withheld for several days with the result that hyperglycaemia is pronounced. Administration of

human growth hormone restores the diabetes to its former state. Furthermore human growth hormone given to hypophysectomized non-diabetic subjects induces fasting hyperglycaemia and in some cases ketonuria after one or two days which ceases when growth hormone is discontinued.

HYPOPITUITARISM

This was considered a common event in the course of diabetes in older reports. Those diabetic patients who developed hypopituitarism in most instances did so acutely. The commonest causes were arteriosclerosis and parturition although in some no obvious cause could be found. Fatalities were quite common, usually within 3 months of onset of hypopituitarism, often with terminal hypoglycaemia. Insulin sensitivity may be extreme and hypoglycaemia intractable in spite of adequate restoration with glucose. Pituitary insufficiency does not prevent the development of diabetes as in the case recorded by Frey (1964). I know of at least one more patient in London, whom I had the good fortune to meet during the membership examination of the Royal College of Physicians.

Knowledge of the effects of hypopituitarism on diabetes have been greatly expanded by experience with hypophysectomy. Attempts to influence diabetes by irradiation of the pituitary were made sporadically before 1939, notably by R. T. Woodyatt of Chicago, the object being to enhance insulin sensitivity. Luft and Olivecrona (1953) began to perform hypophysectomy for advanced retinopathy and renal disease before the report of Poulsen (1953) that a diabetic patient who developed hypopituitarism experienced a great improvement in her advanced retinopathy. Subsequently this work was continued in many centres by various techniques until superseded by local treatment of retinopathy with the introduction of photocoagulation.

DIABETES INSIPIDUS AND DIABETES MELLITUS

This infrequent combination can be part of the DIDMOAD syndrome including optic atrophy and deafness. Spontaneous associations of the two types of diabetes do occur although the difficulties of recognizing pathological thirst are compounded by a previous diagnosis of diabetes mellitus. For this reason minor degrees of diabetes insipidus must be overlooked.

DIABETES AND THE SEX HORMONES

The age of menarche is considered by most writers to be normal or near normal in diabetic girls whether the disease starts before or after sexual maturity. Savage, Lee and Stewart-Brown (1986), in a small group of diabetic girls, confirmed a small delay, with menarche at a mean age of 14 years compared with 13.2 years in a control population. Menstrual function seems to be also abnormal in diabetic women, particularly at times of poor control. In a large Danish study (Kjaer *et al.*, 1992) nearly 20% of young diabetic women reported some disturbance of menstruation compared with 13% of a control group. In addition, 6.7% had periods of secondary amenorrhoea compared with 2% of controls. Amenorrhoea is the rule in untreated severe diabetes or following an attack of ketosis, when it may persist for several months. The probable mechanism is through disruption of GnRH pulsatility (Sherman *et al.*, 1991).

Diabetic control fluctuates perceptibly in some girls and women through the menstrual cycle. Insulin requirements seem to be lowest in the middle of the cycle (7–21 days) and then rise gradually to a maximum at about the time that menstruation begins.

In women, increased testosterone levels and low levels of sex-hormone-binding globulin are associated with hyperinsulinaemia and glucose intolerance, although this association is less clear in men. In men insulin sensitivity correlates with testosterone and SHBG concentrations (Haffner *et al.*, 1994).

OVULATORY SUPPRESSANTS

The reduction in dose of oestrogen in drugs used for contraception has lowered the effects upon metabolism in normal and diabetic women. High-dose oestrogen preparations had a distinct effect upon glucose tolerance, lowering fasting blood glucose but causing intolerance after a glucose load. In addition, triglycerides were increased. The newer preparations still alter glucose and fat metabolism although in a rather more subtle manner (Singh and Nattrass, 1989). Glucose disposal by peripheral tissues is impaired and ketone body levels are increased. In part these changes are a logical conclusion of those seen during the menstrual cycle. None of these effects are sufficient grounds for denying a request for oral contraceptive agents. Any effect upon diabetic control is readily offset by minor adjustments to insulin dose.

REFERENCES

Addison, T. and Gull, W. (1851) On a certain affection of the skin. Vitiligoidea, A Plana, B Tuberosa. *Guy's Hosp. Med. Rep.*, **7**, 265–276.

de Boer, S. Y., Masclee, A. A. M., Lam, W. F. *et al.* (1994) Effect of hyperglycaemia on gallbladder motility in type 1 (insulin-dependent) diabetes mellitus. *Diabetologia*, **37**, 75–81.

Bouchardat, A. (1883) *De la glycosurie ou diabete sucré; son traitement hygienique*, vol. II, Germer-Baillière, Paris.

Brunzell, J. D. and Bierman, E. L. (1982) Chylomicronemia syndrome. *Med. Clin. N. Am.*, **66**, 455–468.

Dunn, F. L. Pietri, A. and Raskin, P. (1981) Plasma lipid and lipoprotein levels with continuous subcutaneous insulin infusion in type 1 diabetes mellitus. *Ann. Intern. Med.*, **95**, 426–431.

Fantus, I. G., Janjua, N., Senni, H. and Andermann, E. (1991) Glucose intolerance in first degree relatives of patients with Friedreich's ataxia is associated with insulin resistance: evidence for a closely linked inherited trait. *Metabolism*, **40**, 788–793.

Felig, P. (1973) The glucose-alanine cycle. *Metabolism*, **22**, 179–207.

Frey, H. M. (1964) The development of diabetes mellitus during pituitary insufficiency. *Acta Med. Scand.*, **175**, 523–527.

Geffner, M. E., Lippe, B. M., Kaplan, S. A. *et al.* (1984) Carbohydrate tolerance in cystic fibrosis is closely linked to pancreatic exocrine fuction. *Ped. Res.*, **18**, 1107–1111.

Haffner, S. M., Karhappaa, P., Mykkanen, L. and Laakso, M. (1994) Insulin resistance, body fat distribution, and sex hormones in men. *Diabetes*, **43**, 212–219.

Herman, J. B., Medalie, J. H. and Goldbourt, U. (1976) Diabetes, prediabetes and uricaemia. *Diabetologia*, **12**, 47–52

Horowitz, M. and Fraser, R. (1994) Disordered gastric motor function in diabetes mellitus. *Diabetologia*, **37**, 543–551.

Houssay, B. A. and Biasotti, A. (1930) La diabetes pacreatica de los perros hipofisoprivos. *Rev. Soc. Argent. Biol.*, **6**, 251–296.

Johnston, D. G., Alberti, K. G. M. M., Faber, O. *et al.* (1977) Hyperinsulinism of hepatic cirrhosis: diminished degradation or hypersecretion. *Lancet*, **i**, 10–13.

Johnston, D. G. Postle, A. D., Barnes, A. J. *et al.* (1979) The role of cortisol in direction of substrate flow, in *Lipoprotein Metabolism and Endocrine Regulation*, (eds L. W. Hessel and H. M. J. Krans), Elsevier, Amsterdam, p. 117–134.

Khan, R. J. Andermann, E. and Fantus, I. G. (1986) Glucose intolerance in Friedreich's ataxia: association with insulin resistance and decreased insulin binding. *Metabolism*, **35**, 1017–1023.

Kim, H., Kalkhoff, R. K, Costrini, N. V. *et al.* (1971) Plasma insulin disturbances in primary hyperparathyroidism. *J. Clin. Invest*, **50**, 2596–2605.

Kjaer, K., Hagen, C., Sando, S. H. and Eshoj, O. (1992) Epidemiology of menarche and menstrual disturbances in an unselected group of women with insulin-dependent diabetes mellitus compared to controls. *J. Clin. Endocrinol. Metab.*, **75**, 524–529.

Krentz, A. J., Coles, N. H., Williams, A. C. and Nattrass, M. (1990) Abnormal regulation of intermediary metabolism after oral glucose

ingestion in myotonic dystrophy. *Metabolism*, **39**, 938–942.

Krentz, A. J., Williams, A. C. and Nattrass, M. (1991) Insulin resistance in multiple aspects of intermediary metabolism in myotonic dystrophy. *Metabolism*, **40**, 866–872.

Kruszynska, Y. T., Harry, D. S., Bergman, R. N. and McIntyre, N. (1993) Insulin sensitivity, insulin secretion, and glucose effectiveness in diabetic and non-diabetic cirrhotic patients. *Diabetologia*, **36**, 121–128.

Lamey, P. J., Darwazeh, A. M. G. and Frier, B. M. (1992) Oral disorders associated with diabetes mellitus. *Diabetic Med.*, **9**, 410–416.

Lawley, T. J., Hall, R. P., Fauci, A. S. *et al.* (1981) Defective Fc-receptor functions associated with the HLA-B8/DRw3 haplotype. *N. Engl. J. Med.*, **304**, 185–192.

Lecocq, F. R., Mebane, D. and Madison, I. L. (1964) The acute effect of hydrocortisone on hepatic glucose output and peripheral glucose utilization. *J. Clin. Invest.* **43**, 237–246.

Leiber (1985) *Ann. Surg*, **5**, 8–28.

Luft, R. and Olivecrona, H. (1953) Experiences with hypophysectomy in man. *J. Neurosurg.*, **10**, 301–316.

McCulloch, A. J., Nosadini, R., Pernet, A. *et al.* (1983) Glucose turnover and indices of recycling in thyrotoxicosis and primary thyroid failure. *Clin. Sci.*, **64**, 41–47.

Marble, A., White, P., Bogan, I. K. and Smith, R. M. (1938) Enlargement of the liver in diabetic children. *Arch. Intern. Med.*, **62**, 740–750.

Marten, R. H. and Dulake, M. (1957) Hydrocortisone in necrobiosis lipoidica diabeticorum. *Br. J. Dermatol.*, **69**, 395–399.

Mohan, V., Snehalatha, C., Jayashree, R. *et al.* (1984) Serum uric acid concentrations in offspring of conjugal diabetic parents. *Metabolism*, **33**, 869–871.

Molenaar, D. M., Palumbo, P. J., Wilson, W. R. and Ritts, R. E. (1976) Leukocyte chemotaxis in diabetic patients and their non diabetic first degree relatives. *Diabetes*, 25(suppl. 2), 880–883.

Moran, A., Pyzdrowski, K. L., Weinreb, J. *et al.* (1994) Insulin sensitivity in cystic fibrosis. *Diabetes*, **43**, 1020–1026.

Neilly, J. B., Martin, A., Simpson, N. and MacCuish, A. G. (1986) Pruritus in diabetes mellitus: investigation of prevalence and correlation with diabetes control. *Diabetes Care*, **9**, 273–275.

Pfeifer, M. A., Brunzell, J. D., Best, J. D. *et al.*

(1983) The response of plasma triglyceride, cholesterol and lipoprotein lipase to treatment in non-insulin-dependent diabetic subjects without familial hypertriglyceridemia. *Diabetes*, **32**, 525–531.

Pietri, A., Dunn, F. L. and Raskin, P. (1980) The effect of improved diabetic control on plasma lipid and lipoprotein levels. A comparison of conventional therapy and continuous subcutaneous insulin infusion. *Diabetes*, **29**, 1001–1005.

Poulsen, J. E. (1953) The Houssay phenomenon in man: recovery from diabetic retinopathy in a case of diabetes with Simmonds' disease. *Diabetes*, **2**, 7–12.

Robertson, H. D. and Polk, H. C. (1974) The mechanism of infection in patients with diabetes mellitus: a review of leukocyte malfunction. *Surgery*, **75**, 123–128.

Rosenbloom, A. L., Silverstein, J. H., Lezotte, D. C. *et al.* (1981) Limited joint mobility in childhood diabetes mellitus indicates increased risk for microvascular disease. *N. Eng. J. Med.*, **305**, 191–194.

Savage, D. C. L., Lee, T. U. and Stewart-Brown, S. L. (1986) Growth in children with diabetes, in *Recent Advances in Diabetes 2*, (ed. M. Nattrass), Churchill Livingstone, Edinburgh, p. 119–125.

Sherman, L. D., Rogers, D. G., Gabbay, K. H. *et al.* (1991) Pulsatility of luteinising hormone during puberty is dependent on recent glycaemic control. *Adolesc. Pediatr. Gynecol.*, **4**, 87.

Singh, B. M. and Nattrass, M. (1989) Use of combined oral contraceptive preparations alters the insulin sensitivity of fatty acid and ketone metabolism. *Clin. Endocrinol.*, **30**, 561–570.

Soler, N. G. and Khardori, R. (1985) Liver enzyme abnormalities after insulin-induced hypoglycaemic coma. *Br. Med. J.*, **291**, 1541.

Stokes, P. L., Asquith, P., Holmes, G. K. T. *et al.* (1972) Histocompatibility antigens associated with adult coeliac disease. *Lancet*, **ii**, 162–164.

Stone, B. G., Gavaler, J. S. Belle, S. H. *et al.* (1988) Impairment of gallbladder emptying in diabetes mellitus. *Gastroenterology*, **95**, 170–176.

Toonstra, J. (1985) Bullosis diabeticorum. Report of a case with a review of the literature. *J. Am. Acad. Dermatol.*, **13**, 799–805.

Unger, R. H. and Orci, I. (1975) The essential role of glucagon in the pathogenesis of diabetes mellitus. *Lancet*, **i**, 14–16.

Urbach, E. (1932) Beitrage zu einer physiologischen und pathologischen Chemie der Haut; eine neue diabetische Stoffwechseldermatose: Nekrobiosis lipoidica diabeticorum. *Arch. Dermatol. Syph.*, **166**, 273–285.

Walsh, O. H., Soler, N. G. and Malins, J. M. (1975) Diabetes mellitus and primary hyperparathyroidism. *Postgrad. Med. J.*, **51**, 446–449.

Walsh, C. H., Cooper, B. T., Wright, A. D. *et al.* (1978) Diabetes mellitus and coeliac disease: a clinical study. *Q. J. Med.*, **47**, 89–100.

Weinstein, S. P., O'Boyle, E. and Haber, R. S. (1994) Thyroid hormone increases basal and insulin-stimulated glucose transport in skeletal muscle. *Diabetes*, **43**, 1185–1189.

Wilson, R. M. and Reeves, W. G. (1986) Neutrophil function in diabetes, in *Recent Advances in Diabetes 2*, (ed. M. Nattrass), Churchill Livingstone, Edinburgh, p. 127–138.

Wise, J. K., Hendler, R. and Felig, P. (1973) Influence of glucocorticoids on glucagon secretion and plasma amino acid concentrations in man. *J. Clin. Invest.* **52**, 2774–2782.

As if the disease of diabetes mellitus was insufficient in itself, defining a life that is regulated and exacting a price in long-term complications, the diabetic patient must face difficulties in everyday life which to most of us give no cause for concern. Employment, marriage, sport and life insurance are contracts or activities that can be entered into by most people without a second thought but for which the diabetic patient finds obstacles being thrust in the way. This chapter deals with a miscellany of hurdles the diabetic patient faces as s/he attempts to follow the doctor's exhortation to live a normal life.

EMPLOYMENT

There is no good evidence that the working capacity of the diabetic population is different from that of non-diabetics. Where attempts have been made to study the potential problem results have been conflicting. Absences attributable to poorly controlled diabetes in a small irresponsible group are probably balanced by the determination to remain at work of a larger number who are aware that their jobs are vulnerable once it is known that they have diabetes.

Pell and D'Alonzo (1967) reported an absence from work due to infectious illness in 662 diabetic workers. Absence of 10 days or more was recorded in 28% of the workers with diabetes compared with 15% controls. This difference was not statistically significant. Robinson *et al.* (1990), in a survey of eight clinics in the UK, found that the proportion of diabetic employees who reported any time off work through illness in the preceding twelve months was 49%, not

significantly different from the 45% in the control group. When the data were analysed in relation to number of days off work, however, 16% of control workers and 29% of the diabetic employees had lost more than 20 days in the past year, which was a significant difference. Similar findings were reported by Waclawski (1990) and further confirmation was given by a 5-year study of postal workers in the UK (Welch, 1986). Compared with controls diabetic employees had nearly twice as many days off work but this excess appeared to be concentrated in just a few of the diabetic workers.

The attitude of employers was studied in the USA by Beardwood (1957) who found that 69% of the companies who answered his questionnaire did employ known diabetics and 25% did not. No reason for either policy was apparent but on the whole the attitude of large concerns was more enlightened than that of the small companies. There are few studies of the situation in Britain but it is probably similar to that in the USA. In the English Midlands 1945–1965 there was a steady demand for labour and a person of reasonable ability was unlikely to be seriously handicapped by having diabetes. In the less good times that have followed with the decline in heavy industry and manufacturing, the position might be different, although even with the contraction of Britain's industry in the late 1980s I did not hear of undue penalties being placed upon the diabetic seeking work. Nevertheless, some discrimination was reported by the patients of Robinson *et al.* (1990) when 13% of diabetic patients reported difficulties in obtaining employment because of their diabetes while only 2% of the control group reported difficulties because of illness. Although this was a highly significant finding it must be born in mind that only one side of the argument is being heard. In reality, only the employer knows the full reason for not offering a candidate a job. A rejected candidate might be in need of a reason for their non-appointment and their diabetes is conveniently to hand. When only young type 1 diabetic patients were considered employment experiences, and indeed educational achievements, were similar to a matched control group (Lloyd, Robinson and Fuller, 1992).

Obviously, decisions about the suitability of a job are individual, depending upon the severity of the diabetes and the personality of the patient, but there are some general rules. A patient controlled by diet only need not be handicapped in any way. It is necessary to emphasize this, for some employers will remove a man from a responsible position simply on the grounds that he has diabetes. The majority of those who are treated by oral preparations are similarly free from restriction.

A diabetic on insulin, however, must accept some limitations. The general rule to follow is that he or she should not be in a position of work where a sudden disabling attack of hypoglycaemia will place the life of the patient, or the lives of others around him/her, at risk of serious injury or death. Leaving aside driving, which is dealt with below, it becomes clear that certain occupations cannot accept this limitation and therefore cannot employ patients taking insulin. Airline pilots, although they do not seem to fly the plane manually for any great length of time, would not benefit from even mild hypoglycaemia on take-off or final approach. Nor would one want that final approach guided by an air traffic controller at risk of hypoglycaemia. At lesser heights, working on scaffolding or ladders is not appropriate and this should be made clear to the patient. Unfortunately,

while the airline industry is tightly regulated – perhaps too tightly, for I cannot see a sensible objection to a well controlled insulin-taking cabin attendant – self-employed builders abound and the medical staff can only indicate, albeit strongly, the inadvisability of working at heights. Short of going to work with the builder or the decorator we cannot ensure that no ladder is climbed. Working with heavy machinery is less of an obstacle now than in years gone by. Most machinery, other than the potentially lethal motor vehicle, is guarded and is consequently less of a threat. Nevertheless only the company and the patient can make the final judgement on risk.

Some other jobs are generally unsuitable but not necessarily so in a particular individual, and it may be better to leave a man doing work in which he is experienced rather than to add the problem of learning a new trade to the difficulties of diet and insulin. Work with a variable energy output such as farm labouring may cause difficulties because of the need to adjust carbohydrate intake in order to avoid hypoglycaemia.

Shift-work with a change every one or two weeks can present a problem. Firms are understandably reluctant to take men off shift-work on medical grounds. In addition, the work is often well paid and many patients are unwilling to be thought different from their workmates, so that it is worth making some effort to overcome the difficulty of frequent alteration from day to night work and back. Even within our own profession shift-work may be used as the underlying reason for schools of nursing rejecting a diabetic applicant, although I have not heard of medical schools invoking this excuse. In doing so they run contrary to the evidence, which is that nearly 90% of diabetic shift-workers perform to the same or a higher level than their non-diabetic counterparts with regard to reliability and absenteeism (Moore and Buschbom, 1974).

Public service is a most difficult area. Those who work in the police force or for the fire brigade are often wholly dedicated to their line of service. Those applying to join have often wanted such a career since childhood. Both groups are devastated by rejection by the service because of their need for insulin. Nevertheless this approach must surely be correct: the policeman on crowd control cannot be at risk of hypoglycaemia; nor can the departure of the fire engine await the diabetic fireman who is about to consume a meal.

Perhaps the ideal for an insulin-taking patient is work with regular hours and constant energy output, and many office posts fulfil these criteria. All the same, many of our patients are employed in heavy industry, including foundry work and coal-mining, and are not obviously handicapped.

We regard it as a duty to press the claims of our 'good' patients to be considered on an equal footing with the non-diabetic. Generally speaking, we would advise a patient to find employment with one of the very large companies. In our experience their attitude is sympathetic, they offer a wide range of jobs and their medical service is extremely helpful when difficulties arise.

The problem of establishment in a salaried service with superannuation is not easy. A number of company medical officers have the dual responsibility of advising on the medical record of applicants for jobs and assessing claims for a disability pension. In this situation the Chief Medical Officer will not deliberately lay problems for himself or his successor in 10 to 20 years time and will therefore think long and hard before accepting a diabetic applicant for a post. The age at diagnosis of diabetes is the most important single factor and we have to recognize, in fairness to the employers, that the chance of a diabetic diagnosed before the age of 15 giving continuous service to the age of retirement is very slender indeed.

DRIVING

Strict regulations on driving by diabetics are in place in the UK, enforced by the Driver and Vehicle Licensing Authority (DVLA). Minor changes occur from time to time and periodically the situation is updated in a new version of *Medical Aspects of Fitness to Drive*, published by Her Majesty's Stationery Office.

In general terms the Authority recognizes the division into driving for a living and driving for pleasure. For the majority of diabetic patients treated by diet, tablets or insulin wishing to use a private car for pleasure or as a means of getting to and from work there will be no problem with obtaining a driving licence. One thing the regulatory authority cannot do, and is not intended to do, is police the number of miles driven. Thus a licence gives authority to drive 2000 miles per year on weekend outings purely for pleasure or 30 000 miles per year where travel is a means of performing a job. Some advice on the latter case may fall to the doctor and patients on insulin should be discouraged from employment with such a heavy driving commitment. It nearly always means irregular meals, overnight stays where any concept of diet does not exist, or driving that extra 100 miles to get home when it is getting towards meal times.

The licensing authority has the power to suspend or revoke a licence and it will occasionally do that. I have always found a reluctance on the part of the Authority to take this step unless they are of the opinion that continued driving may be hazardous to the public. Particular times in the life of the diabetic that cause the Authority anxiety are: beginning insulin treatment; loss of warning of hypoglycaemia; and when hypoglycaemia is a contributory factor to an accident. The Authority will also be concerned in any diabetic patient if long-term complications have progressed to such an extent that they may interfere with driving. Extensive diabetic neuropathy with loss of sensation in the feet is one example, while retinopathy and/or treatment of retinopathy that diminishes visual acuity, night vision or field is another. The presence of ischaemic heart disease is governed by a further set of regulations.

If all this sounds rather complicated for the doctor giving advice it is not – the position is clearly laid out in the publication although the number of amendments often means that the slim volume doubles in size before a new edition. Considering the amount of useless information sent to doctors it is surprising that such an important and useful document is not automatically sent to every doctor but to date it remains the doctor's task to seek it out.

The basic rules for car driving are: the driver must notify the Authority of his/her diabetes; a licence will normally be issued for up to 3 years, at which time it will be reviewed. If, at review, the questionnaire sent to the patient causes concern to the Authority, they will seek a medical report or less often a medical examination. It should be stressed that the decision as to whether a diabetic can hold a licence is not that of the doctor but lies with the Authority. The doctor does, however, have the responsibility for ensuring that the regulations are complied with and that the patient knows the importance of hypoglycaemia. Despite regular advice on carrying carbohydrate in the car it is surprising how many patients omit to do so. The occurrence of hypoglycaemia is the major worry for the diabetic driver, the public at large and the licensing Authority. Cox, Gonder-Frederick and Clarke (1993), in a rather neat study using a driving simulator, observed virtually no impairment of the ability to drive with mild hypoglycaemia of around 3.6 mmol/l (65 mg/dl). Moderate hypoglycaemia of a blood glucose around 2.6 mmol/l (47 mg/dl), however, affected steering, resulting in significantly more swerving, spinning, time over the midline and time off the road. Interestingly, there was also an element of compensation, with more slow driving.

The extent to which the occurrence of hypoglycaemic attacks contributes to road traffic accidents is debatable. Stevens *et al.* (1989) in over 300 diabetic patients found no increase in crashes per million miles compared to control subjects. In contrast, Hansotia and Broste (1991) found an increased standardized crash ratio when more than 700 diabetic drivers were compared with nearly 30 000 control subjects.

Driving for a living, vocational driving, presents a stricter set of regulations. For lorries classed as heavy goods vehicles or buses classed as public service vehicles these are set out by the Licensing Authority. The situation is different for taxi drivers, where licences are granted locally. Diagnosed diabetics, even if treated by diet or tablets, should be advised against seeking employment that requires a vocational licence. The tendency for diabetes to progress to insulin treatment can result in a difficult clinical situation when instigation of insulin treatment may mean the loss of a licence and hence a job. My own view is that doctors should avoid conspiring with patients to maintain them on tablets despite poor diabetic control simply because transfer to insulin would jeopardize their employment. The image of a poorly controlled diabetic lorry driver speeding down a motorway towards me, possibly with impaired lower limb sensation and almost certainly with some blurring of vision, is not one that I lightly entertain. There is a natural reluctance of the Authority to grant a vocational licence to a driver who is on insulin. This reluctance is being translated into firm action as directives from the European Community are absorbed into local practice. The likelihood of any diabetic on insulin being allowed a vocational licence in the future is very small.

Although private hire and taxi licences are agreed locally they too are likely to change in response to European Community directives. In the meantime we have agreed a local policy with the authority through discussions which were helpful to both sides. We do not encourage diabetic patients to take up such employment but patients diagnosed and on diet or tablets may continue to hold a licence. Transfer to insulin treatment means temporary suspension of the licence (3 months and subject to a medical report). Hypoglycaemic coma while driving results in permanent loss of licence. These agreed conditions have worked well but will probably fall short of EC directives. If the latter lead to improved taxi-driving standards in some foreign capitals, I for one will welcome them!

MARRIAGE

Diabetic patients who contemplate marriage are sometimes concerned of the risk of diabetes in any offspring. This is particularly true when both partners are diabetic at marriage although this situation is comparatively uncommon. Other less well voiced fears are the difficulties of pregnancy for the woman and the likelihood of impotence in the man. Patients can be readily reassured on the first two points and contemplated marriage is hardly the time to discuss impotence unless the question is directly asked.

At this stage in the life of the diabetic it is usually the worry of insulin-dependent diabetes that is of concern. The parent or parents may be given a healthy dose of reassurance. The prevalence of diabetes at the age of 25 when both parents are diabetic is 3.4%, of which 2.4% is insulin-dependent diabetes. When the mother is diabetic and the father not the prevalence is 2.4%, and 1.5% is insulin-dependent (Kobberling and Bruggeboes, 1980).

It should be appreciated that these figures may vary enormously in different ethnic groups.

EXERCISE

With increasing emphasis on regular exercise as part of a plan for 'healthy living' diabetic patients will not want to be left out. Indeed it would be argued that regular exercise with its effect upon metabolism and cardiovascular physiology has more to offer the diabetic individual than the non-diabetic. The majority will exercise for recreational purposes only although the few diabetic athletes who have made it to the very top of their sport serve as a tremendous inspiration to children and adolescents with diabetes.

For any sort of exercise muscle requires a supply of fuel. Glucose and non-esterified fatty acids are the main energy supply for working muscle. Initially muscle glycogen is the source of glucose but these limited supplies are soon exhausted and further energy must be blood-borne. In normal people glucose utilization by muscle is matched by increased hepatic glucose output into the circulation. Insulin plays a major role in regulating glucose output although other factors, particularly catecholamines also contribute. In prolonged exercise there is greater dependence upon non-esterified fatty acids as an energy source which must be released by fat cells. Insulin and catecholamines again dominate the regulation of lipolysis.

Exercise in the insulin-dependent diabetic patient must be considered in the light of this information from normal humans but bearing in mind that changes in blood glucose concentration in response to exercise will not influence the amount of circulating insulin. If too little insulin is present at the start of exercise hepatic glucose output will be allowed to rise in an unrestrained manner leading to hyperglycaemia (Zinman *et al.*, 1977). If too much insulin is circulating, hepatic glucose output will be reduced, leading to a fall in blood glucose concentration and, if exercise is maintained, hypoglycaemia (Zinman *et al.*, 1977). Thus in poorly controlled insulin-dependent patients exercise tends to worsen metabolic control while in those well controlled the tendency is to improve control further, reducing insulin requirements.

Exercise influences absorption of insulin from subcutaneous injection sites. Depending upon the type of insulin and the length of time between taking insulin and commencing exercise an increased circulating insulin concentration can be shown (Berger *et al.*, 1982). This finding is true for all sites of insulin injection and not simply a feature attributable to exercising limbs. Altering the site of injection will not therefore contribute to metabolic homoeostasis during exercise.

To avoid hypoglycaemia during exercise either blood supply of glucose to muscle must be increased by intake of oral carbohydrate or the normal, non-exercising, dose of insulin must be reduced. While these concepts are simple the practical application of them is difficult because of a lack of quantitation – how much extra carbohydrate should be taken, or by how much should insulin dose be reduced? I recall feeling foolish when talking to a young woman who had been a very good junior athlete. At some point in her education she had received the usual advice to have a chocolate bar before a race. Only some years later did I realize in talking to her that in a weekend she would run four 100 metre and four 200 metre races – she was good enough to get to the final of both events. I wonder what her fellow competitors felt as they watched this trained athlete guzzle eight chocolate bars on race days!

Reducing insulin dose to allow exercise would be a more logical approach but is clear that nearly everyone underestimates the magnitude of the reduction in dose needed. Dropping the dose by a couple of units will have little effect upon outcome; Kemmer and Berger (1984) showed that the dose should be reduced by 60% to ensure hypoglycaemia-free exercise.

Despite the theoretical difficulties of imitating normal exercise physiology many insulin dependent diabetics do exercise regularly, some to the highest level. Blood glucose monitoring helps considerably in the athlete's assessment of control during exercise. Patients with non-insulin-dependent diabetes may also want to exercise but here the problems encountered are not of metabolic control but the danger of co-existing cardiovascular disease.

SURGERY AND DIABETES

Diabetics are not immune from any surgical disease of the non-diabetic. They should have a better chance of early diagnosis of chronic disease because they are normally seen by a doctor at least once a year and have the opportunity to mention symptoms – even those which they may consider trivial. Unfortunately neither blood nor urine testing for glucose is a routine at all surgical clinics or with all surgeons. Though nearly every patient is tested immediately before operation a positive finding at that time may involve hurried and imperfect treatment of the diabetes in an acute situation.

The commonest error from failure to test the urine is in relation to boils and carbuncles which may recur for many months without any other diabetic symptom.

Balanitis is a common presentation in middle age and may lead to circumcision being advised and even performed unnecessarily.

Carcinoma of the pancreas often presents to the physician with loss of weight and glycosuria and to the surgeon as a vague abdominal disorder. The diabetes is usually slight but the finding of diabetes with loss of weight out of proportion to its severity should arouse suspicion of pancreatic disease.

The autonomic manifestation of neuropathy in the gastrointestinal tract may suggest malignant disease and need careful evaluation. Anorexia, abdominal discomfort, constipation or diarrhoea are associated with delayed gastric emptying and abnormal motility, increased or diminished, of the intestine. Occasionally, a picture suggestive of high intestinal obstruction with repeated vomiting and mild abdominal distension may be deceptive. Laparotomy is entirely negative.

Particularly important is the abdominal pain and rigidity of ketosis which may be so striking that the possibility of peritonitis is seriously entertained even though the ketosis is recognized. The pain is commonly upper abdominal but may be mainly felt in any quadrant and may radiate to the back. Rigidity is usually generalized.

Of course the greatest problem is the true acute abdominal lesion – appendicitis or perforated peptic ulcer – accompanied by ketosis. The best guide is the history. In diabetic ketosis vomiting will have preceded the pain by several hours, the reverse of the sequence in most abdominal emergencies. White cell counts are not helpful as a leucocytosis of 20 000 or more occurs in ketosis.

EFFECT OF SURGERY ON DIABETES

Stress aggravates diabetes. Not the emotional stress of anticipating an operation but the inbuilt biochemical response to a major illness and/or to the traumatic stress of acute or elective surgery. Haemorrhage and shock raise the blood glucose, through increased secretion of the 'stress' hormones, catecholamines, glucagon, cortisol and growth hormone. When this can be counteracted by an increase in insulin secretion as in normal subjects the end result may not be clinically significant. Where the counteraction of the catabolic response will be inadequate, and this can be predicted in all but the mildest of diabetes, it is as well to assume that the diabetes will deteriorate during the period of operation and insulin should be used.

Healing of wounds seems to proceed normally in diabetics whose control is adequate and who have no obvious arterial disease in the affected area. Diffuse changes in the small vessels are said to occur in the skin even of patients without complications. If they are significant at all they do not seem to interfere with the processes of repair. All

the same, surgeons should be aware of the excessive arterial disease and possible nephropathy in long-standing diabetes.

ANAESTHESIA

In practice any anaesthetic which avoids anoxia can be used with confidence. At his preoperative visit to the patient the anaesthetist should be given a clear statement of the history and treatment of the diabetes. Like the surgeon he should be aware of the possibility of vascular and renal disease. The autonomic effects of neuropathy such as delayed gastric emptying and loss of circulatory reflexes may be relevant. Hypoglycaemia during anaesthesia may be unrecognized and show itself only by unexplained tachycardia.

MANAGEMENT OF THE DIABETES

Patients with diabetes well controlled by diet alone may be submitted to planned minor operations without special precautions. The ease with which blood glucose estimation can be performed makes it sensible to measure blood glucose, as a minimum, preoperatively and on return from the operating theatre.

Those on oral agents and under good control should have their tablets up to and including the day before surgery, omitting them only on the day of operation. This view should be modified if a long-acting sulphonylurea is normal treatment. Chlorpropamide and glibenclamide may need to be omitted for 2 days before surgery, or a short-acting drug may be given instead for the days leading up to the event.

If there is any doubt about likely control over surgery, or if the operation is major and lengthy, or if recovery, particularly to the stage of being able to take carbohydrate orally, is likely to be slow then insulin should be used. In this situation and with all insulin-dependent patients, except those undergoing the most minor operations, a simple regimen using intravenous insulin infusion is safest.

This should be started preoperatively, giving 1–2 units per hour with an intravenous infusion of glucose. The precise rate of infusion of glucose takes into account the clinical state of the patient and how much fluid is to be infused in each 24 hours; and of what composition. Adjustments to the rate of infusion are based on regular blood glucose monitoring. A minimum of 10 g glucose per hour is likely to be necessary.

One freedom of this regimen as opposed to older regimens based on intermittent insulin with glucose boluses is that diabetic patients need no longer be first on the operating list. Indeed there is something to be said for putting them later on the list, thus giving the immediate couple of hours preoperatively for regulating the infusions to achieve normoglycaemia. Our own practice is to err on the side of caution and use this simple regimen when there is any doubt about control over surgery. Problems rise all too quickly if diabetes is handled in a carefree manner. These may be grave, such as ketoacidosis or hypoglycaemia during surgery, but are often more tiresome in their solution than grave.

MORTALITY AND LIFE INSURANCE

At present methods for calculating mortality rates for diabetes are severely flawed. Three main approaches have been used and all depend upon a thoroughness of follow-up that is rarely achieved.

The first method which has been used is the follow-up of patients attending a diabetic clinic. Most diabetologists, however, have no idea of the probable bias introduced into such studies by selective referral to the clinic. It is estimated that in the UK 50% of diabetics are not under the care of the local diabetic clinic and clearly a proportion of these will never have presented themselves for enrolment into a cohort study. Instinctively one feels that when diabetes is perceived as mild, for example diagnosed on a mildly abnormal glucose tolerance test and responsive to

dietary treatment, such patients are less likely to be referred whereas the insulin-dependent diabetic will probably have contact with the clinic at some time, thus making themselves available for study. At the other end of the spectrum is the clinic with a regional, national or international reputation which attracts the more difficult or complicated patient. From such a clinic Deckert, Poulsen and Larsen (1978) reported the follow-up of 289 patients diagnosed before 1933, younger than 31 years at diagnosis and followed up in 1973. The mortality rate was two to six times that of the non-diabetic population; 50% survived with diabetes for 35 years, 40% for 40 years; and of those who died one-third did so from uraemia and one-quarter from myocardial infarction.

The second approach that has been adopted is the population-based cohort study. It is difficult to estimate the reliability of the data obtained from these studies. Most have used self-reporting of diabetes, in other words the participants are simply asked whether they are known to have diabetes. Since it is well recognized that for every diabetic diagnosed there is another undiagnosed this is not entirely satisfactory. Where the alternative approach has been used, to diagnose diabetes at entry via glucose measurement or glucose tolerance test, the revision of diagnostic criteria for diabetes has confused these results.

More problems arise from the total number of diabetics in the cohort. When a disease has a prevalence of only 1–2% a huge number of subjects must be followed for the number of deaths in the small diabetic population to be a reliable estimate of the total diabetic population.

The problem is further accentuated by difficulties in ascertainment. Death itself is a pretty final concept to most people but cause of death is often somewhat arbitrary. This is especially true of sudden death, particularly in the younger age groups. Something has to be written on the death certificate in this situation and since there are few causes of sudden death myocardial infarction is a popular choice. To what degree it is a correct assessment of the cause of death is unknown. At least there is a chance of confirming this on post-mortem, which cannot be said for deaths ascribed to hypoglycaemia where there is no reliable method of confirming this as the cause of death.

Yet further problems are encountered in the identification of the deceased as having diabetes from the death certificate which is only patchy. Estimates of the success of ascertaining that the deceased was a diabetic from the death certificate vary from about one-third to three-quarters.

Despite all these limitations and drawbacks a large number of population-based mortality studies have been performed. Somewhat typical of them is the study of Kleinman *et al.* (1988), who followed a population of civilian non-institutionalized subjects which included diabetic men and women. These were people enrolled in the First National Health and Nutrition Examination Survey (NHANES 1). Enrolment of subjects aged 40–77 years took place from 1971–1975 and 7381 of the original 7886 were followed up in 1982–1984. There were 407 people with diabetes at baseline as ascertained by self-report. The design allowed some oversampling of women of childbearing age, the poor and the elderly, and the diabetics were not matched with the non-diabetics. Thus the diabetic population had a mean age 5 years older than the non-diabetic and more of the diabetics had suffered a previous heart attack. Because of the age difference age-adjusted death rates were calculated and these showed that in both diabetic men and women the rates were twice that of the non-diabetic population. Of the excess mortality 75% in men and 57% in women was accounted for by cardiovascular causes. Further refinement of these figures by adjustment for age, smoking, systolic blood pressure, cholesterol and body mass index

gave a relative risk of 2.3 for men and 2.0 for women.

Some studies have given rates broadly similar to these while others have varied considerably. In the Framingham study the 20-year cardiovascular mortality of diabetics to non-diabetics was 1.7 for men and 3.3 for women (Kannel and McGee, 1979) although it is recognized that this population contained some people labelled diabetic who would now be considered to have impaired glucose tolerance. In Tecumseh, Michigan, where 90% of the population was followed for about 18 years the age-adjusted relative risk of ischaemic heart disease was 3.0 for both men and women (Butler *et al.*, 1985); rates of 2.4 for men and 3.5 for women for mortality from ischaemic heart disease were observed in the suburban middle class retirement community of Rancho Bernado (Barrett-Connor and Wingard, 1983); and in the Chicago Heart Association Detection Project in Industry (Pan *et al.*, 1986) a population of employed whites aged 35–64 with no previous history of myocardial infarction and not on antihypertensive medication had rates of 4.7 for death from ischaemic heart disease in women and 3.8 in men.

Studies in Europe report a broadly similar spread of risk depending to a certain extent on the population studied. After 15 years of follow-up in the Paris prospective study the relative risk of death from all causes in the diabetics was 2.3 (Balkau *et al.*, 1991) while in Gothenburg the figures were 3.5 for deaths from all causes and 4.1 for death from coronary heart disease after 7 years of follow-up (Rosengren *et al.*, 1989).

The third approach adopted by the life insurance industry is to follow up diabetics applying for life insurance. Rarely does this approach qualify as truly experimental, which would necessitate acceptance of all diabetic applicants. Where some are refused life insurance their follow-up, despite being more important in expectation of life terms, is usually lost. This introduction of bias adds to that of self-selection – the make-up of the population that applies for life insurance in the first place.

Several large studies with origins in the life assurance industry or hybrids between a life assurance company and a diabetic clinic have been published. It is self-evident that all mortality studies are out of date by the time they are published yet they are the only basis for the derivation of expectation of life and mortality rates. In an actuarial investigation of data collected by the diabetic clinic at King's College Hospital in London between 1936 and 1945 Steeds (1946) calculated that there was a higher mortality in the 21–40 age group, but a longer life expectation in those aged 41–80.

Two large studies have been performed by insurance companies in America. The Lincoln National Life Insurance Company (Cochran, 1968) covered a large number of insured diabetics between 1946 and 1966 while the Equitable Life Assurance Society of the United States (Goodkin *et al.*, 1974) examined those who applied for life insurance between 1951 and 1970. More than 10 000 diabetic lives were followed up in 1971 and strenuous efforts were made to follow up the patients who were declined life insurance. Although 94% were traced it is notable that the population differed from the general diabetic population in that 89% were male and 41% were under the age of 40.

My predecessors in Birmingham, initially John Malins and later Michael FitzGerald, were involved in an actuarial investigation beginning in 1945 in conjunction with the Wesleyan and General Assurance Company and the Britannic Assurance Company, two large insurance companies with their head offices in Birmingham. In the first study covering the years 1945–1959 all patients diagnosed as having diabetes and who attended the diabetic clinic of the General Hospital, Birmingham more than once were followed up. Non-caucasoid lives were excluded from the investigation. The timing

Table 20.1 Ratio of actual to expected mortality (%) for diabetic men and women by age (*n* = 2278 males and 3727 females); patients entered the study between 1 January 1945 and 31 December 1959 and were followed up to 31 December 1959; expected mortality was obtained from the Registrar General's figures for the West Midlands of England given in the 1951 Census

Attained age (years)	Total years of exposure	Actual deaths	Expected deaths	Mortality ratio (%)
Females				
< 40	2289	17	2.8	601
40–49	1782	13	6.9	190
50–59	5110	109	43.0	254
60–69	7054	294	155.4	189
70+	4813	479	334.3	143
Males				
< 40	2890	10	4.7	213
40–49	1816	21	9.6	219
50–59	2598	59	41.3	143
60–69	2717	139	109.5	127
70+	1652	209	167.9	125

of the beginning of the investigation was important – it corresponded approximately with the end of the Second World War, antibiotics were available and the 1951 census provided the data for the control population. The first results were of patients at 31 December 1959 and the status of patients was traced in 98.8% (Hayward and Lucena, 1965).

It is apparent that diabetics suffer heavier mortality than the general population at all ages (Table 20.1), women fare worse than men and the heaviest excess mortality was in the young patients, although the figures in the young groups are very sensitive to small variations in the number of actual deaths.

These patients were again followed up in 1964 (Shaw, 1974) confirming the extra mortality, particularly in female diabetics. There was also a definite tendency for mortality to increase with duration and, as expected, the actual causes of death showed that the principal risk was death from disease of the circulatory system.

Table 20.2 Ratio of actual to expected mortality (%) for diabetic men and women by age (*n* = 1943 males and 2290 females); patients entered the study between 1 January 1960 and 31 December 1967 and were followed up to 31 December 1975; expected mortality was obtained from the *English Life Tables No. 13*, which represents the mortality rates in England and Wales in 1970–1972

Attained age (years)	Total years of exposure	Actual deaths	Expected deaths	Mortality ratio (%)
Females				
< 40	1951	2	1.2	
40–49	1562	9	4.5	200
50–59	3511	74	24.7	300
60–69	6060	204	102.1	200
70+	6653	576	399.8	144
Males				
< 40	2292	10	2.8	357
40–49	2271	16	10.0	160
50–59	4566	81	59.4	136
60–69	5563	232	183.5	126
70+	2809	314	260.6	121

A second investigation began in 1960 and enrolled patients through to 1967. Table 20.2 shows the mortality by attained age in 2290 female patients and 1943 male patients at 31 December 1975. The results confirmed the earlier study, showing a high excess mortality, particularly at younger ages and in females. On this occasion however, there was a high excess mortality in young males rather than young females as shown pre-

viously. These data were analysed further and are shown in Tables 20.3–20.7.

In all the studies duration since diagnosis, although not independent of age, was suggested as influencing mortality ratios. This was apparently confirmed (Table 20.3), although it is clear that the excess mortality is lighter in the early years after diagnosis. The suggestion that after 5 years mortality has reached its maximum can be found in the figures and indeed if the first 2 years from diagnosis are excluded there is no significant difference between mortalities at different durations.

Analysis of the cohort by treatment was also attempted, although the interpretation is fraught with difficulty. Table 20.4 is an analysis by initial therapy.

The suggestion that diabetics treated only by diet have a lighter excess mortality than the orally- or insulin-treated patients; and particularly that those males on diet have no excess mortality, has to be interpreted in the light of the diagnostic criteria for diabetes in place at that time. Undoubtedly the diet group contains some lives who would now be considered non-diabetic. Analysis by therapy at the end of the follow-up period does not alter these results materially. The main change is for females on insulin (up to 207%) and males on diet (down to 82%).

One of the most interesting features is analysis by cause of death. Death was ascer-

Table 20.3 Ratio of actual to expected mortality (%) for diabetic men and women analysed by age and duration – other details as for Table 20.2

Duration since diagnosis (years)	All ages A	E	A/E	< 60 years A	E	A/E	> 70 years A	E	A/E
Females									
0–4	259	204.8	126	33	16.9	195	164	139.4	118
5–9	419	226.9	185	39	11.4	342	277	175.3	158
10–15	186	102.2	182	13	3.4	382	133	84.1	158
Males									
0–4	193	202.2	95	39	36.3	107	98	101.5	86
5–9	325	214.2	152	51	26.3	194	157	110.2	143
10–15	135	99.8	135	17	9.5	179	70	56.2	125

Table 20.4 Ratio of actual to expected mortality (%) for diabetic men and women analysed by initial therapy – other details as for Table 20.2

	Actual deaths	Expected deaths	Mortality ratio (%)
Females			
Diet	178	136	131
Oral agents	556	325	171
Insulin	107	57.5	186
Males			
Diet	137	146	94
Oral agents	413	306	135
Insulin	82	56	147

tained from death certificates and is therefore prone to error yet it remains the current method for collection of national statistics. In many categories the number of deaths was too small to permit reliable analysis but the analysis shows clearly the expected excess from circulatory disease and no excess from cancer (Table 20.5). Interestingly the mortality ratio is lower for cancer and respiratory disease in males and this was analysed separately (Table 20.6). The decrease for cancer is entirely attributable to a reduction in lung cancer.

Circulatory diseases, as has been shown repeatedly, are the major reasons for the excess mortality in diabetics, with ischaemic heart disease the major cause of death (Table 20.7).

The insurance companies draw on data similar to these in assessing the life risk for diabetic applicants (Goldstone, 1992). In general terms those classed as insulin-dependent diabetics must expect some loading such that they will pay increased premiums compared with their non-diabetic counterparts. The amount depends, of course, upon the type and term of the policy, and there is some individual variation among companies, but it will be heaviest at the younger ages. Paradoxically, although the loading may well be heaviest at a younger age, this can have less effect upon premiums. This situation arises from the fact that if the mortality rate at the age of 30 in the diabetic population is twice

Table 20.5 Ratio of actual to expected mortality (%) for diabetic men and women analysed by cause of death – other details as for Table 20.2

Disease category	Actual deaths	Expected deaths	Mortality ratio (%)
Female			
Infective	4	1.7	
Cancers	99	102.3	97
Diabetes	27	6.7	403
Nervous system	2	4.2	
Circulatory disease	583	296.1	197
Respiratory disease	74	74.5	99
Digestive disease	20	13.6	147
Genito-urinary	13	6.0	
Accidents	7	13.2	
Suicide	2	1.8	
Others	7	12.9	
Males			
Infective	1	3.0	
Cancers	96	129.3	74
Diabetes	19	3.5	543
Nervous system	6	4.2	
Circulatory disease	418	265.3	158
Respiratory disease	57	101.0	56
Digestive disease	15	12.8	117
Genito-urinary	9	7.1	
Accidents	8	8.8	
Suicide	3	2.2	
Others	2	5.7	

Table 20.6 Ratio of actual to expected mortality (%) for diabetic men and women for deaths from cancer and lung disease – other details as for Table 20.2

	Actual deaths	Expected deaths	Mortality ratio (%)
Female			
Lung cancer	6	9.7	
Other cancers	93	92.6	100
Pneumonia	66	50.3	131
Bronchitis	4	7.8	22
Others	4	7.2	
Males			
Lung cancer	27	55.9	48
Other cancers	69	73.4	94
Pneumonia	48	39.2	122
Bronchitis	8	50.4	16
Others	1	8.8	

Table 20.7 Ratio of actual to expected mortality (%) for diabetic men and women for deaths from circulatory diseases – other details as for Table 20.2

	Actual deaths	Expected deaths	Mortality ratio (%)
Female			
Chronic rheumatic heart disease	6	9.6	
Hypertensive disease	21	12.5	168
Ischaemic heart disease	319	118.1	270
Other heart disease	27	31.3	86
Cerebrovascular disease	179	102.1	175
Other circulatory disease	31	23.1	134
Male			
Chronic rheumatic heart disease	3	4.6	
Hypertensive disease	14	10.9	128
Ischaemic heart disease	247	150.5	164
Other heart disease	24	18.0	133
Cerebrovascular disease	98	62.1	158
Other circulatory disease	31	17.4	178

the rate of the non-diabetic population, the actual number of deaths will still be very small.

Non-insulin-dependent diabetic patients also suffer some penalty, although they may be able to get standard rates after middle age. The presence of diabetic complications and other disease will affect the risk assessment. Insurance companies do not like the presence of albuminuria, or of ischaemic heart disease. Nor do they approve of poor compliance or control. Nevertheless the companies are in the business of selling life insurance and do not like to decline applicants. Nor, if all risks are declined, is experience ever gained that allows an assessment of risk. Diabetic patients are likely to be accepted, therefore, albeit paying higher premiums and on some occasions even those considered the worst risk may be offered experimental terms.

REFERENCES

Balkau, B., Eschwege, E., Ducimetiere, P. *et al.* (1991) The high risk of death by alcohol related diseases in subjects diagnosed as diabetic and impaired glucose tolerant: the Paris prospective study after 15 years of follow-up. *J. Clin. Epidemiol.*, **44**, 465–474.

Barrett-Connor, E. and Wingard, D. L. (1983) Sex differential in ischaemic heart disease mortality in diabetics: a prospective population-based study. *Am. J. Epidemiol.*, **118**, 489–496.

Beardwood, J. T. (1957) Analysis of a survey concerning employment of diabetics in some major industries. *Diabetes*, **6**, 550–554.

Berger, M., Cuppers, H. J., Hegner, H. *et al.* (1982) Absorption kinetics and biologic effects of subcutaneously injected insulin preparations. *Diabetes Care*, **5**, 77–91.

Butler, W. J., Ostrander, L. D., Carman, W. J. and Lamphiear, D. E. (1985) Mortality from coronary heart disease in the Tecumseh study. *Am. J. Epidemiol.*, **121**, 541–547.

Cochran, H. A. (1968) Discussion: insured diabetics. *Trans. Assoc. Life Med. Dir. Am.*, **52**, 238.

Cox, D. J., Gonder-Frederick, L. and Clarke, W. (1993) Driving decrements in type 1 diabetes during moderate hypoglycemia. *Diabetes*, **42**, 239–243.

Deckert, T., Poulsen, J. E. and Larsen, M. (1978) Prognosis of diabetics with diabetes onset before the age of thirty-one. *Diabetologia*, **14**, 363–370.

Goldstone, R. L. (1992) Diabetes mellitus, in *Medical Selection of Life Risks*, 3rd edn, (eds R. D. C. Brackenridge and W. J. Elder), MacMillan, London, p. 217–230.

Goodkin, G., Wooloch, L., Gottcent, R. A. and Reich, R. (1974) Diabetes – a twenty year mortality study. *Trans. Assoc. Life Assur. Med. Dir. Am.*, **58**, 217.

386 *Management of the diabetic life*

Hansotia, P. and Broste, S. K. (1991) The effect of epilepsy or diabetes mellitus on the risk of automobile accidents. *N. Engl. J. Med.*, **324**, 22–26.

Hayward, R. E. and Lucena, B. C. (1965) An investigation into the mortality of diabetics. *J. Inst. Actuaries*, **91**, 286–315.

Kannel, W. B. and McGee, D. L. (1979) Diabetes and glucose tolerance as risk factors for cardiovascular disease: the Framingham study. *Diabetes Care*, **2**, 120–126.

Kemmer, F. W. and Berger, M. (1984) Exercise in diabetes: part of treatment, part of life, in *Recent Advances in Diabetes 1*, (eds M. Nattrass and J. V. Santiago), Churchill Livingstone, Edinburgh, pp. 137–143.

Kleinman, J. C., Donahue, R. P., Harris, M. I. *et al.* (1988) Mortality among diabetics in a national sample. *Am. J. Epidemiol.*, **128**, 389–401.

Kobberling, J. and Bruggeboes, B. (1980) Prevalence of diabetes among children of insulin-dependent diabetic mothers. *Diabetologia*, **18**, 459–462.

Lloyd, C. E., Robinson, N. and Fuller, J. H. (1992) Education and employment experiences in young adults with type 1 diabetes mellitus. *Diabetic Med.* **9**, 661–666.

Moore, R. H. and Buschbom, R. L. (1974) Work absenteeism in diabetics. *Diabetes*, **23**, 957–961.

Pan, W. H., Cedres, L. B. and Liu, K. *et al.* (1986) Relationship of clinical diabetes and asymptomatic hyperglycemia to risk of coronary heart disease mortality in men and women. *Am. J. Epidemiol.*, **123**, 504–516.

Pell, S. and D'Alonzo, C. A. (1967) Sickness absenteeism in employed diabetics. *Am. J. Pub. Health*, **57**, 253–260.

Robinson, N., Yateman, N. A., Protopapa, L. E. and Bush, L. (1990) Employment problems and diabetes. *Diabetic Med.*, **7**, 16–22.

Rosengren, A., Welin, L., Tsipogianni, A. and Wilhelmsen, L. (1989) Impact of cardiovascular risk factors on coronary heart disease and mortality among middle aged diabetic men: a general population study. *Br. Med. J.*, **299**, 1127–1131.

Shaw, B. H. (1974) A further report on an investigation into the mortality of diabetics. *J. Inst. Actuaries*, **101**, 405–413.

Steeds, A. J. (1946) An investigation into the mortality of diabetic patients attending the diabetic clinic of King's College Hospital. *J. Inst. Act*, **75**, 94–100.

Stevens, A. B., Roberts, M., McKane, R. *et al.* (1989) Motor vehicle driving among diabetics taking insulin and non-diabetics. *Br. Med. J.*, **299**, 591–595.

Waclawski, E. R. (1990) Sickness absence among insulin-treated diabetic employees. *Diabetic Med.*, **7**, 41–44.

Welch, R. A. (1986) Employment of diabetics in a post office region. *J. Soc. Occup. Med.*, **36**, 80–85.

Zinman, B., Murray, F. T., Vranic, M. *et al.* (1977) Glucoregulation during moderate exercise in insulin treated diabetics. *J. Clin. Endocrinol. Metab.*, **45**, 641–652.

INDEX